℞PG PLAB
Part I Exam

Disclaimer

Medicine is an ever changing science. As new research and clinical experience broaden our knowledge, changes in existing treatment and drug therapies are required. The authors and the publisher of this book have checked with sources believed to be reliable in their efforts to provide information that is complete and generally in accordance with the standards accepted at the time of publication. However, in view of the possibility of human error or changes in medical sciences, neither the authors not the publisher nor any other party who has been involved in the publication of this work warrants that the information contained herein is in every respect accurate or complete, and they disclaim all responsibility for any errors or omissions or for the results obtained from use of the information contained in this book. Readers are encouraged to confirm the information contained herein with other sources. Moreover the authors and the publisher do not claim any responsibility for the accuracy or even existence of any question in this book in the exam quoted. All the questione have been reproduced solely on the basis of the memory of the appearing students and there can be wide variations from the actual questions or their options.

RxPG PLAB
PART I Exam
International Edition

- *Over 1000 exhaustively explained memory based EMQs*
- *All the information about PLAB that you will ever need*
- *Rapid notes of High yield material for PLAB*

Himanshu Tyagi
Maulana Azad Medical College
New Delhi

Ankush Vidyarthi
Maulana Azad Medical College
New Delhi

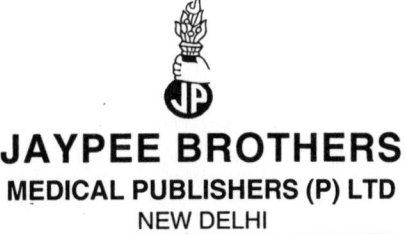

JAYPEE BROTHERS
MEDICAL PUBLISHERS (P) LTD
NEW DELHI

Published by
Jitendar P Vij
Jaypee Brothers Medical Publishers (P) Ltd
EMCA House, 23/23B Ansari Road, Daryaganj
New Delhi 110 002, India
Phones: 3272143, 3272703, 3282021, 3245672, 3245683
Fax: 011-3276490   e-mail: jpmedpub@del2.vsnl.net.in
Visit our website: http://www.jpbros.20m.com

Branches

- 202 Batavia Chambers, 8 Kumara Kruppa Road, Kumara Park East
  Bangalore 560 001, Phones: 2285971, 2382956 Tele Fax: 2281761
  e-mail: jaypeebc@bgl.vsnl.net.in

- 282 IIIrd Floor, Khaleel Shirazi Estate, Fountain Plaza
  Pantheon Road, **Chennai** 600 008, Phone: 8262665 Fax: 8262331
  e-mail: jpmedpub@md3.vsnl.net.in

- 4-2-1067/1-3, Ist Floor, Balaji Building, Ramkote Cross Road
  Hyderabad 500 095, Phones: 6590020, 4758498   Fax: 4758499
  e-mail: jpmedpub@rediffmail.com

- 1A Indian Mirror Street, Wellington Square
  Kolkata 700 013, Phone: 2451926 Fax: 2456075
  e-mail: jpbcal@cal.vsnl.net.in

- 106 Amit Industrial Estate, 61 Dr SS Rao Road, Near MGM Hospital
  Parel, **Mumbai** 400 012, Phones: 4124863, 4104532 Fax: 4160828
  e-mail: jpmedpub@bom7.vsnl.net.in

PG PLAB Part I Exam

© 2003, Himanshu Tyagi and Ankush Vidyarthi

All rights reserved. No part of this publication should be reproduced, stored in a retrieval system, or transmitted in any form or by any means: electronic, mechanical, photocopying, recording, or otherwise, without the prior written permission of the authors and the publisher.

This book has been published in good faith that the material provided by author is original. Every effort is made to ensure accuracy of material, but the publisher, printer and author will not be held responsible for any inadvertent error(s). In case of any dispute, all legal matters to be settled under Delhi jurisdiction only.

First Edition: 2003

Publishing Director: RK Yadav

ISBN 81-8061-030-6

Typeset at   JPBMP typesetting unit
Printed at   Gopsons Papers Ltd., Sector 60, Noida

This book is dedicated to our families, friends and loved ones, who endured and assisted in the task of assembling this guide.

Contents

Preface .... *ix*
Acknowledgements .... *xi*
Why to read this book? .... *xiii*
How to use this book? .... *xv*
How to contribute .... *xvii*

Section 1

Data Base of Information about PLAB

What is PLAB? *3-48*
    Introduction *3*
    PLAB Test Pattern *5*
    Syllabus For PLAB (Ref. GMC) *8*
    List of Eponyms *9*
    How to Approach the Extended Matching Questions Examination *10*
    Part II (OSCE) *13*
    Venue for Examinations *15*
    Recommended Books *17*
    In Short the Whole Process Simplified *19*
    International English Language Testing System (IELTS) *20*
    Routes of Exemption from the PLAB Test *23*
    Overseas Doctors Training Scheme (ODTS) *25*
    Medical Career Structure in The UK *27*
    Visa Matters, Travel and Stay in UK *32*
    Registration and Applying for a Job *33*
    Current Situation of PG Training In UK *38*
    Specialist Training *43*
    Sites for PLAB *48*

Section 2

Data Base of Previous Memory based EMQs with Explanatory Answers

Symbols and Abbreviations *50*

Index: Themes *53*

May—2002 .... *57*
    Questions with Explanatory Answers

March—2002 193
Questions with Explanatory Answers

November—2001 327
Questions with Explanatory Answers

September—2001 461
Questions with Explanatory Answers

July—2001 593
Questions with Explanatory Answers

Section 3
Data Base of High Yield Study Material

High Yield Topic One: Child Immunisation Clinics In UK 733

High Yield Topic Two: What is New in BNF No. 43? 736

High Yield Topic Three: Tumour Markers (Reference 652-OHCM) 737

High Yield Topic Four: Evidence Based Clinical Practice in Psychiatry Guidelines
(Brief Version) 738

High Yield Topic Five: Detection of Deliberate Releases-Cardinal Signs for Case Detection 740

High Yield Topic Six: Asthma Guidelines—Chronic Management 741

High Yield Topic Seven: Fitness To Drive 743

High Yield Topic Eight: Drugs in Pregnancy 744

High Yield Topic Nine: British Nomenclature for Drugs 745

High Yield Topic Ten: GMC Guidelines about Medical Ethics 746

High Yield Topic Eleven: Development (Denver Screening) and Motor Mile Stones 760

Index 761

Preface

The purpose of *First Aid for the PLAB Part I Exam* is to help medical students and international medical graduates review the clinical questions and prepare for the Professional and Linguistics Assessment Board Exam, Part I (PLAB Part I). Preparing for this examination can be a stressful, difficult and costly task. This book helps students make the most of their limited time, money and energy. As is often the case in medical college, we found that the best advice a student can receive is from other medical students. We also recognized that certain clinical topics and situations are 'popular' and appear frequently in examinations. With this in mind, *First Aid for the PLAB Part I Exam* was started in April, 2002.

As we studied for the PLAB Part I Exam, we examined and evaluated scores of books and thousands of sample EMQs. We kept track of useful study strategies, frequently tested facts, and helpful mnemonics through a simple computer database. This book is a culmination of that database.

The title reflects the potential value of this book as the "first" one to get before buying other, and the fact that PLAB exams are stressful and unpleasant experiences that students may "aid" each other in overcoming. We feel that this study guide provides a unique and pragmatic approach to the PLAB Part I and that it contains useful text not found in current PLAB EMQ books.

Throughout the work a conscious motive has been kept by us not to provide solutions to the readers but to make him aware of the direction he or she may need to work into solve any question. Many controversial options or answers have been explicitly been told in the text and the readers are supposed to find or satisfy themselves about the correct answers on their own. We do not believe in spoon feeding as much as we do not believe in letting you wander aimlessly in the wild sea of these questions.

Entries in First Aid for the PLAB Part I Exam originated from hundreds of students who have appeared in previous PLAB exams and reproduced those questions solely on the basis of their memory (Authors did not reproduce any questions themselves, they only solved the material available to them). Because of certain limitations of the method of reproducing question on the basis of memory, there can be wide variations from the actual questions or their options. So we along with the publishers are not claiming any responsibility for the accuracy or even existence of any question in this book in the exam quoted. Still this book is a necessecity as it teaches you to approach the frequently ouccurring PLAB EMQs in a clinical and systematic manner.

We and Jaypee Brothers Medical Publishers (P) Ltd intend to continue updating First Aid for the PLAB Part I Exam so that the book grows in quality and scope and continue to reflect the EMQs asked in the PLAB Part I Exam. If you have any study strategies, high yield facts with mnemonics, book reviews or previous questions of PLAB (should be strictly memory based), please use the forms inside to submit your contributions (See How to contribute, page xvii). Any one who submits material subsequently used in the next edition of First Aid for the PLAB Part I Exam receive personal acknowledgement in the next edition and a handsome cash reward per complete entry.

Good Luck for the PLAB

Dr. Himanshu Tyagi
Dr. Ankush Vidyarthi

Acknowledgements

Dr. Aditya Gupta
Maulana Azad Medical College
Helped us to compile question from the internet: RxPG thanks you for your contribution Adi.

Dr. Vikas Singhal
Maulana Azad Medical College
Helped us to sail past many a difficult questions. RxPG is highly obliged by your invaluable advises "Dosco"!

Dr. Sajat Agarwal
Maulana Azad Medical College
Helped us to develop a system of logical thinking and its practical application to the questions RxPG is grateful for your insights Sajat!

Dr. Mandeep Singh
Maulana Azad Medical College
Helped us to review the proofs of this book. RxPG salutes you for your enthusiasm Mandy!

Piku and Piggy
Our pets! RxPG is indebted to some of your excellent background works, dear!

Dr. M.C. Nath (H.O.D), Dr. Alok, Dr. Swagata and rest of the department, Blood bank
Lok Nayak Hospital
Helped us to complete this book by providing excellent working conditions, while we were busy with this book. RxPG would like to give its heart felt regards to them.

Mr. J.P.Vij, Chairman and Managing Director
Jaypee Brothers Medical Publishers (P) Ltd.
Helped us in this project with his underlying enthusiasm and support for us. RxPG will like to register its gratitude in highest terms for him. Without you this book would never have been possible, sir!

Ms Sunita
Jaypee Brothers Medical Publishers (P) Ltd.
Helped herself in understanding our illegible handwritings, while composing this book. RxPG is looking forward for tougher project with you. Sunita jee!

Why to read this book?

RxPG First Aid for the PLAB Part I Exam has been written keeping in mind the exact quantity and quality of knowledge required by any MBBS graduate to clear PLAB exam. This exam is conducted by General Medical Council (GMC) worldover. GMC has a questions bank of around 2000 questions out of which 200 questions are asked in any PLAB exam. The reason for GMC having such a small question bank is that they have a pains taking method to prepare new questions which are then tested and re-tested on SHOs and students to determine their level of difficulty. All this research consumes time and they are only able to increment their question bank by a few questions each year. Since around ten percent of the total question bank comes as a single question paper of PLAB exam, the frequency of repitition is one in ten, if you solve a single previous year question paper. That means out of 200 questions practised by you, around 20 questions stand a good chance of being repeated. Most of the students, who fail PLAB Part I, do so by a whisker and it is rare to fail by a margin of 20 marks. So practising even one previous question paper can change your fortune. This book contain five previous PLAB papers, i.e. 1000 questions. This is about half of the GMC question bank. So if you practise these five paper in advance you have a chance getting around 100 (20 × 5) repeat questions in your exam. That means you know about 50 percent of the paper in advance after doing this book. This would make not only passing but even scoring high in the PLAB Exam a cake walk. And believe us, when you will only apply for a job in UK. The score will certainly make a difference.

Features of This Book

Textbook type approach: Since passing the PLAB examination requires very specific knowledge about limited topics, we have deliberately kept the textbook type approach throughout to provide you a textbook that is specifically written for PLAB. This also eliminates the need to pains takingly filter bulky textbooks like Kumar and Clarke's for your preparation. Believe us, to pass the PLAB Exam even OHCM and OHCS are not required to be read completely. This exam has a very limited range of topics.

Intelligent format: The idea and the format of this book is based on our research conducting online at www.rxpg.com and offline at Maulana Azad Medical College. Several hundred previous students who have appeared for PLAB examination (including those who've failed it once), have contributed to our research and helped us evolve an intelligent and highly productive format. As per all the books of RxPG series, our format is a trademark for our success.

RxPG analysis: We have included a detailed analysis of every paper and every controversial point or question in this book. This will prove very helpful for those who want to maximize their efficiency and enhance their performance in this highly competitive exam.

Confusa: It is an intergral part of almost all our explanatory answers. This helps you to understand the finer "traps" and "catches" in the question which are usually invisible to untrained minds and accounts for most of the wrong answers. By highlighting there points this book ensures that you won't commit simple mistakes in the actual exam.

Paper-wise approach: The biggest blunder that most of the students appearing for PLAB commit is that they study for it in a subject-wise fashions, i.e. the old Indian way to study for any exam. Studying for PLAB means studying all clinical subjects together and randomly. When you will go through the themes in these previous papers, you will realise that mostly these themes don't represent a subject but a clinical condition that overlaps through many subjects, e.g. in a single theme of acute abdomen, questions can be asked about ectopic pregnancy (Obstetrics), Renal colic (surgery, mesenteric ischaemia (medicine), vertebral column fracture (Orthopaedics) and laxatives (pharmacology). So one need to have an orientation of all the subjects for a single given prospective which is impossible if you study one subject at a time. To validate our hypothesis, we conducted a random case-control study amongst the students of Maulana Azad Medical College who appeared for PLAB April 2002 and July 2002 exams. It was found that students who did integrated study fared better by 5-15% marks than those who preferred the old subject-wise approach. Another significant observation was that subject based preparation gave the students a false feeling of over confidence which proved detrimental in their scores. So RxPG strictly advise you to follow an integrated paper based approach. Subject wise approach is best left for examinations which are based upon reproducibility of facts and figures and PLAB is just not this kind of exam. (Note that even OHCM, in spite of being a book of medicine, has a big section on surgery. It is so because illness don't confine them according to subjects and the question setters of PLAB are more concerned about you having this understanding).

Perfect simulation: RxPG has tried its best to simulate the exact PLAB exam by giving all 200 questions separately and identical answer sheets with them. This helps you to practise marking the answers with speed and precision. This is important because of two reasons. First is that scoring in PLAB exam also depends upon your speed (Three hours are not sufficient for 200 questions). Secondarily, probably you've never came across the whole breath of the paper (usually these are 12-16 option boxes per question). Adjusting to this unique answer sheet takes time and practise, and examination hall is certainly not the first place to learn it. Practise marking with pencil on included answer-sheets and certainly you will be able to limit your "non-educational" mistakes in the actual paper.

Indexing: RxPG circulated a questionnaire, as a part of our offline and online research, among the students preparing PLAB. One of the question in it was "Mention the biggest short-coming of the EMQ books. They are referring to 74 percent of the students wrote "lack of index" or "lack of a table of contents where only the topics of theme are mentioned". RxPG has thus incorporated both these features in this book and certainly this makes RxPG PLAB-years the best buy you can get for PLAB.

Orientation: This book contains total 1000 questions, but the authors have managed to explain 4000. How is it possible? Actually there is a peculiar occurrence our research team has noted while it was going through the previous papers. That is whole themes are often repeated in PLAB exams with the same set of questions, but with a different header, i.e. "Diagnosis of a disease" can change to "Management of a disease". Since there are usually only four types of themes that are asked in PLAB exams (i.e. Diagnosis, Management, Investigation, Treatment), we have included all these four points in almost every explanation. So reading the explanation to one question makes you intelligent four times.

Most authentic questions: Though we are not claiming 100% authenticity, we have put in a lot of time in compiling these papers. Basically we scanned the internet, approached those who've already given the papers and launched a special drive to contribute previous PLAB questions on www.rxpg.com. Since all these three were independent sources with no overlapping between them, we made one complete independent set for each exam from all three sources. Thereafter our research team compared the three sets to reach the most authentic final set of questions. This process was long and tedious, but you will realise the high level of our accuracy in reproducibility, once you'll appear for the PLAB exam.

Online extension: To keep this book alive and interactive, we have an online section dedicated to this book, i.e.

http//www.rxpg.com/plab

Here you'll find any errata or additions to this book, a message board dedicated to PLAB part I and a serious plab e-group. Moreover any information about PLAB is available on www.rxpg.com.

Based exclusively on textbooks for PLAB exam: RxPG had contacted some PLAB coaching institutes about how to study, and all they said is "If you want to clear PLAB, throw all your books away and read only UK textbooks." You all should note that UK adopt quite a different approach about management and treatment of many diseases, so there is lot of unlearning that has to be done (as usually we read USA textbooks like Harrison's). It is true that by reading non-UK books you can indeed easily answer the themes based on "diagnosis", but of late the number of such themes in PLAB exam have consistently fallen and emphasis on "investigation" and "management" has increased. For example most of us crammed throughout our college years that "amyl nitrite" is to be given in case of cyanide poisoning, in UK it is "Dicobalt edetate"- unheard of by most of us. So start un-learning today by following UK textbooks for even the most inconsequential fact. This book will simplify this process for you.

Send us a photocopy of your PLAB I result and get your name in the second edition of this book.

How to use this Book?

QUESTION PAPER SECTION

THEME
Here is the theme of a set of EMQs. It could be a topic, subtopic or a condition. It tells you what the questions are about, in terms of both the clinical problem area, for example chronic joint pain, and the skill required, for example diagnosis. Usually the themes are about only four skills i.e. DIAGNOSIS, INVESTIGATION, MANAGEMENT and TREATMENT.

OPTIONS
Here is the list of options, usually of between 8 to twelve items, each of which is identified by a letter of the alphabet. You should look for the answer to any partcular question under a theme in this list of options. If you cannot find the answer you have thought of, you should look for an option which, in your opinion is the best answer to the problem posed. Marks are not deducted for incorrect answers nor for failure to answer. The total score on the paper is the number of correct answers given. You should, therefore, attempt all items. Each option may be used once, more than once, or not at all. There may be two correct answers for a single question and marking anyone will fetch you the marks.

QUESTIONS
These are several numbered items concerning the theme, usually between three and six. These are the questions—the problems you have to solve. Read them carefully, consider each of the numbered item in the list of options and decide what you think the answer is.

ANSWERS
Here we provide the correct answers to each of the question. We have provided the list of answers after each set of paper.

EXPLANATION SECTION

Here we provide you with text, tables, tips, mnemonics and other material helpful in creating an orientation and grasp of the theme itself. This provide you an advantage of learning a high yield topic in totalty instead of getting partial knowledge by solving the few questions only. It helps you to create a knowledge base on the basis of which you can attempt new questions on this very theme. This is important as themes are repeated more often than the exact questions in the PLAB I exam.

QUESTION
1. Here is the body of the actual question. There are usually three to six such questions under on theme. All this constitute one EMQ.

Diagnosis: Here we provide you with the final diagnosis to the condition in the question.

CLINCHERS
➤ Here we provide the detailed explanations about the answer. We have divided the question stem into a number of parts [clinchers] for the purpose of better explanation and to simplify the process of reaching a final diagnosis. This is important as it will help you cultivate a logical approach to solve the questions.

Confusa: Here we will explain the most confusing aspects of the question that can be responsible for most errors in making the correct diagnosis.

Investigation of choice: Here we give the most important investigation required for the condition in question.

Immediate management: Here we give the most important investigation required for the condition in question

Treatment of choice: Here we give the most important investigation required for the condition in question

How to contribute?

This version of RxPG First Aid for the PLAB Part I exam incorporates hundreds of contributions suggested by faculty and student reviewers of Maulana Azad Medical College. We invite you to participate in this process to bring out a better book next time.

Please send us your suggestions for
- Study and test taking strategies for the PLAB exams (both parts).
- New facts, mnemonics, diagrams, and illustrations which help to simplify the process of learning and cramming for a medical student.
- High yield topics that may reappear in future in above mentioned exams.
- Extended match questions of recent exams.

For each entry incorporated into the next addition, you will receive a hansome cash reward per completed entry, as well as personal acknowledgement in the next edition. Diagrams, tables, partial entries, corrections, and study hints are also appreciated, and significant contributions will be compensated at the discretion of the authors.

The preferred way to submit entries, suggestions, or corrections is via e-mail. Please include name, address, school affiliation, phone number and e-mail address (if different from address of origin). If there are multiple entries, please consolidate into a single e-mail or file attachment. Please send submissions to

Contribute @rxpg.com

Otherwise please send entries, neatly written or typed or on a disk (MS Word), to "RxPG series, **First Aid for the PLAB Part I Exam, Jaypee Brothers Medical Publishers (P) Ltd**, EMCA House, 23/23B Ansari Road, Daryaganj, New Delhi 110 002, India"

Note:
The reward will be given only to the first contributor, however every contributor will get acknowledgement in this book.

Section 1
Data Base of Information about PLAB

What is PLAB?

INTRODUCTION

For an overseas doctor in third world countries the UK degrees in medicine have always had a charm. Having MRCP (UK), MRCS (UK), MRCOG (UK), etc. have always been a ultimate desire for many a doctor. These degrees without any doubt enhance doctors credentials in laymans view compared to his colleagues. Also these degrees enhances one's ability to get better and best job internationally (particularly so in middle east). Having said all these everything boils down to being able to get these degrees. To get ultimately these degrees one has to work in UK (with exceptions in certain specialities). The UK government wants its people get medical services from a qualified doctors with professional knowledge and skill and knowledge of english. So there is the regulatory body for medical profession called general medical council (GMC) (similar to medical council of india). GMC is the body which allows the overseas doctor to practice in United Kingdom after limited registration. To get limited registration one has to pass PLAB test.

Purpose of the PLAB Test
Before granting limited registration to an overseas-qualified doctor, the GMC must be assured that the doctor has the knowledge of english and the professional knowledge and skill which are necessary for medical practice in the United Kingdom. One of the ways in which a doctor can satisfy the GMC that he or she has required abilities is by passing the test conducted by the professional and linguistic assessments board. This is known as the PLAB test. Having said this there are many different ways of obtaining limited registration which is discussed in a separate chapter.

Level of the PLAB Test
The standard required to pass the test is defined by the board in the following terms: "A candidate's command of the english language and professional knowledge and skill must be shown to be sufficient for him or her to undertake safely employment at first year senior house officer (SHO) level in a british hospital".

Qualification and Experience Needed
Admission to the PLAB test is open to doctors whose primary medical qualifications are accepted by the GMC for the purpose of limited registration. These include primary medical qualifications listed in the world directory of medical schools, which is published by the world health organization (WHO). In India it means MBBS degree of yours.

Evidence of Medical Qualification
A candidate will not be asked to provide proof of his/her qualification at the time of applying for admission to the PLAB test. However, before granting limited registration to doctors who have passed the test, the GMC will require the applicants to provide clear evidence that they hold an acceptable primary medical qualification.

The candidate should have a minimum of 12 months postgraduate clinical experience. This experience should be acquired in teaching hospitals or other hospitals which have been approved for internship training by the medical registration authorities concerned.

A doctor, who has not completed such experience, may be allowed by the GMC to enter the PLAB test. However, since the test is set at the level of senior house officer in the NHS, doctors without at least one year's experience of clinical practice are likely to be at a disadvantage. Doctors falling within this category who are able to pass the test will initially be granted limited registration only for employment at the grade of house officer (PRHO of UK), which is the NHS grade occupied by new medical graduates. After an appropriate period of satisfactory service as a house officer, the doctor would be able to apply for registration in respect of posts at a higher grade. The time spent as a House officer would be counted towards the total period of five years which the law permits for practice under limited registration and the number of PRHO is as much as the number of UK graduates, so overseas doctor will find it extremely difficult to obtain these posts. So it is advisable to complete internship and then write PLAB test. The best will be for those who do not want to waste any time after internship can take this exam somewhere in between their internship programme.

For applying for the PLAB test, one should have proved his linguistic capabilities with english as a language and for this one needs to take IELTS test. The minimum score for qualification in speaking: 7.0, listening: 6.0, academic reading: 6.0, academic writing: 6.0 and overall: 7.0. The IELTS is discussed in a separate chapter.

WHAT IT WILL COST

- The fee for taking part I (From 1st April 2001)
  145 pound sterlings
- The fee for taking part II (From 1st April 2001)
  430 pound sterlings
- The fee for checking your original documents when you apply for limited registration which is currently 100 pound sterlings
- The fee for limited registration(From January 2001)
  170 pound sterlings
- Air ticket (Return)
  500 pound sterlings
- Others
  300 pound sterlings

You have to consider the expenses involved in living in UK. Kindly multiply the total amout of money with the rupee value to get the exact amout of money involved in rupees in the process. (exchange rate as on 20 September, 2002 is 1 £ = 76.15 Rupees)

Data Base of Information about PLAB

PLAB TEST PATTERN

This test refers to the whole **PLAB** test which is in **two** parts.

PART-I
An **extended matching questions (EMQ)** examination. The emphasis of this examination is on the clinical management and science as applied to clinical problems. It is confined to core knowledge, skills and attitudes relating to conditions commonly seen by SHO's, to the generic management of life-threatening situations and rarer, but important problems.

The examination paper will contain **200 questions** divided into a nubmer of themes. It will last **3 hours**. As per the GMC information the picture tests, clinical problem solving questions will no more be asked. These have not been asked in the the recent examinations, so student can be quite sure of these being not asked.

Syllabus (as outlined by the GMC in their information brochure).

Part I Assesses the ability to apply knowledge to the care of patients. The subject matter is defined in terms of the skill and of the content.

Skills
Four groups of skills will be tested in approximately equal proportions.
a. *Diagnosis* Given the important facts about a patient (such as age, sex, and nature of presenting symptoms, duration of symptoms) you are asked to select the most likely diagnosis from a range of possibilities.
b. *Investigations* This may refer to the selection or the interpretation of diagnostic tests. Given the important facts about a patient, you will be asked to select the investigation, which is most likely to provide the key to the diagnosis. Alternatively, you may be given the findings of investigations and asked to relate these to a patient's condition or to choose the most appropriate next course of action.
c. *Management* Given the important facts about a patient's condition, you will be asked to choose from a range of possibilities the most suitable course of treatment. In the case of medical treatments, you will be asked to choose the correct drug therapy and will be expected to know about side effects.
d. *Others:* These may include:
   i. Explanation of disease process: The natural history of disease will be tested with reference to basic physiology and pathology.
   ii. Legal/ethical: You are expected to know the major legal and ethical principles set out in the GMC publication- **Duties of a doctor.**
   iii. Practice of evidence based medicine: Questions on diagnosis, investigations and management may draw upon recent evidence published in peer-reviewed journals. In addition, there may be questions on the principles and practice of evidence-based medicine.
   iv. Understanding of epidemiology: You may be tested on the principles of epidemiology, and on the prevalence of important diseases in the UK.
   v. Health promotion: The prevention of disease through health promotion and knowledge of risk factors.
   vi. Awareness of multicultural society: You may be tested on your appreciation of the impact of the practice of medicine of the health beliefs and cultural values of the major cultural groups represented in the UK population.
   vii. Application of scientific understanding to medicine.

FREQUENTLY ASKED QUESTIONS
Below you will find the answers to a number of questions we are often asked.

Which qualifications are accepted? What if mine is not?
These include all the qualifications listed in the World Health Organisation's World Directory of Medical Schools (WHO WDMS). The General Medical Council holds copies and it is a widely available reference book. If your qualification is not in the WDMS, you will probably not be able to apply for registration after passing the PLAB test. The General Medical Council will not lobby the WHO on your behalf and you should contact your medical school or the WHO in Geneva.

What is the format of test?
Before entering Part 1 of the PLAB test, you must have obtained the required minimum scores in the IELTS test. The IELTS test report form is valid for up to two years from the date of the IELTS test to which it relates. The minimum IELTS scores are: Overall 7.0, Speaking 7.0, Listening 6.0, Academic Reading 6.0 and Academic

Writing 6.0. PLAB Part 1 is in Extended Matching Question (EMQ) format. When you have passed PLAB Part 1, you must pass PLAB Part 2—an Objective Structured Clinical Examination (OSCE) within two years.

Can I complete my internship in the UK? Do I need to pass the PLAB test for this?
Yes, you may undertake your internship in the UK, but you must pass the PLAB test first. Because the test is set at SHO level, it will be difficult to pass without any clinical experience.

How can I get a job when I have passed?
You should consult the British Medical Journal Classified Section (www.bmj.com) or get in touch with British Council National Advice Bureau (see Annex G for contact details). The General Medical Council is not linked to the Department of Health or the NHS and we have no information about job vacancies. Passing the PLAB test does not quarantee you a job.

Is Part 1 held overseas different from Part 1 in the UK?
No, they are identical papers, held as far as possible under identical conditions. All papers are marked at the same time in the UK.

How can I prepare for the PLAB test?
We have no recommended texts or specimen papers. There are details about the content and other helpful information for Part 1 in Annex A of this document. We are aware of the existence of preparatory courses, but we do not inspect them and can make no comment on them.

What sort of registration do I get when I pass PLAB and what sort of job can I do?
You may apply for limited registration, which enables you to apply for supervised, educationally approved posts in the NHS. It is granted for individual jobs up to a maximum total period of five years.

How do I get full (permanent) registration?
Full registration allows you to work in unsupervised posts outside the NHS and is not subject to a maximum period. You must have completed at least two years' limited registration before applying for full registration.

Can I have a reduction in the fee because of my special circumstances?
The PLAB test is self-financing and all candidates, except asylum seekers, must pay the full fee for each attempt.

Does a pass in Part 1 of the test entitle me to any sort of registration?
No. You must pass both parts of the test before applying for limited registration.

How long in my IELTS/Part 1 pass/Part 2 pass valid?
You must pass Part 1 within two years of the date of your IELTS report from and you must pass Part 2 within two years of passing Part 1. You do not need a valid IELTS report to take Part 2. At the moment, there is no limit on the time within which you must apply for registration after you have passed Part 2.

What about exemption from the PLAB test?
You may be exempt from the PLAB test in certain circumstances. You should check this by contacting the General Medical Council's Registration Customer Services to ascertan your eligibility for registration.

If I cancel my test place, what happens?
If you want to cancel your place, please give the office which offered you the place as much notice as possible. You must return the letter offering you an Examination place. If you cancel early, we may be able to offer your place to another candidate waiting to take the Examination. You may not pass the letter offering you a place to anyone else.

If you cancel your place, you will be charged a fee. This will normally be deducted from the fee you paid to enter the Examination. The amount charged depends on the amount of notice you give.

Cancellation charges (2002 and 2003)
The current cancellation charges are as follows:

UK centres:

Period of notice	Cancellation charge
Four months or more	£ 70
Between 21 days and four months	£ 100
Less than 21 days	£ 145

If you do not want to re-book a place, we will refund the balance of your fee.

Overseas centres:

Period of notice	Cancellation charge
Before closing date	£ 20
After closing date	No refund

Can I take PLAB Part 2 outside the UK?
No. This is held only in the UK.

What is the pass rate?
There is no set pass rate.

Data Base of Information about PLAB

What happens when I pass/fail Part 1/Part 2?
If you pass Part 1, you will be sent an information pack and an application form for Part 2. If you fail Part 1, we will let you know in writing. We will not give results out over the phone or by fax. We will send you further application papers for Part 1 if you took the test in the UK. If you took the test at an overseas centre, you should contact that centre for another application form (or another centre if you would like to take the Examination in a different place). If you fail Part 2, the General Medical Council will send you a letter detailing your results and a further application form for Part 2. If you pass Part 2, you will be sent an application form and an information pack for limited registration.

What level is the PLAB test set at?
The PLAB test is set at the level of a SHO in a first appointment in a UK hospital. The emphasis of this Examination is on clinical management and science as applied to clinical problems. It is confined to core knowledge, skills and attitudes relating to conditions commonly seen by SHOs, the generic management of life-threatening situations and rarer, but important, problems.

How may times may I take Part 1/Part 2?
There is no limit to the number of times that you may take Part 1, but you must have a valid IELTS report form dated not more than two years before each attempt. You may have four attempts at Part 2, which must be within two years of your Part 1 pass. If you do not pass at your fourth attempt, you must re-take IELTS and Part 1. There are no exceptions to this rule.

SYLLABUS FOR PLAB (REF. GMC)

The content to be tested is, for the most part, defined in terms of patient presentations. Where appropriate, the presentation may be either acute or chronic. questions in part I will begin with a title which specifies both the skill and the content, for example, the management of varicose veins.

You will be expected to know about conditions that are common or important in the United Kingdom for all of the systems outlined below. **Examples** of the cases that may be asked about are given under each heading and may appear under more than one heading.

These examples are for illustration and the list is not exhaustive. Other similar conditions might appear in the examination.

a. **Accident and emergency medicine (to include trauma and burns).**
   Examples: Abdominal injuries, abdominal pain, back pain, bites and stings, breathlessness/wheeze, bruising and purpura, burns, chest pain, collapse, coma, convulsions, diabetes, epilepsy, eye problems, fractures, dislocations, head injury, loss of consciousness, non-accidental injury, sprains and strains, testicular pain.

b. **Blood (to include coagulation defects).**
   Examples: Anaemias, bruising and purpura.

c. **Cardiovascular system (to include heart and blood vessels and blood pressure).**
   Examples: Aortic aneurysm, chest pain, and deep vein thrombosis (DVT), diagnosis and management of hypertension, heart failure, ischemic limbs, myocardial infarction, myocardial ischemia, stroke, varicose veins.

d. **Dermatology, allergy, immunology and infectious diseases.**
   Examples: Allergy, fever and rashes, influenza/pneumonia, meningitis, skin cancers.

e. **ENT and Opthalmology.**
   Examples: Earache, hearing problems, hoarseness, difficulty in swallowing, glaucoma, red eyes, sudden visual loss.

f. **Female reproductive system (to include obstetrics, gynaecology and breast).**
   Examples: Abortion/sterilization, breast lump, contraception, infertility, menstrual disorders, menopausal symptoms, normal pregnancy, post-natal problems, pregnancy complications, vaginal disorders.

g. **Gastrointestinal tract, liver and biliary system and nutrition.**
   Examples: Abdominal pain, constipation, diarrhoea, and difficulty in swallowing, digestive disorders, gastrointestinal bleeding, jaundice, rectal bleeding/pain, vomiting, weight problems.

h. **Metabolism, endocrinology and diabetes.**
   Examples: Diabetes mellitus, thyroid disorders, weight problems.

i. **Nervous system (both medical and surgical).**
   Examples: Coma, convulsions, dementia, epilepsy, eye problems, headache, loss of consciousness, vertigo.

j. **Orthopaedics and rheumatology.**
   Examples: Backpain, fractures, dislocations, jointpain/swelling, sprains and strains.

k. **Psychiatry (to include substance abuse).**
   Examples: Alcohol abuse, anxiety, assessing suicidal risk, dementia, depression, drug abuse, overdoses and selfharm, panic attacks, postnatal problems.

l. **Renal system (to include urinary tract and genitourinary medicine).**
   Examples: Hematuria, renal and urteric calculi, renal failure, sexual health, testicular pain, urinary infections.

m. **Respiratory system.**
   Examples: Asthma, breathlessness/wheeze, cough, hemoptysis, hoarseness, and influenza/pneumonia.

n. **Disorders of childhood (to include non-accidental injury and child sexual abuse; fetal medicine; growth and development).**
   Examples: Abdominal pain, asthma, child development, childhood illness, earache, epilepsy, eye problems, fever and rashes, joint pain/swelling, loss of consciousness, meningitis, non-accidental injury, testicular pain, urinary disorders.

o. **Disorders of the elderly (to include palliative care).**
   Examples: Breathlessness, chest pain, constipation, dementia, depression, diabetes, diarrhoea, digestive disorders, headache, hearing problems, influenza/pneumonia, jaundice, joint pain/swelling, loss of consciousness, pain relief, terminal care, trauma, urinary disorders, vaginal disorders, varicose veins, vertigo, vomiting.

p. **Peri-operative management.**
   Examples: Pain relief, shock.

LIST OF EPONYMS (REF. GMC)

These eponyms may appear in the Examination. The list is for illustrative purposes only, it is not exhaustive. Other eponyms might appear in the Examination.

- Alzheimer's dementia
- Barrett's oesophagus
- Behcet's disease
- Boerhaave's syndrome
- Bornholm disease
- Bowmen's disease
- Budd-Chiari syndrome
- Burkitt Lymphoma
- Charcot-Marie-Tooth disease
- Colles' fracture
- Conn's syndrome
- Coombs' test
- Creutzfeldt-Jakob disease
- Crohn's disease
- Cushing's syndrome
- Down's syndrome
- Duchenne muscular dystrophy
- Epstein-Barr virus
- Fallopian tube
- Fallot's tetralogy
- Fuch's corneal dystrophy
- Gilbert's syndrome
- Goodpasture's syndrome
- Guillain-Barré syndrome
- Hartmann's solution
- Hashimoto's disease
- Henoch-Schönlein syndrome)
- Hirschsprung's disease
- Huntington's chorea
- Kaposi's sarcoma
- Kawasaki disease
- Kleihauer test
- Korsakoff's psychosis
- Kreim test
- Lesch-Nyhan syndrome
- Lewy body dementia
- Mallory-Weiss tear
- Mantoux test
- Meckel's diverticulum
- Meniere's disease
- Munchusen's syndrome
- Paget's disease
- Parkinson's disease
- Perthes disease
- Pick's disease
- Prinzmetal's angina
- Raynaud disease
- Reidel's thyroiditis
- Reiter's syndrome
- Sengstaken-Blakemore tube
- Sjögren's syndrome
- Stokes-Adams attacks
- Swan-Ganz catheter
- Takayasu disease
- Tay-Sachs disease
- Tietze's syndrome
- Tourette syndrome
- Turner syndrome
- von Willebrand's disease
- Wenckeback Phenomenon
- Wernicke's encephalopathy
- Wolff-Parkinson-White syndrome
- Ziehl-Neelsen stain

HOW TO APPROACH THE EXTENDED MATCHING QUESTIONS EXAMINATION

The examination paper will contain 200 questions in the extended matching format, divided into a number of themes.

Each theme has a heading which tells you what the questions are about, in terms both of the clinical problem area (e.g. chronic joint pain) and the skill required (e.g. diagnosis).

Within each theme there are several numbered items, usually between four and six. These are the questions- the problems you have to solve. These are examples below.

Begin by reading carefully the instruction which preceded the numbered items. The instruction is very similar throughout the paper and typically reads. 'For each scenario below, choose the **SINGLE** most discrimination investigation from the above list of options. Each option may be used once, more than once or not at all.'

Consider each of the numbered items and decide what you think the answer is. You should then look for that answer in the list of options (each of which is identified by a letter of the alphabet). If you cannot find the answer in the list you have thought of, you should look for the option which, in your opinion, is the best answer to the problem posed.

For each numbered item, you must choose ONE of the option. You may feel that there are several possible answers to an item, but you must choose the one most likely from the option list. **If you enter more than one answer on the answer sheet you will gain no mark** for the question even though you may have given the right answer along with one or more wrong ones.

In each theme there are more option than items, so not all the options will be used as answer. This is why the instruction says that some options may not be used at all.

A given option may provide the answer to more than one item. For example, there might be two items which contain descriptions of patients, and the most likely diagnosis could be the same in both instances. In these cases, the option would be used more than once.

You will be awarded one mark for each item answered correctly. Marks are **not** deducted for incorrect answers nor for failure to answer. The total score on the paper is the number of correct answers given. You should, therefore, attempt all items. Example of an EMQ:

THEME 1: DIAGNOSIS OF HEARING LOSS

OPTIONS
a. Acoustic neuroma
b. Blast injury
c. Petrous temporal bone fracture
d. Wax impaction
e. Acute otitis media
f. Ototoxicity
g. Fracture base of skull
h. CSOM
i. Glue ear
j. Herpes Zoster
k. Foreign body

*For each presentation below, choose the **most likely dianosis** from the above list of options. Each option may be used once, more than once, or not at all.*

QUESTIONS
1. Man treated with gentamicin for peritonitis for 10 days presents with deafness.
2. Man with poor physical hygiene presents with pain and deafness after taking a shower.
3. Woman presents with deafness and corneal anaesthesia. On MRI, a widened internal auditory meatus is seen.
4. Male, 20 years, with history of head injury, bruising on the side of head complains of hearing loss.
5. A 54-year-old female develops mild fever, malaise and ear pain. 3 days dlater she developed multiple painful vesicles over her early canal and external meatus.

HOW TO STUDY FOR PLAB?

Note
All our conclusions given here are based on our research and feedback received in Maulana Azad Medical College and RxPG.com.

RxPG suggests you to opt for its unique strategy based on 5'P's. These are:
1. Plan
2. Pool
3. Prepare

4. Practise
5. Patience.

Now, these points in some detail are as follows.

Plan

A good plan is very important for your way to success. When you will start preparing for your PLAB exam, you will be more like an amateur in the world of PLAB professionals. By the time you will gain enough experience to play at a level field with them, time will deceive you. So here is where the advices of your seniors come in handy. Approach your seniors in the college, not only who came out with flying colours in the PLAB exam but also those who could not make it. Discuss in detail with the second or third attemptees. This is important as a successful student is usually not aware of the possible blunders anyone could make in their preparation. So do ask everybody about what not to do. Listen to everybody and make your own personalised plan. Do not follow anybody else plan blindly however successful it might have been for that person. This is because only you are the best judge of your shortcomings and plus points.

Pool

The next thing very important for your plan is to find a right kind of student or a pool of students as study partners. Remember if you study alone you are using only 10-20% of your brain faculties. But in a group study the process of gathering the information involves not only your eyes but ears, tongue and perhaps even hands sometimes! So you end up mobilising more of your brain in the same time span and this is very important as you have so little time on your hand. If you can't find a study partner (like if you stay at home in your hometown), then visit http://mediboard.meramamc.com. This page features message boards for PLAB exam from all websites.

Prepare

This needs a lot of consistency and regularity on your part. Believe us, it is not easy. So always have this thing playing in the back of your mind that you have to be regular. Study religiously every day for 5-8 hours. Set some punishments (like studying for more hours next day or mugging that impossible table from OHCM) for yourself if you cannot realise your targets. Set daily goals and allow a little flexibility in your goals and plan. Nothing can go strictly as per schedule, so even if you cannot make it for a few days, does not mean that you should drop the whole plan. Stick to it and see the result yourself. For PLAB, the optimum duration to revise whole syllabi once is 1 month.

Practice

Research showed that attempting mock tests is the best tool to practise for PLAB. Attempting mock tests fine tune your abilities to manage time, work out mistakes, minimising blunders, blunting the anxiety and stress and "gives you a feel" of the real exam. One cannot understand the difference until and unless one gives a mock test. Try these yourself online at
www.RxPG.com

The next most important thing is practise phase is to iron out your mistakes. Attempt tests, analyse your performances, spot the weaknesses, iron them out and then attempt more tests. Remember no one is perfect, but near perfection can be reached only by practise.

Note: You will need to revise selectively and not the whole course again. PLAB EMQs are from a very narrow pool of questions. So instead of wasting time on revising the whole syllabi, do PLAB questions in a retrograde way (like in this book).

Patience

This is the biggest virtue. Remember you will get everything only if you are through will all other 'Ps' and that need loads of patience. Don't be impatient to earn money (so do not do house jobs/residency because even if you get selected while doing them, you would have got a better seat had you opted for not doing it) or to start enjoying the role of a doctor. You are still a student and you are giving these exams as you want to remain as a student for next two/three years. Remember these lines by "Frost" to just keep yourself going:

"The woods are lovely, dark and deep,
But I have promise to keep
and miles to go, before I sleep."

WHAT SHOULD BE YOUR STRATEGY WHILE ATTEMPTING PLAB PART ONE EXAM?

Please read these instructions carefully and devise your own personalised strategy based on it. This strategy has been thoroughly researched and is found to be very effective.

Steps (after sitting on your seat in examination hall)
1. Read and listen to all instructions carefully.
2. Rapidly browse through the paper after opening the seal (when you are told to do so). Going through all the sheets in one minute helps you to:

- Get a feel of the paper and therefore help you concentrate afterwards.
- Check out any missing pages and misprints in the paper.

3. **Take a deep breath and concentrate**
   - If you have any problem in concentration because of anxiety, close your eyes and count backwards from 100 to 1. This is a very effective method to get focussed in a very short time.

4. **Start solving the paper. Take two rounds as follows:**

FIRST ROUND: Answer all the questions as much as possible.
- Clearly mark the one you have left on question paper, (write all the probable options in front of them—this saves time and confusion in second round).
- Keep on tansferring the answers on the answer sheet at the same time. Never leave this for the end as this can be suicidal.
- Answering reflexly here is very important. One can develop these reflexes by practising on as many mock tests as one can. Online mock tests are available at www.rxpg.com.
- Don't do any hard thinking in this round. If you are forced to think long on any question then leave it for the next round. First round should be based on a quantitative approach as 3 hours is actually little time to solve 200 EMQs.
- Note the time taken to finish this round. Ideally you should be able to finish this round in first two hours.

Advantages: 120-130 questions in two third of total time takes off the pressure, thereby you can:

- Relax and work efficiently to provide quality in the tougher questions left
- Not fall in danger of leaving the simple questions unattempted if time runs out.

SECOND ROUND: This round will decide your passing or failing the exam. So gather all your alertness and focus extra hard now. You should:
- Give maximum one minute to each question.
- If still there is confusion, mark the most probable answer according to you and move ahead. Don't get stuck any where.
- Do not leave any question unattempted as there is **No** negative marking.

After these if you still have time, tally your answers on the answer sheet with that of question paper randomly. This helps in exclusion of any inadvertent mistake by you while transferring the answers.

Ideal way to attempt a theme:
- Read the header and imbibe its relevance
- Go through all the options rapidly
- Read instructions before the questions especially what it is asking for i.e. first investigation or most definitive investigation (both of these will result in different answers).
- Attempt questions one by one and simultaneously transfer your answers on answer sheet.
- Think on a SHO level only and never think like a theorist while solving EMQs.

Please note that this strategy is just like an ideal infrastructure on which your final strategy should be based. You should know or find what works best for you and thus fine tune this strategy to get your own customised version.

PART II (OSCE)

You may only enter part II of the test when you have passed part I. **You have to take part II within 2 years of passing part I.** This test is set at the following standard:

A candidate's command on English language and professional knowledge and skill must be shown to be sufficient for him or her to undertake safely, employment at first year Senior House officer level in a British hospital.

This test is a **14 station objective structured clinical examination (OSCE).**

The syllabus and format of this test as given in the GMC information brochure.

Aim
1. The aim of the OSCE is to test your clinical and communication skills. It is designed so that an examiner can observe you putting these skills into practice.

Overall Format
2. When you enter the examination, you find a series of 14 booths, known as 'station'. Each station requires you to undertake a particular task. Some tasks will involve talking to or examining patients, some will involve demonstrating a procedure on an anatomical model. Detail of the tasks are explained below under 'content'.
3. There will also be two rest stations in the circuit. At some tests one of these two station will contain instruction asking you to perform certain tasks as if you were at a real station. These are pilot stations and the results will not count towards your overall OSCE grades.
4. You will be required to to perform all tasks. You will be told the number of the station at which you should begin when you enter the examination room. Each task will last five minutes.
5. Your instruction will be posted outside the station. You should read these instructions carefully to ensure that you follow them exactly. An example might be:
'Mr McKenzie has been referred to you in a rheumatology clinic because he has joint pains. Please take a short history to establish supportive for a differential diagnosis.
6. A bell will ring. You may then enter the station. There will be an examiner in each station. However, unlike in the oral examination, you will not be required to have a conversation with the examiner; you should only direct your remarks to him or her if the instructions specifically ask you to do so. You should undertake the task as instructed. A bell will ring after four minutes 30 seconds to warn you that you are nearly out of time. Another bell will ring when the five minutes are up. At this point you must stop immediately and go and wait outside the next station. If you finish before the end, you must wait inside the station but you should not speak to the examiner or to the patient during this time.
7. You will wait outside the next station for minute. During this time you should read the instructions for the tasks in this station. After one minute, a bell will ring. You should then enter the station and undertake the task as instructed.
8. You should continue in this way until you have completed all 14 tasks. You will then have finished the OSCE.

Content of the Station
9. Each station consists of a scenario. An examiner will be present and will oserve you at work.
10. The scenario could be drawn from any medical speciality appropriate to a senior house officer (SHO).
11. Although the tasks you will be instructed to do will not necessarily be tested in the order given here. Under each skill area, you will find some examples. Please note that these are only examples; other topics will be tested.The main skills tested in OSCE examination are—**History taking, clinical examination skills, practical skills, communication and examination skills.**

A. History Taking
Your candidate instructions will set the scene. You will be asked to take a history from an actor pretending to be a patient (a stimulated patient). The actor will have been given all the necessary information to be able to answer your questions accurately. You should treat him or her as you would a real patient.

Eg: Diarrhoea, wheeze, vaginal bleeing, palpitations, abdominal pain, headache, anxiety.

B. Clinical Examination
You will be asked to examine a particular part of the body. You may have to examine a stimulated or real

patient or perform the examination on an anatomical model. Although you should talk to the patient as you would to a patient in real life. You should only take a history or give a diagnosis if the instructors require you to do so. You may be asked to explain your actions to the examiner as you go along.

Examples: Breast examination, cardiovascular examination, examination of abdomen, hip examination, knee examination, pervaginal examination, perrectal examination.

C. Practical Skills/Use of Equipment
This is to assess some of the practical skills an SHO needs. The stations concerned will normally involve anatomical models rather than patients.

Examples: IV cannulation, cervical smear, suturing, blood pressure.

D. Emergency Management
These stations will test whether you know what to do in an emergency situation. You may have to explain what you are doing to the patient or to the examiner. Your instructions will make this clear.

E. Communication Skills
There will be a communication skill element in most stations. However, in some stations this skill will be the principal skill tested. Areas tested may include interviewing (including appropriate questioning, active listening, explaining clearly, checking understanding) and building rapport (including showing empathy and respect, sensitivity to other's emotions and coping with strong emotions in others).

Examples: Instructions for discharge from hospital, explaining treatment, consent for autopsy, ectopic pregnancy explanation.

Data Base of Information about PLAB

VENUE FOR EXAMINATIONS

You can take **part I** of the test in:
- The UK (Birmingham, Edinburgh, Glasgow, London).
- Bangladesh (Dhaka).
- Egypt (Cairo).
- India (Kolkata, Chennai, New Delhi, Mumbai).
- Pakistan (Islamabad, Karachi).
- Sri Lanka (Colombo).

Part II of the test is available only in UK in London, Edinburgh, Leeds and Liverpool.

Details of dates are set out by the GMC at regular intervals the candidates are advised to get in contact with the office of the nearest British Council Divisions.

NOTIFICATION OF RESULTS

The part I paper is marked by computer. At the end of the part I test, you will be told the date on which your results will be available. Usually it takes about 4 weeks for the declaration of results.

For part II, you will be given grades for each station. However, the overall result of the examination is either pass or fail and this result is usually sent out 2 weeks after the date of the examination.

PLAB test dates and contacts

Part 1 and Part 2

Note: Due to the high demand for places, you are strongly advised to allow at least four months from the time of submitting an application to getting a place. You may not hold a place in more than one examination.

Part 1

Tests for which places are currently available are listed below. Candidates for tests held outside the UK should apply to the local British Council office. Applications presented in person will not be given preference. For information about accommodation in the UK, visit the British Tourist Authority website.

NB: We are reviewing the test schedule after March 2003 in light of increasing demand. Further dates will be available shortly.

Date	Country	City
14/11/2002		London
09/01/2003		London
12/03/2003		Manchester
14/05/2003	UK	London
09/07/2003		Birmingham
17/09/2003		London
12/11/2003		Manchester

Note: on the following dates the test is held at **all** the following overseas centres:

Date	Country	City
	Bulgaria	Sofia
	Dubai	Dubai
14/11/2002	Egypt	Cairo
12/03/2003	India	Chennai, Kolkata, Mumbai, New Delhi
09/07/2003	Nigeria	Lagos
12/11/2003	Pakistan	Islamabad, Karachi
	Sri Lanka	Colombo

The closing date for receipt of application forms tests overseas is six weeks before the test. If you wish to enquire about availability for test dates please fax +44 (0)20 7 915 3565 or telephone +44 (0)20 7915 3630. Applications presented in person will not be given preference.

Local British Council contacts

Country	City	Contact & email	Tel	Fax
Bulgaria	Sofia	Nadya Ogorelkova	359 2 9424200	359 2 9424306
Dubai	Dubai	Lorraine Sequeira	971 4 3370109	971 4 3370703
Egypt	Cairo	Magda Mohie El Din	203 4846630	203 4820199
India	Kolkata	Suchitra Mukherjee	033 282 9108	033 282 4804
	Chennai	Nirupa Fernandez	044 852 5002	044 852 3234
	Mumbai	Vivek Singh	022 282 3560	022 282 2024
	New Delhi	PV Chaary	011 371 1401	011 371 0717
Nigeria	Lagos	Mrs Bimbola Fashola	01 269 2188	01 269 2193
Pakistan	Islamabad	Shahnaz Farooq	92 51 111 424 424	92 51 276 683
	Karachi	Karima Kara	92 21 111 424 424	92 21 5685694
Sri Lanka	Colombo	R B Nedumaran	1 581171	1 587079

Part 2

Tests with available places are listed below, although these may be filled before the closing date shown. From time to time Part 2 tests are added to or removed from the list of available dates. We may allocate you a place on any day within a block of consecutive tests at the same test centre.

Please note that if you have a confirmed booking on a test and wish to change to an earlier test which has been added to the list, you will still be charged a cancellation fee.

Due to the high demand for Part 2 places, you are strongly advised to allow at least four months from the time of submitting an application to getting a place. You should take this into account when applying for Part 2, which you must pass within two years of passing Part 1.

Maps of test locations appear below. For information about accommodation in the UK, visit the British Tourist Authority website.

PLAB Part 2 Schedule for 2002-2003 (as on 20th Sep, 2002)

Date	City	Closing date
09/10/2002	London	full
10/10/2002		full
26/11/2002	London	full
27/11/2002		full
27/11/2002	Edinburgh	full
28/11/2002		full
17/12/2002		
18/12/2002	London	
15/01/2003	London	20/12/2002
16/01/2003		
15/01/2003	Liverpool	20/12/2002
16/01/2003		
19/02/2003	London	31/01/2003
20/02/2003		
27/02/2003	London	07/03/2003
28/02/2003		
30/04/2003	London	11/04/2003
01/05/2003	London	11/04/2003
25/03/2003	London	07/03/2003
30/04/2003	Edinburgh	11/04/2003
01/05/2003	Edinburgh	11/04/2003
04/06/2003	Leeds	16/05/2003
05/06/2003		

RECOMMENDED BOOKS

MEDICINE
- OHCM, 5 edn—read it thoroughly with at least two revisions
- Kumar and Clark, 5 edn—Only for reference purposes.
- Lecture notes in emergency medicine—read selected topics from it like
  - Poisonings
  - Abdominal pain
  - Head injury

SURGERY
- OHCM, 5 edn—thorough reading
- Lecture notes, surgery—thorough reading with at least one revision
- Bailey and Love—Strictly for reference purposes

GYNAECOLOGY AND OBSTETRICS
- Lecture notes—thorough reading
- Ten teachers (Obs and Gynae) and Shaw's (Gyn)—Strictly for references

PSYCHIATRY
- Kumar and Clark, 5 edn + OHCS

ORTHOPEDICS
- OHCS, 5 edn

DERMATOLOGY
- Kumar and Clark, 5 edn + OHCS

OTHER
OHCS, 5 edn, Read tohroughly with at least one revision

EMQ
Nothing except fischtest and this book.

This is a review of books which we feel necessary for preparing for PLAB.

Medicine
1. "Oxford Handbook of Clinical Medicine" (OHCM) and 'Oxford Handbook of Clinical Specifications'(OHCS) published by the Oxford University Press are very important books for PLAB. They are like your bible(or bhagvadgita!). Go through them at every single opportunity and learn them cover to cover. The years of experience of PLAB writing students is that this itself is enough to get you through the exam.
2. Davidson or Kumar and Clarke should form the basic textbook to prepare for medicine. There is no need to try and go through both of these books. A candidate should be thorough with either of the two books. It is better to go through the book one has read during his UG studies though some feel Kumar and Clarke is better option.
3. "Lecture Notes on Clinical Medicine". This book is optional. You may briefly go through this book. You do not have to read this book thoroughly if you have done the above reading for medicine.
4. Large textbooks of medicine and surgery like the Oxford Textbook of Medicine, Harrison's Principles of Internal Medicine and Sabiston's Textbook of Surgery are too large for study for this exam. However, these volumes are ideal for referring when one is solving EMQs.
5. "French Index of Differential Diagnosis" is a good reference book.

Paediatrics
6. Oxford handbooks cover this subject adequately, but "Essential Paediatrics" by David Hull published by Churchill Livingstone can be referred for important topics.

Dermatology
7. Go through OHCM and for very important topics please go through "Lecture Notes in Dermatology".

Surgery
8. Bailey and Love is very useful book containing all the information needed regarding for surgery
9. "Lecture Notes on General Surgery" is a good book for surgery reading.
10. Oxford handbooks contribute good supplementary reading, especially the "OHCM".
11. Orthopaedics is well covered in the "OHCM" but if time allows one should also read "Lecture Notes on Orthopedics" or Concise System of Orthopaedics and Fractures by Apley.

ENT and Ophthalmology
12. OHCS does contain ENT and Ophthalmology, ENT and Ophthalmology constitutes a very

small portion of the PLAB test. The small coverage of this topic in this books is quite adequate to prepare for the PLAB test.
13. Lecture Notes in ENT and Ophthalmology can be referred to for some selected important topics.

Obstetrics and Gynaecology
13. Ten Teachers by is the one, which is commonly referred to by most of the students.
14. Lecture Notes on Obstetrics and Gynaecology can be another option but these subjects are also very well covered in the OHCS.

Psychiatry
15. The OHCM should suffice. For further reading one is advised to go through Davidson or Kumar and Clarke.

IN SHORT THE WHOLE PROCESS SIMPLIFIED

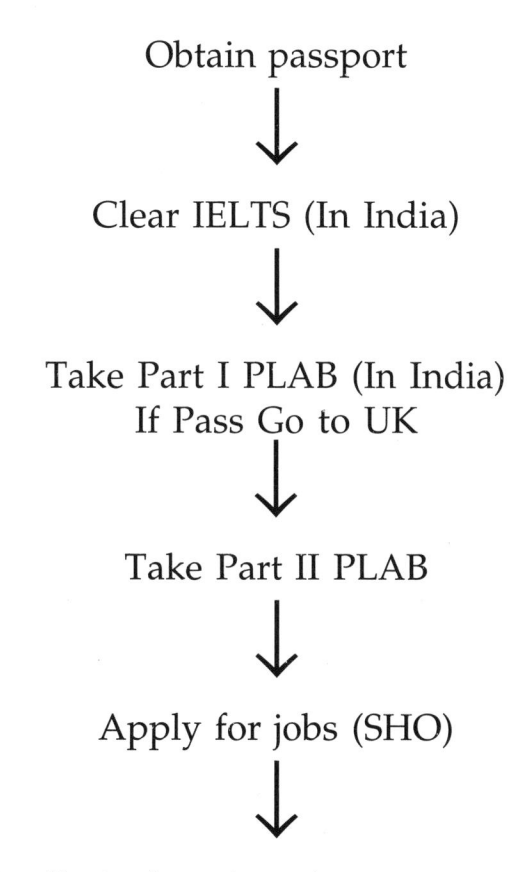

Obtain passport
↓
Clear IELTS (In India)
↓
Take Part I PLAB (In India)
If Pass Go to UK
↓
Take Part II PLAB
↓
Apply for jobs (SHO)
↓
Apply for limited registration once you get a job

INTERNATIONAL ENGLISH LANGUAGE TESTING SYSTEM (IELTS)

Before attempting PLAB one has to prove his linguistic ability in English by getting adequate score in academic module of international english language testing system (IELTS). GMC has decided that adequate score in IELTS is a necessary prerequisite for attempting PLAB. IELTS is now an integral part of the PLAB and therefore no other english proficiency test is acceptable. PLAB and IELTS application forms should have identical details, especially the name and address as the two results will be joined together. So IELTS is the first hurdle one has to clear before attempting PLAB. The british council (which administers IELTS) requires ones identity. The only identify british council accepts valid PASSPORT or A NATIONAL IDENTITY CARD WITH A NUMBER. **Having a valid PASSPORT is the prerequisite for attempting IELTS so get a passport as the first step towards UK.**

INTRODUCTION
IELTS is a test of english language proficiency. It is a way of assessing the english of non-native speakers who want to study or train using english. The test is offered on demand and measures general language skills and also the skills needed for studying and training.

When can one take the Test?
Test centres have their own testing days in response to local demands. You have to apply 3-4 months in advance to be assured of a date of your choice.

What does the test consist of?
The candidates are tested in communication (written as well as oral) skills in the IELTS exam.
PLAB candidates shoud sit for the academic module. The test format is as follows:

I. *Listening*
   4 sections, around 40 items
   30 minutes

II. *Academic Reading*
   3 sections, around 40 items
   60 minutes

III. *Academic Writing*
   2 tasks (150 to 250 words)
   60 minutes

IV. *Speaking*
   10-15 minutes

More details regarding each component of the exam is detailed in IELTS hand book which you will get when you apply for the test.

How long does it take to get the Result and What does it Mean?
- Your results are sent to you and can be sent direct to the GMC within two weeks of taking the test.
- Scores are recorded on a test report form.
- All scores are given on a scale ranging from 1 to 9; i.e. from non-user to expert user with fully operational command of the language.
- The GMC requirement is a minimum of Band 7.0 on the IELTS on a scale of 9 Bands.

Doctors taking PLAB need to get an overall IELTS score of at least 7 but must not score less than 6 in any section of the test. From June 2000 candidates must, in addition, score a minimum of 7 in the speaking section of the test.

Doctors with exemption from PLAB must not score less than 7 in any section of the test.

How can one Prepare for the Test?
An IELTS specimen material pack is available in british council and library. This includes a full practice test with a cassette and an answer key. One can gain experience in the format of the test and get an idea of ones competence. Another book called 'How to prepare for IELTS' is designed to help candidates prepare for the test. This book is available from the british council.

A study pack called 'Cambridge Practice Tests for IELTS T by Vanessa Jackman and Clare Mc-Dowell is available at the british library for reference.

Useful Tips
Instead of buying these expensive books, one may spend time at the british library reading the books for 3 to 5 days. One could also photocopy important sections from one's friend's copy. It is wise to go through these practice packs prior to taking the test (even if one thinks one is proficient with english language).

How do you Apply for IELTS?
One should write to the nearest test centre which is given below and ask them for an application form and IELTS Handbook. The names of test centres in UK, India, Pakistan, Bangladesh and Shrilakna is given below:

Data Base of Information about PLAB

Address
Bridgewater House
58 Whitworth Street
Manchester,
United Kingdom, M1 6BB
Tel: 44 1619577218
Fax: 441619577029
E-mail: ed@britcoun.org

India
In India there are 12 centres currently which offer IELTS. They are in Delhi, Mumbai, Kolkata, Chennai, Bangalore, Thiruvanthapuram, Hyderabad, Pune, Ahmedabad, Bhopal, Lucknow, Patna.

In North India
Examination Services Manager
New Delhi

Address
Name: Sanjay Patro
British High Commission
British Coundil Division
17 Kasturba Gandhi Marg
E-mail:sanjay.patro@in.britishcouncil.org. New Delhi 110 001
Tel: 91-3710111/37 10555
Fax: 91-3710717

The British Library
Mayfair Building,
Hazratganj
Lucknow 226 001
Telephone + 91 (0)522 22 2144
Fax + 91 (0)522 27 5426
E-mail bipin.kumar@in.britishcouncil.org.

The British Library
Guru Teg Bahadur Complex
Roshanpura Naka,
Bhopal 462 003
Telephone +91 (0)755 55 3767
Fax+91 (0)755 57 2797
E-mail girish.kunkur@in.britishcouncil.org.

In South India
Examination Services Manager
Chennai

Address
Name:Nirupa Fernandez
British Deputy High Commission
British Council Division
737 Anna Salai
E-mail:nirupa.fernandez@in.britishcouncil.org.
Chennai 600 002
Tel: 91-44-852-5002
Fax: 91-44-852-3234

The British Library
39, St. Mark's Road
Banglore 560 001
Telephone +91(0)80 2240763,
221 3485
Fax + 91(0) 80 224 0767
E-mail iqbal.jahagirdar@in.britishcouncil.org.

The British Library
Sarovar Centre, 5-9-22
Secretariat Road,
Hyderabad 500 063
Telephone+91(0)40 230774, 210267
Fax: +91(0)40 329 8273
E-mail sudhakar.goud@in.britishcouncil.org.

The British Library
YMCA Building,
Thiruvananthapuram 695 001
Telephone +91(0)471 330716
Fax +91(0)471 33 0717
E-mail tk.subramoni@in.britishcouncil.org.

Examination Services Manager
Kolkata

Address
Name: Suchitra Mukherjee
British Deputy Commission
British Council Division
5 Shakespeare Sarani
E-mail:suchitra.mukherjee@in.britishcouncil.org.
Kolkata 700071
Tel: 91-33-282-9108/9144
Fax: 91-33-282-4808

The British Library
BP Koirala Marg (Bank Rd.), Patna 800 001
Telephone +91(0)612 22 4198
Fax +91 (0)612 23 0798
E-mail dipak.goswami@in.britishcouncil.org.

Examinatination Services Manager
Mumbai

Address
Name: Kamal Taraparevala
British Deputy High Commission
British Council Division
Mittal Tower 'C' Wing
Nariman Point
Mumbai 400021
E-mail:kamal.taraporevala@in.britishcouncil.org.
Tel: 91-22-222-3560
Fax: 91-22-285-2024

The British Library
Bhaikaka Bhawan,
Law Garden Road,
Ahmedabad 380 006
Telephone +91(0)79 646 4693
Fax- +91 (0)79 646 9493
E-mail satish.deshpande@in.britishcouncil.org.

The British Library
917/1,
Fergusson College Road,
Pune 411 004
Telephone +91 (0)20 565 4352
Fax +91 (0)20 565 4351
E-mail.anil.bakshi@in.britishcouncil.org.

Pakistan
Examination Services Manager
Karachi

Address
Name: Irum Fawad
The British Council
20 Bleak House Road,
Near Cant's Station
E-mail:Irum.Fawad@bc-karachi.bcouncil.org.
(PO Box 10410), Karachi
Tel: 92215670391-7
Fax: 92215682694

Examination Services Manager
Islamabad

Address
Name: Shahnaz Farooq
The British Council
Block 14, Civic Centre   Tel: 9251111424424
G-6   Fax: 9251276683
E-mail:shahnaz.farooq@bc.islamabad.bcouncil.org.
Islamabad

Bangladesh
Examination Services Manager
Dhaka

Address
Name: Saidur rahman
The British Council   Tel: 8802868905-7
5 Fuller Road,   Fax: 8802863375
PO Box 161
E-mail:srhman@The British Council.net
Dhaka 1000

Sri Lanka
Examination Services Manager
Colombo

Address
Name: Ethel Nanayakkara   Tel:941581171
The British Council   Fax: 941587079
49 Alfred Gardens
E-mail:ethel.nanayakkara@britcoun.lk
(PO Box 753) Colombo 3
Sri Lanka

Data Base of Information about PLAB

ROUTES OF EXEMPTION FROM THE PLAB TEST

INTRODUCTION
Doctors with a primary medical qualification accepted for limited registration must either have passed the PLAB test (a test of proficiency in the English language and knowledge of medicine), or be exempted from it before limited registration may be granted. Doctors may be granted exemption from the test if they qualify through one of the following routes. These doctors are not normally required to pass the test **unless they have previously failed it.** That means **once one attempts PLAB one cannot get limited registration through other routes.**

1. SPONSORSHIP ROUTE
This is for doctors who are sponsored for approved postgraduate training in the UK by one of the approved sponsoring bodies or the head of a university department.

To be eligible for restricted exemption a doctor must be sponsored for approved postgraduate training in the UK by one of the approved sponsoring bodies. The approved sponsoring bodies in the UK are the medical royal colleges, the faculty of public health medicine, the british council, the commonwealth scholarship commission and the department of health (on behalf of the WHO).

Doctors who may be sponsored by the university head of department, are those who wish to undertake clinical duties in connection with or as a supplement to their academic training. In order to apply for such exemption the head of the university department should write to the GMC on behalf of the doctor setting out details of the post.

All doctors applying for exemption from the test by the sponsorship route must fulfil the following experience requirements. They must
- have completed overseas an acceptable internship of not less than twelve months, or other experience which the GMC regard as equivalent; and
- thereafter have completed not less than two years in medical practice overseas, of which not less than one year must have been spent in the specialty in which he or she wished to pursue further training in the UK; and
- the doctor must have been appointed, normally before arrival in the United Kingdom, either within the national health service to a supervised training post at the grade of senior house officer or higher or within a university, or comparable research body, to an appointment as lecturer or above, or to a clinical research position of equivalent status. In such cases there must be an honorary national health service contract and
- **he/she must have a minimum overall scale of 70 in IELTS academic modules with not less than 7.0 in each band.**

2. Higher Qualification Route
This is for doctors who, in addition to their primary overseas medical qualification, and 12 months internship also either hold or have passed all the examinations for a higher qualification granted by one of the medical royal colleges or faculties in the United Kingdom or the republic of Ireland (such as the MRCP (UK), FRCO path or FRCS Ireland) or have passed or been exempted from the primary examinations for the MRCPath or the FRCR. These doctors may be granted restricted exemption from the PLAB test in relation only to supervised appointments in the specialty or group of specialities covered by the higher qualification. A doctor applying for limited registration by this roue must first be offered a post for which limited registration may be granted, as explained above. They must meet the IELTS requirement described before.

3. Senior Doctor Route
The GMC will also accept an application from a doctor who has been qualified and has practised overseas for at least 10 years and reached consultant grade or equivalent. To be eligible a doctor should be intending to settle permanently in the UK and must have the support of UK consultant who can offer or arrange a post for which limited registration may be granted. The UK consultant must also be prepared to provide the necessary assurances as to the doctor's linguistic and professional ability as required by section 22 of the Medical Act 1983. For further information the consultant should write to the GMC enclosing the doctor's full curriculum vitae.

4. UK Qualification Route
Doctors who, in addition to their primary overseas medical qualification plus 12 months internship, also hold or have passed all the examinations for one of the following primary medical qualifications set by the united examining board:
- LRCS England, LRCP London
- LMSSA London

- LRCP Edinburgh, LRCS Edinburgh, LRCPS Glasgow are eligible for exemption from the PLAB test.

5. Irish Qualification Route

This is for doctors who are not EEA nationals and who qualified in the Republic of Ireland and have normally completed a one year internship.

Following a decision by overseas comittee non EEA nationals with Irish qualifications will, with effect from 1, January 2000, Cease to be except from the PLAB test solely by virtue of their primary qualifications. From this date, such doctors who wish to apply for limited registration will be required either to pass the PLAB test or to provide other objective evidence of their capability for medical practice in UK.

6. Temporary Full Registration: Visiting Overseas Doctors

Doctors who have a primary medical qualification and 12 months internship which is accepted for limited registration may under section 29 of the Medical Act 1983 apply for temporary full registration as a visiting overseas doctor. This type of registration is intended for doctors who are coming to the UK to demonstrate or provide specialist services in short term appointments as visiting consultants or professors or at a similar academic level in a teaching hospital or medical school. Doctors wishing to apply should arrange for their prospective employer to write to the GMC for further details enclosing a full curriculum vitae and providing details of the post for which registration is required. All such initial applications are determined by a committee of the GMC.

7. Primary Medical Qualification Recognised for full/Provisional Registration

Doctors are exempt from the PLAB test because they qualified as follows:
a. in Australia, New Zealand, the West Indies; or
b. at the Universities of Cape Town, Natal or the Witwatersrand in South Africa; or
c. at certain universities in Hong Kong, or Singapore where the language of instruction is english; or
d. at the University of Malaya on or before 31 December 1987.

As from 1 January 1999, doctors who hold a qualification from the countries listed in sections a) to d) will be required to pass the IELTS test with a minimum overall score in 7.0 in the Academic module with not less than 7.0 in each band.

For further information and whether they qualify for these the candidates are advised to write to GMC directly.

Data Base of Information about PLAB

OVERSEAS DOCTORS TRAINING SCHEME (ODTS)

What is the ODTS?

The overseas doctors training scheme (ODTS) is a formalised double sponsorship scheme initiated jointly by the department of health and the royal colleges and administered by the relevant royal college. The scheme grants acceptable candidates exemption from the professional and linguistic assessment board (PLAB) examination.

The scheme provides very able overseas-qualified doctors with postgraduate training posts to enable them to continue or complete their specialist training in the UK before returning home. It is not intended that overseas doctors remain in the UK on completion of their specialist training.

Why was the ODTS set up?

The royal colleges felt that a formalised scheme of this nature was needed to provide supervised specialist training of a consistently high standard for overseas-qualified doctors of quality who wished to complete their training in the UK. The aim of the scheme is to ensure that the training is of a high standard in order to prepare the overseas doctor for a specialist career in medicine in his/her own country.

Who is eligible?

The requirements are as follows

From January 1998, all overseas doctors must have passed the academic version of the IELTS test (international english language testing system) to be granted limited registration by the general medical council. Doctors with exemption from PLAB must score a minimum of 7 in each of the four bands of the test. This includes doctors from english speaking countries; USA, Australia New Zealand, Canada, South Africa, West Indies).

A primary medical qualification acceptable to the GMC for limited registration; plus one year's post-qualification experience (normally referred to as internship).

At least two years experience in the relevant speciality in which they wish to practice. An aceptable post graduation qualification and/part-1 of the relevant royal college examination.

Canditates who do not meet the above requirements, would not be eligible for the ODTS scheme. Also excluded from applying would be the following:
- applicants who have previously failed the PLAB test.
- applicants who do not hold Part 1 of the relevant royal college examination.
- applicants qualified in and/or nationals of an EEA country, or those with enforceable EC rights.
- applicants already working or who are resident in the UK, or another member state of the EU.

Which ODTS schemes exist?

Summary of recent information received from the royal colleges on the ODTS.

We have summarised below the current situation from information collected by the individual royal colleges. The situation is fluid and liable to change. **It is therefore important that you contact the relevant royal college for information and advice, before coming to the UK.**

The authors want the reader to write to respective royal college to know the latest status.

Royal College of Anaesthetists

ODTS double-sponsorship scheme. The initial approach must be made by a senior medical practitioner from the UK. All appointments must be to substantive, approved training posts. Applications will also be considered from individual doctors whose medical background meets the criteria of the royal college. They would be required to apply for advertised, approved training posts, in open competition.

Royal College of Obstetricians and Gynaecologists

The overseas doctors training scheme and double ended sponsorship scheme organised by the RCOG was abolished from February 2000. Requirements of a new unified scheme have been approved by the college council but the college is still waiting a final report from the department of health, reviewing of all the sponsorship schemes, before the RCOG will be in aposition to omplement the new scheme. It is hoped that the new scheme will involve interviewing doctors overseas and numbers will be restricted to ensure that there is always a training programme available for every successful candidate (i.e. no waiting list). Until such time when the requirements for the new scheme are approved by department of health, the college will not be able to sponsor new doctors for exemption from the GMC's PLAB test. In the mean time the doctors who wish to apply for the new sponsorship scheme, should contact the college the details will be sent to them as soon as they become available.

E-mail:– cwood@rcog.org.uk

Royal College of Ophthalmologists

Dual sponsorship scheme is in operaiton. All posts must be approved for training by the college and postgraduate dean. Honorary SHO posts will be longer be accepted unless they have the approval of the postgraduate dean. For further information contact the royal college. E-mail enquiries to **education@rcophth.btinternet.com**. Information can also be had from colleges website address.

Royal College of Paediatrics and Child Health

Double sponshorship scheme: overseas sponsor and UK sponsor. The college will sponsor doctors for supernumerary posts that have been approved by the postgraduate dean and for approved substantive training posts. International Paediatric Training Scheme; information about the scheme is being updated, contact the royal college for advice.

Royal College of Physicians of Edinburgh

The college has temporarily suspended the overseas doctors training double sponsorship scheme. Please contact the royal college for updated information.

Royal College of Physicians and Surgeons of Glasgow

The college has advised that there are difficulties in placing people applying for the ODTS. Docotrs applying must be funded/supported by their home country. Please contact the royal college for updated information.

Royal College of Physicians of London

The royal college of physicians overseas doctors training scheme is closed. The college is awaiting the rsult of the current review of overseas doctors training being carried out by the department of health, before making a final decision on the development of any revised scheme. The college will consider applicantions for sponsorship for PLAB exemption from physicians who have been awarded an official scholarship or bursary for clinical training in the UK. Overseas training enquiries, telephone +44(0) 207935 1174;fax- +44(0)20 74864034
E-mail:international@rcplondon.ac.uk

Royal College of Psychiatrists

ODTS is closed indefinitely. Consultant assisted sponsorship scheme; Doctors applying for this scheme must have a UK sponsor who should be a consultant in the NHS and a member of the royal college of psychiatrists. Your UK sponsor must be able to offer you a training post within their own training scheme, which should be fully approved by the college. Your UK sponsor is also required to provide written confirmation that they know your overseas sponsor personally. For further information contact the royal college of psychiatrists.

Royal College of Radiologists

The initial application must be made by the UK Sponsor, not the trainee. An overseas sponsor is also required. The UK training post must be within a training scheme recognised by the royal college of radiologists, and a salaried, substantive NHS training post. For further information contact the royal college of radiologists.

Royal College of Edinburgh

The ODTS double sponsorship scheme is the only scheme operated at present. It is the responsibility of the overseas sponsor to set up a post for the application in the UK, in partnership with a UK consultant. The first contact with the Royal college must be made by the UK consultant who is offering the post.

Royal college and Surgeons of England

Applicants must be nominated by an approved sponsoring body in their home country. The royal college of surgeons of England will act as the UK sponsoring body. The college is not able to arrange training posts for sponsored doctors at present. Trainees must have an appointment arranged in the UK before applying to the college for double sponsorship. For further information, please contact the college.

Overview

- Applications direct from candidates will not be accepted by the royal colleges; only appropriate sponsors may apply on their behalf.
- Many more applications are received than there are training posts available.
- Detailed information on a particular overseas doctors training scheme is provided by the relevant college. If further information is required, please contact the college at the address given **in useful addresses chapter.** Applications from sponsors should be sent to the same address.

Data Base of Information about PLAB

MEDICAL CAREER STRUCTURE IN THE UK

Contents:
1. Entry to Medical School
2. The Medical School Training
3. House Jobs
4. Senior House Officer
5. General Practice Vocational Training
6. The General Practitioner (GP)n
7. Middle Grade Hospital Posts
8. Consultants
9. The Pay Review Body
10. Analysis

1. Entry to medical school

The UK education system is often spoken of as divided into Primary Education (5-12), Secondary Education (12-18) and Higher Education (18+). Education is compulsory up until the age of 16, and there is a national exit exam at this stage, formerly known as 'O' Levels, now known as GCSEs. There is a National Curriculum in place, laid down by the Department of Education, which closely determines the content and scope of education up to this point. Students who chose to complete Secondary Education then confine their studies to 3 or (occasionally) 4 subjects, in which they will have final exit examinations at the age of 18. These are known as 'A' Levels. The grades scored in these examinations, and the nature of the subjects studied, determines and limits the choice of subject that may be studied in Higher Education and the quality of the institution where such study may be undertaken. There are about 30 Medical Schools in the UK. Most have an annual intake of around 100 new students, whom they train over the period of a five-year course. Entry to Medical School is normally made at the age of 18, following on immediately from 'A' Levels. However, all UK Medical Schools appear to accept a small number of mature students annually as part (5%) of their intake. Students applying to medicine require three or four high grade 'A' Level passes, and will usually have studied at least three out of Mathematics. Further Mathematics, Physics, Chemistry or Biology. Some Medical Schools run one-year 'Pre-Medical' courses for students who have non-science 'A'-Levels in order to convert.

2. The medical school training

There is some variability in the length and approach of the training of doctors, which is undertaken by different UK Medical Schools. The 'Classical' approach has been a five-year course, broken into two distinct segments:

Pre-clinical
Two years of theory: Anatomy, Physiology, Biochemistry, Pharmacology, Pathology, Genetics, Sociology, Psychology, Bacteriology, and Embryology.

Clinical
One year of half-and-half theory (more Pathology) and early clinical experience, followed by one year of full time hospital-based experience, shadowing 'real' doctors, followed by the final year, which is basically one long revision course.

But the lack of early clinical experience, and the predominance of overtechnical theory in the Pre-clinical phase have come under criticism. Some Medical Schools have adopted what they believe to be a more integrated course structure.

3. House jobs

Following qualification, doctors in the UK hold only provisional registration and license to practice. All such licenses are granted by the UK doctors' regulatory body, the General Medical Council (GMC). A provisional license entitles the holder to practice medicine only under supervision by a fully licensed practitioner. Full registration is obtained upon satisfactory completion of an approved, supervised apprenticeship of one-year duration, which must contain at least 4 months each of Hospital Medicine and Hospital Surgery.

Out of these regulations were born the 'Junior House Jobs', equivalent to the US internship. Although the stipulation is only for 4 months, in practice 99.9% of UK graduates undertake two 6-month contracts, one in Medicine and the other in Surgery. Accreditation for such posts towards full registration is granted by the Medical School. Although clearly intended to oblige the new doctor to get a broad practical grounding in the bread and butter of medicine, the staffing requirements of the hospitals has historically forced considerable bending of this intent, so that it is entirely possible for a doctor to become fully registered having done six months of Neurology and six months of Neurosurgery, having never seen an Appendicitis or a Coronary.

A Junior House Officer (JHO) typically works an average of 72 hours a week, based on a full 40-hour working week and cover for every 4th night and weekend. Such a regular rota results in a regularly repeating four week working cycle of 104, 56, 72 and 56 hours respectively with the longest continuous shift being 56 hours (9 am Saturday until 5 pm Monday).

Basic starting salary for a House Doctor is £16145 annually for the basic 40-hour week, and the additional On-Call duties are paid at half (50%) this hourly rate. Thus, a House Doctor on a 1:4 rota works an average of 32 additional hours each week, for whcih they receive an additional £6458 annually before deductions. Malpractice Insurance for this period is nil: the State pays any costs.

4. Senior house officer

Following completion of the House Jobs, and acquisition of Full Registration, UK doctors may begin specialist training. In the initial phase, this involves seeking further six-month contracts in appropriate specialities at the grade of Senior House Officer (SHO). Over a period of two to four years, a prospective specialist will change jobs (and frequently hospital) every six months so as to gain experience in and around their chosen subject. What counts as appropriate is determined semi-explicitly by the various Royal Colleges, who exercise responsibility for the Post-Registration training of all UK Doctors. During this period of time, it is common (well, effectively mandatory) to sit the relevant examination of the Royal College, since advancement to the next grade of training is virtually impossible without this. By the completion of the SHO phase, the doctor is usually 4 years out of Medical School.

SHO hours of duty are very similar to that of the JHO, and although they often have a JHO whom they supervise, they are often very much in the front line. Remuneration is calculated in exactly the same way, from a starting basic salary of £20135 rising to £24200 after four years. Additional duty hours (On-Call) are also calculated at 50% of the normal hourly rate. Malpractice insurance remains covered by the State.

5. General practice vocational training

In parallel with hospital training, doctors who aspire to become General Practitioners (Family Doctors) also undertake a period of hospital-based experience, working as SHOs for two years. The two years must include not less than six months in each of two of Medicine, Geriatrics, Accident and Emergency, Paediatrics, Psychiatry and Obstetrics and Gynaecology. The remaining year is commonly made up of another two from the list, although other options (e.g. Orthopaedics) are permitted. These posts are specifically accredited for General Practice training by the Royal College of General Practitioners, but in practice are virtually indistinguishable from speciality training posts. Many Hospitals, partly in order to solve recruitment difficulties and effort, offer GP training scheme contracts of two years duration at SHO grade during which time the doctor will work in a variety of specialities as required by the RCGP for accreditation. It is not obligatory to gain training accreditation by means of a hospital scheme; indeed approximately 30% of doctors who gain GP accreditation do so via a 'DIY' scheme. Terms and Conditions of Service, hours of work, remuneration and Malpractice arrangements are as for speciality training SHOs.

Following the prescribed hospital two years, Vocational Trainees for General Practice undertake a year working in an approved General Practice Partnership under the guidance and instruction of an approved GP Trainer. During this time, the Trainee gradually gains in experience until working with the same freedom and responsibilities towards the patients as the Partners.

The Trainee year is characterized by compulsory attendance at a weekly full day-release vocational training course, during which topics as diverse as Practice Finance, Man Management, Transactional Analysis and Group Dynamics might be taught. Therapeutics and more clinical skills are often left to the recommended additional 3 hours a week dedicated one-on-one teaching with the Trainer. Malpractice insurance is arranged privately by the individual Trainee, current cost is approximately £1100 annually. Working hours are probably about 72 hours a week. Remuneration is less than for hospitals, being 122% of the basic salary for an SHO of the same seniority (the 15% is a flat rate payment for all On-Call) and a further £3928 for the Car expenses.

At the end of the Trainee year, it is common to take the examination of the Royal College of General Practitioners by way of an exit examination. This is not a necessary requirement (yet) of acquiring full accreditation for completion of GP training. Having completed this training vocationally trained GPs are free to apply for posts as a partner in General Practice whenever and wherever the vacancies appear. Malpractice Insurance remains the responsibility of the individual GP, and costs upwards of £1500 annually (I think...).

6. The general practitioner

Individual General Practitioners in the UK currently have, on average, about 1800 patients registered under their care. They almost universally work within a business structure, being contracted by the State to provide certain core medical services for the patients on their list. A typical GPs day usually takes the form of a 2-3 hour surgery in the morning, and another in the afternoon. These surgeries may be by appointment, or open access at the GPs choosing. On average, each patient spends between 5 and 8 minutes with the GP at each such consultation. After morning surgery, UK GPs usually perform home visits, to which patients have a right. On average, there are around four of these, per GP, per day. Following this most GPs now run special clinics of one form or another during the afternoon: diabetic, hypertensive, child surveillance, ante natal clinics and so on. The core service also includes an obligation to provide 24 hour, 7 days a week, 365 days a year emergency medical services, at the patient's home should they so require. GPs may delegate some or all of this 'On-Call' commitment to colleagues, or deputies, but remain ultimately medico-legally responsible for the actions of their stand-in. On average, a GP works around 70 hours a week in 1995. Malpractice Insurance remains the responsibility of the individual GP, and costs £2165 in 1999.

Remuneration of GPs is complex. General Practitioners, as they did before the NHS, generally work in partnerships of some 3-5 doctors. The greater part of a partnership's income now derives from fulfillment of their NHS contract. The bulk of the income comes from multiplying the total number of patients cared for by a fee per patient (known as the capitation fee):

Capitation Fees (March 1999 figures):
Patient under 65 years of age: £17.65
Patient between 65 and 75: £23.25
patient over 75: £45.05

...and then adding on the Basic Practice Allowance which is linked to the absolute number of patients:
Basic Practice Allowance (March 1999 Figures)
For first 400 patients (minimum qualifying list) £3,440 lump sum
Next 401-600 patients £8.60 per patient
Next 601-800 patients £6.88 per patient
Next 801-1000 patients £5.16 per patient
Next 1001-1200 patients £3.44 per patient
More than 1200 nil extra

Capitation fees and Basic Practice Allowance alone would give a GP with a typical age: sex mix and list size an income of around £51,000 gross a year. In addition to this income, however, almost all practices elect to provide a range of optional additional services (not compulsory under the contract) for which there are additional payments available from the state on a fee-per-item basis. For example, some of the more common 'extras' and the payment GPs received in March 1999 for each patient so treated:

Contraceptive advice ro treatment £16.40 per year per patient
Complete antenatal and intrapartum care £205 per pregnancy
Minor Surgery £128.25 per five cases
Child Health Surveillance £12.75 per child under five years old
Temporary Resident (up to 15 days) £10.40 per patient
Temporary Resident (more than 16 days) £15.60 per patient
Training Grant (for training GP Trainees) £5,645 per Trainee

There are also a number of Health Promotion activities for which GPs receive payments provided they reach various uptake targets in their population:
Childhood Immunizations (higher target) £2,580 (lower target) £860
Pre-school Boosters (higher target) £765 (lower target) £860
Cervical Cytology (higher target) £2,865 (lower target) £955

...and then there are deprivation payments, if your practice area is considered to be particularly poor (and the morbidity consequently higher), Rural Practice Allowance (to cover the additional costs of driving around remote areas), Seniority Payments etc. etc. etc. This baroque arrangement requires much chasing of paper, and permanent uncertainty regarding your final income. A significant number of GPs intermittently question whether it would be simpler to become a salaried service, directly employed (rather than contracted) by the State in the same way as Consultants. Opponents of this idea say that it would prevent keen, dynamic GPs from being able to increase their individual incomes through hardwork.

From this grand total of income from all sources, the expenditure of the practice such as on buildings and staff must first be deducted, and the remainder is incoem for the Partners. GPs can also earn additional money through private, i.e. non-government, medical work (e.g. Occupational Health for a local Industrial Employer, medicals for insurance companies). Some practices share equally the pooled private incomes of all the partners, whereas in other practices the individual partners retain whatever they earn in addition to NHS income.

This payment scheme suggests that the more work GPs do, the more they earn over and above the capitation fee payment. Whilst this is broadly true for an individual practice, it is not true for the combined income of all GPs - the total amount earned annually by all GPs in the NHS. This is because the money paid out each year - both for honouring the contract and as fees for all the optional sections - actually comes out of one big, but finite, pot of money. The size of this pot is calculated precisely in advance, on an annual basis, by choosing a sum of money which is considered an appropriate annual income for an average GP inthe coming year. This 'average gross intended remuneration' figure is then multiplied by the number of GPs in the country to arrive at the total budget for GP services which the Government expects to pay during the following year. All the various fees - capitation, basic practice allowance, item of service fees etc. - are then reverse-engineered from this sum.

The 1999 figure for average gross intended remuneration stands at £75,892. This figure often appears in the popular press as evidence that GPs are fabulously well paid, considering they spend all day on the golf course. Of course, this gross figure is before the GP has paid any of their staff.

In 1999 the Department of Health reckons that it costs £24,700 per GP in a practice to cover the practice expenses, a figure calculated by the Dept. of health randomly selecting a small group of 'typical' practices annually and, from their accounts, calculating an average expenditure. Thus the total practice income, before expenses, should be the number of GPs multiplied by £75,892. After the expenses are met, however, the Government intends each GP to take home an average net intended remuneration of £50,760 on which the GP subsequently pays income tax and so forth (currently about 30%).

A digest of the 1992-1993 workload survey of General Practitioners, an annual study used as part of the process of deciding centrally what GPs should be paid, is here.

7. Middle grade hospital posts
The posts of Registrar, Senior Registrar and Specialist Registrar grade make up the middle grade hospital medical staff.

Entry to the middle grades of Junior Hospital Doctor is now regulated by a strict quota system. It was recognized inthe early 1970s that the medical career ladder had a significant bottle neck developing in it such that, without action, there would soon be large numbers of doctors who had completed their sepcialist training, but for whom Consultant Posts did not exist. It was felt that this would be detrimental to the morale of the profession and the well being of the public (see the Snow report). As a result, a committee named JPAC sits annually to decide on exactly how many Registrar and Senior Registrars there will be that year nationally in each of the variouis specialities. Thus, all Registrars and Senior Registrars are assigned a number, and no further middle grade appointments may be made unless a number becomes free (unless the doctor is from overseas, and not intending to settle in the UK).

In theory, this quota system was supposed to control matters while a 2% compound annual increase in Consultant numbers gradually relieved the need for it. It is a matter of considerable debate as to whether this expansion has taken place, and whether JPAC has done its job properly. Cynical Juniors argue that it is not in the Consultants' interest to expand Consultant numbers at this increases competition for their Private Practice Income, nor is it in their interest to decrease the numbers of Juniors, who do all the NHS work on behalf of the Consultants when they are busy in their Private Practice.

Middle Grade posts are usually of three-year tenure, although there is commonly rotation between firms and sub-specialities within and between hospitals during this time. Further Royal College Examinations - usually of a more clinical bent than previously - are undertaken during this time. Because of the persistence of the bottleneck, it is also becoming common (verging again on obligatory) to undertake some form of research work as a Registrar in order to further your chances of succeeding in an application for a Senior Registrar post.

Registrar and Senior Registrar hours of duty are notionally also no more than an average 72 hour week, but since there are relatively fewer of them it is probable that many are still on 83 hours or more. Most, if not all, are shielded from the front line of duty by virtue of having an SHO and/or a JHO working beneath them. Some of them even get to sleep! Basic remuneration for these posts is £22510 rising to £32830 after 9 years. Additional Duty Hours are calculated as before. Malpractice Insurance is still covered by the State.

8. Consultants
The average age of appointment is probably about 32 overall, tending to be somewhat higher in the Surgical Specialities. Most Consultants contract part-time with the NHS in order to build and maintain a Private Practice in addition; typically they work for the NHS three and a half days a week, and spend the rest of the tiem in Private Practice. Private diagnostic or Inpatient services are generally provided by commercial hospitals, run by organizations such as BUPA or AMH.

NHS salaries for Consultants commence at £45740 rising to £59040 after five years. Consultants on part time salaries will earn proportionately less from NHS work. The State provides malpractice cover arising out of any work performed on the NHS, but the Consultant must make separate arrangements for any claims arising out of Private Practice.

9. The pay review body

Fairly early on in the history of the NHS it was recognized that the position of the government is effectively a monopoly employer made pay bargaining somewhat tricky, and potentially unfair. A similar problem was identified for other professions, such as Nurses and Teachers. In order to avoid any unseemly rows between gentlemen, the government instituted a system of independent pay review bodies. The idea was that, on an annual basis, the government and doctors would put to a panel of independent reviewers their views as to what doctors should be paid. It was expected that, more often than not, both sides would usually, as gentlemen do, suggest more or less identical pay levels. Only when a minor disagreement arose, say every decade or so, would the Review Body has to actually do any arbitrating. Whatever figure was agreed would be universally binding to all state hospitals.

The reality has been rather different. The Pay Review bodies for medical and dental practitioners have never received 'joint' (i.e. concordant) evidence, and in some years have actually had to arbitrate more than once. The government, especially in recent years, has often overruled the arbitrated decision, or agreed to fund half of a recommended increase centrally, insisting that the rest of the pay increase be met locally by individual hospitals making savings from their service provision.

Needless to say, neither side is particularly happy with the way things have turned out. However, the profession seems even less thrilled at the direction the government seems to be taking now: Trust hospitals will soon acquire the right to ignore any centrally agreed pay scales, and will begin local pay bargaining. This is a move the government supporters, and wants to take even further with pay settlements both nationally and locally having an element of performance related pay built into them.

10. Analysis

The description above attempts to give an overview of the various training requirements for doctors working in the UK. The mechanisms to ensure appropriate experience also presuppose appropriate supervision at all stages. Whilst there has always been an understanding that complete supervision was unrealistic, in recent years it is widely felt that quantity of experience has been relied on too heavily as a substitute for quality. Consultants, nominally the supervisors of the continuing education of the Junior and Middle Grade Staff on their firm, have always been obliged to balance the pressures to maintain the service against the expenditure of time in training activities. As hospitals became more intensive places to work, the balance was tipped against supervision and quality of experience. The demands for improved patient throughput on reduced budget that have arisen with the NHS reforms have only served to strengthen these pressures.

VISA MATTERS, TRAVEL AND STAY IN UK

Decide first whether you want to take part I in India or in UK, if you decide to take part I in India and after passing part I, after receiving hall ticket for part II, go to the British Embassy at Madras (Chennai) (for candidates from South India), Mumbai (for candidates from West Zone). Kolkata (East Zone), New Delhi for all others. There, one will be applying for a visa for a period of six months. One has to take these documents to be on the safe side.

1. PLAB hall ticket with passport.
2. Sponsor's letter from UK.
3. Bank statement showing finances of atleast Rs. 2-2.5 lakhs.
4. A leave note from your present employer.

Visa Facts

1. Prior to october 2nd 2000, single entry VISA's were isued for 6 months, generally as a "tourist" or "for PLAB". Since then VISA's are being issued for upto 1 year or even 2 years, and are multiple-entry. This means that you can travel between India and UK as many times as you want, without having to get a new VISA.
2. The cost of the VISA is Rs.2300/- for a 6 month single entry but these are subject to change and should be found out from the British High Commission at the time of visa application.
3. On getting a job, you change your VISA to "permit free" VISA. Only then you can begin work in the hospital and be paid for it. The change of VISA happens within a day as soon as you produce the GMC registration and take it and your passport to the immigration office.
4. If you do not get a job in the first 6 months, your VISA has expired, you could extend it for another 6 months within the UK.

Experiences with Getting VISA from India

VISA is not a big problem, unlike the US VISA, only a few are refused VISA. The VISA form is available beforehand and you may fill it and take it with you. The officer mainly wants to confirm that you can fend for yourself in the months leading upto the examination and beyond before you get a job. They also would like to hear that you will return back to India when you are done with your training. You can show that you have reasons to return back (such a property in india, a promise of a job, etc.).

A PLAB admit card is almost a must. You do not need "no objection certificates" from anyone.

On some occasions the VISA officers have allegedly asked (unbecoming) questions, possibly due to a basic ignorance of the special VISA doctors have, to work in the UK. You should point out that doctors and dentists do not need a "work permit", they can work on a "Permit free training" type VISA. At heathrow, the VISA is but a formality, only those with forged documents are sent back.

The common mistakes doctors make:

1. Lying for anything to a VISA officer is a problem.
2. Do not produce any forged or wrong documents.
3. If they ask how long do you want to stay in UK, tell honestly that after the exam, I will be looking for a training post, and the earliest I return could be months or even a year odd.
4. No taking proper support letter from UK and PLAB entry letter is not helpful.
5. Refusal of VISA by the US on your passport is often counterproductive.

The cost of an air tickets to UK at present, is approximately Rs. 20000-30000 depending on the Air line (one-way). While travelling, take most of your clothing as buying these will entail extra expenses in England.

Pack lots of warm clothing, like thermal undergarments and sweaters. Take along packets of 'sambhar' powder and chilli powder to aid you in cooking.

Take a couple of blazers and ties along with formal showes. In hosptials in the UK, senior house officers wear formal outfits with a tie and the consultants wear suits. However, when you appear for PLAB part 2, you will have to wear a suit, preferably black. You will not need your white coats or your medical instruments when you appear for Part 2.

Before landing in England, have full knowledge of the place where you will be staying. It would be pertinent to note that paying guest accomodation in eastham is most suitable for Indian students. These houses are occupied by India families who will help in every way.

After landing in England and getting place of boarding, one would be benefitted immensely by joining the MMC flats (madras medical college alumni flats). Here make a down payment of 100 pounds and use the material in the files for extensive revision. There is no need to pay for any subsequent attempts. The only disadvantage of this place is that one cannot xerox the files kept there.

REGISTRATION AND APPLYING FOR A JOB

The results of PLAB II (OSCE) examination will be declared within two to three weeks of the test. It will be either PASS or FAIL.

If one passes the OSCE one will be sent forms and details about applying for limited regisrtation. Before you are granted limited registration your primary qualification must be checked. After passing the examination one will register with the general medical council after paying a registration fee. Then you should look for job opportunities in classified section of the BMJ and British Journal of Hospital Medicine.

The addresses and websites for looking for job is given in the end of the book.

Limited Registration
The information in this chapter will apply if one has taken and passed the PLAB test and hold a primary medical qualification accepted by the GMC for limited registration.

Applications, original documents and payments may be sent by post or submitted in person between 09:00 am and 16:30 pm monday to friday at the general medical council, reception, 5th floor, north entrance, 178 great portland street, London W1N 6 JE, please note that it is not possible for the reception staff to indicate whether or not registration will be granted.

The GMC authorities are not in position to answer questions relating to work permits or visas. One should direct such enquiries to the home office, immigration department, lunar house, wellesley road, Croydon Surrey.

Similarly, if one needs advice about postgraduate training, how to apply for jobs or clinical attachments one should contact the national advice centre for postgraduate medical education, central information service. The british council, Medlock Street, Manchester M15 4PR which is given separately.

BASIC REQUIREMENTS FOR LIMITED REGISTRATION
Qualifications
You must hold or have passed the final qualifying examinations for a primary medical qualifications accepted for limited registration. The GMC authorities normally accept primary medical qualifications awarded at universities listed in the world directory of medical schools published by the world health organisation as well as qualifications and universities which are not in the directory but which have, in the past, been accepted by the GMC. There are about 1400 universities awarding primary medical qualifications which are currently accepted.

Selection for Employment
By law, one must have been selected for employment before GMC can grant, one limited registration for the first time. Registration will normally be granted only for supervised employment in posts which afford education and training approved by a royal college or faculty or joint higher committee or, in scotland, by a regional postgraduate committee. The GMC authorities understand that normally only posts in the national health service training grades of senior house officer (SHO), specialist registrar (SpR) are educationally approved in this way, Positions such as a staff grade or consultant posts are not so approved.

Good Character
The medical act requires that the GMC is satisfied that an applicant for limited registration is of good character. One is asked to complete a declaration on the form and one should tell the GMC if one has any convictions or have had any restrictions placed on one's practice in another country.
Other types of employment one can hold under limited registration.

Honorary Posts
Limited registration may also be granted for an honorary, supernumerary or non established hospital post which is not itself educationally approved but only if there is an equivalent established post in exactly the same grade and speciality which is educationally approved in the manner described above.

Clinical Assistant Posts
Limited registration may also be granted for a hospital post at clinical assistant grade. but only if the post is approved for training programmes under the auspices of a university faculty or university clinical department, and documentary evidence or this is provided by the head of the faculty or department concerned.

Posts at House Officer Level or in Family Planning Clinics
Please contact the board for individual advice if you wish to work in these posts.

Note-If one has taken the PLAB test without first completing a 12 month's internship, or its equivalent one will have to complete the balance of experience in house officer posts, either in the UK or overseas. One can then apply to work at senior house officer level or higher.

Scope of Limited Registration

Once limited registration has been granted the board will send a certificate of limited registration which sets out the description of the employment which one may undertake. It you work in one post which are not covered by the description on one's certificate one may be practising illegally. It is one's responsibility to ensure that one holds registration which is appropriate to the employment in which one is engaged. Further advice on the scope of limited registration is given in the booklet 'limited registration' which will be sent with certificate of limited registration.

Guidance on the duties of a doctor will be sent with the first certificate issued. Additional specific guidance will be sent concerning the scope of limited registration.

Five Year Maximum Period

By law the maximum total period of limited registration which can be granted to a doctor is five years.

Limited registration will expire on the terminal date of registration shown on certificate of limited registration.

How to make an Application for Registration

Once one has passed the PLAB test a form LR/PLAB will be sent. One should complete part 1 oneself, and then ask an authorised officer of the autority or institutiion in which one is to be employed to complete part 2. This will normally be the medical, staffing officer, unit medical officer, personnel officer or cosultant in administrative charge.

If one is applying for a further period of limited registration one also needs to complete part 1, of form LR/PLAB. However, part 2 of the form need only be completed if one intends to renew or extend one's registration for employment as a house officer or clinical assistant.

Registration of Names

One will be registered in the names which appears on one's original diploma of qualification (or an english translation of it). Additional documentary evidence of your names may be required if:

a. One wishes to be registered in a name which is different from that which appeares on one's diploma; or
b. One submits any other documents in support of one's application which refers by a name which does not appear on the original diploma.

One should bear in mind that, although initials can appear in doctor's entries in the limited register, all names must be shown in full in the 'main' register. If one was subsequently to apply for full registration at a later date, therefore, it may be necessary to provide further evidence of full names at that stage.

Where additional documentary evidence of a doctor's name is required the following is normally accepted provided that the document is original and gives in full both his name in which one wishes to be registered:

a. A further certificate from the university at which you obtained your primary medical qualification confirming the the person who graduated and the person applying for registration are one and the same;
b. As evidence of a change of name on marriage, a marriage certificate.

One should give an address for entry in the register which is reliable and effective so that communications from the GMC can reach you without delay. Failure to maintain a reliable address may lead to delay in future grants of limited registration or to erasure from the register. Changes of address can be notified in writing (letter or fax) or by telephone.

Evidence of Qualifications

One will need to send original documentary evidence of one's primary medical qualification if not already produced. This evidence should comprise:

a. The original diploma issued by the university or other body which granted the medical qualification; or
b. An original certificate from that university or body stating the date on which the medical qualification was granted; or
c. An original certificate from that university or body stating that one passed the examinations and completed the curriculum necessary for obtaining the qualification and that one is eligible to receive the qualification.

Any certificate as described at a or b should bear the stamp or insign of the university or body by which it was first issued or give other acceptable evidence of authenticity. It should also be signed by a person whose name and official position at the university or body are clearly identified.

The GMC authorities accept only original documents: duplicate copies of university diplomas, including attested copies and photocopies are not accepted. If one cannot provide original documents, one should inform in writing of the circumstances why this is so. The candidate will be advised on what other arrangement, if any, can be made.

Documents not in English must be accompanied by the original of a translation certified as correct by a government authority or an official translator.

Fees
The fees for an initial application for limited registration for up to 12 months and seven days is £ 300. In addition a scrutiny fee of £ 100 is also payable (making a total of £ 400) unless one has already paid this fee when applying to take the PLAB test. The fees for further grants of limited registration are as follows:
 a. Renewal of limited registration for up to 12 months and seven days for the same description or range of employment as that or which limited registration was previously granted: £ 70.
 b. Extension of limited registraion for up to 12 months and seven days for a different or additional description or range of employment from that for which limited registration was previously granted: £ 140.
 c. Each additional year or part of a year, if more than 12 months and seven days registration is required at one time: £ 70 .

One can pay by cash, cheque, banker's draft or traveller's cheque provided that they are issued in sterling. Euro cheques up to a maximum value of £ 700 are also accepted.

How to Stop your Registration
Voluntary Erasure
The main advantage of voluntary erasure is to avoid using portions of the total period of five years, limited registration during periods when one does not need to be registered.

If one wishes to remove one's name from the register before the date on which one's limited registration expires one should complete the form on the back of all current certificates of limited registration.

If one proposes to apply for voluntary erasure while holding a contract of employment as a medical practitioner in the United Kingdom one is advised to discuss the matter with one's employing authority.

Voluntary erasure is not granted retrospectively. One should not assume that one's name has been removed from the register until one has received a letter confirming this.

No fee is charged for voluntary erasure but no refund is made for unused periods of limited registration, nor is credit given for registration.

When one wishes one's name to be returned to the register following voluntary erasure an application should be made on form LR/PLAB.

Notes on Moving from Limited to Full Registration
Please use of this chapter to help to make your application to move from limited to full registration.

Please note that these does not apply if one has requalified in the United Kingdom by obtaining one or more of the following qualifications:
 1. LRCS England, LRCP London, LMSSA London; or
 2. LRCP Edinburgh, LRCS Edinburgh, LRCPS Glasgow;

Please contact the GMC for the appropriate application form and guidance.

About this Guidelines
This guidelines is divided into the following sections:
A. What one should know about full registration.
B. Guidences used in deciding and application.
C. Other ways to move from limited to full registration.
D. What happens to an application.
E. How to make application.
F. Unsuccessful applications.

A. What one Should know about Full Registration
- The guidelines the board uses to decide whether one can move from limited to full registration are decribed in detail.
- The GMC authorities understand that the grant of full registration does not of itself have an effect an status under the immigration rules.
- If one's experience does not meet the guidelines please contact the authorities for advice before making an application.

B. Applications which do not Meet the Guidelines
1. Applications which do not meet the guidelines will be determined by the GMC's overseas committee.
2. However, it is open to apply if one has held limited registration with preserved rights that is, one's limited registration is not restricted to maximum of five years in aggregate and one has.
 a. At least 10 years continuous service in the NHS in predominantly substantive or long-term (longer than six months) locum posts.
 b. Recent clinical practice in the UK (at least two years practice during the previous three years) Plus.
 c. Favourable reports from the UK consultants who have supervised one during the most recent two years practice.

The authorities will need to refer to the GMC's overseas committee applications from doctors with 'preserved rights' whose experience falls outside these guidelines.

One should inform if one has been offered a post as trainee in general practice and has obtained hospital experience accepted by the joint committee on postgraduate training for general practice as fulfilling the relevent requirments of the vocational training regulations. The Board will then tell what further documents one will need.

The overseas committee has indicated that, except in exceptional circumstances, it does not wish to consider applications where an applicant's experience falls substantially short of the guidelines. If one feels that one's circumstances are exceptional one must provide details of one's reasons for applying early.

E. How to make your Application
1. As the board has to gather a number of items to enable it to process one's application, one should make it well in advance of the date on which on would like full registration to begin.
2. Your application should consist of:
a. A completed application form to move from limited to full registration (Form LRFR);
b. A fee of £500 if one is making first application or £250 if one is re-applying;
c. The documents described in paragraphs D4 (if not already submitted) D6, and D10;
3. Please send application to the GMC. If one done not with to send original documents or payments through the post, one may bring them between 9.00 hours and 16.30 hours monday to friday to the GMC's reception on the fifth floor at 178 great portland street, London WIN6JE.

Documents Required
Primary Medical Qualifications
The GMC will normally have seen evidence of one's primary medical before one was the prefix 'p.e.' on one's certificate of limited registration this means that the GMC has received evidence only that one has passed the examinations for one's primary medical qualification. In this case, please submit additional evidence that the qualification was subsequently conferred. The orignal diploma issued by the university or body stating the qualification and the date on which it was formally conferred. Such a certificate should bear the stamp of the university or body. It should also be signed by a person whose name and official position at the university body are clearly identified.

The board accepts only documents as evidence of one's primary qualification, not copies or photocopies. The evidence does not have diploma itself. It may be an original letter from the university or an original certificate. If one cannot provide original documents, please write and provide with details as to the reasons why. If the document is not in english, please provide an original translation certified as correct by a government authority or an offcial translator.

Evidence of Basic Specialist Training
If appropriate, please provide a document from the training body to confirm that one has completed basic specialist training. Photocopies and faxed copies are acceptable for this purpose.

Completing the Application Form
Applicant's name for entry in the register.

This will usually be the same as shown in the limited register (initials cannot be included in your register entry see d. below). If it is diferent you should send additional documentary evidence of the change. The following evidence is acceptable.
a. A further original certificate from the university at which you obtained your overseas primary medical qualification showing both the name in which you graduated and the name which you wish to be entered in the register of medical practitioners, with all names shown in full.
b. An original marriage certificate accompanied by a translation if necessary, provided that the certificate shows the name in which you have held limited registration and in full, the name which you are now using.
c. An affidavit or statutory declaration sworn before a notary public or oath commissioner.
d. Your passport as evidence of a name previously recorded by the GMC as an initial.

Address for Entry in the Register
It is important to choose for entry in the register of medical practitioners. It is reliable and effective. The board sends all communication to your registered address. If you do not respond to them, this may in certain circumstances lead to the erasure of your name from the register. You may wish to bear in mind that the whole of your register entry including your address is public information and, for this reason, you may prefer not to use your professional or private address for registration purposes.

While your application is being considered the board may wish to contact you by telephone. It would, therefore be helpful if you could provide a daytime telephone and/or fax number. These will not form part of your register entry and will not be disclosed.

Consultant's Reports

You will need to provide in form LRFR the names and addresses of the consultants who have supervised you in every post at least for 3 months duration held in the UK during the last three years. Please forward to each of them a copy of the enclosed consultant report form (CRF) asking them to complete it and return it direct to the GMC. Further CRGs may be provided if required. Please do not ask your consultants to give their reports to you, the reports should be sent direct to the GMC.

Declaration

As an applicant for full registration you must satisfy the registrar of the GMC that you are of good character. You must declare on form LRER whether you gave been convicted or found guilty by a court of law and whether you have been suspended or disqualified or prohibited from practicing medicine, or from being registered as a medical practitioner, in any country.

Information About Fees

The fee for an initial application is £ 500 pounds payable in advance. If the board does not approve your application, £ 250 pounds will be retained by the GMC to cover the cost of considering and determining your application; the remainder of the fee paid will be refunded to you. The fee for any subsequent application is £ 250 pounds.

Cheques or money orders for the appropriate fee should be made payable to the general medical council. Payments sent from overseas should be by bank draft or money order payable in sterling in the United Kingdom or by a cheques on an account in the UK.

The board will send you a refund of any fees paid for whole years of unused limited registration which remain to you at the date on which full registration is granted.

Outcome of Your Application

If your application meets the guidelines, the board will send you a certificate of full registration and information booklet about full registration and a copy of the publication of duties of a doctor. When you are fully registered, your name will appear in the prinicipal list of the register of medical practitioners. You will need to pay an annual fee of 80 £ on the anniversary of your date of full registration.

Not all applications received by the GMC meet the guidelines and you should not, therefore work in any post for which full registration is required until the board have informed you that your application has been granted. If you currently hold limited registration for your present employment in the UK and are eligible to apply for it to be extended or renewed, you should do so if you need further registration while your application for full registration is being considered.

If your application is refused the board will notify you by letter as soon as the overseas committee has made its decision and the board will refund £ 250.

If you have held limited registration for a period of at least three years and six months at the time of the GMC's decision to refuse your application for full registration, you may apply to the review board for overseas qualified practitioners for a review of the decision. If you are eligible to apply to the board you will be given further information about this in the letter notifying you of the outcome of your application.

CURRENT SITUATION OF PG TRAINING IN UK

"Whether I will get a training post in the UK. After passing the PLAB".

"Whether I get the the speciality of my choice after passing the PLAB in UK".

These are the questions which haunts any overseas doctor, however well versed he may be with the UK and NHS. This is the most importanrt factor which demotivates an overseas doctor from writing the PLAB test for fear of not getting the job after the PLAB test. The information given below will be of help in knowing ones possibility of getting jobs after passing the PLAB test.

The Opportunity

Every year there are possible opportunities for up to 3,000 doctors who are not UK graduates to obtain training positions in the NHS. There is no overall control on the numbers coming to the UK to seek these posts. There is currently strong competition for most hospital posts.

1. HOW TO USE THIS CHAPTER

1. Read the notes below to understand the training grades of:
    - Pre-registration House Officer (PRHO)
    - Senior House Officer (SHO)
    - Specialist Registrar (SpR)
2. Study the tables within these pages on the number of posts in your chosen speciality which are held by overseas doctors.
   From this information you can draw some conclusions about your chances of gaining a post.
3. Be clear about the relationship between general medical council (GMC) registration and training posts.

Some doctors are able to obtain sponsorship for exemption from the PLAB test. Sponsorship is linked to a training post. Doctors are only sponsored if they have been offered a post.

Many doctors obtain limited registration by passing the professional and linguistic assessment board (PLAB) test which is set by the UK licensing body. The general medical council (GMC).

It is important that doctors understand that passing the PLAB in no way guarantees employment in an NHS training post. There is no link between PLAB test places and the number of training places which will become available.

Registration of non UK graduates with the General Medical Council

Grants of Registration to EEA doctors	1994	1995	1996	1997	1998	1999
Full Registration	1444	1779	2084	1860	1590	1392
Grants of Full Registration to Overseas Qualified Non EEA Doctors						
Transfer from Limited Registration without re-qualification in the UK	994	1639	1894	1981	1885	1796
Doctors holding recognised overseas qualifications	1530	1630	1976	1634	1419	977
Grants of Limited Registration to Overseas Qualified Non EEA Doctors						
Initial grants	2335	2727	2959	2659	2098	2149
Renewals and Extensions	6760	6615	6085	5981	5474	5989

These figures are provided to give an idea of the number of overseas doctors gaining registration each year.

The most useful figures are those for grants of limited registration because this is only granted to doctors appointed to training posts at SHO and SpR grades. Initial grants of limited registration last for a maximum of one year renewals and extensions represent doctors continuing their training for a second and subsequent years in the same or a different institution.

Doctors granted full registration may be taking up training posts, career posts or not taking any post at all.

4. Note that it is uncommon for an overseas doctors to be appointed directly to Type I SpR programmes which lead to the award of a Certificate of Completion of Specialist Training. Many doctors will wish to undertake a short period of training in the SHO grade prior to seeking entry to higher specialist training.
5. The postgraduate deans are responsible for the management of all postgraduate training in the NHS. There are 20 deans covering the UK. Posts which have not been approved by the dean and the relevant royal college are not training posts and fall outside the scope of the permit free arrangements in the immigration rules.

6. Further guidance on your chances of obtaining a training post can be obtained by studying the positive and negative factors listed below.

Positive Factors	Negative Factors
Age under 35	Age over 35
Postgraduate experience in a teaching hospital before coming to the UK	Only internship experience
Success in local or UK	No examination success at postgraduate examinations postgraduate level
Clearly expressed training objective	Vague training objective or expression of interest in more than one speciality
Willingness to go anywhere in the UK	Requirement for one UK location only
Initial experience in locum (short term) posts (only available to doctors who have passed PLAB) in the UK	No locum experience in the UK
Link between home department and the UK	No link with UK

Each dean has a designated member of staff to advise on the special needs of overseas doctors. Training posts must be approved by the postgraduate dean's department. Postgraduate deans ensure the delivery of training in their area and the annual review of trainees progress.

7. The royal colleges and faculties publish appropriate syllabuses and handbooks, conduct appropriate tests, assessments and examinations, and visit and inspect training programmes and placements. Their approval is essential to ensure that where required training posts are accepted for royal college examinations and specialist registration.

2. TRAINING POSTS IN THE NATIONAL HEALTH SERVICE

The purpose of this section is to outline the types of position and the requirements for entry into each training grade. In addition, the section contains information regarding the job opportunities available in each grade. This latter information is liable to change with time, possibly quickly and therefore caution is necessary in interpretation of the figures.

Pre-registration House Officer Posts (PRHO)

These are posts held by doctors **who have just received their medical degrees.** All graduates of British medical schools are required to complete one year of satisfactory service in house officer posts before full registration can be offered by the GMC. The posts are offered by NHS trust hospitals and supervised by the medical schools who must certify that the doctor's performance is satisfactory before acceptance by the GMC for full registration.

Overseas qualified doctors are strongly advised to complete their pre-registration (Internship) in their own country. This is because in most countries the period of internship is designed to complement and build on their undergraduate training. The number of PRHO posts available in the UK is related to the number of doctors graduating from UK medical schools and opportunities are, therefore, limited.

In September 1999 there were 3,543 PRHOs in post of which

UK medical school graduate	3122	88.1%
European economic area graduates	367	10.4%
Overseas graduates	54	1.5%

The permit free rules do allow for a year as a house officer in addition to four as an SHO.

Basic Specialist Training: Senior House Officer (SHO) Posts

These posts are designed to offer basic specialist training in the main specialities.

The minimum duration of an SHO post is six months but many SHO posts are organised into rotations through various specialities. During these posts doctors decide on their broad area of specialisation and enter into the early years of speciality experience.

The period of time spent in SHO posts varies. It must be a minimum of two years, but 3-4 years is common, allowing the doctors to take the first postgraduate qualifications of one of the royal colleges and increasingly a period of one or two years is being spent in a research position leading to a thesis for a higher university degree.

Concern has been expressed about the numbers of SHO posts which offer unsatisfactory training and thus poor career progression for those holding the posts. A recent GMC initiative has addressed this problem by advising criteria by which all posts must be judged. Together with the attention now being paid to these posts by postgraduate deans, the training potential is increasing. All posts are approved for educational purposes by the postgraduate dean.

Nearly all non-EEA doctors will start at SHO level and because of the smaller number of SpR posts many of these will spend the whole of their limited period in the UK in this grade. Non-EEA doctors who are successful in obtaining an SHO post will be offered work permit free status in the UK by the home office. This status is granted yearly for upto 4 years depending on satisfactory progress being made.

Entry into the grade is by an equal opportunities competitive process with the degree of competition varying according to the speciality. For the more popular specialities it is common to have 100 applications for each available post. This does not mean that only one in a hundred doctors gets a post. It does mean, however, that doctors have to make many applications and some do not get a post when they want it.

Study following Table to see the number of SHO posts being offered to overseas doctors.

Vacant SHO posts are advertised in medical journals such as the BMJ, lancet and hospital doctor.

Vacancies in the NHS are often advertised on a website www.doctors.net.uk

Higher Specialist Training; Specialist Registrar (SpR) Grade
Entry into this grade is highly competitive. The length of training varies according to the speciality but is usually between five and six years. The posts usually rotate between approved hospitals and are approved by the relevant higher speciality training committee via speciality advisory committees. The numbers of specialist registrars are controlled by the postgraduate deans.

Type 1 Specialist Registrar Training
This training is designed to equip the trainee with the skills needed to practice as a specialist and meet the formal requirements for specialist registration.

At the end of the training, a certificate of completion of specialist training (CCST) is awarded. Increasingly this will only be awarded if the trainee has been successful in a speciality exit examination conducted by an intercollegiate examination board. Possession of a CCST certificate is now required for entry to the specialist register. Specialist registration is in turn necessary for appointment to a consultant post.

These posts can only be held by doctors who are eligible for a national or visiting training number (NTN or VTN) explanation of training numbers is given in the next pages.

Type II Specialist Registrar Training (FTTA)
Also known as fixed term training appointments (FTTA), Type II SpR appointments are training of fixed duration (normally 6 months to 2 years) to meet a specific identified training goal. It is possible for doctors to be appointed directly to these posts without the need to go through competitive procedures and therefore

Senior House Officers by Speciality and Country of Qualification as at 30th September 1999 in England.

Speciality	UK	Rest of EEA	Elsewhere	Total
Accident and Emergency	1252	60	210	1,522
Anaesthetics	687	89	443	1,219
Cardiology	169	11	30	210
Cardio-thoracic Surgery	105	9	34	148
Child and Adolescent Psychiatry	44	7	17	68
Clinical Oncology	97	7	14	118
Dermatology	48	3	9	60
Gastroenterology	62	4	10	76
General Medicine	1221	104	413	1,738
General Surgery	592	51	230	873
Genito-urinary Medicine	53	4	5	62
Geriatric Medicine	477	34	137	648
Haematology	77	4	23	104
Medical Oncology	54	3	11	68
Neurological Surgery	80	2	29	111
Neurology	98	9	8	115
Obstetrics and Gynaecology	716	145	514	1,375
Ophthalmology	195	45	167	407
Orthopaedic Surgery/Trauma	548	79	343	970
Otolaryngology	182	36	140	358
Paediatric Surgery	48	7	20	75
Paediatrics	1021	141	523	1,685
Plastic Surgery	96	15	26	137
Psychiatry	738	160	577	1,475
Psychiatry of Old Age	69	18	52	139
Renal Disease	119	6	11	136
Respiratory Medicine	84	7	20	111
Rheumatology	64	7	13	84
Urology	136	11	47	194

Note the 26 specialities with fewer than 50 SHOs or fewer than 10 overseas SHOs have been excluded for simplicity.

overseas doctors have the opportunity to gain specialist skills without the intense competition for type I posts. Holders of these posts will be given an FTN (fixed training number).

Type II training does not lead to the award of a CCST although doctors who are subsequently appointed to type I training following a period spent in type II may be some or all of that training recognised for CCST purposes.

Locum Appointment for Training (LAT)
This is an appointment within the specialist registrar grade where it is decided that CCST training experience can be offered and this training can count towards a CCST if the trainee is subsequently appointed to an SpR post with a training number.

Data Base of Information about PLAB

Locum Appointment for Service (LAS)
These are shorter term appointments of upto three months within the specialist registrar grade which do not offer structured training. They do not carry training approval and cannot be held under the permit free scheme.

The Numbers Game; Training nubmers explained

National Training Number (NTN)
The NTN can only be issued to doctors who have competed and been accepted for a type 1 training programme which may lead to a certificate of completion of specialist training (CCST).
An NTN can only be awarded to doctors who
  a. benefit from European community rights; or who
  b. have overseas nationality but who have right of indefinite residence or settled status in the United Kingdom.

Visiting Training Number (VTN)
This number is only issued to doctors who have competed and been accepted for a type 1 training programme which may lead to the award of a CCST.
A VTN can only be awarded to doctors who
  a. do not benefit from European community rights; or who
  b. have overseas nationality but have no right of indefinite residence or settled status in the United Kingdom.

Fixed Term Training Number (FTN)
The FTN is only issued to doctors who have competed and/or who have been accepted for a type II training programme otherwise known as a fixed term training appointment (FTTA). An FTN can only be awarded to:
  a. doctors who benefit from European community rights, other than UK nationals; or
  b. doctors who do not have a right of indefinite residence or settled status in the United Kingdom; or
  c. exceptionally, where there is an identified service need, doctors who hold a UK CCST and who benefit from European community rights or have a right of indefinite residence or settled status in the United Kingdom and who wish to pursue a sub-speciality training programme within the grade. Such doctors will be the exception since most sub-speciality training will be done before the award of a CCST.

Training numbers are issued to all doctors entering the SpR grade including those holding honorary contracts but not those entering either a locum appointment service (LAS) or a locum appointment training (LAT).

Specialist Registrars by Speciality and Programme Type
(All Deaneries in England and Walses, March 2000)
Important; See note below on variation of definition from SHO statistics.

Speciality	National Training Number	Visiting Training Number	Fixed Term Nubmer EEA	Fixed Term Number Elsewhere
Accident and Emergency	279	28	0	1
Anaesthetics	1266	273	4	59
Cardiology (Cardiovascular Disease)	225	7	0	7
Cardio-thoracic Surgery	63	5	3	62
Child and Adolescent Psychiatry	163	13	0	0
Clinical Oncology (Radiotherapy)	164	29	0	2
Clinical Radiology (Diagnostic Radiology 1)	519	100	2	11
Dermatology	100	5	0	4
Endocrinology and Diabetes Mellitus (Endocrinology 2)	156	36	0	4
Gastroenterology	254	28	0	10
General (Internal) Medicine	9	2	0	2
General Surgery	516	84	3	98
Geriatric Medicine (Geriatrics)	281	88	0	6
Haematology	175	21	0	4
Immunology	23	1	0	0
Medical Microbiology and Virology	102	22	0	2
Medical Oncology	77	8	0	2
Histopathology	166	65	0	1
Neurosurgery	65	10	0	29
Neurology	112	2	0	5
Obstetrics and Gynaecology	514	64	5	285
Ophthalmology	250	18	0	5
Oral and Maxillofacial Surgery	84	1	0	4
Trauma and Orthopaedic Surgery (Orthopaedic Surgery)	563	30	0	140
Otolaryngology (ENT)	158	7	2	25
Paediatric Cardiology	10	4	1	3
Paediatric Surgery	33	3	1	10
Paediatrics	775	216	1	39
Plastic Surgery	117	5	0	12
General Psychiatry (Mental Illness)	335	38	0	2
Old Age Psychiatry (Psychiatry)	157	29	0	0
Public Health Medicine	294	25	0	0
Rehabilitation Medicine	35	18	0	0
Renal Medicine (Nephrology)	130	12	0	4
Respiratory Medicine	179	23	0	10
Rheumatology	166	15	0	11
Genito-urinary Medicine(Venereology)	76	21	0	1

Competition
All SpR posts for typeI training must be filled by open competition. It is not a requirement that FTTA posts be advertised.
See above table for the numbers of overseas doctors being offered SpR posts.

Definition
The SHO figures in Table on page 40 are compiled by country of medical qualification. The registrar figures

in Table 8.3 are compiled on the basis of right of residence in the UK. A doctor with British nationality obtaining a medical degree outside the EEA will count as Overseas in the SHO table and will, if appointed to a type 1 SpR programme, be awarded an NTN.

While not exactly comparable the figures do give an approximate indication of the opportunities available in the specialist registrar grade. There are significant numbers of non EEA doctors in type II training with FTNs. It is more likely that this number will rise rather than fall in the next few years.

1. Diagnostic Radiology
Note there are no SHO posts in this discipline.

2. Endocrinology and Histopathology
Not included in SHO table because there are very few SHO posts.

3. General Medicine
Note there are few posts at SpR grade in General Medicine. Most SHOs proceed to subspecialities such as endocrinology, cardiology and others proceed to other specialities including general practice.

Subjects excluded from list.

The following subjects have been excluded from the SpR list because there are no EEA or overseas doctors employed.

Audiological Medicine
Chemical Pathology
Clinical Cytogenetics
Clinical Immunology
Clinical Neurological Physiology
Psychotherapy
Communicable Diseases
Forensic Psychiatry
Occupational Health
Palliative Medicine
Learning Disabilities

The National Advice Centre for
Postgraduate Medical Education
The British Council, Bridgewater House,
58 Whitworth Street, Manchester M1 6BB
Tel 44(0)161-957-7218, Fax:44(0)161-957-7029
E-mail nacpme@britishcouncil.org.

SPECIALIST TRAINING

In order to become a trained specialist in the hospital service in the United Kingdom (UK) doctors must obtain qualification and experience in addition to their primary medical qualification (first degree in medicine). This is achieved in two stages.
- basic specialist training (At senior house officer [SHO] grade)
- higher specialist training (At specialist register [SpR] grade)

The successful specialist completion of training will take at least six to eight years (Two years SHO and four to six years in specialised register grade). A doctor can then apply to the specialist training authority (STA) of the medical royal college for a certificate of complertion of specialist training (CCST). When this certificate has been awarded, the doctor may then apply to the general medical council (GMC) for inclusion in the specialist register after which doctors may become candidates for substantive and honorary consultant posts in the NHS. This procedure became a legal requirement at the beginning of 1997.

This chapter explain two basic stages in general terms. Overseas qualified doctors wishing to continue or complete their specialist training in the UK should contact the postgraduate dean of the national health service (NHS) region in which they are wish to be established. The dean will, in consultation with the appropriate royal college or faculty establish the UK equivalence of whatever specialist training and experience they may have already acquired in their own country and will then advice on appriorate training in Britain. Some doctors initiate their training programmes in the UK by writing to the royal colleges. Once in a post in the UK, doctors may also seek advice on training and courses through their local postgraduate medical centre (i.e. from the royal college regional adviser).

Entry to higher specialist training is very competitive. Posts are divided into those open to EEA nationals, (or those with enforceable EC rights), and those only open to overseas (non EEA) nationals. The posts open to non EEA nationals are called visiting specialist register (VSpR). Training in CCST level is only possible through a VSpR post. Overseas doctors who wish to obtain specialist experience without proceeding to the CCST may apply for fixed term training appointment (FTTA) posts.

European economic area doctors do not require work permits for any type of post.

Permit- Free Training

Overseas doctors (non-EEA) seeking postgraduate basic specialist/ general professional training in hospital and who intend to return home after their training will be eligible for an initial grant of up to three years permit free training and extention may be available up to an aggregated maximum of four years.

Doctors in higher specialist training will be eligible to apply for an initial grant of three years permit free training on first entering the United Kingdom or after completing basic specialist training, (where this is appropriate), with provisions for further extensions of stay each not exceeding three years, dependent on the requirement of their training programme. The amount of time be closely allied to the training programme enabling doctors to proceed to a certificate of completion of specialist training (CCST) where this is appropriate.

The revised arrangement do provide for doctors to move from basic to higher specialist training. If a doctors is moving to higher to specialist training, then he/she will be eligible to apply for an extension of up to three years and/further extension as appropriate. If he/she is moving during an existing permit free period, then that period would continue until expiry at which time an application could be made for an extension of upto three years and thereafter further extension as appropriate.

'All extension request must have the support of the postgraduate dean'.

In order to qualify for permit free training in the UK an overseas doctors must satisfy the immigration authorities upon arrival in Britain of the following— that he or she:
- intends to undergo postgraduate training in a hospital;
- is currently registered, or is eligible to apply for registration with GMC (having passed or been exempted from the PLAB test)
- intend to leave the UK after completing their training.

1. Specialities

The following is a list of CCST specialities:
- Accident and emergency medicine, allergy, anaesthetics, audiological medicine,
- Cardiology (also known as cardio-vascular disease),
- Cardio-thoracic surgery (also known as thoracic surgery), chemical pathology,

- Child and adolescent psychiatry, clinical cytogenetics and molecular genetics, clinical genetics,
- Clinical neurophysiology, clinical oncology (also known as radiotherapy),
- Clinical pharmacology and therapeutics,
- Clinical radiology (also known as diagnostic radiology and formerly known as radiology),
- Dermatology, endocrinology and diabetes mellitus, forensic psychiatry, gastro-enterology,
- General adult psychiatry (also known as general psychiatry and formerly known as mental illness),
- General internal medicine (also known as general medicine), general surgery,
- Genito-urinary medicine (also known as venereology), geriatric medicine (also known as geriatrics), haematology, histopathology (also known as morbid anatomy and histopathology), immunology (also known as immunopathology),
- Infectious diseases (also known as communciable diseases),
- Intensive care medicine,
- Medical microbiology and virology (also known as medical microbiology), medical oncology,
- Medical ophthalmology, neurology, neurosurgery (also known as neurological surgery),
- Nuclear medicine, obstetrics and gynaecology, occupational medicine, old age psychiatry,
- Ophthalmology, oral and maxillo-facial surgery,
- Otolaryngology (also known as ENT surgery), paediatric cardiology, paediatric surgery, paediatrics,
- Palliative medicine, plastic surgery, psychiatry of learning disability, psychotherapy,
- Public health medicine (also known as community medicine), rehabilitation medicine,
- Renal medicine (also known as renal disease and formerly known as nephrology),
- Respiratory medicine (also known as thoracic medicine), rheumatology,
- Trauma and orthopaedic surgery (also known as orthopaedic surgery), tropical medicine, urology
- There is also a specialist training certificate in general practice (see number 3 later in text).
- Doctors should be aware that appointment to post is competitive although from time-to-time and for varying reasons, the degree of competition may change, i.e. posts may become more or less freely available.

2. Training

Training is carried out in two stages:
- Basic specialist training at senior house officer grade (SHO)
- Higher specialist training at specialist registrar grade (SpR)

Basic Specialist Training

This usually takes place during the two or three years after registration. In practice the period may be longer due to shortages of suitable vacancies in certain popular specialities at the higher level. Basic specialist training is controlled by the various royal colleges and faculties. The extent and nature of the training will vary according to the speciality.

During this period, doctors obtain three or four training posts approved by the postgraduate dean in the senior house officer grades. These posts are advertised in the british medical journal, The lancet and other journals. Posts are filled in open competition and doctors are usually required to attend an interview. These posts, which are salaried, serve to broaden their experience. In-service training and short courses are arranged by the hospital to supplement the working experience. At the same time doctors should be aware that in order to be eligible to sit the exams of particular royal colleges or faculties and thus to be able to go on to higher specialist training, appropriate clinical experience in certain specialities may be obligatory.

Specialist training in almost all specialities is controlled by the various royal colleges and faculties. These regulate their own examinations and it is therefore important that prospective candidates contact them as early as possible to ensure they have (or will acquire) the correct qualification and experience to be eligible to sit the examinations. Most of these examinations are in two or three parts. Some of the examinations, or parts of them, may be taken overseas.

Listed below is a selection of qualifications that may be obtained during basic specialist training. The MRCP (UK) is considered essential for doctors aiming at higher specialist training in a medical speciality and is also a useful additional qualification for those wishing to enter other specialities. Doctors intending to make a career in surgery initially take the MRCS/AFRCS examinations (two to three years). For other specialities, the doctor takes the examinations appropriate to those areas. For full details of examination regulations please contact the appropriate institutions directly.

MRCP (UK) – Membership of the Royal College of Physicians

MRCS – Membership of the Royal College of Surgeons

AFRCS – Associate Fellow of the Royal College of Surgeons

MRCOG	–	Membership of the Royal College of Obstetricians and Gynaecologists
MRCGP	–	Membership of the Royal College of General Practitioners
FRCA	–	Fellowship of the Royal College of Anaesthetists
MRCPath	–	Membership of the Royal College of Pathologists (parts 1 and 2)
AFOM	–	Associateship of the Faculty of Occupational Medicine

The second parts of the MRCPath and the membership examinations of the faculty of occupational medicine (MFOM), fellowship of the faculty of public health medicine (FPHM) and the intercollegiate examinations in the surgical specialities are taken during the period of higher specialist training.

Past examination papers can normally be obtained from the royal colleges and faculties and from commercial organisations such as pass test who also produce revision books for the most popular examinations. Some, but not all, royal colleges and faculties may also issue lists of recommended textbooks.

There are also opportunities to study for postgraduate degreres and diplomas, for example.

Doctor of Medicine (MD)
Master of Surgery (ChM or MS)
Diploma in Tropical Medicine and Hygiene (DTM and H)
MSc in cardiovascular Studies
MSc in Immunology
MSc in Haematology or Chemical Pathology or Medical Microbiology

Information on courses available can be found in the **guide to postgraduate degrees, diplomas and courses in medicine**, in **British qualifications** and in **graduate studies.** Doctors should check with the appropriate royal college or faculty to as certain whether these postgraduate degrees and diplomas give exemption from any part of their examinations.

Once appointed to a training post a doctor should be able to benefit from the facilities provided by the national health service (NHS) for in-service training and courses. Many medical centres throughout the UK hold part-time and short courses suitable for doctors preparing for examinations. Doctors in hospital training posts who are interested in attending such courses should seek advice from their own consultant, the clinical tutor at the local postgraduate centre or the regional postgraduate dean. Courses are also listed in the guide to postgraduate degrees, diplomas and courses in medicine, available at most British Council offices and at the BMJ book shop in London. Some courses are also advertised in journals such as the british medical journal and the lancet. Courses that the doctor wishes to take in addition to training provided by the hospital will usually have to be arranged and paid for by the doctor.

Higher Specialist Training
Higher specialist training follows basic specialist training and normally lasts for a period of four to six years, depending on the speciality. It is frequently the case that a higher qualification will already have been obtained during basic specialist training as a prerequisite for proceeding to higher specialist training.

During higher specialist training, doctors, in discussion with the postgraduate dean, will undertake a specialist training programme. This will involve working in three or four approved training posts in one speciality or groups of closely related specialities, supplemented by courses; in some specialities they may be required to do a period of laboratory work or research.

Higher specialist training is overseen by various joint training committees (and other equivalent committees). In most specialities these committees will recommend the award of a **CCST** to the STA to doctors who have successfully completed higher specialist training programmes. Details of higher specialist training programmes are available from the relevant royal college.

In surgery, trainees must pass the intercollegiate board examination in the appropriate speciality as a mandatory prerequisite to the award of CCST. The examination may not be taken until trainees have satisfactorily completed the fourth year of higher surgical training.

Some examinations may only be taken during higher specialist training, e.g. the intercollegiate board examination in surgery and the FRCR (fellowship of the royal college of radiologists).

3. General practice
Higher specialist training is not required for doctors wishing to enter general practice. The requirement is to complete three years of approved postgraduate training placements, at least 12 months of which must be spent in SHO posts in relevant specialities such as obstetrics and gynaecology, paediatrics, psychiatry, general medicine, general surgery or geriatrics. At least 12 months must also be spent as a GP registrar in an approved UK NHS training practice. After this, a certificate of prescribed experience, or of equivalent experience in issued by the joint committee on postgraduate training

for general practice. Full GMC registration is always required for the period of training as a GP registrar, but only limited registration is necessary for the hospital component of the training programme.

Some doctors who intend to become GPs may wish to study for the examinations of the royal college of general practitioners (MRCGP). However this is not obligatory. Others may wish to obtain the MRCP, or MRCOG, or other specialist qualifications as a useful addition to their training. Please note there are additional immigration regulations for overseas doctors wishing to enter general practice.

Overseas doctors contemplating training a general medical practice in the UK should note that, except in limited circumstances, no funding will be made available for salary, expenses or the trainers grant through the GP registrar scheme. Doctors in doubt as to their entitlement should seek advice from their course organiser or the director of postgraduate GP education.

4. Certificates of Completion of Specialist Training European Economic Area (EEA) Doctors

EEA member states must recognise specialist qualifications or training obtained by EEA nationals in other EEA countries that conform to, or are equivalent to, the requirements laid down in directive 93/16.

There are four types of certificate. The type issued depends on whether the specialist training was completed before or after december 1976 and how far it complies with the requirements of Directive 93/16.
 – Certificate of Completion of Specialist Training
 – Certificate of Equivalence
 – Certificate of Specialist Practice
 – Certificate of Training in a Speciality

Eligibility for the CCST is determined solely in relation to a doctor's specialist medical training; the fact that he or she may not be a national of a member state of the EEA or hold a primary medical qualification granted in the EEA has no relevance. It will, of course, be a mtter for other European member states a to whether they recognise UK CCSTs awarded to non-EEA qualified, non-EEA nationals.

The STA issues CCSTs to doctors who have been appointed to a type I specialist registrar programme and who have completed satisfactorily, specialist training, based on assessment of competence, to a standard compatible with independent practice and eligibility for consideration to a consultant post.

CCSTs perform the dual function of marking the end point of a specialist training programme in the career structure in the UK. They also fulfil the UK's obligation in relation to the issue of specialist certificates for European purposes. possession of a CCST, or of a designated specialist qualification awarded in another EEA member state, entitles its holder to be included in the GMC's specialist register (SR).

OBSERVER ATTACHMENTS AND SUPERNUMERARY (UNPAID) TRAINING POSTS

Contents
1. Observer attachments
2. Supernumerary (unpaid) training posts
3. How to arrange an observer attachment or a supernumerary training post
4. Useful publications
5. Useful addresses

If, as an overseas doctor, you do not wish to, or have been unable to, obtain a salaried training post, you may wish to consider the alternatives of an observer attachment or a supernumerary (unpaid) training post. It is important that you understand the difference between these two forms of training.

Observer attachments
A doctor on an observer attachment will only watch medical practice and will not be permitted to do anything concerned with the treatment of patients. Such attachments are of use for short periods to become familiar with the UK National Health Service or to see new procedures, e.g. when preparing for PLAB. Observer attachments will not count towards the experience required for a doctor to be eligible to sit any examinations set by the Royal Colleges and equivalent bodies. An overseas doctor does not require registration with the UK General Medical Council (GMC) to undertake an observer attachment.

Supernumerary (unpaid) training posts
Postgraduate training in the SHO and Specialist Registrar grades is controlled by the Postgraduate Deans. As a general rule the Deans will not give permission for supernumerary (honorary) training posts though permission may still be given for exceptional reasons. Special arrangements have been made to facilitate training for doctors who are holders of a Scholarship, awarded by an organisation/funding body within their own country, for clinical studies in the UK. Details about the scheme are available from the Health Department of the British Council.

Where a supernumerary post has been offered this will deopend on registration with the GMC. The GMC will not grant registration for a supernumerary SHO or

Registrar post unless there is a letter of support from the Postgraduate Dean. These posts offer the opportunity to obtain clinical experience but this is unlikelly to be accepted for the experience required for a doctor to be eligible to sit the examinations set by the Royal Colleges or equivalent bodies. A doctor offered a supernumerary post would, after a period of adaptation, be fully involved in the work of the department including taking part in the on-call rota.

Obviously the consultant responsible will have to be satisfied that the doctor has the ability and the necessary experience to carry out the work competently. A supernumerary post will not be affected until the employing Health Authority has offered an honorary contract of employment.

How to arrange an observer attachment?
Doctors must arrange observer status themselves by writing directly to hospitals as there is no formal mechanism.

Hospital addresses are given in the Health Services Year Book and the Medical Directory which are available for consultation at most British Council offices. When writing to hospitals, doctors should address their letter to the 'Clinical Director' of the appropriate department or 'The Hospital's Clinical Tutor'. Doctors should expect a large number of negative responses since only a few hospitals will be in a position to take doctors for observer attachments.

Doctors should also be aware that some hospitals may charge a fee for observer attachments.

Useful publications
Health Services Year Book (Annual)
Published by FT Healthcare
Directory of trust and other organizations involved in a whole range of health services in the UK.

Medical Director (Annual)
Published by FT Healthcare
An alphabetical listing of doctors in the British Isles who are provisionally and fully registered with the GMC. The Directory also has details of UK hospitals, medical faculties of universities, medical research institutions and other professional bodies. Also available on CD-Rom.

Useful addresses
FT Healthcare
Maple House, 149 Tottenham Court Road, London W1P 9LL
Tel: +44 (0) 207 896 2409
General Medical Council
178 Great Portland, London W1N 6JE
Tel: +44 (0) 207 580 7642

Health Department, The British Council
Bridgewater House, 58 Whitworth Street, Manchester M1 6BB
Tel: +44 (0) 161 957 7474
Fax: +44 (0) 161 957 7029
Email: **uma.bradshaw@britishcouncil.org**

SITES FOR PLAB

1. **www.mcqs.com** (paid site, $ 35 lifetime access useful EMQ and discussion board)
2. **www.onexamination.com** (free site, free EMQ access and discussion board)
3. **www.medicbyte.com** (free site offers paid online coaching and useful info)
4. **www.fischtest.co.uk** (free site and very useful information)
5. **www.plabpass.i-p.com** (free site with sample EMQ)
6. **www.plab.co.uk** (free site with information for part 1 coaching)
7. **www.pastest.co.uk** (pastest is known for its reputation)
8. **www.plabmaster.com** (YBES—useful tips)
9. **www.medical-library.org** (paid site £ 10 per year; very useful eading material given in form of themes and ideal preparatory material for PLAB 1 exam)
10. **www.bmj.com** (free site useful information on latest developments)
11. **www. overseasdoctors.com** (free with useful information but has to be updated)
12. **www.RxPG.com** (semi-paid, contains more than 15,000 EMQs)
13. **www.bnf.org** (must visit a week before PLAB exam to get aware about recent changes and developments)
14. **www.gmc-uk.org** (the GMC website).

Section 2

Data Base of Previous Memory based EMQ's with Explanatory Answers

Symbols and Abbreviations

Other abbreviations are given on pages where they occur: consult the index.

ABC	airway, breathing, and circulation: basic life support
ABG	arterial blood gas measurement (PaO_2, $PaCO_2$, pH, HCO_3^-)
ABPA	allergic bronchopulmonary aspergillosis
ACE (i)	angiotensin-converting enzyme (inhibitors)
ACTH	adrenocorticotrophic hormone
ADH	antidiuretic hormone
ADP	adenosine diphosphate
ADL	activities of daily living
AF	atrial fibrillation
AFB	acid-fast bacillus
AFP	(and α-FP) alpha-fetoprotein
Ag	antigen
AIDS	acquired immunodeficiency syndrome
alk phos	alkaline phosphatase (also ALP)
ALL	acute lymphoblastic leukaemia
AMA	antimitochondrial antibody
AMP	adenosine monophosphate
ANA	antinuclear antibody
ANCA	antineutrophil cytoplasmic antibody
APTT	activated partial thromboplastin time
ARDS	acute respiratory distress syndrome
ASD	atrial septal defect
ASO(T)	antistreptolysin O (titre)
AST	aspartate transaminase
ATN	acute tubular necrosis
ATP	adenosine triphosphate
AV	atrioventricular
AVM	arteriovenous malformation(s)
AXR	abdominal X-ray (plain)
azt	zidovudine
Ba	barium
BAL	bronchoalveolar lavage
BCR	British comparative ratio (≈ INR)
bd	*bis die* (twice a day)
BKA	below-knee amputation
BMJ	*British Medical Journal*
BNF	*British National Formulary*
BP	blood pressure
bpm	beats per minute (eg pulse)
ca	carcinoma
CABG	coronary artery bypass graft
cAMP	cyclic adenosine monophosphate (AMP)
CAPD	continuous ambulatory peritoneal dialysis
CBD	common bile duct
CC	creatinine clearance
CCF	congestive cardiac failure (i.e. left and right heart failure)
CCU	coronary care unit
CHB	complete heart block
CHD	coronary heart disease (related to ischaemia and atheroma)
CI	contraindications
CK	creatine (phospho)kinase (also CPK)
CLL	chronic lymphocytic leukaemia
CML	chronic myeloid leukaemia
CMV	cytomegalovirus
CNS	central nervous system
COC	combined oral contraceptive, ie (o)estrogen + progesterone
COPD	chronic obstructive pulmonary disease
C-OTM	*Concise Oxford Textbook of Medicine* (OUP 1e, 2000)
CPAP	continuous positive airways pressure
CPR	chronic renal failure
CRP	cardiopulmonary resuscitation
CRF	C-reactive protein
CSF	cerebrospinal fluid
CT	computer tomography
CVP	central venous pressure
CVS	cardiovascular system
CXR	Chest X-ray
d	day(s) (also expressed as x/7)
DC	direct current
DIC	disseminated intravascular coagulation
DIP	distal interphalangeal
dL	decilitre
DoH (or DH)	Department of Health (United Kingdom)
DM	diabetes mellitus
DU	duodenal ulcer
D&V	diarrhoea and vomiting
DVT	deep venous thrombosis
DXT	deep radiotherapy
E-BM	evidence-based medicine (& its journal published by the BMA)
EBV	Epstein-Barr virus
ECG	electrocardiogram
Echo	echocardiogram
EDTA	ethylene diamine tetraacetic acid (eg in full blood count bottle)
EEG	electroencephalogram
ELISA	enzyme linked immunosorbant assay
EM	electron microscope
EMG	electromyogram
ENT	ear, nose, and throat
ERCP	endoscopic retrograde cholangiopancreatography
ESR	erythrocyte sedimentation rate
EUA	examination under anaesthesia
FB	Foreign body
FBC	full blood count
FDP	fibrin degradation products
FEV_1	forced expiratory volume in first second
FFP	fresh frozen plasma
F_IO_2	partial pressure of O_2 in inspired air
FROM	full range of movements
FSH	follicle-stimulating hormone

Data Base of Previous Memory based EMQ's

FVC	forced vital capacity	LMN	lower motor neurone
g	gram	LP	lumbar puncture
GA	general anaesthetic	LUQ	left upper quadrant
GAT[sandford]	Sanford *guide to antimicrobial therapy* ISBN 0-933775-43-1 www.sandfordguide.com	LV	left ventricle of the heart
		LVF	left ventricular failure
GB	gall bladder	LVH	left ventricular hypertrophy
GC	gonococcus	µg	microgram
GCS	Glasgow coma scale	MAI	*Mycobacterium avium intracellulare*
GFR	glomerular filtration rate	MAOI	monoamine oxidase inhibitors
GGT	gamma glutamyl transpeptidase	mane	morning (derived from the latin)
GH	growth hormone	MCV	mean cell volume
GI	gastrointestinal	MDMA	3,4-methylenedioxymethamphetamine
GP	general practitioner	ME	myalgic encephalomyelitis
G6PD	glucose-6-phosphate dehydrogenase	MET	maximal exercise test
GTN	glyceryl trinitrate	mg	milligram
GTT	glucose tolerance test (also OGTT: oral GTT)	MI	myocardial infarction
GU	genitourinary	min(s)	minute(s)
h	hour	mL	millilitre
HAV	hepatitis A virus	mmHg	millimetres of mercury
Hb	haemoglobin	MND	motor neurone disease
HBsAg	Hepatitis B surface antigen	MRI	magnetic resonance imaging
HBV	hepatitis B virus	MRSA	methicillin resistant *Staphylococcus aureus*
Hct	Haematocrit	MS	multiple sclerosis (do not confuse with mitral stenosis)
HCV	hepatitis C virus		
HDL	high-density lipoprotein	MSU	midstream urine
HDV	hepatitis D virus	NAD	nothing abnormal detected
HHT	hereditary haemorrhagic telangiectasia	NBM	nil by mouth
HIDA	hepatic immunodiacetic acid	ND	notifiable disease
HIV	human immunodeficiency virus	NEJM	*New England Journal of Medicine*
HOCM	hypertrophic obstructive cardiomyopathy	ng	nanogram
HONK	hyperosmolar nonketotic (diabetic coma)	NG(T)	nasogastric (tube)
HRT	homrone replacement therapy	NICE	National[UK] Institute for Clinical Excellence (www.nice.org.uk)
HSV	Herpes simplex virus		
ICP	intracranial pressure	NIDDM	noninsulin-dependent diabetes mellitus
IDA	iron-deficiency anaemia	NMDA	N-methyl-D-aspartate
IDDM	insulin-dependent diabetes mellitus	NNT	number needed to treat, for 1 extra satisfactory result
IFN-α	alpha interferon		
IE	infective endocarditis	NR	normal range—the same is reference interval
Ig	immunoglobulin	NSAID	nonsteroidal anti-inflammatory drugs
IHD	ischaemic heart disease	N&V	nausea and/or vomiting
IM	intramuscular	od	*omni die* (once daily)
INR	international normalized ratio (prothrombin ratio)	OD	overdose
IPPV	intermittent positive pressure ventilation	OGD	oesophago gastro duodenoscopy
ITP	idiopathic thrombocytopenic purpura	OGS	oxogenic steroids
ITU	intensive therapy unit	OGTT	oral glucose tolerance test
iu	international unit	OHCS	*Oxford Handbook of Clinical Specialties*, 5e, OUP
IVC	inferior vena cava	om	*omni mane* (in the morning)
IV(I)	intravenous (infusion)	on	*omni nocte* (at night)
IVU	intravenous urography	OPD	out-patients department
JAMA	*Journal of the American Medical Association*	ORh-	blood group O, Rh negative
JVP	jugular venous pressure	OT	occupational therapist
K	potassium	OTM	*Oxford Textbook of Medicine* (OUP 3e, 1996)
KCCT	kaolin cephalin clotting time	OTS	*Oxford Textbook of Surgery* (OUP 2e, 2000)
kg	kilogram	P_2	pulmonary component of second heart sound
kPa	kiloPascal	P_aCO_2	partial pressure of carbon dioxide in arterial blood
L	litre	PAN	polyarteritis nodosa
LBBB	left bundle branch block	P_aO_2	partial pressure of oxygen in arterial blood
LDH	lactate dehydrogenase	PBC	primary biliary cirrhosis
LDL	low density lipoprotein	PCP	*Pneumocystis carinii* pneumonia
LFT	liver function test	PCR	polymerase chain reaction (DNA diagnosis)
LH	luteinizing hormone	PCV	packed cell volume
LIF	left iliac fossa	PE	pulmonary embolism
LKKS	liver, kidney (R), kidney (L), spleen	PEEP	positive end-expiratory pressure

PERLA	pupils equal and reactive to light and accommodation	SLE	systemic lupus erythematosus
PEFR	peak expiratory flow rate	SOB	short of breath (SOB(O)E short of breath on exercise)
PID	pelvic inflammatory disease	SR	slow-release (also called modified-release)
PIP	proximal interphalangeal	stat	*statim* (immediately as initial dose)
PL	prolactin	STD/STI	sexually-transmitted disease or sexually-transmitted infection
PMH	past medical history	SVC	superior vena cava
PND	paroxysmal nocturnal dyspnoea	SXR	Skull X-ray
PO	*per os* (by mouth)	Sy(n)	syndrome
PPF	purified plasma fraction (albumin)	T°	temperature
PPI	proton pump inhibitor, eg omeprazole, lanzoprazole, etc	$T_{½}$	biological half-life
PR	*per rectum* (by the rectum)	T3	triiodothyronine
PRL	prolactin	T4	thyroxine
PRN	*pro re nata* (as required)	TB	tuberculosis
PRV	polycythaemia rubra vera	tds	*ter die sumendus* (to be taken 3 times a day)
PSA	prostate specific antigen	TFTs	thyroid function tests (eg TSH)
PTH	parathyroid hormone	TIA	transient ischaemic attack
PTT	prothrombin time	TIBC	total iron binding capacity
PUO	pyrexia of unknown origin	tid	*ter in die* (3 times a day)
PV	*per vaginam* (by the vagina)	TPR	temperature, pulse and respiration count
qds	*quater die sumendus* (to be taken 4 times a day)	TRH	thyroid-releasing hormone
qid	*quater in die* (4 times a day): qqh: *quarta quaque hora* (every 4h)	TSH	thyroid-stimulating hormone
		U	units
R	right	UC	ulcerative colitis
RA	rheumatoid arthritis	U&E	urea & electrolytes and creatinine in plasma, unless stated otherwise
RAD	right axis deviation on the ECG		
RBBB	right bundle branch block	UMN	upper motor neurone
RBC	red blood cell	URT	upper respiratory tract
RFT	respiratory function tests	URTI	upper respiratory tract infection
Rh	Rh; not an abbreviation, but derived from the rhesus monkey	US(S)	ultrasound (scan)
		UTI	urinary tract infection
RIF	right iliac fossa	VDRL	venereal diseases research laboratory
RUQ	right upper quadrant	VE	ventricular extrasystole
RVF	right ventricular failure	VF	ventricular fibrillation
RVH	right ventricular hypertrophy	VMA	vanillyl mandelic acid (HMMA)
R_x	recipe (treat with)	V/Q	ventilation/perfusion ratio
S or sec	second(s)	VSD	ventriculo septal defect
S1,S2	first and second heart sounds	WBC	white blood cell
SBE	subacute bacterial endocarditis (IE, *infective endocarditis*, is better)	WCC	white cell count
		wk(s)	week(s)
SC	subcutaneous	WR	Wassermann reaction
SD	standard deviation	yr(s)	year(s)
SE	side effect(s)	ZN	Ziehl-Neelsen (stain for acid-fast bacilli, eg mycobacteria)
SL	sublingual		

Themes

MAY-2002

1. The diagnosis of non-accidental injury
2. The treatment of visual impairment
3. The treatment of septicemia
4. Investigation of neurological complaints
5. Complications of blood dyscrasias
6. Differential diagnosis of ectopic pregnancy
7. Management of an injured patient
8. Differential diagnosis of hypertension
9. Investigation of hoarseness
10. Differential diagnosis of developmental delay
11. Management of coma
12. Management of depression
13. Investigation of hemoptysis
14. The diagnosis of shock
15. The management of head injury
16. Diagnosis of stroke/TIA
17. The prevention of jaundice/hepatitis
18. The management of earache
19. The types of skin cancer
20. Management of drug dependency
21. Causes of pneumonia
22. Differential diagnosis of rectal lesions
23. Investigation of joint pain
24. Diagnosis of central chest pain
25. Investigation of miscarriage
26. The disease process in asthma
27. Management of meningitis
28. Important side effects of common drugs
29. Investigation of acute abdomen
30. Tests in diabetes
31. Treatment of anxiety disorders
32. Diagnosis of vaginal discharge
33. Management/investigation of limb ischemia
34. Investigation of trauma
35. Management of infertility
36. Diagnosis of acute chest pain
37. Differential diagnosis of abdominal pain in a woman.
38. The management of hypertension in pregnancy
39. Diagnosis of visual loss
40. The painful hip in children

MARCH-2002

1. Diagnosis of hearing loss
2. Diagnosis of epistaxis
3. Mechanism of action of drugs
4. Drugs used in management of asthma
5. Diagnosis of electrolyte disturbances
6. Diagnosis of unconscious patients
7. Investigation of unconscious patients
8. Management of burns
9. Vaccines
10. Investigations in postoperative patients
11. Contraception
12. Dementia diagnosis
13. Side effects of antipsychotic drugs
14. Dementia diagnosis
15. Diagnosis in trauma patients

16. Cranial nerve palsies
17. Management of fractures
18. Child care
19. Diagnosis of confusion
20. Management of eczema
21. Investigations of inectious diseases
22. Mechanisms of hypertension
23. Differential diagnosis of hemoptysis
24. Complications of myocardial infarction
25. Investigations of neurological complaints
26. Investigation of complications of prostatic carcinoma
27. Diagnosis of altered bowel habit
28. Management of epilepsy
29. Diagnosis of gynaecological conditions
30. Feeding
31. Pain relief
32. Palliative care
33. Anaemia investigations
34. Management of gynaecology conditions
35. Management of varicose veins
36. Investigations in jaundice
37. Investigation of scrotal pain
38. Diagnosis of abdominal conditions
39. Differential diagnosis of thyroid disorders
40. Complications of breast carcinoma

NOVEMBER-2001

1. Diagnosis of personality disorders
2. Diagnosis of diabetic complications
3. Diagnosis of pneumonia organisms
4. Diagnosis of sudden visual loss
5. Differential diagnosis of dementia
6. Prescribing and renal failure
7. Immediate management in trauma
8. Treatment of asthma in childhood
9. Diagnosis of complications of cholecystectomy
10. Postoperative complications
11. The diagnosis of abdominal pain
12. Diagnosis of hip pain
13. The management of red eye
14. The diagnosis of weakness and ill health
15. Pharmacology and toxicology
16. Diagnosis of malabsoption and diarrhoea in children
17. Management of pain in labour
18. The diagnosis of facial pain
19. The diagnosis of difficulties with micturition
20. Investigation of breast disease
21. The management of patients in a coma
22. Transmission of disease
23. ECG interpretation
24. Dizziness fits and confusion
25. Non-accidental injury
26. Differential diagnosis of angina
27. The immediate management of meningitis
28. Prescription and disease
29. Clinical management of hypertension in pregnancy
30. Diagnosis of constipation
31. Human immunodeficiency virus
32. Diagnosis of renal disease
33. Risk factors for deep vein thrombosis (dvt)
34. Diagnosis of a rash
35. Association of skin lesions and specific disease
36. Natural history cervical cancer
37. Diagnosis of common genetical disorders
38. Management of acute chest pain
39. Investigations of patient with haemoptysis
40. Antibiotic prophylaxis of surgical patients

Data Base of Previous Memory based EMQ's

SEPTEMBER 2001

1. Investigation of red eye
2. Management of sudden visual loss
3. Diagnosis of head injury
4. Poisoning management
5. Drugs
6. Investigation in gastro-intestinal disease
7. Differential diagnosis of dysphagia
8. Diagnosis of hepato-biliary disease
9. Diagnosis of scrotal pain
10. Diagnosis of diabetic complications
11. Investigations of thyroid disorders
12. Investigation of abdominal pain in a woman
13. Management of renal disease
14. Iimmediate management of electrocyte disturbances
15. Investigation of pulmonary diseases
16. Diagnosis of pulmonary diseases
17. Management of acute chest pain
18. Complications of breast carcinoma
19. The diagnosis of non-accidental injury
20. Investigation of neck lumps
21. Immediate management of burns
22. Developmental milestones
23. Anatomical localisation of multiple sclerosis
24. Role of immunization and in prevention in liver diseases
25. Diagnosis of hearing loss
26. Investigation of painful joints in children
27. Etiology of anaemia
28. Management of epistaxis
29. Immediate management of common haematological complications
30. First investigation of thromboembolic disease
31. Investigation of complications of prostatic carcinoma
32. Prescribing for pain relief
33. Diagnosis of gynaecological conditions
34. Vaginal bleeding medical traetment
35. Diagnosis of visual impairment
36. Rheumatology diagonsis
37. First step in management of mi complications
38. Fluid resuscitation in children
39. Antibiotic prophylaxis of surgical patients
40. Immunization in children

JULY-2001

1. Prescription and renal failure
2. Investigation/ management of cystitis
3. Differential diagnosis of vomiting in children
4. Differential diagnosis of acute dyspnoea (data interpretation—CO_2, Oxygen, Chest X-ray, ECG
5. Management of multiple trauma
6. Differential diagnosis of altered bowel habit
7. Differential diagnosis of acute urinary retention
8. Investigation/management of meningitis
9. Differential diagnosis of shock
10. Investigation of aortic aneurysm
11. Investigation/differential diagnosis of abdominal pain
12. Different diagnosis of fractures in children
13. Multiple sclerosis-anatomical sites involved
14. Differential diagnosis of chronic neurological diseases
15. immediate management of burns
16. Differential diagnosis of hearing tests
17. Biostatistics
18. Epidemiology in cardiac conditions
19. Management of myocardial infarction
20. Causation of diseases
21. Management and investigations of speech disorders

22. Transmission of diseases
23. Management of acute psychoses
24. Management of anxiety
25. Basics of poisoning
26. Investigation of anaemia-
27. Management of asthma
28. Initial management/investigation in eye conditions
29. Management/investigation of head injury
30. Differential diagnosis of joint disease
31. Causes of confusion in the elderly
32. Investigation of vaginal bleeding
33. Investigation of thyroid disease
34. Diagnosis/management of lumps of the head and neck
35. Postoperative complications
36. Mode of inheritance
37. Progression of carcinoma breast
38. Prescribing for pain relief
39. Differential diagnosis of acute abdominal pain in a young woman
40. Ethical practice of medicine in uk.

May—2002

RxPG Analysis
Total themes: 40
Repeat themes: 9
Repeat themes with a different header: 7

May–2002

May—2002

THEME 1: THE DIAGNOSIS OF NON-ACCIDENTAL INJURY

OPTIONS
a. Accidental injury
b. Emotional abuse
c. Physical abuse
d. Sexual abuse
e. Child neglect
f. Osteogenesis imperfecta
g. ITP
h. Normally present in a child.
i. Elderly abuse
j. Henoch-Schönlein purpura
k. Immune thrombocytopenia purpura

*For each presentation below, choose the **single most likely diagnosis** from the above list of options. Each option may be used once, more than once, or not at all.*

QUESTIONS

1. A 16-year-old mother brings her baby for immunization. The nurse notices the baby has multiple bruises along both arms and legs. The baby is crying excessively. The house officer notices multiple fractures and that the baby has blue sclerae.

2. A 70-year-old man is receiving treatment for Alzheimer's disease. He is looked after by a 23-year-old grand daughter. He has recently developed fecal incontinence. The SHO notices bruises on both wrists and back.

3. An anxious mother brings her 6-year-old daughter who is bleeding per vaginum. Six months prior to this presentation the girl had a confirmed streptococcal sore-throat infection. She is otherwise normal.

4. A 4-day-old girl is brought to casualty by the maternal grandparent who is worried about two dark bluish patches on the child's buttocks. Child's mother is white and the father is black.

5. An 8-year-old girl is noted to have fresh bloody staining of her pants. She also suffers from enuresis. She has recently started horse-riding lessons.

THEME 2: THE TREATMENT OF VISUAL IMPAIRMENT

OPTIONS
a. Intra-ocular steroids
b. Intravenous steroids
c. Oral steroids
d. Laser treatment
e. No treatment required
f. Tropicamide
g. Amethocaine
h. Timolol
i. Pilocarpine
j. Vitrectomy
k. Tetracycline ointment
l. ECCE with PCIOL

*For each presentation below, choose the **single most appropriate treatment** from the above list of options. Each option may be used once, more than once, or not at all.*

QUESTIONS

6. A 73-year-old complains of a severe right-sided headache associated with an acute loss of right-sided vision. Urgent treatment is needed to prevent left sided vision loss.

7. A 75-year-old has difficulty watching television complaining of a peripheral constriction of vision. On examination, there is cupping of both optical discs.

8. A 50-year-old with a history of SLE complains of loss of vision. On examination, he is found to have multiple opacity in the lens of his eyes.

9. A diabetic on oral hypoglycemics complains of sudden deterioration in vision of his right eye. On examination, he is found to have bilateral proliferative retinopathy with retinal hemorrhage on the right side.

10. An 80-year-old has markedly decreased visual acuity. On fundoscopy, she is found to have bilateral macular pigmentation.

THEME 3: THE TREATMENT OF SEPTICEMIA

OPTIONS
a. Percutaneous drainage
b. Ventilatory support + IV fluids
c. Stent
d. Acyclovir
e. Open surgical debridement
f. Resection of superficial tissue with wide margin
g. Oral cefuroxamine
h. IV corticosteroids
i. Laparotomy
j. Intravenous catecholamines
k. Flucloxacillin

*For each presentation below, choose the **single most appropriate treatment** from the above list of options. Each option may be used once, more than once, or not at all.*

QUESTIONS

11. A 28-year-old woman after cholecystectomy following a perforated gallbladder has a raised right diaphragm with a temperature of 38°C and a pulse of 120 beats per minute.

12. A febrile 39-year-old woman with hypertension, has a history of recurrent urinary tract infections. Abdominal ultrasound showed a dilated calyx.

13. A 32-year-old woman has chickenpox. She scratches herself excessively and develops a blue discoloration on the abdomen. She has a history of not passing urine in the last 24 hours. She continues to scratch herself and the discolouration increases in size.

14. A middle-aged man with acute pancreatitis develops hypotension. On CT, he is found to have peripancreatic fluid and a lack of enhancement of the pancreatic tail.

15. Following a perforated bowel, a middle-aged man develops severe shock and septicemia as well as a central dark discoloration on his abdomen, which is growing larger.

THEME 4: INVESTIGATION OF NEUROLOGICAL COMPLAINTS

OPTIONS
a. Twenty-four hour holter monitor
b. EEG
c. Serum calcium
d. Random glucose
e. CT scan
f. MRI spine
g. Lateral cervical spine radiograph
h. Carotid doppler
i. ESR
j. MRI skull
k. None required

*For each presentation below, choose the **single most helpful investigation** from the above list of options. Each option may be used once, more than once, or not at all.*

QUESTIONS

16. A 16-year-old girl suddenly collapses after standing for a while. Her limbs are flaccid and she is not incontinent. Following 30 seconds she recovers fully.

17. An 82-year-old has five episodes of loss of consciousness with no convulsions.

18. A 50-year-old male wakes up with a tingling and numbness in his right hand. This is accompanies by slurring of speech which recovers following about four hours complications and associations of blood dyscrasias.

19. A 34-year-old woman has 6 month history of on and off hemiparesis which resolves with no neurological deficits.

20. A 55-year-old woman treated for breast cancer with chemotherapy and radiotherapy presented with a history of confusion, tiredness, weakness and polyuria. On examination no neurological deficits were found.

May—2002

THEME 5: COMPLICATIONS OF BLOOD DYSCRASIAS

OPTIONS
a. Splenomegaly
b. Hepatomegaly
c. Generalized lymphadenopathy
d. Gingival hypertrophy
e. Macroglossia
f. Meningitis
g. Petechial rash
h. Subarachnoid hemorrhage
i. Intracerebral hemorrhage
j. Bone pain
k. Thrombophilia

*For each presentation below, choose the **single most common complication of given blood dyscrasias** from the above list of options. Each option may be used once, more than once, or not at all.*

QUESTIONS

21. A 51-year-old is lethargic and found to be anemic. his blood picture is found to have a granulocytic tendency with an increase in the platelet count.

22. A 5-year-old with generalised lymphadenopathy develops fever and neck stiffness and headache. he is found to have a lot of lymphoblasts in the blood picture.

23. 55-year-old man with history of hypertension untreated presents with hemiparesis.

24. A 72-year-old is having a routine examination. he is found to have a mild lymphocytosis and splenomegaly.

25. A 38-year-old woman presents with cervical lymphadenopahty. Mature lymphoblasts are seen on the blood film. Examination reveals a mild splenomegaly. She is on phenytoin for epilepsy.

THEME 6: DIFFERENTIAL DIAGNOSIS OF ECTOPIC PREGNANCY

OPTIONS
a. Appendicitis
b. Inevitable abortion
c. Missed abortion
d. Septic abortion
e. PID
f. Diverticular disease
g. Torsion of an ovarian mass
h. Irritable bowel syndrome (IBS)
i. Toxic shock syndrome
j. Inflammatory bowel disease
k. Incomplete abortion

*For each presentation below, choose the **single most likely diagnosis** from the above list of options. Each option may be used once, more than once, or not at all.*

QUESTIONS

26. A pregnant woman with an LMP of 9 weeks and a positive home pregnancy test presents with an enlarged tender uterus and bright red bleeding per vagina. On examination her cervical os is fully open.

27. A 16-year-old with right iliac fossa pain has a vaginal ulatrsound which demonstrates an echogenic cystic mass just superior ro the right fornix.

28. An 18-year-old girl is doing her exams and is very stressed. she has missed her last period. Her pregnacy test is negative. She complains of a three month hsitory of generalised abdominal pain and bloating.

29. A 22-year-old girl with a hitory of two terminations complains of right iliac fossa pain, a water y brownish vaginal discharge and fever. She is found to have an elevated white cell count. She uses tampons.

30. A 27-year-old girl reliably on oral contraceptives develops a high white cell count, fever and a malodourous vaginal discharge young woman with 9 weeks pregnancy presents with heavy bleeding and passage of clots. USG shows fetal heart activity. How to manage?

THEME 7: MANAGEMENT OF AN INJURED PATIENT

OPTIONS
a. Diagnostic needle thoracocentesis
b. CT scan
c. X-ray femur
d. Splinting of the femur
e. Auscultation
f. Chest X-ray
g. Fluid challenge
h. Blood transfusion
i. Suprapubic cystostomy
j. 500 ml IV mannitol
k. Walk around

*For each presentation below, choose the **single most likely diagnosis** from the above list of options. Each option may be used once, more than once, or not at all.*

QUESTIONS

31. A young man involved in a motorcycle accident is stable in the casulaty department. His neck is cleared but when he sits up he develops sudden shortness of breath. His breath sounds are dimished on the right side.

32. A young man involved in a motorcycle accident has a secure airway and a normal Glasgow Coma scale. He is noted to have a swollen right thigh.

33. A young man involved in a motorcycle accident has a secure airway, is ventilated, immobilsed and anesthesized after admission with a Glasgow Coma Scale of 9. He is noted to have a swollen right thigh.

34. A man involved in a mining accident presents with oliguria and passing dark brown urine.

35. A 23-year-old man who sustained a pelvic fracture is unable to pass urine. On examination he has abdominal tenderness and fullness and blood on the uretheral meatus.

THEME 8: DIFFERENTIAL DIAGNOSIS OF HYPERTENSION

OPTIONS
a. Conn's disease
b. Cushing's disease
c. Co-arctation of the aorta
d. Exerbation of chronic hypertension
e. Renal artery stenosis
f. Carcinoid syndrome
g. Essential hypertension
h. Phaeochromocytoma
i. Acromegaly
j. Addison's disease
k. Cushing's syndrome

*For each presentation below, choose the **single most likely diagnosis** from the above list of options. Each option may be used once, more than once, or not at all.*

QUESTIONS

36. A 17-year-old girl with hypertension of 160/100 is found to have a femoral pulse delay.

37. A 40-year-old with a blood pressure of 180/115 is found to have a loud bruit in his right upper abdomen.

38. A 50-year-old male complains of flushing, tremor, palpitations. He is found to have a fluctuating blood pressure of 200/120.

39. A middle aged woman with a blood pressure of 160/110 is found to have abdominal striae and facial hirsutism.

40. A 42-year-old patient with prominent jaw and supraorbital ridges.

THEME 9: INVESTIGATION OF HOARSENESS

OPTIONS
a. Fibre-optic bronchoscopy
b. CT scan
c. Laparoscopic mediastinotomy
d. Surgical mediastinotomy
e. Laryngoscopy
f. No further investigation required
g. Chest X-ray
h. Throat swab
i. TSH
j. MRI
k. Sputum culture

*For each presentation below, choose the **single most appropriate investigation** from the above list of options. Each option may be used once, more than once, or not at all.*

QUESTIONS
41. A patient is suspected of having bronchiectasis.

42. A patient with an area of consolidation and fever on his chest X-ray is treated with antibiotics. His fever resolves but four weeks later he still has a large area of consolidation.

43. A singer has a six month history of hoarseness.

44. A 55-year-old smoker complains of shortness of breath and a cough. Laryngoscopy is normal.

45. A 30-year-old complains of hoarseness since he came back from a football match the day before.

THEME 10: DIFFERENTIAL DIAGNOSIS OF DEVELOPMENTAL DELAY

OPTIONS
a. Birth dysphyxia
b. Fragile X syndrome
c. Duchenne muscular dystrophy
d. Storage disorder
e. Hnter's disease
f. Hypothyroidism
g. Meningitis
h. Constitutional delay
i. Treatment of hyperthyroidism
j. Prematurity
k. Normal finding

*For each presentation below, choose the **single most likely** diagnosis from the above list of options. Each option may be used once, more than once, or not at all.*

QUESTIONS
46. A four-year-old boy walks with a prominent lordosis. He has good speech, can build objects using blocks and has good social awareness.

47. A nine-month baby born at term has a weight in the 97th percentile. His development is delayed.

48. A nine month baby born at term has a weight in the 3rd percentile. His development is delayed. His head and body size are both small.

49. A nine-year-old girl has difficulty with speech. She has recently been hospitalised for a medical reason. Her speech before hospitalisation was completely normal.

50. A four-year-old boy has delayed speech. Both his father and paternal uncle has the same problem.

THEME 11: MANAGEMENT OF COMA

OPTIONS
a. 50% dextrose drip
b. 5% dextrose drip
c. Naloxone
d. Direct intravenous insulin
e. Insulin through a drip
f. One litre of normal saline
g. Naltrexone
h. IV CaCl$_2$
i. IV bicarbonate
j. Calcium resonium
k. Dobutamine
l. CT scan

*For each presentation below, choose the **single most appropriate management** from the above list of options. Each option may be used once, more than once, or not at all.*

QUESTIONS

51. A middle-aged woman remains unconcious 12 hours following a cholecystectomy. On examination both pupils are seen to be pinpoint.

52. A young diabetic is admitted in a comatose state. His plasma glucose level is 2 mmols.

53. A young diabetic is admitted in a comatose state. his plasma glucose level is 17mmols and he is dehydrated.

54. A 37-year-old alcoholic is found wandering in a park. His partner says he has had a number of falls recently and in the A and E the patient is confused. The blood sugar level is normal.

55. A 25-year-old found deeply unconscious is brought to the accident and emergency (A and E) department. He has an abrasion over his left temple and puncture marks on his left forearm.

THEME 12: MANAGEMENT OF DEPRESSION

OPTIONS
a. ECT
b. Amitryptaline
c. Tricyclies
d. Imipramine
e. Psychoanalysis
f. Marital counselling
g. Lithium
h. St. John's Wart
i. MAO inhibitors
j. Fluoxetine
k. Lorazepam

*For each presentation below, choose the **single most likely diagnosis** from the above list of options. Each option may be used once, more than once, or not at all.*

QUESTIONS

56. A middle-aged woman has had several admissions for severe depression. She now turns up with a very severe depression despite all treatment.

57. A woman has bouts of depression alternating with bouts of mania. She has had first line anti-depressants but they have not worked.

58. A young dentist, successful at work lacks confidence in himself. He finds that he is unable to socialise properly and has early morning waking. He is on no treatment.

59. A 44-year-old has repeated episodes of depressed mood in response to feeling rejected, and a craving for sweets and chocolate. These reactive mood changes are accompanied by lethargy and increased appetite, particularly with a preference for carbohydrates.

60. A 20-year-old previously healthy girl is waiting for her college exam result. The result is arriving that day by post and she is suffering from acute anxiety due to the importance of the results for her future career. Her mother consults their general practitioners.

THEME 13: INVESTIGATION OF HEMOPTYSIS

OPTIONS
a. CT
b. MRI
c. Laryngoscopy
d. Sputum culture
e. Sputum cytology
f. Ventilation perfusion scan
g. Thoracoscopy
h. Pulmonary angiogram
i. Selective arteriogram
j. Mediastinoscopy
k. Fine needle aspiration
l. Fibreoptic bronchoscopy

*For each presentation below, choose the **single most definitive diagnosis investigation** from the above list of options. Each option may be used once, more than once, or not at all.*

QUESTIONS

61. Carcinoma of the right main bronchus.

62. Pulmonary embolism.

63. Bronchial carcinoid.

64. Bronchiectasis.

65. Tuberculosis.

THEME 14: THE DIAGNOSIS OF SHOCK

OPTIONS
a. Anaphylaxis
b. Septic shock
c. Cardiogenic shock
d. Hypovolemic shock
e. Pulmonary embolism
f. Disseminated intravascular coagulation
g. Neurogenic shock
h. Spinal shock
i. Acute renal failure (ATN)
j. Third space sequesteration
k. CHF

*For each presentation below, choose the **single most likely diagnosis** from the above list of options. Each option may be used once, more than once, or not at all.*

QUESTIONS

66. A middle-aged man has recently been operated after sustaining a perforated gallbladder. He becomes increasingly comatose and on examination is noted to have peripheral warming.

67. Following a motorcyle accident a young man has a pulse rate of 110 and a blood pressure that falls to 90/50. On examination of the CXR he is noted to have fractures of the lower ribs on the left.

68. A 64-year-old patient on the surgical ward has been operated on for a hernia, he presents with warm extremities and a blood pressure of 90/60 mm Hg.

69. A woman had a caesarean section done in the morning presented with a blood pressure of 80/65 mmHg and pulse rate of 120 beats/min.

70. A 23-year-old man is brought into the accident and emergency department from the local park, with a read swollen arm. He is found to have a blood pressure of 100/60 mm Hg.

THEME 15: THE MANAGEMENT OF HEAD INJURY

OPTIONS
a. CT scan
b. Neck collar
c. MRI
d. Skull X-ray
e. Discharge home with head injury instructions
f. Admit overnight for observation
g. Suction of skull vault
h. Antibiotics
i. Intracranial pressure monitoring
j. Burr holes
k. IV mannitol

*For each presentation below, choose the **single most appropriate management** from the above list of options. Each option may be used once, more than once, or not at all.*

QUESTIONS

71. Following an alcoholic binge a 36-year-old male falls and comes to casualty with a cut in his temporal region his Glasgow Coma Scale is normal and his neck is cleared by the orthopedic SHO.

72. An 8-year-old boy falls off a swing at his school. He is brought to casualty by one of his teachers. He has a bruise over his right eye but the examination is otherwise normal. He is fully conscious with no history of blackouts since the accident. A skull X-ray is performed, which is normal.

73. A young woman is involved in an RTA and is brought in with a Glasgow Coma Scale of 6. A CT scan shows evidence of diffuse cerebral oedema but no evidence of haemorrhage. She has bilateral papilledema.

74. A young man is involved in a fight and suffers a blow to the back of the head. A skull X-ray reveals a depressed fracture of the occiput. His Glasgow Coma Scale on admission is 14 but falls rapidly within an hour.

75. A 24-year-old patient presents with RTA. The pupil on the left side is dilated and the patient is obtunded. CT scan of the head reveals a biconvex hyperdense lesion on the temporal region.

THEME 16: DIAGNOSIS OF STROKE / TIA

OPTIONS
a. Carotid artery stenosis
b. Cerebellar hemorrhage
c. Cerebral embolus
d. Cerebral hemorrhage
e. Cerebral vasculitis
f. Migraine
g. Subarachnoid hemorrhage
h. Subdural hematoma
i. Temporal arteritis
j. Vertebrobasilar TIA
k. Polymyalgia rheumatica (PMR)

*For each presentation below, choose the **single most likely diagnosis** from the above list of options. Each option may be used once, more than once, or not at all.*

QUESTIONS

76. A 27-year-old woman has a long-standing history of headaches associated with nausea and vomiting. On this occasion she present with sudden loss of vision in the right half of the visual field. By the time you see her it has improved considerably.

77. An 82-year-old woman complains of increasing weakness and muscle pain to the point where she is finding it difficulty to brush her hair and get out of a chair. She now presents with sudden loss of vision in her left eye.

78. A woman previously in good health, presents with sudden onset of severe occipital headache and vomiting. Her only physical sign on examination is a stiff neck.

79. A 74-year-old woman had a fall two weeks ago. She is brought into the A and E department with slowly increasing drowsiness. On examination you find mild hemiparesis and unequal pupils.

80. A 73-year-old man presents with hemianopia, hemi-sensory loss, hemiparesis and aphasia of 16 hr duration.

THEME 17: THE PREVENTION OF JAUNDICE/HEPATITIS

OPTIONS:
a. Hepatitis A
b. Hepatitis B
c. Hepatitis C
d. Cirrhosis
e. Hepatocellular carcinoma
f. Sclerosing cholangitis
g. Infectious mononucleosis
h. Lyme disease
i. Leptrospirosis
j. Sclerosing cholangitis
k. Chronic active hepatitis

*For each presentation below, choose the **single most effective prevention** from the above list of options. Each option may be used once, more than once, or not at all.*

QUESTIONS

81. Immunization of health workers who are in contact with body fluid.

82. Mass immunization of hepatitis B, besides preventing hepatitis B also prevents.

83. Avoidance of alcohol for six months after hepatitis A..

84. Counselling for intravenous (IV) drug users to use needle exchange facilities.

85. Immunization of sewage workers.

THEME 18: THE MANAGEMENT OF EARACHE

OPTIONS
a. Removal of foreign body by suction under GA
b. Removal of foreign body using forceps under GA
c. Amoxycillin
d. Amoxicillin with clavulanic acid
e. Aciclovir
f. No specific treatment required
g. Paracetamol
h. Antibiotic against otitis externa
i. Metronidazole
j. Cefuroxime
k. Gentamycin
l. Myringotomy

*For each presentation below, choose the **single most appropriate management** from the above list of options. Each option may be used once, more than once, or not at all.*

QUESTIONS

86. A 7-year-old has right sided earache and rhinorrhea. On examination his right sided tympanic membrane appears pink in colour.

87. A 4-year-old with right sided earache is examined using otoscopy. This reveals a red bulging tympanic membrane

88. An 8-year-old boy who has been playing outside now complains of right sided earache. On inspection a green bead is seen protruding into his ear canal. The walls of the canal are red.

89. A 9-year-old girl with a history of recurrent otitis media now complains of left sided earache. On examination the right sided tympanic membrane appears scarred. On examination of the left ear, pus is seen throughout the ear canal

90. A 54-year-old female develops mild fever, malaise and ear pain. 3 days dlater she developed multiple painful vesicles over her early canal and external meatus.

THEME 19: THE TYPES OF SKIN CANCER

OPTIONS

a. Kaposi's sarcoma
b. Lentigo maligna
c. Squamous cell carcinoma
d. Basal cell carcinoma
e. Melanoma
f. Keratosis
g. Acanthoma
h. Neurofibroma
i. Leukoplakia
j. Mycoses fungoides
k. Bowen's disease

*For each presentation below, choose the **single most likely diagnosis** from the above list of options. Each option may be used once, more than once, or not at all.*

QUESTIONS

91. A fair 18-year-old girl has had dark black facial patches, one of which is now growing rapidly in size.

92. A 70-year-old bald gardener has had a brownish patch on his scalp which has been slowly growing for the last 30 years.

93. A young HIV positive man develops raised patches in his skin and in his mouth.

94. A builder has been exposed to sun for long periods of time devlops an ulcerated lesion on his face.

95. An 18-year-old girl with moles on her back of different colour and sizes.

THEME 20: MANAGEMENT OF DRUG DEPENDENCY

OPTIONS

a. Disulfiram
b. Methadone
c. Needle exchange programme
d. Intravenous vitamin B and thiamine
e. Gradual reducing course of diazepam
f. Outpatient referral to drug dependency team
g. Chlormethiazole
h. Chlordiazepoxide
i. Naloxone
j. Group psychotherapy
k. Hospital admission
l. Inform police

*For each presentation below, choose the **single most appropriate management** from the above list of options. Each option may be used once, more than once, or not at all.*

QUESTIONS

96. A 70-year-old woman has taken 20 mg of temazepam at night for the last 30 years. She has begun to suffer with falls and has agreed that the temazepam might be contributing to the falls.

97. A 26-year-old heroin addict is worried because her partner has been diagnosed as having HIV infection. She is HIV negative. She does not feel able to stop using heroin currently.

98. A 40-year-old man has become increasingly dependent on alcohol since his wife died last year. He admits that he has a problem and wishes to stop drinking. He does not with to take antidepressants.

99. A 63-year-old retired surgeon is admitted with a short history of bizarre behaviour. He claims that GMC are investigating him for murder and have hired a private detective to follow him. He has evidence of a coarse tremor, horizontal nystagmus and an ataxic gait. His wife says that the story about GMC is untrue but is worried about the amount of gin that her husband has drunk since retirement.

100. A 37-year-old retired professional footballer admits of using cocaine and heroin for the last three years. He has recently signed a contract to present a sports show on television and wishes to 'clean his life up' first. His wife and family are very supportive of this.

May—2002

THEME 21: CAUSES OF PNEUMONIA

OPTIONS
a. Bronchiectasis
b. *Haemophilus influenzae*
c. *Mycoplasma pneumoniae*
d. *Staphyloccus aureus*
e. *Streptococcus pneumoniae*
f. *Pneumocystis carinii*
g. Acid fast bacillus
h. Candidiasis
i. *Legionella pneumophila*
j. *Chlamydia psittaci*
k. *Chlamydia trachomatis*

*For each presentation below, choose the **single most likely** diagnosis from the above list of options. Each option may be used once, more than once, or not at all.*

QUESTIONS

101. A middle-aged woman develops a purulent cough with some hemoptysis. A chest X-ray reveals right upper lobe consolidation.

102. A young woman with no relevant medical history develops a severe purulent cough. A chest X-ray reveals multiple cavitating bilateral lung lesions.

103. A young male prostitute develops a dry cough. A chest X-ray reveals bilateral interstitial infiltrates.

104. A young man has recently suffers from a bout of influenza. He now develops a purulent cough.

105. Man comes back from a holiday in Malaysia and he develops malaise, fever and dry cough.

THEME 22: DIFFERENTIAL DIAGNOSIS OF RECTAL LESIONS

OPTIONS
a. Amebic dysentery
b. Pseudomembranous colitis
c. Crohn's involvement of the colon
d. Ulcerative Proctitis
e. Ulcerative pancolitis
f. Diverticular disease
g. Cecal carcinoma
h. Sigmoid carcinoma
i. Condyloma accuminatum
j. Anal fissure
k. Sigmoid volvulus

*For each presentation below, choose the **single most likely** diagnosis from the above list of options. Each option may be used once, more than once, or not at all.*

QUESTIONS

106. A businessperson has just returned from a business trip to Asia. He now develops copious watery and bloody diarrhea.

107. A middle-aged man develops constipation with overflow diarrhea and bright red bleeding per rectum. A barium enema reveals an ulcerated stricture in the sigmoid colon.

108. A young man develops bloody diarrhea. A rigid sigmoidoscopy examination revealed granular ulceration in the sigmoid colon with proximal sparing.

109. A middle-aged woman has been on several antibiotic treatments recently because of a persistent pneumonia. She now develops a severe watery diarrhea. Colonoscopy reveals whitish plaques scattered throughout the colon.

110. An elderly woman is found anemic. As part of her examination, she has a barium enema, which reveals a mass lesion in the ascending colon.

THEME 23: INVESTIGATION OF JOINT PAIN

OPTIONS
a. Serum uric acid
b. Joint fluid uric acid crystals
c. Plain radiograph of the knee
d. Plasma rheumatoid factor
e. Joint fluid rheumatoid factor
f. ESR
g. Antinuclear DNA antibody
h. Joint fluid culture
i. Joint fluid crystal examination
j. Plain radiograph of hip
k. Blood culture
l. X-ray femur

*For each presentation below, choose the **single most likely investigation** from the above list of options. Each option may be used once, more than once, or not at all.*

QUESTIONS
111. A middle-aged woman with a history of rheumatoid arthritis develops sudden swelling in one of her knees. This knee is swollen and hot to touch.

112. An elderly man with recently diagnosed heart failure has been treated with diuretics. He now develops severe joint pain in his left ankle with swelling and redness.

113. A 78-year-old woman complains of a stiff left hip joint after walking some distance. This is most evident when she attempts to abduct the hip joint with limited abduction.

114. A 34-year-old woman complains of bilateral stiff and painful joints in her hands and feet.

115. A 67-year-old woman complains of right hip pain. On examination the right hip is adducted, externally rotated and flexed.

THEME 24: DIAGNOSIS OF CENTRAL CHEST PAIN

OPTIONS
a. Dissecting aortic aneurysm
b. Myocardial infarction
c. Osteochondritis
d. Achalasia
e. Pericarditis
f. Pulmonary embolism
g. Reflux oesophagitis
h. Lung fibrosis
i. Spontaneous pneumothorax
j. Pleural effusion
k. Tension pneumothorax
l. Oesophageal candidiasis

*For each presentation below, choose the **single most likely diagnosis** from the above list of options. Each option may be used once, more than once, or not at all.*

QUESTIONS
116. A tall 34-year-old man develops severe central chest pain radiating to his back. He soon develops a dense hemiplegia.

117. An elderly gentleman suffers a sudden severe crushing central chest pain radiating to his neck

118. A middle-aged man has severe chest pain. Repeated St elevation patterns are seen and a Pericardial rub is heard.

119. A woman 10 days following hysterectomy complaints of severe left sided chest pain and breathlessness. Chest X-ray and ECG failed to relieve any abnormality.

120. A young homosexual man complains of central chest pain. On examination of his mouth, he has white granular lesions on the buccal mucal which is red.

THEME 25: INVESTIGATION OF MISCARRIAGE

OPTIONS
a. Serum HCG levels
b. Lupus plasma marker
c. Hysteroscopy
d. Colposcopy
e. Ultrasound examination
f. MRI
g. Hysterosalpingogram
h. Abdominal X-ray
i. Cardiotocogram
j. Serum AFP levels
k. Kliehauer's test

*For each presentation below, choose the **single most likely** investigation from the above list of options. Each option may be used once, more than once, or not at all.*

QUESTIONS

121. A woman in the eight-week of her pregnancy develops bright red bleeding of four hours duration. On examination her cervical os is completely closed.

122. A woman in the twelfth week of her pregnancy develops bright red bleeding of four hours duration with large clots. On examination the cervical os is wide open.

123. A woman in the tenth week of her pregnancy develops bright red bleeding of one day duration. Her Gp organises an ultrasound examination which reveals heart contractions.

124. A 23-year-old woman has a history of a termination of pregancy at 12 weeks. She subsequently suffers a spontaneous misacarriage aftr 22 weeks of pregnancy. She has a history of DVT.

125. A young lady had a miscarriage in her second trimester following which she bleed profusely, needing 6 units of blood and had to be taken for surgical evacuation of her uterus. She needed medical treatment as she had milk secretion for a few days, but since she has had no periods.

THEME 26: THE DISEASE PROCESS IN ASTHMA

OPTIONS
a. IgA
b. IgM
c. IgE
d. IgG
e. T cells
f. Histamine
g. Improvement of FEV of 5% after treatment
h. Improvement of FEV of 15% after treatment
i. Vital capacity
j. Antigen provocation test
k. Raised eosinophil count
l. Beta-2 receptors

*For each presentation below, choose the **single most likely** cause from the above list of options. Each option may be used once, more than once, or not at all.*

QUESTIONS

126. This test of lung function is characteristically not involved in asthmatic patients.

127. This substance is released by mast cells and causes flushing.

128. This substance is characteristically found in the saliva of most asthma patients IgE.

129. This test is done as a diagnostic test for asthma.

130. Blocking of these can cause worsening of asthma.

THEME 27: MANAGEMENT OF MENINGITIS

OPTIONS

a. Lumbar puncture
b. CT skull
c. X-ray
d. Immunisation
e. Immediated hydration
f. Rifampicin prophylaxis
g. Immediate hydration
h. Contact tracing
i. Isoniazid prophylaxis
j. Transfer to ITU
k. Reassure
l. Serum urate

*For each presentation below, choose the **single most appropriate management** from the above list of options. Each option may be used once, more than once, or not at all.*

QUESTIONS

131. An HIV patient develops a severe headache and confusion. She is discovered to have bilateral papilloedema.

132. An 8-year-old boy with acute leukemia is admitted in a comatose state. He is found to have lymphoblast depletion prevention.

133. A 14-year-old boy presents with drowsiness and generalised headache. He is recovering from a bilateral parotitis. His CT scan is normal.

134. An intravenous drug abuser presents with suspected meningitis. The organism is confirmed in the CSF by India ink preparation.

135. An anxious mother called you to say that her son's best friend in school has caught meningitis.

THEME 28: IMPORTANT SIDE EFFECTS OF COMMON DRUGS

OPTIONS

a. Impotence
b. Wasting
c. Deep vein thrombosis
d. Bronchospasm
e. Pseudomembranous colitis
f. Haemorrhagic cystitis
g. Constipation
h. Retrobulbar neuritis
i. Endometrial carcinoma
j. Stevens-Johnson syndrome
k. Retroperitoneal fibrosis

*For each presentation below, choose the **single most important side effects** from the above list of options. Each option may be used once, more than once, or not at all.*

QUESTIONS

136. Cimetidine.

137. Cyclophosphamide.

138. Diamorphine.

139. Amoxicillin.

140. Oral contraceptive pill.

May—2002

THEME 29: INVESTIGATION OF ACUTE ABDOMEN

OPTIONS
a. Serum amylase levels
b. CT scan
c. Ultrasound
d. Erect chest X-ray
e. Plain film of the kidneys, ureter and bladder
f. Stent
g. Barium enema
h. Sigmoidoscopy
i. Diagnostic laparoscopy
j. Arterial blood gases
k. Urgent operation

*For each presentation below, choose the **single most appropriate investigation** from the above list of options. Each option may be used once, more than once, or not at all.*

QUESTIONS
141. Middle-aged man with hematuria and colicky left loin pain.

142. An elderly gentleman with left iliac fossa pain and tenderness and rectal bleeding.

143. A middle-aged woman with recurrent right upper abdominal pain radiating to the right shoulder. She is tender in this region.

144. Middle-aged chronic alcoholic presents with severe pain in upper abdomen, radiating to the back.

145. A fit 17-year-old man present with a 12 hour history of central abdominal pain localising to his right iliac fossa. He is pyrexical with tenderness, guarding and rebound tenderness in the right iliac fossa.

THEME 30: TESTS IN DIABETES

OPTIONS
a. Glucose tolerance test
b. Random glucose level
c. Fasting glucose level
d. Determination of diurnal steroid level pattern
e. Serum insulin levels
f. Hemoglobin Ac
g. Dietary adjustment
h. Twice daily long/short mixed insulin injections
i. Subcutaneous insulin sliding scale
j. Insulin tolerance test

*For each presentation below, choose the **single most likely diagnosis** from the above list of options. Each option may be used once, more than once, or not at all.*

QUESTIONS
146. A 35-year-old female with a high blood glucose level is noted to be obese and has abdominal striae.

147. An elderly gentleman with frequency is found to have a raised random blood glucose level.

148. An elderly gentleman with polyuria is found to have a raised fasting blood glucose level.

149. A known diabetic on treatment has several episodes of hypoglycemia.

150. A 27-year-old woman was found to have glycosuria at a routine antenatal clinic visit. A glucose tolerance test confirmed the diagnosis of gestational diabetes. What will be your like of action.

THEME 31: TREATMENT OF ANXIETY DISORDERS

OPTIONS
a. Fluoxetine
b. Amitryptaline
c. Tricyclics
d. Behaviour therapy
e. Marriage counselling
f. Psychoanalysis
g. ECT (electro convulsive therapy)
h. Desensitisation
i. Counselling
j. Systemic relaxation
k. No treatment required
l. MAO inhibitors

*For each presentation below, choose the **single most appropriate treatment** from the above list of options. Each option may be used once, more than once, or not at all.*

QUESTIONS

151. A female lawyer is becoming increasing anxious when she has to speak in front of people. This is affecting her work as she needs to speak out in court.

152. A student approaching her secondary level exams is becoming increasingly anxious a few days ahead of her exam.

153. A 20-year-old woman attends A and E complaining of sudden breathlessness and anxiety. She describes palpitations and paresthesiae of her hands, feet and lips. ECG shows sinus tachycardia and O_2 saturation is normal.

154. This treatment is very effective in endogenous anxiety and phobias.

155. A 25-year-old woman finds it difficult to leave her house. She becomes very agitated in supermarkes and describes palpitations and difficult breathing when in crowds.

THEME 32: DIAGNOSIS OF VAGINAL DISCHARGE

OPTIONS
a. Cervical epithelial conversion (cervical erosion)
b. Candidiasis
c. Herpes simplex
d. Gonorrhea
e. Syphilis
f. *Chlamydia*
g. Endometriosis
h. Endometritis
i. Gardnerella vaginalis
j. Bacterial vaginosis
k. Pelvic inflammatory disease

*For each presentation below, choose the **single most likely diagnosis** from the above list of options. Each option may be used once, more than once, or not at all.*

QUESTIONS

156. A pregnant woman has a vaginal discharge. The Ph is 2 and mycelia are seen.

157. A woman has a vaginal discharge. The Ph is 8 and clue cells are seen.

158. A woman has severe right sided abdominal pain and fever. She has a foul smelling vaginal discharge. She has a palpable right sided firmness.

159. A woman on the contraceptive pill for several years has a slight whitish vaginal discharge. On inspection she is found to have a pinkish coloration of the outer cervix.

160. A middle-aged woman with a vaginal disharge is found to have several ulcers at the vaginal introitus.

May—2002

THEME 33: MANAGEMENT/INVESTIGATION OF LIMB ISCHEMIA

OPTIONS
a. Amputation
b. Arteriography
c. Bypass graft
d. Intra-arterial vasodilator
e. Femoral embolectomy
f. Advise stop smoking and exercise
g. Fasciotomy
h. Venography
i. Compartmental manometry
j. Ankle-branchial index measurement (ABPI)
k. None of the above

*For each presentation below, choose the **single most appropriate answer** from the above list of options. Each option may be used once, more than once, or not at all.*

QUESTIONS
161. Man involved in road traffic accident is found to have comminuted fractures of the tibia and fibula. He develops rapid swelling of the lower limb below the knee. Arterial pulses are absent below the knee.

162. An elderly male develops pain in his thigh and leg when walking for approximately 20 metres. This pain resolves with rest. He is a long-time smoker. In examination his dorsalis pedis pulse on the affected side is absent.

163. A 70-year-old with known atrial fibrillation on treatment dvelops a sudden cold leg. Pulses are absent in the level at and below the knee.

164. A 67-year-old male with a history of peripheral vascular disease develops sever ulceration and cellulitis in his left foot and extending up his left leg above the left ankle. The popliteal pulse is absent on that side. He has a history of ulceration on the contralateral side which resolved following a bypass graft operation on that side.

165. A 55-year-old man complains of intermittent pain in his toe on walking. He says that in addition it looks 'white'.

THEME 34: INVESTIGATION OF TRAUMA

OPTIONS
a. Chest X-ray
b. CT head scan
c. Lateral cervical spine X-ray
d. Lumbar spine X-ray
e. MRI thoracolumbar spine
f. Shoulder X-ray
g. Skull X-ray
h. USG abdomen
i. MRI skull
j. Peritoneal lavage
k. Nerve conduction studies

*For each presentation below, choose the **single most helpful investigation** from the above list of options. Each option may be used once, more than once, or not at all.*

QUESTIONS
166. A 33-year-old boxer who complains of left sided weakness 24 hours after a boxing match.

167. An 18-year-old man who has sustained stab wounds to his abdomen and trunk. His respiratory rate is 23 breaths/min, his breath sounds appear normal but his pulse is 142/min and his BP is only 80/40 mm Hg.

168. A 48-year-old woman complains of left shoulder and neck pain after having fallen off her bicycle. She has a graze on her forehead and also complains of tingling in her left ring and little fingers [digits IV and V].

169. A 28-year-old motorcyclist has been involved in an accident and complains of loss of sensation below the umbilicus and paralysis of both legs. His BP is 80/50 mm Hg with a pulse rate of 72/min.

170. A 55-year-old roofer complains of lower back pain radiating into the right leg having fallen from a scaffold. He has no loss of power or sensation when examined.

THEME 35: MANAGEMENT OF INFERTILITY

OPTIONS
a. Bacteriological examination of urine
b. Day 21 progesterone
c. Semen analysis
d. Tubal patency test
e. Wait and see
f. Karyotyping
g. TSH
h. USG abdomen
i. Serum prolactin
j. Urinary B-HCG
k. Urinary FSH/LH

*For each presentation below, choose the **single most appropriate management** from the above list of options. Each option may be used once, more than once, or not at all.*

QUESTIONS

171. A couple aged 25 years have been trying for a baby for six months.

172. Useful in determining ovulation.

173. An essential investigation for all heterosexual infertile couples.

174. This investigation is of little value in infertility.

175. It is an essential investigation of the female partner.

THEME 36: DIAGNOSIS OF ACUTE CHEST PAIN

OPTIONS
a. Acute pancreatitis
b. Angina pectoris
c. Aortic dissection
d. Trigeminal neuralgia
e. Herpes zoster
f. Lobar pneumonia
g. Ruptured oesophagus
h. Herpes simplex
i. Acute myocardial infarction
j. Spontaneous pneumothorax
k. Acute cholecystitis
l. Bornholm disease
m. Tietze's syndrome
n. Oesophageal spasm
o. Fracture rib

*For each presentation below, choose the **single most likely diagnosis** from the above list of options. Each option may be used once, more than once, or not at all.*

QUESTIONS

176. A 23-year-old woman develops an acute pain in her right chest radiating to her right shoulder associated with a fever. She is vomiting and has mild yellowing of her skin.

177. A tall young man developed sharp chest pain on his right, following a road traffic accident. On palpation, this area is tender. A chest X-ray shows his lungs are not injured.

178. A 23-year-old male prostitute develops severe chest pain. This area of chest pain corresponds to an area with an erythematous rash.

179. A 69-year-old man develops crushing chest pain associated with nausea and profuse sweating radiating to the neck. By the time he gets to the hospital [quarter of an hour later] the pain is gone.

180. Minutes after upper GI endoscopy a 57-year-old man develops chest pain. When you examine him, he has a crackling feeling under the skin around his upper chest and neck.

May—2002

THEME 37: DIFFERENTIAL DIAGNOSIS OF ABDOMINAL PAIN IN A WOMAN.

OPTIONS
a. Uterine rupture
b. Ulcerative colitis
c. Twisted ovarian mass
d. Threatened miscarriage
e. Irritable bowel syndrome
f. Pelvic inflammatory disease
g. Renal colic
h. Endometriosis
i. Appendicitis
j. Acute pancreatitis
k. Ectopic pregnancy
l. Septic abortion
m. Break through bleeding
n. Inevitable miscarriage
o. Missed abortion
p. Bowel carcinoma

*For each presentation below, choose the **single most likely diagnosis** from the above list of options. Each option may be used once, more than once, or not at all.*

QUESTIONS

181. A 35-year-old woman complains of abdominal discomfort relieved by passing flatus or defecation. Over the last 6 months she has had episodes of diarrhoea and constipation, but denied she had lost weight.

182. A 37-year-old woman presents with a sudden onset of severe left iliac fossa pain. On vaginal USG, 2 cm echogenic masses are seen in the broad ligament. She says this pain seems to come on every month.

183. A 23-year-old woman just had an intrauterine device fitted. She complains of a watery brown vaginal discharge and abdominal pain.

184. An 18 weeks pregnant female presents with lower abdominal pain and tenderness, with offensive vaginal discharge. She has high grade fever since last two days.

185. A 32-year-old woman who conscientiously uses the oral contraceptive pill, has experienced monthly vaginal bleeding. On abdominal examination she is uncomfortable. Her temperature is 37°C. She is otherwise healthy.

THEME 38: THE MANAGEMENT OF HYPERTENSION IN PREGNANCY

OPTIONS
a. Low dose aspirin
b. A period of observation for blood pressure
c. Twenty-four hours urinary protein
d. Fetal ultrasound
e. Retinoscopy
f. Induction of labour
g. Renal function tests
h. Intravenous antihypertensive
i. Intravenous benzodiazepine
j. Magnesium hydroxide
k. Oral antihypertensive
l. Oral diuretic
m. Recheck blood pressure in seven days
n. Complete neurological exam
o. Immediate caesarian section

*For each presentation below, choose the **single most appropriate action** from the above list of options. Each option may be used once, more than once, or not at all.*

QUESTIONS

186. A patient in her third pregnancy presents to her GP at 12 weeks gestation. She was mildly hypertensive in both of her previous pregnancies. Her BP is 150/100 mm Hg. Two weeks later at the hospital antenatal clinic her BP is 150/95 mm Hg.

187. A 22-year-old Nigerian woman has an uneventful first pregnancy to 30 weeks. She is then admitted as an emergency with epigastric pain. During the first two hours her BP rises from 150/105 to 170/120 mmHg. On dipstick she is found to have 3+ proteinuria. The fetal cardiotocogram (CTG) is normal.

188. At an antenatal clinic visit at 38 weeks gestation, a 36-year-old multiparous woman has a BP of 140/90 mmHg. She has no proteinuria and is otherwise well.

189. At 32 weeks, a 22-year-old primigravida is found to have a BP of 145/100 mmHg. She has no proteinuria but is found to have edema of her knees.

190. At 34 weeks, a 86 kg woman complains of persistent headaches and 'flashing lights'. There is no hyperreflexia and her BP is 150/100 mmHg. Urinalysis is negative but she has finger edema.

THEME 39: DIAGNOSIS OF VISUAL LOSS

OPTIONS
a. Acute glaucoma
b. Central retinal vein occlusion
c. Central retinal artery occlusion
d. Cranial arteritis
e. Uveitis
f. Occipital lobe infarct
g. Direct trauma
h. Retrobulbar neuritis
i. Retinal detachment

*For each presentation below, choose the **single most likely** cause of visual loss from the above list of options. Each option may be used once, more than once, or not at all.*

QUESTIONS

191. A 35-year-old man presents with pain in the right eye, vomiting and loss of vision.

192. A 55-year-old known diabetic and hypertensive wakes up in the morning with diminished vision.

193. A 25-year-old man presents to the accident and emergency department with pain in the right eye associated with backache.

194. An elderly woman presents with a history of visual loss and scalp soreness.

195. An elderly man who is an inpatient (for hypertension) wakes in the morning note that he cannot see his breakfast. He has no other complaints. He has a carotid bruit.

THEME 40: THE PAINFUL HIP IN CHILDREN

OPTIONS
a. Developmental dysplasia of the hip (CDH)
b. Irritable hip syndrome
c. Osteomyelitis
d. Perthes' disease
e. Septic arthritis
f. Slipped upper femoral epiphysis (SUFE)
g. Osteogenesis imperfecta
h. Fracture femur
i. Osteogenic sarcoma
j. Ewings sarcoma
k. Juvenile rheumatoid arthritis

*For each presentation below, choose the **single most likely** condition from the above list of options. Each option may be used once, more than once, or not at all.*

QUESTIONS

196. A six-year-old boy complains of intermittent hip pain for several months. Hematological investigations are normal. X-rays show flattening of the femoral head.

197. A two-year-old girl with one day history of increasing hip pain has become unable to weight bear. Her WCC is 21/fl, with an ESR of 89 mm/hr and a CRP of 300 mg/l. A radiograph of the hip shows a widened jaoint space.

198. A 12-year-old boy with left groin pain for 6 weeks is noticed to stand with the left leg externally rotated. Examination reveals negligible internal rotation of the hip.

199. A four-year-old boy complains of right hip pain a few days following an upper respiratory tract infection. Blood tests are as follows: WCC 12/fl, ESR 10 mm/hr and CRP 2 mg/l

200. A five-year-old girl complains of progressively increasing severe pain in her left hip and upper leg for 6 days. She is able to walk but limps visibly. Blood tests are as follows: WCC 19/fl, ESR 72 mm/hr and CRP 94 mg/l. X-rays and ultrasound scans of the hip are normal.

May—2002

General Medical Council PLAB Test Part 1

DO NOT WRITE IN THIS SPACE

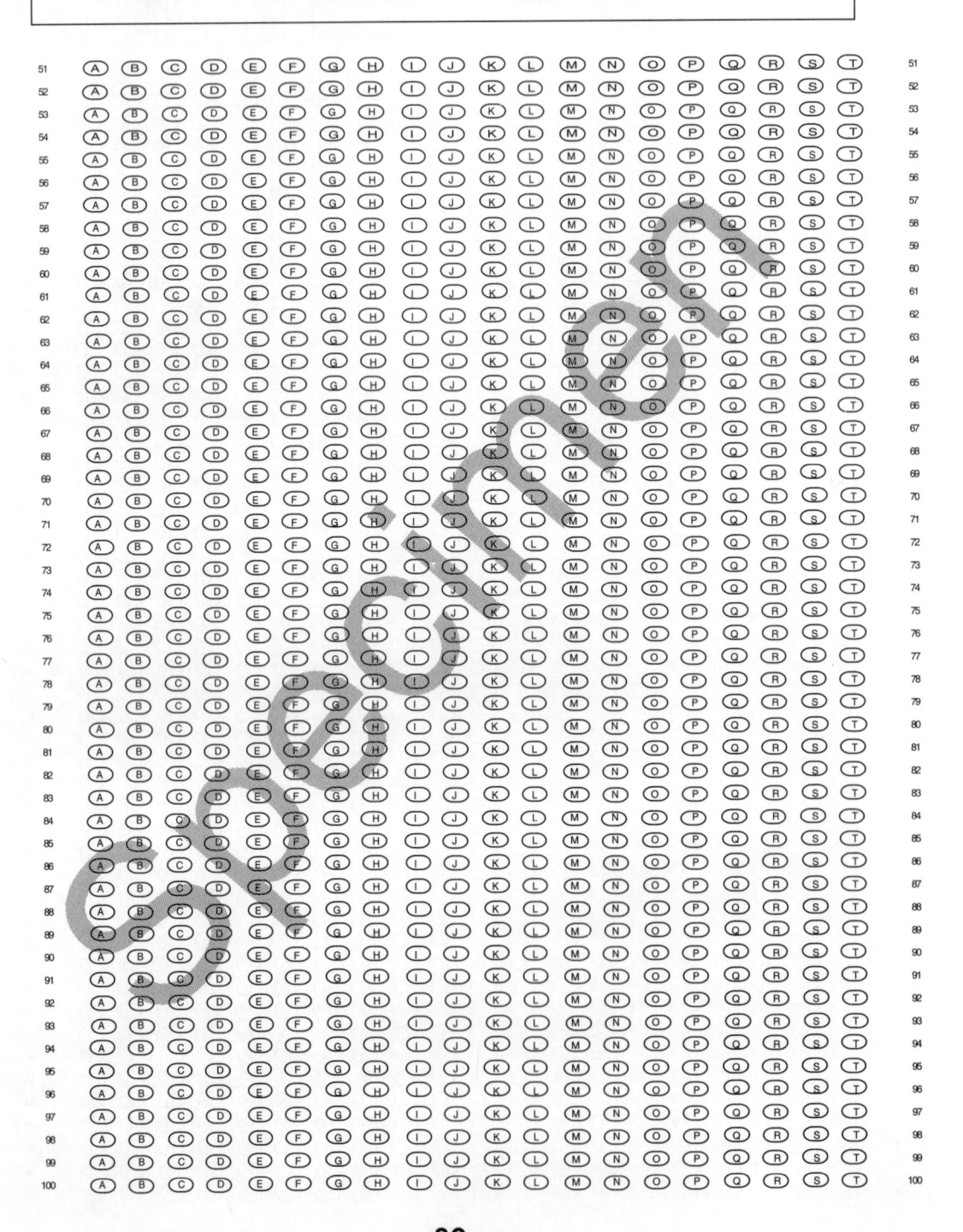

May—2002

DO NOT WRITE IN THIS SPACE

DO NOT WRITE IN THIS SPACE

May—2002

Answers

1	f	Osteogenesis imperfecta
2	g	Elderly abuse
3	d	Sexual abuse
4	c	Physical abuse
5	a	Accidental injury
6	b	IV steroids
7	h	Timolol
8	l	ECCE with PCIOL
9	J	Vitrectomy
10	d	Laser treatment
11	a	Percutaneous drainage
12	a	Percutaneous drainage
13	k	Flucloxacillin
14	b	Ventilatory support + IV fluids
15	i	Laparotomy
16	k	None required
17	a	24 hours holter monitor
18	h	Carotid doppler
19	j	MRI skull
20	c	Serum calcium
21	k	Thrombophilia
22	f	Meningitis
23	i	Intracerebral haemorrhage
24	a	Splenomegaly
25	d	Gingival hypertrophy
26	b	Inevitable abortion
27	g	Torsion
28	h	IBS
29	e	PID
30	i	Toxic shock syndrome

31	a	Diagnostic needle thoracocontesis
32	d	Splinting
33	d	Splinting
34	g	IV mannitol
35	i	Suprapubic systostomy
36	c	Coarctation of aorta
37	e	Renal artery stenosis
38	h	Phacochromocytoma
39	k	Cushing's syndrome
40	i	Acromegaly
41	b	CT scan
42	a	Fibre-optic bronchoscopy
43	e	Laryngoscopy
44	g	Chest X ray
45	e	Laryngoscopy
46	c	Duchenne muscular dystrophy
47	f	Hypothyroidism
48	h	Constitutional delay
49	g	Meningitis
50	k	Normal finding
51	c	Naloxone
52	a	50% Dextrose drip
53	e	Insulin through a drip
54	l	CT scan
55	c	Naloxone
56	a	ECT
57	g	Lithium
58	c	Tricyclics
59	j	Fluoxetine
60	k	Lorazepam

61	l	Fibreoptic bronchoscopy		93	a	Kaposi's sarcoma
62	h	Pulmonary angiogram		94	c	Squamous cell carcinoma
63	a	CT		95	e	Melanoma
64	a	CT		96	e	Gradual reducing course of dizepam
65	d	Sputum culture		97	c	Needle exchange programme
66	b	Septic shock		98	j	Group psychotherapy
67	d	Hypovolaemic shock		99	d	IV vitamin B and thiamine
68	b	Septic shock		100	f	Outpatient referral to dry depending team
69	d	Hypovolaemic shock		101	e	Streptococcus
70	a	Anaphylaxis		102	d	Staphylococcus
71	d	Skull X-ray		103	f	Pneumocystis carinii
72	f	Admit overnight for observation		104	d	Staphylococcus
73	k	IV mannitol		105	i	Legionella
74	a	CT scan		106	a	Amoebic dysentery
75	j	Burr holes		107	h	Sigmoid carcinoma
76	f	Migraine		108	c	Crohn's involvement of colon
77	k	PMR		109	b	Pseudomembranous colitis
78	g	Subarachnoid haemorrhage		110	g	Caecal carcinoma
79	h	Subdural haematoma		111	i	Joint fluid crystal examination
80	a	Carotid artery stenosis		112	b	Joint fluid uric acid crystals
81	b	Hepatitis B		113	j	Plain radiograph of hip
82	e	Hepatocellular carcinoma		114	d	Plasma rheumatoid factor
83	d	Cirrhosis		115	j	Plain radiograph of hip
84	b	Hepatitis B		116	a	Dissecting aortic aneurysm
85	a	Hepatitis A		117	b	Myocardial infaction
86	g	Paracetamol		118	e	Pericarditis
87	l	Myringotomy		119	f	Pulmonary embolism
88	a	Removal of foreign body by suction under GA		120	g	Reflux oesophagitis
89	d	Amoxicillin with clavulinic acid		121	e	USG
90	e	Aciclovir		122	e	USG
91	b	Lentigo maligna		123	d	Colposcopy
92	f	Keratosis		124	b	Lupus plasma marker

125	f	MRI
126	i	Vital capacity
127	f	Histamine
128	k	Raised eosinophil count
129	h	Improvement of FEV, of 15% after treatment
130	l	Beta-2-receptors
131	b	CT skull
132	l	serum urate
133	a	Lumbar puncture
134	a	Lumbar puncture
135	k	Reassure
136	a	Impotence
137	f	Haemorrhagic cystitis
138	g	Constipation
139	j	Stevens-Johnson syndrome
140	c	Deep vein thrombosis
141	e	Plain film of kidneys, ureter and bladder
142	h	Sigmoidscopy
143	c	USG
144	a	Serum amylase levels
145	i	Diagnostic laparoscopy
146	d	Determination of diurnal steroid level pattern
147	c	Fasting glucose
148	a	GT T
149	f	Haemoglobin A/C
150	a	GT T
151	h	Desensitization
152	j	Systemic relaxation
153	k	No treatment required
154	l	MAO inhibitors
155	d	Behaviour therapy
156	b	Candidiasis
157	j	Bacterial vaginosis
158	k	PID
159	a	Cervical erosion
160	c	Herpes simplex
161	i	Compartmental manometry
162	b	Arteriography
163	e	Femoral embolectomy
164	a	Amputation
165	j	ABPI
166	b	CT head scan
167	h	USG abdomen
168	c	Lateral cervical spine X-ray
169	e	MRI thoracolumbar spine
170	d	Lumbar spine X-ray
171	e	Wait and see
172	b	Day 21 progesterone
173	c	Seman analysis
174	a	Bacteriological examination of urine
175	d	Tubal patency test
176	k	Acute cholecytitis
177	o	Fracture rib
178	e	Herpes zoster
179	b	Anjina pectoris
180	g	Ruptured oesophagus
181	e	IBS
182	h	Endometriosis
183	f	PID
184	l	Septic abortion
185	m	Break through bleeding
186	k	Oral antihypertensive
187	h	IV antihypertensive
188	b	A period of observation for BP

189	d	Fetal USG
190	c	24 hours urinary protein
191	a	Acute glaucoma
192	i	Retinal detachment
193	e	Uveitis
194	d	Cranial arteritis

195	f	Occipital lobe infarcts
196	d	Perthes' disease
197	e	Septic arthritis
198	f	SUFE
199	b	Irritable hip syndrome
200	c	Osteomyelitis

May—2002

EXPLANATIONS

1. A 16-year-old mother brings her baby for immunization. The nurse notices the baby has multiple bruises along both arms and legs. The baby is crying excessively. The house officer notices multiple fractures and that the baby has blue sclerae.

Diagnosis: Osteogenesis imperfecta.

Clinchers
- *16-year-old mother:* Not of much significance except the fact that battered baby condition is more prevalent among teenage mothers.
- *Multiple bruises along both arms and legs:* Because of connective tissue involvement, the skin scars extensively.
- *Crying excessively:* Because of pain induced by fractures and generalised illness.
- *Multiple fractures:* It is the hallmark of severe osteogenesis imperfecta. But these are also found in battered baby syndrome (non-accidental injury).
- *Blue sclerae:* It is the differentiating feature from non-accidental injury as blue sclerae are almost pathognomic of osteogenesis imperfecta with this clinical profile.

CONFUSA
Non-accidental injury is the main differential diagnosis in this case. Other thing to be noted is that osteogenesis imperfecta is known by many different names and they can appear in the options as such, i.e. fragilitas ossium, brittle bone syndrome, Adair-Dighton syndrome.

Investigation of choice
Screening: X-ray (decrease in bone density)
Definitive: Absorptiometry (X-ray/photon)

Immediate management
Symptomatic treatment (i.e. fractures—traction followed by light cast).

Treatment of choice
Judicious exercise programme to prevent loss of bone mass secondary to physical inactivity.

Your notes:

---

2. A 70-year-old man is receiving treatment for Alzheimer's disease. He is looked after by a 23-year-old granddaughters. He has recently developed fecal incontinence. The SHO notices bruises on both wrists and back.

Diagnosis: Elderly abuse.

Clinchers
- *70-year-old:* Proves that he is an elderly person!
- *Alzheimer's disease:* Such patients are usually very difficult to look after and one usually requires the services of a trained nurse to care for such demented persons.
- *Fecal incontinence:* Must have compounded the problems of the young granddaughters who was looking after him.
- *Bruises on both wrists and back:* Bruises on both wrists strongly suggest towards use of handcuffs on him, (which his granddaughter might have used to prevent him from wandering aimlessly and getting lost—a frequent occurrence in dementia). The bruises on the back could result either from direct assaults or from the violent attempts of the patient to get free from the handcuffs (thereby bruising his back against wall/bed/chair).

CONFUSA
This is a straight forward question with only a mild confusion between some terminologies in the options. It can qualify as a physical abuse alos, but elderly abuse is more specific and his children rather than the granddaughter are more responsible for his condition.

Investigation of choice
Detailed history.

Immediate management
Admission in hospital and inform social services.

Treatment of choice
Rehabilitation.

Your notes:

3. An anxious mother brings her 6-year-old daughter who is bleeding per vaginum. Six months prior to this presentation the girl had a confirmed streptococcal sore-throat infection. She is otherwise normal.

Diagnosis: Sexual abuse.

Clinchers

> *6-year-old:* Usually such a young child cannot give a proper history of sexual abuse.
> *Bleeding per vaginum:* A common finding in children's sexual abuse. Other common finding is presence of veneral disease before puberty.
> *Confirmed streptococcal sore throat six months back:* This is important as it can be a precipitating factor of Henoch-Schölein purpura. However, it usually does not occur after so long as six months as it is IgA mediated. It usually presents within 2-6 weeks.
> *Otherwise normal:* Rules out any systemic disease.

CONFUSA
The main differential diagnosis in this case is HSP. However, the main finding in HSP is a purpura on extensor surfaces which is excluded in this question (as the child is otherwise normal). So it is safe to answer as a childhood sexual abuse. (Also do not forget the theme is non-accidental injury).

Investigation of choice
Forensic specimens (pubic hair, vaginal swabs) by an expert.

Immediate management
Inform social services.

Treatment of choice
Follow local guidelines of the region.

Your notes:

4. A 4-day-old girl is brought to casualty by the maternal grandparent who is worried about two dark bluish patches on the child's buttocks. Child's mother is white and the father is black.

Diagnosis: Battered baby.

Clinchers

> *Brought to casualty by the maternal grandparent.* Always suspect abuse if accompanying adult is not a parent.
> *Two dark bluish patches on the child's buttocks.* Injury to buttocks is one of the most common finding in battered baby syndrome.
> *Child's mother is white and the father is black.* Inter-racial marriages are often a risk factor for battered baby syndrome.

CONFUSA
The main differential diagnosis in this case is 'birth marks' or congenital nevus. But they are usually present either at birth or after seven days (Strawberry angioma). Here the socio-cultural history is also raising suspicious of battered baby syndrome.

Investigation of choice
Detailed history from accompanying adult + complete physical examination.

Immediate management
Inform social services.

Treatment of choice
Follow local guidelines of region/hospital.

Your notes:

5. An 8-year-old girl is noted to have fresh bloody staining of her pants. She also suffers from eneuresis. she has recently started horse-riding lessons

Diagnosis: Accidental injury.

Clinchers

> *Fresh bloody staining of her pant:* Most probably from trauma as the history given in question does not potray any illness.
> *She also suffers from eneuresis:* Bedwetting occurs on most nights in 15% of 5-year-olds, and is still a problem in upto 3% of 15-year-olds (usually from delayed maturation of bladder control). So it is probably normal.
> *She has recently started horse-riding lessons:* It can be reason for trauma, most probably rupture of hymen, which is common in horse riding training for adolescent girls.

CONFUSA
GMC has tried to mislead us by putting the history of eneuresis in this question. But eneuresis has nothing to do with bleeding anywhere. So the question is still straight enough.

Investigation of choice
For bleeding: Local examination.

For eneuresis: Test for UTI, GU abnormality and DM.

Immediate management
Reassurance.

Treatment of choice
Desmopressin nasal spray.

Your notes:

6. A 73-year-old complains of a severe right sided headache associated with an acute loss of right sided vision. Urgent treatment is needed to prevent left sided vision loss

Diagnosis: Giant cell arteritis (GCA).

Clinchers

> *73-year-old:* Cranial arteritis is common after 55 years of age (60 years according to Kumar and Clark).
> *Severe right sided headache:* Headache is almost invariable in GCA. Pain is felt over the inflamed superficial, temporal or occipital arteries. Though the disease process ultimately involves arteries bilaterally, in the initial stages it is usually unilateral.
> *Associated with an acute loss of right sided vision:* Visual loss owing to inflammation and occlusion of the ciliary and/or central retinal artery occurs in 25% of cases and untreated GCA. It is characteristically sudden, painless, partial or complete, uniocular visual loss. Amaurosis fugax may precede total visual loss.
> *Urgent treatment is needed to prevent left sided vision loss:* Urgent GCA patients need to have an ESR and high dose. Oral steroids immediately. However if visual symptoms are present, give higher doses IV as it could be sight saving.

CONFUSA
Other forms of arteritis, such as SLE and PAN, can occasionally present with similar features (but PLAB questions on GCA are usually straight forward). Also note that GCA is closely related to polymyalgia rheumatica and these can occur in the same patient.

Investigation of choice
- *Screening:* ESR.
- *Definitive:* Temporal artery biopsy (skip lesions occur, so repeat any negative biopsy if there are strong clinical pointers)

Immediate management
Two things are to be done immediately"
1. ESR
2. High dose oral steroids (IV if visual symptoms).

Treatment of choice
Prednisolone, 40-60 mg/24h, PO
- Dose is reduced as ESR falls/is increased if symptoms recurs.
- Headache subsides within hours of first large dose.
- Remission in 2 years usually.
- Steroid treatment is the main cause of death in long-term in GCA patients.

7. A 75-year-old has difficulty watching television complaining of a peripheral constriction of vision. On examination there is cupping of both optical discs

Diagnosis: Chronic simple glaucoma (CSG).

Clinchers
- *75-year-old:* CSG risk increases with increasing age.
- *Difficulty watching television:* CSG can produce intermittent blurring of vision or peripheral constriction of visual field, both of which can interfere in sight.
- *Complaining of a peripheral constriction of vision:* Characteristic of CSG. Nasal and superior fields are lost first with the last vision remaining in the temporal field. Since the central field is intact, good acuity is maintained.
- *On examination there is cupping of both optical discs:* Intraocular pressure >21 mmHg causes optic disc cupping ± capillary closure, hence nerve damage, with sausage-shaped field defects (scotomata) near the blind spot, which may then coalesce to form major defects. Normal optic cups are similar in both eyes in shape and occupy < 50% of optic disc. In glaucoma these enlarge (widens and deepens) and optic disc pales (atrophy).

CONFUSA
Simple glaucoma is asympatomatic until visual fields are severely and irreversibly impaired. Some people may get glaucoma with normal intraocular pressure (IOP).

Investigation of choice
IOP measurement + perimetry.

Immediate management
Dorzolamide (if IOP ↑)

Treatment of choice
- Medical reduction of IOP (i.e. timolol)
- Surgery if medical intervention fails (flap valve trabeculectomy)

Note: In older patient (like this case) Argon laser trabeculoplasty is preferred over surgery.

Your notes:

8. A 50-year-old with a history of SLE complains of loss of vision. On examination he is found to have multiple opacities in the lens of his eyes

Diagnosis: Cataract.

Clinchers
- *History of SLE:* SLE is nonorgan specific due to immune disease in which antinuclear antibodies (ANA) occurs. There is no direct relationship between SLE and opacities in the lens. Though retinal exudates are sometimes seen in SLE patients.
- *In this question, since it is a diagnosed case of SLE:* We presume that patient is on treatment. Steroids are the most commonly prescribed drugs in SLE. This question could be explained on this basis (corticosteroid induced cataract).
- *Multiple opacities in the lens of his eyes:* These are associated with the use of topical as well as systemic steroids. Prolonged use of steroids may result in cataract formation.

CONFUSA
Since the patient is 50-year-old, it can well be a senile cataract also.

Immediate management
- Decrease the dose of steroids.
- Low dose steroids have value in chronic disease.

Treatment of choice
For cataract: ECCE with PCIOL.

Your notes:

9. A diabetic on oral hypoglycemics complains of sudden deterioration in vision of his right eye. On examination he is found to have bilateral proliferative retinopathy with retinal hemorrhage on the right side.

Diagnosis: Vitreous hemorrhage.

Clinchers

- *Diabetic:* The most common and characteristic form of involvement of eye in diabetes is retinopathy. Diabetes is the leading cause of blindness in UK in those aged 20-65.
- *On oral hypoglycemics:* Oral hypoglycemics does not have any specific visual side effects.
- *Complains of sudden deterioration in vision of his right eye:* The cause of it must be vitreous hemorrhage.
- *Bilateral proliferative retinopathy with retinal hemorrhage on the right side:* High retinal blood flow induces a microangiopathy in capillaries, precapillary arterioles and venules, causing occlusion and leakage. Occlusion causes ischaemia which leads to new vessel formation in the retina, the optic disc and on the iris, i.e. proliferative retinopathy. New vessels can bleed, causing vitreous hemorrhage. Rupture of micro-aneurysms causes retinal hemorrhages, flame hemorrhages when at nerve root level, blot hemorrhage when deep in retina.

CONFUSA

Although retinal detachment (which is also common in diabetic retinopathy) can present with same picture, it will be evident on fundoscopy which has been done in this case.

Investigation of choice

Fundus fluorescein angiography to elucidate areas of neovascularisation, leakage and capillary non-perfusion.

Immediate management

Control of hypertension (usually associated and can deteriorate a case of vitreous hemorrhage) + refer urgently to ophthalmologist.

Treatment of choice

If vitreous hemorrhage is massive and does not clear, surgical vitrectomy may be needed. Otherwise do photocoagulation.

Your notes:

10. An 80-year-old has markedly decreased visual acuity. On fundoscopy she is found to have bilateral macular pigmentation.

Diagnosis: Senile macular degeneration (SMD).

Clinchers

- *80-year-old:* As the name suggests it occurs in elderly people. It is the most common cause of registrable blindness in UK. Usually it occurs above 65 years age.
- *Markedly decreased visual acuity:* Loss of central vision (hence visual acuity) is the main presenting complaint in SMD. Visual fields are unaffected.
- *Bilateral macular pigmentation:* SMD is a bilateral disease. The disc appears normal but there is pigment, fine exudate and hemorrhage at the macula. It is of two types—exudative and nonexudative. Drusen of Bruch's membrane is one of the earliest findings in the macula, varying in size, shape and colour. Drusen need not result in visual loss, and visual impairment may occur associated with a generalised pigmentary granularity and/or with atrophy of retinal pigment epithelium, photoreceptors and choriocapillaries.

CONFUSA

Though it is a bilateral disease, the fellow eye may appear quite different in its fundus appearance. Macula holes are an uncommon type of macula degeneration, which may present with distorted vision as well as visual loss.

Investigation of choice

Fundoscopy by an expert.

Immediate management

None except counselling.

Treatment of choice

For most there is no effective treatment (especially for nonexudative SMD).

Laser photocoagulation is indicated in patients with exudative SMD having foveal choroidal neovascularisation to prevent further loss of vision.

Your notes:

11. A 28-year-old woman after cholescystectomy following a perforated gallbladder has a raised right diaphragm with a temperature of 38°C and a pulse of 120 beats per minute.

Diagnosis: Subphrenic abscess (right sided).

Clinchers
- *Woman:* The incidence of cholelithiasis (which sometimes lead to perforated gallbladder) in much more in females. Although its maximum incidence is seen in forties (fair, fat, fertile female in forties).
- *Perforated gallbladder:* Usually the underlying cause of subphrenic abscess is a peritonitis involving the upper abdomen, i.e. leakage following biliary or gastric surgery or perforation.
- *After cholecystectomy:* Subphrenic infection usually follows general peritonitis after 10-21 days, although if antibiotics have been given as abscess may be disguised and may only become manifest weeks or even months after the original episode.
- *Raised right diaphragm:* It occurs if the abscess is of a significant size.
- *Temperature of 38°C:* Along with a mild persisting/swinging pyrexia, other features can be anemia, malaise, nausea and loss of weight. Tachycardia usually occurs in response to pyrexia (as is in this case).

CONFUSA
There may be no localising symptoms of a subphrenic abscess if it is small enough (hence the aphorism—pus somewhere, pus nowhere, pus under the diaphragm).

Investigation of choice
- *Screening:* Ultraound/Chest X-ray.
- *Definitive:* CT scan (it also locates any other peritoneal collections of pus).

Immediate management
Broad spectrum antibiotics.

Treatment of choice
- Percutaneous drainage (USG/CT guided)
- Surgical drainage is done if:
  - Percutaneous drainage fails
  - Abscess is loculated

Your notes:

---

12. A febrile 39-year-old woman with hypertension, has a history of recurrent urinary tract infections. Abdominal ultrasound showed a dilated calyx.

Diagnosis: Pyonephrosis.

Clinchers
- *Febrile:* It signifies a purulent infection.
- *39 years old:* Pyonephrosis is most commonly secondary to an obstructing ureteral stone. It produces hydronephrosis which in turn gets infected (especially by Proteus) due to stagnation of urine. The peak age of incidence is 20-50 years.
- *Woman:* The incidence of renal calculi in females is four times less than males. In this case there is history of recurrent UTI which can produce a benign ureteral stricture/functional obstruction to produce an infected hydronephrosis (pyonephrosis).
- *Dilated calyx:* It is due to back pressure due to obstruction and is a characteristic finding in hdyronephrosis.

CONFUSA
The contentious feature in this case can be the presence of hypertension. It could be totally unrelated to this condition or due to scarring by previous episodes of nephritis secondary to UTI.

Investigation of choice
IVU
- Little or no function
- Enlarged renal shadow

DMSA scintigraphy—will quantify residual function in the kidney after treatment.

Immediate management
Antipyretics.

Treatment of choice
- Urgent drainage by percutaneous nephrostomy.
- If no residual renal function—nephrectomy.

Your notes:

13. A 32-year-old woman has chickenpox. She scratches herself excessively and develops a blue discoloration on the abdomen. She has a history of not passing urine in the last 24 hours. She continues to scratch herself and the discoloration increases in size.

Diagnosis: Toxic epidermal necrolysis (TEN)

Clinchers

- *Chickenpox:* The most common infectious complication of varicella is secondary bacterial superinfection of the skin, which is usually caused by *Streptococcus pyogenes* or *Staphylococcus aureus*.
- *Scratches herself:* This complication mostly results from excoriation of skin lesions after scratching. About 3% of the general population harbour the toxin producing *Staphylococcus aureus* on their skin.
- *32-year-old woman:* TEN occurs predominantly in middle-aged and elderly women. More commonly it is due to drug reactions but infections causes are also prevalent.
- *Blue discoloration on abdomen:* There is erythroderma with extensive desquamation and in places blistering and erosions.
- *History of not passing urine in last 24 hrs:* TEN produces rapid dehydration and sickness. The patient need to be nursed as though they had extensive burns.

CONFUSA
Staphylococcal scalded skin syndrome presents with similar symptoms but is usually a disease of newborns (In older patients the same disease is termed as TEN). Gas gangrene can be a diagnosis in this case if there had been any mention of crepitus.

Investigation of choice
Pus or staphylococcal organisms are not present in the lesion so the diagnosis has to be totally clinical.

Immediate management
Fluid resuscitation + systemic steroids + antibiotics (flucloxacillin).

Treatment of choice
Debridement of nectoric tissue + flucloxacillin.

Your Notes:

---

14. A middle-aged man with acute pancreatitis develops hypotension. On CT he is found to have peripancreatic fluid and a lack of enhancement of the pancreatic tail

Diagnosis: Hypotensive shock secondary to acute pancreatitis.

Clinchers

- *Middle-aged man:* Most common cause of acute pancreatitis in a middle-aged is alcohol. In females it is gallstones. (Note: But alcohol more commonly is responsible for chronic pancreatitis).
- *With acute pancreatitis:* The usual symptoms are epigastric pain which radiates to back between the scapulae. The pain vary from mild discomfort to excruciating in severe disease. It is usually accompanied by nausea and vomiting. Sitting forward may help.
- *Develops hypotension:* It is because of third space accumulation of fluid in the peripancreatic region early in the disease. It can produce hypotensive shock which may be compounded by episodes of vomiting. So fluid resuscitation is of utmost importance.
- *Peripancreatic fluid and a lack of enhancement of the pancreatic tail:* Contrast enhances dynamic CT scanning is the most valuable technique in diagnosis of acute pancreatitis. It can detect swelling of the pancreas and the presence of pancreatic necrosis, peripancreatic fluid collections or diffuse inflammatoy changes in the retroperitoneum (which explains the lack of enhancement of the pancreatic tail).

CONFUSA
If there is doubt about the diagnosis, explorative laparotomy must be performed in all but mild cases to excluded a potentially fatal but treatable non-pancreatic lesion.

Investigation of choice
- *Screening:* Serum amylase (five times increase).
- *Definitive:* USG/CT/ERCP.

Immediate management
- Fluids (plasma expander + normal saline)
- Analgesia (pethidine + prochlorperazine)
- Monitoring of vitals

Treatment of choice
- Conservative if mild
- ERCP + gallstone removal if progressive jaundice
- A recent study using the platelet activating factor antagonist (lexipafant) showed a reduction in complications and overall mortality if given within 48 hours.

15. Following a perforated bowel, a middle-aged man develops severe shock and septicemia as well as a central dark discoloration on his abdomen, which is growing larger.

Diagnosis: Generalised peritonitis.

Clinchers
- *Severe shock and stepticemia:* Any delay in treatment of peritonitis secondary to a perforation produces profound toxaemia and septicemia. Since this stage takes some time to develop, it means that perforation is 10-15 hours old.
- *Central dark discoloration on his abdomen, which is growing larger:* This is a feature of generalised peritonitis which is by chemical irritation due to leakage of intestinal contents and superadded infection by E. coli and bacteroides. Basically it rules out localised peritonitis in this patient and hence rules out any need for conservative management only.

CONFUSA
Conservative treatment is indicated, at least initially, where the infection has been localised (appendix mass), or where the primary focus is irremovable (pancreatitis). Surgery is indicated if the source of infection can be removed or closed, e.g. the repair of a perforated ulcer or removal of a gangrenous, perforated appendix.

Investigation of choice
- Chest X-ray (erect)
- Findings: Free gas under diaphragm

Immediate management
Morphine + fluids + antibiotics.

Treatment of choice
Generalised peritonitis is always treated surgically after adequate resuscitation with the re-establishment of a good urinary output.

Your Notes:

16. A 16-year-old girl collapses after standing for a while. Her limbs are flaccid and she is not incontinent. Following 30 seconds she recovers fully

Diagnosis: Vasovagal syncope.

Clinchers
- *16-year-old girl:* Vasovagal syncope is the simple faint which the majority of the population suffer at some time, particularly in childhood, in youth or in pregnancy.
- *Collapses after standing for a while:* Prolonged standing, fear, pain, or venesection are common precipitation.
- *Her limbs are flaccid:* This differentiation it from epilepsy though some jerky movements can occur in vasovagal attacks, the limbs are never tonic-clonic.
- *She is not incontinent:* Incontinence of urine is rare and there is never incontinence of faeces in a vasovagal syncope.
- *Following 30 seconds she recovers fully:* In vasovagal syncope, the subject fallts to ground and is unconscious for less than two minutes. Recovery is rapid and there is no postictal confusion or amnesia.

CONFUSA
The main points to differentiate between syncope and pathological causes of loss of consciouness in the presence and absence of postictal confusion and duration of the episode.

Investigation of choice
Syncope can usually be distinguished on the basis of clinical history alone. Investigate fully if in doubt.

Immediate management
Lie flat + elevate lower limbs + record pulse.

Treatment of choice
Vasovagal syncope do not require any specific treatment except prophylactic avoidance of precipitants.

Your Notes:

17. An 82-year-old has 5 episodes of loss of conciousness with no convulsions in a single day.

Diagnosis: Stokes-Adams attacks.

Clinchers

- *82-year-old:* Stokes-Adams attacks are important causes of recurrent episodes of loss of consciousness, particularly in the elderly.
- *5 episodes of loss of conciousness:* Attacks may happen severe times a day and in any posture.
- *With no convulsions:* Convulsions are typically absent in Stokes-Adams attacks. A few clonic jerks may occur if an attack is prolonged.

CONFUSA

The question does not provide a specific picture of Stokes-Adams attacks which is palpitations → collapse + paleness + flushing → recovery (within seconds). However, other conditions can be easily excluded by age and recurrence.

Investigation of choice
ECG (24 hours Holter monitoring).

Immediate management
Lie flat + elevate lower limbs + record pulse.

Treatment of choice
Permanent pacemaker (even when asymptomatic)

Your Notes:

---

18. A 50-year-old male wakes up with a tingling and numbness in his right hand. This is accompanies by slurring of speech which recovers following about four hours complications and associations of blood dyscrasias.

Diagnosis: Transient ischaemic attack (TIA) in carotid territory.

Clinchers

- *50-year-old male:* TIA is more common after the age of 40 as the incidence of its predisposing diseases is more after this age.
- *Wakes up with a tingling and numbness in his right hand:* Contralateral weakness/numbness is characteristic of carotid territory ischaemia. On the other hand, in vertebrobasilar territory ischaemia hemiparesis and hemisensory loss, bilateral weakness or sensory loss are features.
- *This is accompanied by slurring of speech:* Dysarthria is a feature of both carotid and vertebrobasilar territory ischaemia but dysphasia is present in only carotid territory ischaemia.
- *Which recovers following about four hours complications:* By definition, a TIA has to fully resolve within 24 hours.
- *Associations of blood dyscrasias:* Hematological disease (polycythaemia, sickle cell, multiple myeloma) can cause TIA (though emboli from heart are the most common).

CONFUSA

Always keep in mind the differential diagnosis of TIA, which are:
- *Migraine:* Symptoms spread and intensify over minutes, often with visual scintillations before headache (headache is rare in TIA)
- *Focal epilepsy:* Symptoms spread over seconds and often include twitching and jerking

Investigation of choice
Carotid doppler.

Immediate management
Antiplatelet drug (aspirin if no peptic ulcer).

Treatment of choice
Carotid endarterectomy.

Your Notes:

19. A 34-year-old woman has 6 month history of on and off hemiparesis which resolves with no neurological deficits.

Diagnosis: Multiple sclerosis (MS).

Clinchers
- *34-year-old woman:* MS has a female preponderence with mean age of onset as 30 years.
- *6 months history of on and off hemiparesis which resolves with no neurological deficits:* First presentations of MS are usually monosymptomatic: unilateral optic neuritis (pain on eye movement and rapid deterioration in central vision) numbness or tingling in the limbs, leg weakness or brainstem or cerebellar symptoms such as diplopia or ataxia. Less often there may be more than one symptom. Symptoms may be worsened by heat (e.g. a hot bath) or exercise. The early picture is usually one of relapses followed by remissions with full functional recovery. With time, remissions, become incomplete and cause accumulation of progressive disability.

CONFUSA
Isolated neurological deficits are never diagnostic, but may become so if a careful history is taken to reveal previous episodes. Nevertheless the diagnosis of MS is always clinical, requiring demonstration of lesions disseminated in time and space, unattributable to other causes.

Investigation of choice
- None is pathognomic.
- MRI for plaque demonstration in occipital lobe.

Immediate management
Methylprednisolone (shortens relapses)

Treatment of choice
β-interferon 16.

Your Notes:

20. A 55-year-old woman treated for breast cancer with chemotherapy and radiotherapy presented with a history of confusion, tiredness, weakness and polyuria. On examination no neurological deficits were found.

Diagnosis: Hypercalcemia.

Clinchers
- *55-year-old woman:* The age is conducive with the incidence of breast malignancies.
- *Chemotherapy and radiotherapy treatment:* It means that the tumor is inoperable with metastatic spread out palliative treatment is being given. Breast cancer commonly metastasize to bone (lytic metastases), brain and liver.
- *Confusion, tiredness, weakness and polyuria:* These are a characteristic group of symptoms in hypercalcemia. Other features can be anorexia, polydipsia, nausea, constipation, dehydration, etc. These signs and symptoms are most obvious with serum calcium more than 3 mmol/L.

CONFUSA
A brain metastases might also produce similar symptoms and signs. But since on examination no neurological deficits are found, it can be safely excluded.

Investigation of choice
Serum calcium.

Immediate management
Rehydrate with 3-4 litres of 0.9% saline IV over 24 hours.

Treatment of choice
- Bisphosphonate IV
- Best treatment is control of underlying malignancy
- In resistant hypercalcemia consider calcitonin.

Your Notes:

21. A 51-year-old man is lethargic and found to be anemic. His blood picture is found to have a granulocytic tendency with an increase in the platelet count.

Diagnosis: Myelofibrosis.

Clinchers

- *51-year-old man:* Usually it occurs in older patients.
- *Lethargic:* The disease presents insidiously with lethargy, weakness and weight loss. Patients often complains of a fullness in the upper abdomen due to splenomegaly.
- *Anemic:* Anemia with leucoerythroblastic features is present. Poikilocytes and red cells with characteristic tear-drop forms are seen. The WBC count may be over $100 \times 10^9/L$, and the differential WBC count may be very similar to that seen in CML; later leucopenia may develop.
- *His blood picture is found to have a granulocytic tendency with an increase in the platelet count:* The platelet count may be very high but in later stages, thrombocytopenia occurs. The granulocytic tendency is due to increased WBC counts (see above) with many granulocyte precursors in the peripheral blood.

CONFUSA
The major diagnostic difficulty is the differentiation of myelofibrosis from CML as in both conditions there may be marked splenomegaly and a raised WBC count with many granulocyte precursors in the peripheral blood. The main distinguishing features are the appearance of the bone marrow and the absence of the Philadelphia chromosome in myelofibrosis. Fibrosis of the marrow, often with a leucoerythroblastic anemia, can occur secondarily to leukemia or lymphoma, tuberculosis or malignant infiltration with metastatic carcinoma, or to irradiation.

Investigation of choice
Bone marrow trephine biopsy (show markedly increased fibrosis and megakaryocytes).

Immediate management
Blood transfusion (as he is anemic).

Treatment of choice
- Support blood count + folate + analgesics + allopurinol
- Hydroxyurea/busulfan to reduce high metabolic acitivity and WBC and platelet levels
- Chemotherapy and radiotherapy to reduce spleen size.

22. A 5-year-old boy with generalised lymphadenopathy develops fever and neck stiffness and headache. He is found to have a lot of lymphoblasts in the blood picture.

Diagnosis: Acute lymphoblastic leukemia (ALL)

Clinchers

- *5-year-old boy*
  cALL—2-4 yrs old
  tALL—10-12 yrs old
  ALL is predominantly a disease of children.
- *Generalised lymphadenopathy:* In addition the other usual signs and symptoms are bone pain, arthritis, splenomegaly, thymic enlargement and cranial nerve palsies. Marrow failure produces anemia, infection and bleeding.
- *Fever and neck stiffness and headache:* These are the signs of leukemic meningitis (CNS is also a potential site of relapse ALL, other such sites are testes).
- *Lot of lymphoblasts in the blood picture:* ALL manifests as a neoplastic proliferation of lymphoblasts which is evident in peripheral blood picture.

CONFUSA
Fever per se is absent in ALL (characteristically present in AML). The fever in this case may be due to secondary infections which are usually viral, but Candida, Pneumocystis pneumonia and bacterial septicemia can also occur. Neck stiffness can be feature of subarachnoid haemorrhage and shigella dysentry apart from its most common cause meningitis (leukemic meningitis in this case). But beware of the fact that neck stiffness is usually absent in neonatal meningitis.

Investigation of choice
- *Screening:* Peripheral blood smear.
- *Definitive:* Bone marrow aspiration/biopsy.

Immediate management
- Blood and platelet transfusions
- IV antibiotics at first sign of infection
- Prophylactic neutropenic regimen

Treatment of choice
Chemotherapy (under UK national trials).

Your notes:

23. A 55-year-old man with history of hypertension untreated presents with hemiparesis

Diagnosis: Intracerebral haemorrhage.

Clinchers
- *55-year-old man:* Elderly person are more prone to hypertensive complications especially if it is left-untreated. Incidence of hypertension in males is more.
- *History of hypertension untreated:* Intracerebral haemorrhage occurs typically in patients with untreated hypertension. SAH is also associated with hypertension but its association is not so typical and usually present with severe headache and neck stiffness.
- *Presents with hemiparesis:* Focal neurological deficits are more common with intracerebral bleeds (cf SAH) which occurs at well-defined sites (basal ganglia, pons, cerebellum and subcortical white matter) due to rupture of Charcot-Bouchard aneurysms.

CONFUSA
- Hemiplegia/hemiparesis
  - Early—suggests formation of an intracerebral hematoma
  - Late—suggests vasospasm and ischaemia
- Clinically thre is no entirely reliable way of distinguishing between intracerebral hemorrhage and thromboembolic infarction, as both produce a sudden focal deficit. Intracerebral hemorrhage, however, tends to be dramatic and accompanied by a severe headache (but still less severe than that of SAH).

Investigation of choice
Visualized reliably by immediate CT (contrast from infarction).

Immediate management
Urgent neurosurgical evacuation of the clot should be considered when an intracerebral hematoma behaves as an expanding mass, causing deepening coma and coning.

Treatment of choice
Unlike thromboembolism antiplatelet drugs are contraindicated. Surgery is indicated if conservative measures fail.

Your notes:

24. A 72-year-old man is having a routine examination. He is found to have a mild lymphocytosis and splenomegaly.

Diagnosis: Chronic myeloid leukemia (CML).

Clinchers
- *72-year-old:* Though it occur most commonly in middle age, old age is no exception for it.
- *Is having a routine examination:* 10% cases of CML are detected by chance. Its symptoms are mostly chronic and insidious, e.g. weight loss, tiredness, gout, fever, sweats, bleeding or abdominal pain.
- *He is found to have a mild lymphocytosis and splenomegaly:* Splenomegaly (often massive) is characteristic of CML (Note: that AML and CML are characterised by early megaly'-spleno and/or hepato-). In the chronic phase of CML, there is only mild lymphocytosis.

CONFUSA
It might be a little difficult to rule out other conditions with such a meagre information but it is safe to diagnose CML. In CLL splenomegaly is a late presentation, i.e. even after the disease can be diagnosed from blood film but in CML the splenomegaly is positive even on presentation.

Investigation of choice
Blood film ± bone marrow aspiration/biopsy.

Immediate management
Hydroxyurea 0.5-2 g/24 h PO.

Treatment of choice
- Allogenic transplantation of bone marrow

Note: But it is attempted only if:
- Patient < 55 years
- Patient is in chronic phase.
- Since the age of this patient is 72 years it will not be attempted.

Your notes:

25. A 38-year-old woman presents with cervical lymphadenopathy. Mature lymphoblasts are seen on the blood film. Examination reveals a mild splenomegaly. She is on phenytoin for epilepsy.

Diagnosis: Phenytoin side effects.

Clinchers
- *Cervical lymphadenopathy:* It can occur as a syndrome of hypersensitivity to phenytoin. It includes rashes, DLE and neutropenia. It is rare but requires discontinuation of therapy.
- *Mature lymphoblasts.* It is also a component of the above mentioned hypersensitivity syndrome. It manifest as leukocytosis often with atypical lymphocytes and eosinophils.
- *Mild splenomegaly:* Can occur in phenytoin treatment as a response to various blood dyscrasias phenytoin causes as side effects.

CONFUSA
Acute myeloid leukemia can be excluded as the presenting cells are not myeloblasts. Plus it need bone marrow biopsy for definitive diagnosis. Nevertheless, gum hyperplasia can occur in this condition also in addition to phenytoin therapy. (So even if you are confused, you would not be wrong). Acute lymphoblastic leukemia is characterised by immature lymphoblasts and not mature lymphoblasts (as in this case).
Note: Cyclosporin also causes gum hypertrophy.

Investigation of choice
Phenytoin blood levels (Normal: 40-80 µmol/L).

Immediate management
Systemic steroids to reduce symptoms.

Treatment of choice
Discontinue phenytoin.

Your Notes:

26. A pregnant woman with an LMP of 9 weeks and a positive home pregnancy test presents with an enlarged tender uterus and bright red bleeding per vaginum. On examination her cervical os is fully open.

Diagnosis: Inevitable abortion.

Clinchers
- *Pregnant woman with an LMP of 9 weeks:* Inevitable abortion in first trimester presents with bleeding. In second trimester, however, it may start with rupture of membranes or intermittent lower abdominal pain (mini labour).
- *Positive home pregnancy test:* Proves that her amenorrhoea is due to pregnancy only. This rules out other causes of vaginal bleeding.
- *Presents with an enlarged tender uterus:* Pain appears usually following hemorrhage (bleeding is usually painless). Most common presentation is with painful (colicky) or tender lower abdomen with a dull backache.
- *Bright red bleeding per vaginum:* The bleed is usually bright red and contains fetal and placental parts which the patient may describe as thick dark red blood clots.
- *Her cervical os is fully open:* This is the only feature that differentiates between threatened (os remains closed) and inevitable abortion.

CONFUSA
Incomplete abortion is a difficult entity to differentiate from inevitable abortion. The diagnosis of incomplete abortion is only possible after a detailed clinical examination (small for date uterus, retained products, patulous os), so it is safe to term as such cases as inevitable abortion before the clinical examination.

Investigation of choice
Complete clinical examination.

Immediate management
Morphine IM + Methergin

Note: Methergin not to be give in second trimester inevitable abortion.

Treatment of choice
- *First trimester:* Dilatation and evacuation followed by curettage under GA.
- *Second trimester:* Oxytocin drip.

27. A 16-year-old girl with right iliac fossa pain has a vaginal ultrasound which demonstrates an echogenic cystic mass just superior ro the right fornix.

Diagnosis: Torted ovarian cyst.

Clinchers
- *16-year-old girl:* Although there is no particular age incidence, usually it is seen in teenage girls.
- *Right iliac fossa pain:* Torted right ovarian cyst can mimic appendicits and ectopic pregnancy. Twisting occludes the venous return but arterial supply continues to engorge the cyst and cause great pain.
- *Echogenic cystic mass just superior to the right fornix:* This is the typical position of an ovarian cyst. Also it appears as a cystic mass on USG (24% of all ovarian tumors are functional cysts).

CONFUSA
The main differential diagnosis in this question is ectopic pregnancy which can be safely ruled out as there is no given history of any amenorrhoea. Note that neither USG nor bimanual examination can confirm the difference between ectopic pregnancy/appendicitis or torted cysts.

Investigation of choice
Only laparoscopy can distinguish a cyst from an ectopic pregnancy or appendicitis (contraindicated in malignancy).

Immediate management
FNAC to rule out malignancy.

Treatment of choice
Urgent laparotomy.

Your notes:

---

28. An 18-year-old girl is doing her exams and is very stressed. She has missed her last period. Her pregnancy test is negative. She complains of a three months history of generalised abdominal pain and bloating.

Diagnosis: Probable irritable bowel syndrome (IBS).

Clinchers
- *18-year-old girl:* Patients are usually 20-40 years old and females are more frequently affected than males.
- *Doing her exams and is very stressed:* Symptoms of IBS are exacerbated by stress, menstruation or gastroenteritis.
- *She has missed her last period:* It might be reason for her stress in addition to her exams. On the other hand, it could also be secondary to anorexia induced by IBS.
- *Her pregnancy test is negative:* Proves that her amenorrhoea is not due to pregnancy.
- *She complains of a three month hsitory of generalised abdominal pain and bloating:* Generalised abdominal pain and bloating are features of IBS. But IBS is diagnosed only if symptoms persist for >6 months. (The abdominal pain can also be central or lower).

CONFUSA
Coeliac disease also present with generalised abdominal pain and bloating. It could be a diagnosis in this case and should be ruled out by proper investigations. Basically IBS is a diagnosis of exclusion. But IBS < 6 months and presence of anorexia (as in this case) are usually markers of an organic disease.

Investigation of choice
- *For young patients with a classical history:* do FBC, ESR, LFT, urinalysis, sigmoidoscopy and rectal biopsy.
- *If any marker of organic disease is present:* do either barium enema or colonoscopy.

Immediate management
Careful explanation and reassurance.

Treatment of choice
Symptomatic (see pg 237, OHCM, 5th edn).

Your notes:

29. A 22-year-old girl with a history of two terminations complains of right iliac fossa pain, a watery brownish vaginal discharge and fever. She is found to have an elevated white cell count. She uses tampons.

Diagnosis: Pelvic inflammatory disease (PID).

Clinchers
- *22-year-old girl:* Sexually active women under 25 years of age have the highest prevalence of PID (especially Chlamydia).
- *History of two terminations:* PID can cause repeated abortions ectopic pregnancy and tubal infertility.
- *Right iliac fossa pain:* An adnexal mass and iliac fossa pain (either side) may be present in 20% of woman, usually those who are most systemically unwell (as is this case).
- *Watery brownish vaginal discharge:* A watery brown vagnal discharge always signifies endometrial inflammation (endometritis). So it is more in favour of PID rather than an ectopic.
- *Fever:* In more severe cases of PID, pyrexia, a raised neutrophil count and a raised ESR can be present.
- *Elevated white cell count:* Due to severe infection as explained above. This episode is most probably an "acute on chronic PID."

CONFUSA
Ectopic pregnancy can be the main confusing diagnosis in this question but is ruled out as its patient usually present with a hyperacute history, amenorrhoea and shock. Moreover, it is not there in the list of options.

Investigation of choice
Gold standard: Laparoscopy.

Immediate management
Urine pregnancy test to rule out ectopic.

Treatment of choice
Antibiotics (after proper culture)
- Endocervical swabs
  - *Chlamydia*
  - *Neisseria*
- High vaginal swabs
  - *Trichomonas*
  - *Bacterial vaginosis*

Your Notes:

30. A 27-year-old girl reliably on oral contraceptives develops a high white cell count, fever and a malodourous vaginal discharge.

Diagnosis: Staphylococcal toxic shock syndrome (TSS)

Clinchers
- *27-year-old girl:* Tampon use is more prevalent in 20's and 30's when active life style is more common.
- *Reliably on oral contraceptives:* OCP reduces the overall risk and incidence of PID (except monoilial vaginitis, whose risk it may increase).
- *High white cell count:* It signifies a systemic dissemination of the infection (It is absent in monoilial vaginitis until and unless the patient is immunocompromised).
- *Fever:* It also suggest a systemic dissemination of infection which is always present in TSS.
- *Malodourous vaginal discharge:* A retained tampon almost always produce an offensive discharge (In monoilial vaginitis there may be a yeasty smell).

CONFUSA
It is a somewhat tricky question and the best answer among in given options is TSS. But it could be a severe episode of simple PID also (remember OCP's reduce its incidence but not nullify it, i.e. they can occur).

Investigation of choice
Blood culture/tampon culture.

Immediate management
Resuscitation should commenced immediately with oxygen and fluids.

Treatment of choice
Antistaphylococcal therapy (flucloxacillin).

Your notes:

31. A young man involved in a motorcycle accident is stable in the casualty department. His neck is cleared but when he sits up he develops sudden shortness of breath. His breath sounds are dimished on the right side.

Diagnosis: Simple right sided pneumothorax.

Clinchers
- *Young man:* Young man usually have uncomplicated pneumothoraces as they have no add on lung pathologies.
- *Involved in a motorcycle accident:* Motorcycle accident injuries are mostly sustained on head, chest (rib fractures) and legs.
- *Is stable in the casualty department:* Rules out any life-threatening injury.
- *His neck is cleared:* It gives him a reason to sit straight. The overworked SHO might have missed the rib fractures.
- *When he sits up he develops sudden shortness of breath:* Traumatic pneumothorax may follow rib injury which might produce it in the proces of sitting up.
- *Breath sounds are dimished on the right side:* In pneumothorax there are diminished breath sounds on the affected side (plus there is hyperresonance to percussion).

CONFUSA
Tension pneumothorax should be differentiated from simple pneumothorax by presence of tracheal deviation, impaired cardiac output, distended neck veins and cyanosis (late).

Investigation of choice
Chest X-ray (except in tension pneumothorax where the first thing to do is needle thoracocentesis).

Immediate management
High concentration O_2 by mask
+
Monitor SaO_2, BP and ECG
+
Consider early analgesia

Treatment of choice
Needle aspiration
↓ if fails
Chest drain
- Other indications for chest drain
  - Recurrence within 24 hours
  - Haemopneumothorax
  - IPPV

32. A young man involved in a motorcycle accident has a secure airway and a normal Glasgow Coma Scale. He is noted to have a swollen right thigh.

Diagnosis: Right femoral shaft fracture.

Clinchers
- *Young man involved in a motorcycle accident:* Most of the motorcycle accident victims are young moles who are out to take an adventurous ride.
- *Has a secure airway:* That means that immediate management of ABC (airway, breathing and circulation) has been done.
- *Normal Glasgow Coma Scale:* This rules out any head injury (except subdural hematoma).
- *Swollen right thigh:* This could be soft tissue injury or a fracture femur. However, fracture femur is more common in a motorcycle accident.

CONFUSA
This is a simple question which is testing your knowledge of basic rules of management of trauma. These are divided into primary survey and secondary survey. Primary survey is based on ABC approach and AVPU scoring is done. Glasgow scoring is done only in secondary survey. Since it has been done in this patient it means secondary survey has been done and hence it is time for splinting.

Investigation of choice
Femoral shaft fracture should be clinically evident without immediate resort to radiographs. X-rays are mainly used to excluded other injuries and to check the position of bone after application of a splint.

Immediate management
Effective analgesia. Initially nitrous oxide mixture and then IV opiates—if not contraindicated—or femoral nerve block.

Treatment of choice
Thomas or other traction splint.

Your notes:

33. A young man involved in a motorcycle accident has a secure airway, is ventilated, immobilsed and anesthesized after admission with a Glasgow Coma Scale of 9. He is noted to have a swollen right thigh.

Diagnosis: Right femoral shaft fracture with moderate head injury.

Clinchers
- *Young man involved in a motorcycle accident:* Young men are more often victims of two wheeler accidents.
- *Has a secure airway:* It means that primary survey is over.
- *Ventilated, immobilsed and anesthesized:* It means that secondary survey is also over.
- *Glasgow Coma Scale of 9:* It denotes moderate head injury (GCS range 9-12).
- *Swollen right thigh:* It is most probably femoral shaft fracture as it is very common in such accidents.

CONFUSA
Now the question boils down to what next to do? Like in the preveious question, we shall have to follow a sequential management. Anaesthesia is usually not given in a case of head injury except when femoral fracture needs to splinted (Entonox) or cranial hematoma is to be evacuated. Since there are no given symptoms/signs of a cranial hematoma, it has to be the reduction of femoral fracture.

Investigation of choice
Femoral shaft fracture should be clinically evident without immediate resort to radiographs. X-rays are mainly used to excluded other injuries and to check the position of bone after application of a splint.

Immediate management
Effective analgesia. Initially nitrous oxide mixture and then IV opiates—if not contraindicated—or femoral nerve block.

Treatment of choice
Thomas or other traction splint.

Your notes:

---

34. A man involved in a mining accident presents with oliguria and passing dark brown urine.

Diagnosis: Acute tubular necrosis secondary to rhabdomyolysis.

Clinchers
- *Mining accident:* Mining accident can produce urinary symptoms commonly in two ways:
  1. Direct urethral injury (due to pelvic fracture)
  2. Rhabdomyolysis secondary to crush injury.
- *Oliguria:* Oliguria in this case can be due to either:
  1. Urethral trauma and hence rentention
  2. ATN
- *Dark brown urine:* It is due to appearance of myoglobin (a muscle protein) in urine. It is released on muscle injury (crush injury) or necrosis or reperfusion of an ischaemic limb.

CONFUSA
Dark urine which is positive for blood on dipstick but without RBCs on microscopy can be confusing, but it is a characteristic finding in rhabdomyolysis. Urethral trauma can be safely excluded as there will be retention and fresh red blood on meatus.

Investigation of choice
Dipstick test and microscopy for urine.

Immediate management
Large volumes of IV fluids
  +
IV mannitol/IV bicarbonate

Treatment of choice
Hemodialysis/filtration if required.

Your notes:

35. A 23-year-old man who sustained a pelvic fracture is unable to pass urine. On examination he has abdominal tenderness and fullness and blood on the urethral meatus.

Diagnosis: Injury to membranous urethra.

Clinchers
- *Pelvic fracture:* Membranous urethra is most commonly injured in pelvic fractures, especially those involving dislocation of a portion of the pelvis. It is usually form at its junction with the prostatic urethra.
- *Abdominal tenderness and fullness:* It signifies distended bladder which can be painful and tender. It is due to discontinuity of the outflow system due to injury.
- *Blood on the urethral meatus:* The presence of bleeding from the meatus, or a fracture of the pelvis, combined with urinary retention, should alert to the possibility of extravasation of urine which could lead to secondary infection.

CONFUSA
Injury to bulbous urethra is usually not associated with pelvic fractures and is commonly seen after direct blows to perineum. It is characterised by severe perineal pain, bruising and fresh blood dripping from external meatus. In any suspected urethral injury, a Foley's catheter should never be passed before obtaining an urethrogram.

Investigation of choice
Urethrogram with water soluble contrast (to identify any extravasation, loss of continuity and to localise site of injury).

Immediate management
Per rectal examination to palpate prostate. An absent or high prostate implies a complete rupture of the membranous urethra and warrants urgent exploration.

Treatment of choice
Suprapubic catheterisation
  +
Repair

36. A 17-year-old girl with hypertension of 160/100 is found to have a femoral pulse delay.

Diagnosis: Coarctation of aorta.

Clinchers
- *17-year-old girl:* Coarctation of aorta is often asymptomatic for many years. Headaches and nose bleeds (due to hypertension) and claudication and cold legs (due to poor blood flow in lower limbs) may be present. It is associated with Turner's syndrome. Primary amenorrhoea must be present if that is the case. But it must be noted that coarctation is twice as common in males as in females.
- *Hypertension of 160/100:* Hypertension is typically present in the upper limbs. Decreased renal perfusion can lead to the development of systemic hypertension that persists even after surgical correction.
- *Femoral pulse delay:* Weak and delayed (radiofemoral delay) pulses are characteristically present in the legs.

CONFUSA
Aortic stenosis or sclerosis are basically the disease of the aortic valve and not of aorta itself. However, in 80% of cases coarctation of aorta is associated with a bicuspid (an potentially stenotic) aortic valve.

Investigation of choice
- *Screening:* Chest X-ray.
- *Findings:* Dilated aorta indented at the site of coarctation (shaped like a figure of 3). Rib notching in adults.
- *Definitive:* Aortography.

Treatment of choice
Surgical excision of coarctation and end-to-end anastomosis of aorta:
- *Extensive coarctation:* prosthetic vascular grafts.
- *Childhood operation:* prevents renal systemic hypertension
- *Alternative:* Balloon dilatation

Your notes:

May—2002

37. A 40-year-old man with a blood pressure of 180/115 is found to have a loud bruit in his right upper abdomen.

Diagnosis: Right renal artery stenosis.

Clinchers
- *40-year-old:* The most common causes of renal artery stenosis is atherosclerosis. It is common in age > 50 years though cases may be seen in younger ages (as in this case). Fibromuscular dysplasia is another cause seen in younger females (20-30 yrs).
- *Blood pressure of 180/115:* Unilateral renal ischaemia results in reduction in the pressure in afferent glomerular arterioles. This leads to an increase in the production and release of renin from the juxta-glomerular apparatus with a consequent increase in angiotensin II. This leads to systemic hypertension.
- *Loud bruit in his right upper abdomen:* It is due to stenosis in the involved renal artery. Coexistent carotid or femoral bruits are present if the cause is atherosclerosis. Leg pulses may be absent due to coexistent peripheral vascular disease.

CONFUSA
The presence of a loud bruit in right upper abdomen clinches the diagnosis here. But if there is no mention of it in a question with suggestion towards renal hypertension, then the only other differential (for unilateral disease) is reflux nephropathy.

Investigation of choice
- *Screening:* Spiral CT/MRI
- *Definitive:* Renal angiography (Gold standard)

Immediate management
Hypotensive therapy (ACE inhibitors contraindicated).

Treatment of choice
Percutaneous transluminal renal angioplasty or surgery.

Your notes:

---

38. A 50-year-old male complains of flushing, tremor, palpitations. He is found to have a fluctuating blood pressure of 200/120.

Diagnosis: Phaeochromocytoma.

Clinchers
- *50-year-old male:* Phaeochromocytomas occur at all ages but are most common in young to mild adult life. They are usually associated with MEN type II syndromes. Sometimes they are inherited (autosomal dominant).
  There is a slight female preponderance, but this fact is not proven in meta-analyses.
- *Flushing, tremor, palpitations:* Either pallor or flushing may occur during the attack paroxysmal symptoms occur which may mimic a seizure disorder or panic attack. Other symptoms can be headache, sweating, pulsatile scotomas, etc. They are precipitated by stretching, sneezing, stress, sex, smoking, surgery, parturition of cheese, alcohol or tricyclices.
- *Fluctuating blood pressure of 200/120:* Hypertension is the most common sign and is episodic (NOTE). It resonds poorly to traditional antihypertensive treatment. It might be sustained in a significant proportion of patients but even in these there are distinct crises.

CONFUSA
The main differential diagnosis is from essential hypertension with hyperadrenergic features (sweating, tachycardia, increased cardiac output), but GMC has never asked such a question. One can be confused with carcinoid syndrome which does not produce such hypertensive episodes and diarrhoea (recurrent, watery) is pathognomically present in them.

Investigation of choice
- *Screening:* 24 h urine collection for
  - HMMA
  - VMA
  - Total/free meta-adrenalines
- *Definitive*
  - Adrenal tumor (90%)—MRI
  - Extra-adrenal (10%)—MIBG scan

Treatment of choice
- Surgery
- Careful BP control for 2 weeks preoperative (α-blocker before β-blockers).

39. A middle-aged woman with a blood pressure of 160/110 is found to have abdominal striae and facial hirsutism.

Diagnosis: Cushing's syndrome

Clinchers
- *Middle-aged:* Peak age—30-50 years.
- *Woman:* More common in women (only for pituitary dependent adrenal hyperplasia). But the most common cause of Cushing's syndrome is iatrogenic (exogenous steroid administration).
- *Blood pressure of 160/110:* Hypertension is common (>150/90) as are other effects of glucocorticoid excess like truncal obesity, increased body weight, water retention, osteoporosis, etc.
- *Abdominal striae:* Purple abdominal striae especially on abdomen are pathognomic and occur only with ACTH dependent causes. These are secondary to weakening and rupture of collagen fibers in dermis coupled with truncal obesity.
- *Facial hirsutism:* In women, increased levels of adrenal androgens can cause acne, hirsutism, and oligomenorrhea or amenorrhoea.

CONFUSA
Cushing's syndrome can be easily diagnosed from the clinical picture. The tough job is to differentiated between ectopic ACTH tumor or pituitary disease which is causing the syndrome. Severe hirsutism/virilization suggests an adrenal tumor. Specific diagnosis is possible only by localization tests like plasma ACTH, CRH test (Read pg 301, OHCM, 5th edn).

Investigation of choice
- *Screening:* Overnight dexamethasone suppression test
- *Definitive:*
  - 48 h DST
  - Circardian rhythm of cortisol
  - Secretion (lost in Cushing's syndrome)
- *Localisation*
  - Plasma ACTH
  - High dose DST
  - CRH test
- *Others*
  - Pituitary—MRI
  - Adrenal—CT/MRI

Immediate management
Remove source if iatrogenic.

Treatment of choice
Surgery after control of cortisol hypersecretion (Iatrogenic cases usually resolve on removal of source).
- Radiotherapy if surgery not possible

40. A 42-year-old patient with prominent jaw and supraorbital ridges.

Diagnosis: Acromegaly.

Clinchers
- *42-year-old:* It usually presents between the ages of 30 and 50 years. Its onset is insidious.
- *Prominent jaw and supraorbital ridges:* Most of the features of acromegaly are due to growth of soft tissues. Main features are:
  - Large tongue
  - Prominent supraorbital ridge
  - Prognathism
  - Increased teeth spacing
  - Increased shoe size
  - Thick spade like hands

Other features are: Coarse, oily skin, deepening voice, arthralgia, kyphosis, proximal muscle weakness, paraesthesiae—due to carpal tunnel syndrome, progressive heart failure, goitre, sleep apnoea.

CONFUSA
In acromegaly, isolated growth hormone measurement may show riased scretion, but levels vary with the time of the day and other factors so random measurement are not diagnostic.

Investigation of choice
Oral glucose tolerance test (OGTT) with growth hormone measurement is diagnostic.

Immediate management
Obtain old photos to compare. Take new photographs of full face, torso, hands on chest.

Treatment of choice
Trans sphenoidal surgery.

Note: For older patients (or failed surgery)—external irradiation.

Your notes:

May—2002

41. A patient is suspected of having bronchiectasis.

Diagnosis: Bronchiectasis (as given in the question).

Clinchers
- *Suspected of having bronchiectasis:* Bronchiectasis does not cause hoarseness per se. It can be secondary to:
  1. *Persistent and recurrent cough:* Which may produce laryngeal trauma to produce hoarseness.
  2. *Steroid inhaler use:* Which have a direct effect on laryngeal musculature to produce hoarseness. Or it can predisposes to laryngeal candidiasis on prolonged use which may produce hoarseness. Steroid inhalers (or oral steroids) can decrease the rate of progression of bronchiectasis by acting as anti-inflammatory agents.

CONFUSA
The only confusion in this question is whether to first confirm the diagnosis of bronchiectasis or to seen for laryngeal pathology secondary to bronchiectasis (as described above). It will be safe to go for the confirmation of the diagnosis first as the second option is dependent on it.

Investigation of choice
High resolution CT scan.

Immediate management
- Bronchodilators if demonstrable airflow limitation.
- Antibiotics if infection is present.

Treatment of choice
- *Conservative* i.e. postural drainage + antibiotics + bronchodilators + steroids
- *Surgery*
  - In localised disease (left lower lobe and lingual are most common sites for localised disease)
  - To control severe hemoptysis.

Your notes:

---

42. A 58-year-old man with fever and an area of consolidation on his chest X-ray is treated with antibiotics. His fever resolves but four weeks later but he still has a large area of consolidation.

Diagnosis: Bronchial carcinoma.

Clinchers
- *58-year-old man:* Elderly males with lung symptoms should be investigated to rule out lung cancer especially if they have history of smoking.
- *Fever:* This is because of the secondary pneumonia. Carcinoma causing partial obstruction of a bronchus interrupts the mucociliary escalator, and bacteria are retained within affected lobe.
- *An area of consolidation on his chest X-ray:* Secondary pneumonia due to above described mechanism appears as a lobar consolidation on CXR.
- *Is treated with antibiotics:* Treatment with antibiotics usually clears the pneumonia and resolves the fever within few days.
- *His fever resolves but four weeks later:* Any opacity secondary to inflammation should have been resolved in four weeks.
- *He still has a large area of consolidation:* Any opacity persisting beyound this time should make one strongly suspicious of a neoplastic lesion in this age group.

CONFUSA
The only confusion in this question can exist if one overlook the age of the patient and remain focussed only on the complications of pneumonia.

Investigation of choice
- *Screening:* CXR (already done in this case)
- *Definitive:* Bronchoscopy with biopsy.

Immediate management
Assess operability.

Treatment of choice
- Non-small cell tumors: Surgery (avoided in > 65 yrs with metastatic disease as rate of mortality is more than expected five-year survival)
- Radiotherapy: For bronchial obstruction (as in this case).

Your notes:

43. A singer has a six months history of hoarseness.

Diagnosis: Vocal nodules.

Clinchers
- *Singer:* These can be two causes of hoarseness in singers that are attributable to their profession
  1. Vocal nodules
  2. Vocal cord trauma
- *Six months history of hoarseness:* A six month history rules out trauma of vocal cords as it presents acutely and there is almost always a history of prolonged rehearsals (usually happens just before a show in amateur singers). A prolonged hisotry points towards vocal nodules.

CONFUSA
The only confusion is between nodules and trauma which can be safely distinguished by presentation and duration. However, note that it is vocal cord trauma and consequent submucosal haemorrhage that fibrose into a vocal nodule.

Investigation of choice
Indirect laryngoscopy.

Immediate management
Vocal rest to prevent further trauma.

Treatment of choice
Early cases of small nodules can be managed conservatively by education of patient in proper use of voice. With this treatment many nodules in children disappear completely. But this case will require surgery because of his profession (singing). Other indications for surgery are large nodules and nodules of long standing.

Your notes:

44. A 55-year-old smoker complains of shortness of breath and a cough. Laryngoscopy is normal.

Diagnosis: Suspected bronchial carcinoma.

Clinchers
- *55-year-old smoker:* A 55-year-old smoker would have been smoking for about 30-35 years and that makes him a high-risk case for bronchial carcinoma.
- *Shortness of breath:* It can be a presenting complaint of a bronchial carcinoma but is only for less than 5% cases. Other symptoms that can occur as a presenting complaint in < 5% cases are chest infection, malaise, weight loss, hoarseness and distant spread.
- *Cough:* It is the most common presenting symptom of bronchial carcinoma. Other common presenting complaints are hemoptysis and chest pain.
- *Laryngoscopy is normal:* This rules out any laryngeal pathology resulting in this presentation, i.e. carcinoma of larynx which is also common in male smokers (carcinoma larynx presents as dysphagia and hoarseness).

CONFUSA
Because of their common aetiology COPD is also frequently present in elderly smokers. So it always need to be ruled out preoperatively by lung function tests and gas transfer tests.

Investigation of choice
- *Screening:* CXR is the most valuable test.
- *Definitive:* CT chest.

Immediate management
Symptomatic.

Treatment of choice
Surgery (see Q 42).

Your notes:

45. A 30-year-old complains of hoarseness since he came back from a football match the day before.

Diagnosis: Vocal cord trauma

Clinchers
- *30-year-old:* This is quite a young age which rules out any neoplasia in larynx or lungs. Moreover many other chronic diseases will only present symptomatically after fourth decade of life. So the cause of haorseness has to be acute.
- *Hoarseness since he came back from a football match the day before:* The person would have been involved in persistent screaming and shouting while cheering up his side in the football match. Excessive vocal use may cause laryngeal trauma or temporary hoarseness.

CONFUSA
Other causes of traumatic hoarseness are excessive vomiting, coughing or inhaling fumes. If the hoarseness persist over one week, it suggest some laryngeal pathology (e.g. vocal nodules) and demand immediate laryngoscopy.

Investigation of choice
Laryngoscopy if hoarseness persists.

Immediate management
Vocal rest.

Treatment of choice
Symptomatic.

Your notes:

46. A four-year-old boy walks with a prominent lordosis. He has goood speech, can build objects using blocks and has good social awareness.

Diagnosis: Duchenne muscular dystrophy (DMD).

Clinchers
- *Four-year-old boy:* DMD is present at birth, but the disorder usually becomes apparent between ages 3 and 5. It occurs exclusively in boys as it is a X-linked recessive disease.
- *Walks with a prominent lordosis:* Contractures of the heel cords and iliotibial bands forces the child to walk on toes, thereby producing a lordotic posture (This happens before the progressive loss of muscle strength makes him wheelchair bound).
- *He has goood speech, can build objects using blocks, has good social awareness:* Intellectual development in DMD is common, the average IQ is approximately one standard deviation below the mean. Impairment of intellectual function appears to be nonprogressive and performance is least affected.

CONFUSA
Bilateral congenital dysplasia/dislocation of hip (CDH) can be a confusing option in this case but it can be safely excluded by the fact that CDH is 6 times more common in girls and usually diagnosed well before 4 years. Although the findings in bilateral CHD can be similar, i.e. lordosis and wide perineum. Becker muscular dystrophy can be a clinical differential, especially because of less incidence of mental retardation in it, but it usually presents after 5 years of age.

Investigation of choice
- *Screening:* Serum creatine phosphokinase (CK)
- *Definitive:* EMG and biopsy (abnormal fibres surrounded by fat and fibrous tissues).

Immediate management
Screen for any chest infection (usually present in DMD) and treat if present.

Treatment of choice
- Prednisolone 0.75 mg/kg
- Aim to keep boy walking by using knee-ankle-foot orthoses
- Spinal fixation (Luque operation) or bracing reduces scoliosis.

47. A nine-month-baby born at term has a weight in the 97th percentile. His development is delayed.

Diagnosis: Hypothyroidism.

Clinchers
- *Nine-month-baby:* Hypothyroidism can be easily diagnosed at this age as before this age it manifest as very nonspecific features, i.e. excessive sleeping, inactivity, slow feeding and little crying.
- *Born at term:* There may be no signs at birth, the first sign is often prolonged neonatal jaundice. A term delivery in this case also exclude prematurity as a cause of developmental delay.
- *Has a weight in the 97th percentile:* Hypothyroidism produces a decrease in BMR, thereby resulting in weight gain.
- *His development is delayed:* Delayed growth and mental development, hypotonia and slowly relaxing reflexes are characteristic in hypothyroidism. Other features are coarse dry hair, flat nasal bridge, protruding tongue, umbilical hernia and slow pulse. Other late signs: IQ decrease, delayed puberty (occasionally precocious), short stature and delayed dentition).

CONFUSA
Differential diagnosis of large tongue are
- Hypothyroidism
- Amyloidosis
- Storage disorders

Investigation of choice
- *Screening:* Heel prick test (filter paper blood spots at 5-7 days of age)
- *Definitive:* TSH/wrist X-ray (bone age is less than chronological age).

Treatment of choice
Thyroxine 10 µg/kg/day ($\leq$ 50 µg/day)—infants
100 µg/day—5 years age
- Start adult doses at 12 years
- Adjust according to growth rate and clinical response.

Your notes:

---

48. A nine-month-baby born at term has a weight in the 3rd percentile. His development is delayed. His head and body size are both small.

Diagnosis: Constitutional delay.

Clinchers
- *Nine-month-baby:* Earliest possible age to make a diagnosis of constitutional delay.
- *Born at term:* Rules out any growth delay due to prematurity.
- *Has a weight in the 3rd percentile:* Third percentile is the lowest cut off of weight in normal range (highest is 97th percentile). This signifies a delay in weight gain although he is considered normal.
- *His development is delayed:* There could be many causes for delayed development which could not be ascertained here because of lack of detailed history and information in the question.
- *His head and body size are both small:* Since both head and body are small, there is a uniform all round delay—by definition this is constitutional delay. He might have been a small for gestation age baby.

CONFUSA
Microcephaly is a feature of many congenital disorders resulting in developmental delay (e.g. fetal alcohol syndrome, intrauterine infections, chromosomal disorders, etc.). But in it body size is usually normaly.

Investigation of choice
Detailed work up to find a cause.

Immediate management
Ensure proper nutrition.

Treatment of choice
Depends upon cause, otherwise no treatment required as he is in normal range.

Your notes:

49. A nine-year-old girl has difficulty with speech. She has recently been hospitalised for a medical reason. Her speech before hospitalisation was completely normal.

Diagnosis: Meningitis.

Clinchers

- *Nine-year-old girl:* Hemophilus influenzae commonly causes meningitis in < 5 years age. Afterwards pneumococcal and meningococcal meningitis are more common.
- *Difficulty with speech:* Meningitis can produce focal neurological signs such as this. Many false localising signs may also be present because of increased intracranial tension.
- *She has recently been hospitalised for a medical reason:* Meningitis requires hospital admission.
- *Her speech before hospitalisation was completely normal:* This tell that the rise in ICT is progressive and immediate intervention is required.

CONFUSA

"Treatment for hyperthyroidism" can be a confusing option as carbamazepine (used as a first line drug) can produce agranulocytosis → sore throat → speech difficulty. But it can be safely excluded as hyperthyroidism per se does not warrant hospital admission and sore throat does not chiefly present as speech difficulty. Although the typical case of childhood hyperthyroidism is a prepubertal girl.

Investgation of choice

Lumbar puncture is contraindicated in the presence of focal signs. If purpura are present along with fever do blood culture, otherwise CT to find out the pressure effects of increased ICT.

Immediate management

Benzyl penicillin after taking blood sample + high flow O_2.

Treatment of choice

Antibiotic according to culture report.

Organism	Antibiotic	Second choice
• Unknown pyogenic	Cefotaxime	Benzyl penicillin+ Chloramphenicol
• Meningococcus	Benzyl penicillin	Cefotaxime
• Pneumococcus	Cefotaxime	Penicillin
• Hemophilus	Cefotaxime	Chloramphenicol

50. A four-year-old boy has delayed speech. Both his father and paternal uncle has the same problem.

Diagnosis: Familial occurrence (i.e. normal finding here).

Clinchers

- *Four-year-old boy:* Normally sequence of speech development is
  - At 1 year: Few words may be used meaningfully
  - At 1½ years: 2 word utterances ("Mommy come")
  - At 2 years: Subject-verb-object sentences
  - At 3½ years: Mastered thought, language, obstruction and elements of reason
- *Delayed speech:* If a child reaches 3 years age with < 50 words vocabulary, suspect some abnormality.
- *Both his father and paternal uncle has the same problem:* Since there are two people in the family with the same features, it is strongly suggestive of a familial occurrence.

CONFUSA

If the father and uncle now have good speech and their problem is only a delayed development of speech, then the child's parents should be reassured (after excluding deafness and other common ailments that hampers speech development).

Investigation of choice

Evaluation by a speech therapist to classify the type of problem.

Immediate management

Refer to speech therapist.

Treatment of choice

Wait and watch (if no other abnormality is found).

Your notes:

First Aid for the PLAB

51. A middle-aged woman remains unconcious 12 hours following a cholecystectomy. On examination both pupils are seen to be pinpoint.

Diagnosis: Opiate overdosage.

Clinchers

➤ *Middle-aged woman:* Maximum incidence of gallstones is in middle-aged women. In the UK they are found in approximately 10% of women in their forties increasing to 30% after the age of 60 years. They are about half as common in men (aphorism: fair, fat, fertile, females of forty).

➤ *Remains unconcious 12 hours following a cholecystectomy:* Opiate overdosage (prescribed postoperatively for analgesia) can produce coma, respiratory depression and acidosis.

➤ *Both pupils are seen to be pinpoint:* Pinpoint pupils are seen in opiate overdose and hence our suspicion is confirmed.

CONFUSA
The other common etiology of pinpoint is pontine hemorrhage. But that is very unlikely in postoperative middle-aged patient. Moreover no indication of any hypertensive disease is given in this question (Hypertension is associated with pontine hemorrhage).

Investigation of choice
Respiratory rate.

Immediate management
Respiratory support (oxygen/IPPV)

Treatment of choice
Immediate reversal by naloxone.

Your notes:

---

52. A young diabetic is admitted in a comatose state. His plasma glucose level is 2 mmols/L

Diagnosis: Hypoglycemia

Clinchers

➤ *Young diabetic:* The most common cause of hypoglycemia is insulin or sulfonylurea treatment in a known diabetic. It can also be due to insufficient food or change in routine of insulin (i.e. site of injection, type of insulin, new syringe size). It is more so in younger patients because there is usually no set lifestyle.

➤ *Comatose state:* Initially, a hypoglycemic patient is restless and agitated but, if untreated, rapidly becomes unresponsive. There is pallor profuse sweating and a bounding pulse. Aggression can be such that the patient arrives in police custody and may be thought to be intoxicated. False neurological signs are sometimes seen.

➤ *His plasma glucose level is 2 mmols:* Hypoglycemia by definition is < 2.5 mmol/L.

CONFUSA
The other two conditions which can produce comatose state in a diabetic are:
- Nonketotic (HONK) coma
- Diabetic ketoacidosis (DKA)

Investigation of choice
- Venous blood glucose
- In case of unexplained hypoglycemia
  - Liver function tests
  - Insulin assay
  - C peptide assay
  - Toxicology (paracetamol) screen

Immediate management
Start treatment after taking blood sample.

Treatment of choice
- 50 ml of 50% dextrose solution (adults)
- 2-5 ml/kg of 10% dextrose solution (child)
- If venous access is delayed:
  - Glucagon 1-2 mg IM (20 µg/kg for children)
- 50% dextrose harms veins, so follow by 0.9% saline flush.
- If there is no prompt recovery after treatment, give dexamethasone 4 mg/4h IV to combat cerebral edema after prolonged hypoglycemia.
- Once conscious, give sugary drinks.

53. A young diabetic is admitted in a comatose state. His plasma glucose level is 17 mmols and he is dehydrated.

Diagnosis: Diabetic ketoacidosis (DKA).

Clinchers

- *Young diabetic:* DKA coma only cocurs with type I diabetes, so it is more common in young diabetics (as type I diabetes usually presents in childhood).
- *Comatose state:* Apart from coma other symptoms are polyuria, polydipsia, lethargy, anorexia, hyperventilation, ketotic breath (smells like peach), dehydration, vomiting, abdominal pain, etc.
- *Plasma glucose level is 17 mmols:* Normal range of blood glucose is 3.5-5.5 mmol/l. Usually in DKA it is > 20 mmol/L. But 17 mmol/l is also a very high value.
- *Dehydrated:* Gross hyperglycemia causes an osmotic diuresis, decreased tissue perfusion and circulatory collapse. It produces dehydration. Dehydration is more life-threatening than any hyperglycemia—so its correction takes precedence.

CONFUSA

Some students get confused between DKA and HONK coma (hyperglycemic hyperosmolar nonketotic coma).

DKA	HONK
1. Occurs only in IDDM	1. Occurs only in NIDDM
2. History of 2-3 days	2. Longer history (eg 1 wk)
3. Glucose usually > 20 mmol/l	3. Glucose >35 mmol/l
4. Acidosis present (pH <7.3)	4. Acidosis absent
5. Ketotic breath present	5. No ketotic breath
6. Younger patients	6. Patient often old
7. Insulin given immediately in treatment	7. Insulin is given late, cautiously and in lower dosage

Investigation of choice
Plasma osmolality (2[Na$^+$] + [urea] + [glucose])

Immediate management
IV access and stard fluid (0.9% NS) immediately.

Treatment of choice
Fluid replacement (0.9%NS) + 10U soluble insulin IV (if plasma glucose > 20 mmol/L).
↓
Insulin sliding scale.

Your notes:

54. A 37-year-old alcoholic is found wandering in a park. His partner says he has had a number of falls recently and in the A and E the patient is confused. The blood sugar level is normal.

Diagnosis: Head injury (probable).

Clinchers

- *Alcoholic:* Subdural hematomas are commonly seen in alcoholics. There may be no apparent injury. The first sign may be a failure to wake up after an episode of heavy drinking.
- *History of number of falls recently:* Frequent falls weaken the bridging veins which traverse the subdural space. They can bleed to give rise to subdural hematomas. This mechanism is responsible for their frequent incidence in alcoholics. Subdural hematomas are also common among elderly and HIV patients. But in them the pathogenesis is cerebral atropy → shrinkage of brain → stretching of bridging veins → rupture → hematoma.
- *Confused:* A CT scan is indicated in all cases of clouding on consciousness or low GCS in an alcoholic, as the clinical assessment is difficult in an intoxicated patient.

CONFUSA
A normal blood sugar rules out hypoglycemia which is a more common cause of confusion in an alcoholic. On the other hand this patient could be plainly showing only the features of intoxication, but CT scan is still essential from medicolegal point of view in UK.

Investigation of choice
CT scan (subdural hematoma—inner concave border).

Immediate management
Admit in hospital (at least overnight).

Treatment of choice
Depends on CT findings.

Your notes:

55. A 25-year-old found deeply unconscious is brought to the accident and emergency (A and E) department. He has an abrasion over his left temple and puncture marks on his left forearm.

Diagnosis: Narcotic overdose.

Clinchers

- *25-year-old:* Maximum incidence of drug addiction in UK is in teens and twenties.
- *Deeply unconscious:* Opiates the most common drugs of abuse which produces unconsciousness. Other drugs are:
  - Barbiturates
  - Solvents
  - Benzodiazepines
- *Abrasion over his left temple:* It might be sustained secondarily due to a fall on being knocked out of consciousness by the "kick" of the drug of abuse.
- *Puncture marks on his left forearm:* It suggests IV drug abuse. There will be several puncture marks varying ages along the line of veins. Since most people are right handed, it is usual to find out such marks on left forearm. Next most common site is feet.

CONFUSA

Abrasion over his left temple could suggest an intracranial injury also. But first priority will always be to give Naloxone IV (flumazenile if BZD abuse suspected) and then to evaluated for head injury.

Investigation of choice
Pupil size (pinpoint pupil in opiate overdose).

Immediate management
Naloxone IV.

Treatment of choice
According to local guidelines for drug abusers, i.e.
- If willing to leave the habit—refer to local deaddiction centre
- If not willing—enrol in needle exchange programme.

Your notes:

56. A middle-aged woman has had several admissions for severe depression. She now turns up with a very severe depression despite all treatment.

Diagnosis: Refractory depression.

Clinchers

- *Middle-aged woman:* Middle-aged females are most prone to depression.
- *Has had several admissions for severe depression:* This proves that the depression is persistent and many different treatment approaches have been tried.
- *She now turns up with a very severe depression despite all treatment:* This means that the depression is severe and refractory to drug treatment. The condition can lead to a serious risk of health and may be the patient can go into a depressive stupor if left untreated.

CONFUSA

ECT is the treatment of choice in depression where,
- The patient is dangerously suicidal
- Delay in treatment represents a serious health risk
- The patient is refusing food and drink
- Patient is in depressive stupor

Investigation of choice
Preanaesthetic checkup (as patient will be given ECT under GA, usually thiopental).

Treatment of choice
Electroconvulsive therapy (ECT).

Your notes:

57. A woman has bouts of depression alternating with bouts of mania. She has had first line antidepressants but they have not worked.

Diagnosis: Manic depressive illness (MDI) (Bipolar affective disorder)

Clinchers
- *Woman:* Depression is more common in females especially those in middle-age group.
- *Bouts of depression alternating with bouts of mania:* This fulfils the criteria to be diagnosed as MDI. Usually there is also a history of MDI in a close relative.
- *She has had first line antidepressants but they have not worked:* In MDI antidepressants work only in the depressive phases. For prophylaxis lithium is required.

CONFUSA
Cyclothymic disorders is less severe manic depressive illness (i.e. instead of manic episodes, there will be euphoric or hypomanic episodes. Note: Mania has delusions as a sign, hypomania does not). Cyclothymia is basically cyclical mood swings without the more florid features.

Investigation of choice
Plasma creatinine and TSH (to exclude kidney or thyroid disease, necessary before starting lithium therapy).

Immediate management
Sedation if manic (chlorpromazine or benzodiazepine).

Treatment of choice
Lithium prophylaxis.

Your notes:

58. A young dentist, successful at work lacks confidence in himself. He finds that he is unable to socialise properly and has early morning waking. He is on no treatment.

Diagnosis: Mild depression

Clinchers
- *Young dentist:* Mild episodes of depression are very common among young professionals. The usual precipitants in them are overrealisation of thier shortcomings in their professional field.
- *Successful at work:* It proves that the depression is not major as it is not interfering with his work and efficiency.
- *Lacks confidence in himself:* This signifies a personality problem and can be a reason for his depression.
- *He finds that he is unable to socialise properly:* It is a feature of a personality disorder and could be the precipitating cause of depression.
- *Early morning waking:* It is a pathognomic feature of depression.
- *He is on no treatment:* It means that first line anti-depressant therapy can be used in this case.

CONFUSA
The main confusion in this question lies in choosing the answer. Since he has a personality disorder, it needs to be corrected for complete cure of his depression. But a definitive indication for antidepressant therapy is present (early morning awakening), so it has to be initiated first. Psychoanalysis and counselling will follow it.

Investigation of choice
Detailed history.

Immediate management
Trycyclic antidepressants (presence of biological features or stressful life events suggests a good response to antidepressants). Give imipramine as it is more effective for early moring awakening as it less sedating—less interference with work).

Treatment of choice
Tricyclic antidepressants + psychoanalysis.

Your notes:

59. A 44-year-old has repeated episodes of depressed mood in response to feeling rejected, and a craving for sweets and chocolate. These reactive mood changes are accompanied by lethargy and increased appetite, particularly with a preference for carbohydrates.

Diagnosis: Depression.

Clinchers

➤ *44-year-old:* Depression is most common among middle-aged people (especially females).
➤ *Repeated episodes of depressed mood in response to feeling rejected:* It proves that the depression is recurrent and has a basis, i.e. it is not endogenous depression.
➤ *Craving for sweets and chocolate:* Usually depression causes poor appetite and weight loss, but in some rare cases it may produce increased appetite.

CONFUSA

Bulimia nervosa is characterised by binge eating and vomiting afterwards. Depression is a feature in it also but it typically follows the episodes of vomiting and is absolutely never precipitate by feeling of rejection. MAO inhibitors are the antipsychotics which stimulate appetite and help in gaining weight (by increasing a craving for carbohydrates, fluoxetine is an antidepressant which helps in losing weight and hence is preferred in obese patients with depression.

Investigation of choice
Detailed history.

Immediate management
Cognitive therapy (for feeling of rejections).

Treatment of choice
Fluoxetine.

Your Notes:

60. A 20-year-old previously hearlthy girl is waiting for her college exam result. The result is arriving that day by post and she is suffering from acute anxiety due to the importance of the results for her future career. Her mother consults their general practitioners.

Diagnosis: Acute anxiety neurosis.

Clinchers

➤ *Previously healthy:* Rules out any past history of any psychiatric or organic disorder.
➤ *College exam result due:* Causes of acute anxiety are usually stress and life events (e.g. gaining a spouse, losing a job, moving a house, results, etc).
➤ *Mother consults their general practitioner:* Acute anxiety before such an important event is normal. It remains physiological until it does not affect one's performance or social life. If her mother has consulted a GP for the anxiety, it must be significant and affecting her life/personality in some way. Since anxiety neurosis is characterised by a response out of proportion to the stress that precipitates them (an exaggeration of personality), this case seems more as a neurosis rather than a normal response.

CONFUSA

• Before diagnosing a neurosis, always rule out any underlying depression
• Panic attacks (hyperventilation syndromes) are also common in young females but are not precipitated usually by any obvious cause and have a totally different symptomatic profile.

Investigation of choice
Detailed psychiatric history.

Immediate management
Symptom control (best way is through simple listening and reassurance).

Treatment of choice
Behaviour therapy + diazepam/lorazepam.

Your notes:

61. Carcinoma of the right main bronchus.

Diagnosis: Already stated as the question.

Clinchers

Hemoptysis is the second most common symptom of presentation of a bronchial carcinoma, occurring in 70% of cases. (The most common symptom is cough, occurring in 80%).

Bronchial carcinoma is a frequent carcinoma asked in PLAB exams. So let us seen some most frequently occurring clinchers in such questions
- Elderly
- Smoker
- Male
- Cough
- Hemoptysis
- Dyspnoea
- Chest pain
- Recurrent/slowly resolving pneumonia
- Anorexia
- Weight loss
- Clubbing
- Hypertrophic pulmonary osteoarthritis (wrist pain)
- Supraclavicular or axillary lymphadenopathy.

CONFUSA
Most of the neurological signs caused by a bronchial carcinoma are due to brain metastases. Nonmetastatic neurological signs do occur and can be confusing, there are: confusion, fits, cerebellar syndrome, proximal myopathy, peripheral neuropathy, polymyositis, Eatan-Lambert syndrome.

Investigation of choice
- *Screening:* CXR (often normal).
- *Definitive:* Fibreoptic bronchoscopy (as it gives a histological diagnosis also and can assess operatibility)

Treatment of choice

Depends on stage: Surgical excision in operable cases, otherwise palliative radiotherapy.

Your notes:

62. Pulmonary embolism.

Diagnosis: Already stated as the question.

Clinchers

Since the question, has not given any clinical profile, let us see the most common 'clinchers', that GMC uses in their exams for this condition.
- *Precipitants:* Air travel, recent operation, pregnancy, OCP, hormone replacement therapy, disseminated malignancy, DVT.
- *Symptoms:* Acute breathlessness, pleuritic chest pain, haemoptysis.
- *Signs:* Tachypnoea, tachycardia, hypotension, raised JVP, pleural rub.
- *CXR:* Usually normal (in GMC questions).
- *ECG:* Usually normal (in GMC questions), $S_I Q_{III} T_{III}$ pattern, sinus tachycardia, right bundle branch block.

CONFUSA
Pulmonary embolism produces central cyanosis due to decreased oxygen saturation which is produced by only three other common conditions, i.e.
- Pulmonary oedema
- Severe respiratory disease
- Congenital cyanotic heart disease.

Investigation of choice

Investigation of pulmonary embolism is a point of major confusion in PLAB examination. Consider following points while choosing the investigation for PE:
- *Screening*
  - V/Q scan—only if the patient is stable and not severely breathless
  - Spiral CT with contrast—if facilities are available patient's general state do not allow a V/Q scan to be done
- *Definitive:* Pulmonary angiogram—but not usually done because of risk of complications and it being an invasive test.

Note: Always look in the "instructions" to the theme about the type of investigation being asked for, i.e. is it "definitive" or "screening". It is important as the answer is usually different for both and you will end up losing marks for something you know.

Immediate management

Anticoagulation with LMW heparin (Dalteparin 200 U/kg/24 hr SC; max dose 18,000 IU/24h)
- Stop when INR > 2

Treatment of choice

Oral warfarin 10 mg for minimum 3 months.

63. Bronchial carcinoid.

Diagnosis: Already stated as the question.

Clinchers
Questions about bronchial carcinoids are a rarity in PLAB exam. Still let us review some salient features of them.
- Usually follow a benign course
- May secrete other hormones, effects of whom constitute the common presenting complaints of this condition. They can secrete
  - ACTH
  - Arginine vasopressin
- Carcinoid syndrome is only produce when any carcinoid has liver metastases. It is characterised by:
  - Cutaneous flush
  - Bronchoconstriction
  - Diarrhoea.

> **CONFUSA**
> Bronchial carcinoids and small cell carcinoma both develops from the same cells (kulchitsky cell in bronchial epithelium). But carcinoid can be differentiated by presence of carcinoid syndrome (only in presence of liver metastases) and cardiac valvular lesions—both of these are absent in small cell carcinoma of lung. Paraneoplastic syndromes are not a criteria for differentiation as both can cause them (especially ACTH).

Investigation of choice
- *Screening:* 24 hour urine 5HIAA increase.
- *Definitive:* CXR/CT—usually done only if liver metastases are absent as only then a curative resection is possible.

Immediate management
High dose octreotide for crises + careful fluid balance.

Treatment of choice
- Crises—Octreotide
- Flushing—Ketanserin
- Diarrhoea—Loperamide/cyproheptadine
- Hepatic metastases—embolisation
- Bronchial obstruction—surgical debulking

Your notes:

64. Bronchiectasis.

Diagnosis: Already stated as the question.

Clinchers
Bronchiectasis is a frequent question in PLAB exam. The most frequent 'clinchers' used by GMC to describe this condition are:
- *Secondary to:* Cystic fibrosis, kartageneger's syndrome, pertussis in the childhood, allergic bronchopulmonary aspergillosis.
  "Non-GMC" conditions—Young's syndrome (primary ciliary dyskinesia), measles, bronchiolitis, pneumonia, TB, HIV, bronchial obstruction (tumour, foreign body), hypogammaglobulinaemia, rheumatoid arthritis, ulcerative colitis, idiopathic.
- *Symptoms:* Persistent cough, copious purulent sputum, intermittent hemoptysis.
- *Signs:* Finger clubbing, coarse inspiratory, crackles, wheeze.
- *Complications:* Pneumonia, pleural effusion, pneumothorax, hemoptysis, cerebral abscess, amyloidosis.

> **CONFUSA**
> Spirometry is bronchiectasis shows an obstructive pattern. Reversability should be assessed to differentiate from asthma.

Investigation of choice
- *Screening:* CXR—Tramline and ring shadows.
- *Definitive:* High resolution CT chest—to assess extent and distribution.

Immediate management
Antibiotics if infection (usually pseudomonas) is present.

Treatment of choice
Postural drainage + bronchodilators (if asthma, COPD, cystic fibrosis, ABPA present) + steroids (if ABPA present).

Indications for surgery are:
- Localized bronchiectasis
- To control severe hemoptysis.

Your notes:

65. Tuberculosis.

Diagnosis: Already stated as the question.

Clinchers
GMC usually does not ask such one word questions. Most probably the person who has recapitulated these questions could not remember the clinical situations. Anyway, tuberculosis is a frequent topic and is almost invariably associated with south east asian immigrants (only in GMC questions). The other GMC 'clinchers' that appear routinely are:
- *Skin TB:* (lupus vulgaris), apple jelly nodules especially on face and neck.
- *Addison's disease:* Secondary to TB.
- *TB meningitis:* Subacute, CSF protein increase, fever
- *Bazin's disease:* Skin TB with localized areas of fat necrosis with ulceration and an indurated rash, characteristically on adolescent girl's legs.
- *Pulmonary TB:* Cough, sputum, hemoptysis, pleural effusion, chronic symptoms.

CONFUSA
Contact lens staining is an indirect and confusing side effect of antitubercular therapy. It occurs due to orange discoloration of tears (and other body fluids like sweat and urine) by rifampicin.

Investigation of choice
- *Screening:* Mantoux test.
- *Definitive:* Sputum culture (AFB +)

Immediate management
Rule out any immunodeficiencies (i.e. HIV, malignancy, DM, steroid treatment, debilitation).

Treatment of choice
First 8 weeks: Rifampicin + Isoniazid + Pyrazinamide ± Ethambutol
Then for 4 months: Rifampicin + Isoniazid
- Give pyridoxine throughout treatment
- Give steroids also in meningeal and pericardial TB.

Your notes:

66. A middle-aged man has recently been operated after sustaining a perforated gallbladder. He becomes increasingly comatose and on examination is noted to have peripheral warming.

Diagnosis: Hyperdynamic (warm) septic shock

Clinchers
- *Middle-aged man:* Gallbladder perforation can be due to gallstones or trauma. Irrespective of etiology, the thing to be kept in mind is that bile is not a sterile fluid and contains many bacteria (Ref: Love and Bailey, 23rd edn, pg 1300).
- *Recently been operated after sustaining a perforated gall-bladder:* Peritonitis or suppurative biliary conditions predispose to serious gram-negative infections leading to hyperdynamic septic shock.
- *Becomes increasingly comatose:* Generalised capillary leakage and other fluid losses lead to severe hypovolemia with reduced cardiac output, tachycardia and vasoconstriction. The systemic infection induces cardiac depression, pulmonary hypertension, pulmonary edema and hypoxia and make him increasingly drowsy.
- *Have peripheral warming:* Initially the patient has abnormal or increased cardiac output with tachycardia and a warm, dry, skin.

CONFUSA
The patient can become cold and clammy, if severe sepsis or endotoxaemia is allowed to persist. In that case the condition may be overlooked by untrained minds.

Investigation of choice
Blood cultures.

Immediate management
High concentration O_2 + vigorous fluid resuscitation.

Treatment of choice
Antibiotics IV.

Your notes:

67. Following a motorcyle accident a young man has a pulse rate of 110 and a blood pressure that falls to 90/50. On examination of the CXR he is noted to have fractures of the lower ribs on the left.

Diagnosis: Splenic rupture

Clinchers
- *Motorcyle accident:* The main injuries in a motorcycle accident are sustained on head, thorax and legs.
- *Young man:* Young men are more involved in motorcycle accidents.
- *Pulse rate of 110:* A pulse >100 and systolic BP < 100 signifies hypovolemic shock.
- *Blood pressure falls to 90/50:* This signifies a massive blood loss.
- *Fractures of the lower ribs on the left:* Fracture of ribs does not lead to a significant fall in BP as the blood loss is very minimal. It could fall to 90/50 only if there is rupture of spleen which lies beneath lower left ribs.

CONFUSA
Hemothorax can present with same profile but that would be visible on CXR.

Investigation of choice
- Peritoneal lavage if patient is shocked
- Otherwise USG

Immediate management
Fluid resuscitation + cross-match.

Treatment of choice
Urgent laparotomy (with splenic preservation wherever possible).

Your Notes:

---

68. A 64-year-old patient on the surgical ward has been operated on for a hernia, he presents with warm extremities and a blood pressure of 90/60 mm Hg.

Diagnosis: Septic shock.

Clinchers
- *Operated on for a hernia:* Gram-negative shock is common after colonic, biliary and urological surgery and with infected severe burns.
- *Warm peripherals:* The principal effect of endotoxins is to cause vasodilatation of the peripheral circulation together with increased capillary permeability. Initially this produces warm peripheries but later on the peripheries can be cold (thereby making the differentiation difficult).
- *BP 90/60 mmHg:* Any shock results in inadequate organ perfusion. Sepsis induces hypotension usually results from a generalised maldistribution of blood flow and blood volume and from hypovolemia due to diffuse capillary leak. In septic shock the BP is < 90 mmHg systolic or 40 mmHg less than patient's normal BP and is unresponsive to fluid resuscitation.

CONFUSA
Risk factors for gram-positive bacteremia include the presence of intravascular catheters or mechanical devices, burns and IV drug use.

Investigation of choice
Blood culture and Gram stain.

Immediate management
Colloid/crystalloids IVI + refer to ITU for monitoring ± ionotropes (e.g. dopamine in 'renal' dose of 2-5 µg/kg/min IVI).

Treatment of choice
This is a case of intra-abdominal sepsis. The standard treatment for it is,
    Cefuroxime + metronidazole (both IV)

Your Notes:

69. A woman had a caesarean section done in the morning presented with a blood pressure of 80/65 mmHg and pulse rate of 120 beats/min.

Diagnosis: Hypovolemic shock.

Clinchers
- *Caesarean section:* It is a major operation and may lead to hypovolemia if the patient has bleed extensively during the surgery or postoperative intrauterine bleeding due to uterine atonia (common after a caesarean section).
- *BP of 80/65 mmHg:* Reduction in circulating blood volume results in a reduction fo stroke volume and cardiac output. BP is initially maintained (as in cardiogenic shock), with increased sympathetic activity raising the peripheral vascular resistance leading to the clinical picture of a cold, clammy patient with a tachycardia (and hence a pulse rate of 120 bpm). As volume losses increase, the blood pressure falls. So most probably the patient is still bleeding (most probably intrauterine).

(Note: There is no tachycardia in a spinal shock).

CONFUSA
In young and fit, the systolic BP may remain normal, although the pulse pressure will narrow, with upto 30% of blood volume depletion.

Investigation of choice
BP/CVP/urine output.

Immediate management
If bleed already—Colloid.
If bleeding—Blood.

Treatment of choice
Treatment of underlying cause.

Your notes:

70. A 23-year-old man is brought into the accident and emergency department from the local park, with a red swollen arm. He is found to have a blood pressure of 100/60 mm Hg.

Diagnosis: Anaphylactic shock secondary to bee sting.

Clinchers
Brought from local park, with a red swollen arm: This situation is pointing towards a bee sting sustained in the park. Normally bee stings do not produce swelling and redness of the whole arm until and unless a component of anaphylaxis is there. Time to onset is variable, but symptoms usually occur within seconds to minutes of exposure to the offending antigen.

Symptoms of anaphylaxis are usually:
- *Respiratory:* Mucous membrane swelling (lips, larynx), hoarseness, stridor, wheezing.
- *CVS:* Tachycardia, hypotension (in this case BP is 100/60 mmHg)
- *Cutaneous:* Pruritus, urticaria, angioedema

Since anaphylaxis is a type I IgE mediated response, this person must have had a previous exposure to the bee sting.

CONFUSA
Anaphylactoid reactions are different from anaphylaxis as they result from direct release of mediators from inflammatory cells, without involving antibodies (anaphylaxis is IgE mediated), usually in response to a drug, e.g. N-acetylcysteine.

Investigation of choice
Check for laryngeal edema as it can be fatal.

Immediate management
- Secure airway + 100% O_2
- Intubate if respiratory obstruction is imminent

Treatment of choice
Adrenaline IM (0.5 ml of 1:1000)

Note: Adrenaline is not given IV unless the patient is severely ill, or has no pulse.

Prophylaxis can be effectuated by desensitization to hymenoptera venom.

Your Notes:

71. Following an alcoholic binge a 36-year-old male falls and comes to casualty with a cut in his temporal region his Glasgow Coma Scale is normal and his neck is cleared by the orthopedic SHO.

Diagnosis: Superficial head injury.

Clinchers
- *Following an alcoholic binge*: Alcoholics warrants overnight admission in the hospital as they cannot be assessed properly on presentation for head injury. This is applicable even if the GCS is normal. Other patients warranting admission in spite of normal GCS are children and postictal (confused) patients.
- *Falls:* Most probably it is the reason for the cut in the temporal region. Note that alcoholics are more prone to develop subdural hematomas due to weakening of bridging veins because of repeated falls.
- *A cut in his temporal region:* It must be a simple laceration if there is no associated fracture of temporal bone. It requires prompt suturing to maintain hemostasis.
- *Glasgow Coma Scale is normal:* Rules out any immediate brain damage/hematoma. But not that it is difficult or even misleading in an alcoholic.
- *His neck is cleared by the orthopedic SHO:* It rules out any spinal injury.

CONFUSA
The main confusion is about whom to admit or discharge in a case of head injury. The criteria are:

Criteria for admission in a case of head injury
- Difficult to assess
  - *Child*
  - *Postictal*
  - *Alcohol intoxication*
- CNS signs
- Severe headache or vomiting
- Fracture
- Smelling of alcohol with GCS < 15

Criteria for discharge with written advise (all criteria must be fulfilled)
- Fully conscious on presentation
- No abnormal neurological signs
- Loss of consciousness < 5 min
- Post-traumatic amnesia < 5 min
- No severe headache
- No vomiting
- No skull fracture
- No bleeding disorder
- Good home conditions

Note: Get an X-ray skull in all suspected medicolegal cases (like this one) even if you suspect no bony injury.
Other main confusion is about anterograde and retrograde amnesia. Note the only the extent of anterograte amnesia correlates with severity of injury (admit if > 5 min). Retrograde amnesia does not correlate well with severity. Also retrograde amnesia never occurs without anterograde amnesia. Anterograde amnesia (also known as post-traumatic amnesia—PTA) if under one hour, means mild injury whereas > 24 years denotes severe injury. OHCM has stated on the contrary and thus created this confusion. But refer Kumar and Clark, pg 1084, 4th edn and lecture notes in emergency medicine, pg 36 second edition.

Investigation of choice
X-ray skull (CT in an alcoholic is only indicated if GCS falls).

Immediate management
Suturing of laceration.

Treatment of choice
Monitoring and discharge with written advise after a time period.

Your notes:

May—2002

72. An 8-year-old boy falls off a swing at his school. He is brought to Casualty by one of his teachers. He has a bruise over his right eye but the examination is otherwise normal. He is fully conscious with no history of blackouts since the accident. A skull X-ray is performed, which is normal.

Diagnosis: Insignificant head injury.

Clinchers

- *8-year-old boy:* Children are difficult to assess for head injury and their admission for monitoring is indicated.
- *Falls off a swing at his school:* A common mode of injury to a school going child. But the most common head injury is by RTA.
- *Brought to casualty by one of his teachers:* That means that no adult member of family is with him—a contraindication for discharge.
- *Bruise over his right eye:* Usually children do not suffer from fracture of skull bones as these are more pliable.
- *Examination is otherwise normal:* Rules out any cerebral injury GCS scoring should be done on adult scale and children. GCS if for < 5 years.
- *Fully conscious:* Also in favour of any cerebral injury but not that young children lose consciousness less readily that adults. Significant brain injury can occur without a history of loss of consciousness.
- *No history of blackouts since the accident:* Also a good prognostic sign.
- *Skull X-ray is normal:* Rules out any fracture which commands admission. But one should be aware of suture lines and normal anatomical variants while interpreting the X-rays.

CONFUSA
Assessment of consciousness in a child can be difficult. The best judge for minor alteration in consciousness in children are their parents.

Investigation of choice
Skull X-ray (already done in this case).

Immediate management
Antiseptic dressing of the bruise.

Treatment of choice
Admit and monitor.

Your notes:

---

73. A young woman is involved in an RTA and is brought in with a Glasgow Coma Scale of 6. A CT scan shows evidence of diffuse cerebral oedema but no evidence of haemorrhage. She has bilateral papilledema.

Diagnosis: Vasogenic cerebral edema

Clinchers

- *Involved in an RTA:* RTA usually produces vasogenic cerebral edema (i.e. increased capillary permeability).
- *Glasgow Coma Scale of 6:* Because cranium defines a fixed volume, brain swelling quickly results in increased ICP which may produce a sudden clinical deterioration. If untreated the GCS may fall further and the patient may be in a risk of brain herniation.
- *CT scan shows evidence of diffuse cerebral oedema but no evidence of haemorrhage:* This rules out any focal pathology which might be responsible for increased ICT and hence rules out any surgical intervention (craniotomy/burr hole).
- *Bilateral papilledema:* It signifies raised ICT.

CONFUSA
Papilloedema is an unreliable sign, but venous pulsation at the disc may be absent (Note: it is absent in about 50% of normal people, but loss of it is a useful sign).

Investigation of choice
ICT monitoring (as cerebral edema peaks in two-three days).

Immediate management
IV dexamethasone (controversial).

Treatment of choice
IV mannitol + restriction of free water.

Your Notes:

74. A young man is involved in a fight and suffers a blow to the back of the head. A skull X-ray reveals a depressed fracture of the occiput. His Glasgow Coma Scale on admission is 14 but falls rapidly within an hour.

Diagnosis: Subdural hematoma.

Clinchers
- *Is involved in a fight:* This makes it a medicolegal case and thereby warrant at least a skull X-ray (in UK).
- *Suffers a blow to the back of the head:* A blow to the back of head, if strong enough to produce a fracture in skull, will be invariably associated with neck injury. So exclude any cervical spine injury.
- *Skull X-ray reveals a depressed fracture of the occiput:* The principle local complications of skull fractures are:
  - Meningeal artery rupture, causing an extradural hematoma
  - Dural vein tears, leading to subdural hematoma.
- *Glasgow Coma Scale on admission is 14 but falls rapidly within an hour:* Since there is no lucid interval, the suspicion is more towards a subdural hematoma (Note: *Subdural* hematomas often have *subdued* onset, i.e. after sometime—hours to days).

CONFUSA
Linear skull fractures usually do not need any surgical intervention but depressed fractures almost always need surgical elevation and debridement. Cerebral contusions may result in a similar clinical picture to subdural hematoma, with a delayed recovery from trauma.

Investigation of choice
CT scan (since GCS is falling).

Immediate management
Inform neurosurgery after starting resuscitation.

Treatment of choice
Surgical elevation of fracture and evacuation of clot.

Your notes:

---

75. A 24-year-old patient presents with RTA. The pupil on the left side is dilated and the patient is obtunded. CT scan of the head reveals a binconvex hyperdense lesion on the temporal region.

Diagnosis: Extradural hemorrhage.

Clinchers
- *History of RTA:* Road traffic accidents produces maximum mortality due to head injuries.
- *Pupil on left side is dilated:* In cases of intracranial hematomas localising neurological symptoms (e.g. ipsilateral pupil dilatation, hemiparesis) occurs late (average 63 days in case of subdural hematoma). So the patient is in a critical stage warranting urgent surgical decompression).
- *Obtunded:* Deteriorating level of consciousness is caused by a rising ICP (due to the expanding hematoma).
- *Biconvex hyperdense lesion on the temporal region:* Fresh bleed on CT appears hyperdense. A binconvex hematoma is characterisitc of an extradural hematoma (lens-shaped). Its most common site is temporal region.

CONFUSA
In subdural hematoma, the CT appearance is usually concave on the inner side, most commonly in parietal region. Midline shift may be present.

Investigation of choice
CT scan (already done in this patient).

Immediate management
Urgent evacuation of the clot through multiple burr holes (as the patient is very critical and there is no spare time for transfer to a neurosurgical unit/centre).

Treatment of choice
Identification and ligation of the bleeding vessel (usually middle meningeal vessels).

Your notes:

76. A 27-year-old woman has a long-standing history of headaches associated with nausea and vomiting. On this occasion she present with sudden loss of vision in the right half of the visual field. By the time you see her it has improved considerably.

Diagnosis: Migraine

Clinchers

- *27-year-old woman has a long-standing history of headaches:* Onset of migraine is usually in childhood, adolescence or early adulthood; however, initial attack may occur at any age. It is more frequent in women, family history is often positive.
- *Headaches associated with nausea and vomiting:* Classic triad of migraine is:
    1. Premonitoring visual (scotoma or scintillations), sensory or motor symptoms
    2. Unilateral throbbing headache
    3. Nausea and vomiting
- *Sudden loss of vision in the right half of visual field:* Visual symptoms of migraine can be visual chaos (cascading, distortion, melting and jumbling of print lines, dots, spots, zig-zag fortification specta) and hemianopia.
- *By the time you see her it has improved considerably:* Visual symptoms in migraine last for about 15 minutes and then improved. It is generally followed by the headache within one hour.

CONFUSA
TIAs can mimic migraines visual symptoms of migraine.

Investigation of choice
Carotid doppler to rule out TIA.

Immediate management
Dispersible high dose aspirin.

Treatment of choice
Migraine prophylaxis (if attacks > twice/month) with pizotifen.

Note:
- Premenstrual migraine may respond to diuretics or depot oestrogens.
- Contraceptive pill need not be discontinued if migraine is causing no focal pathology.

Your notes:

77. An 82-year-old woman complains of stiffness and muscle pain to the point where she is finding it difficult to brush her hair and get out of a chair. She now presents with sudden loss of vision in her left eye.

Diagnosis: Polymyalgia rheumatica (PMR)

Clinchers

- *82-year-old:* The patient of PMR is always over 50 years.
- *Weakness and muscle pain:* PMR causes a sudden onset of severe pain and stiffness of the shoulders and neck, and of the hips and lumbar spine (a limb girdle pattern).
- *Finding it difficult to brush her hair:* This implies a shoulder girdle weakness as she has difficulty lifting her hand overhead.
- *Difficulty getting out of chair:* This implies a hip girdle weakness.
- *Sudden loss of vision in her left eye:* PMR is associated with temporal arteritis in 25% of people (the patient may have current PMR, a history of rencet PMR, or be on treatment for PMR). Involvement of the ophthalmic arteritis in temporal arteritis causes sudden painless temporary and permanent visual loss.

CONFUSA
It is often difficult to remember the differentiating clinical features of common 'PLAB' myopathies. Here is a refreshes:
Polymyositis—proximal pain and weakness
PMR—Proximal morning stiffness and pain
Myopathy—No pain, no stiffness, only weakness

Investigation of choice
ESR and/or CRP.

Immediate management
Ophthalmology referral urgently.

Treatment of choice
Prednisolone high dose IV immediately.

Your Notes:

78. A woman previously in good health, presents with sudden onset of severe occipital headache and vomiting. Her only physical sign on examination is a shift neck.

Diagnosis: Subarachnoid haemorrhage (SAH)

Clinchers
- *Woman:* Females have a slightly higher incidence of SAH. Lack of estrogen in the postmenopausal females has been cited as a reason.
- *Previously in good health:* Rules out any other medical disorder. Also most of the patient of SAH present with a sudden and spontaneous occurrence with no preceeding disorder. The typical age for SAH is 35-65 years.
- *Sudden onset:* It's onset is sudden (within a few seconds). Some patient may earlier experience a sentinal headache due to small warning leaks from the offending aneurysm.
- *Severe occipital headache:* SAH presents with a devastating headache which the patients usually describe as "the worst headache of my life" or "I thought I had been kicked in the head". It is most commonly occipital. Vomiting may accompany.
- *Stiff neck:* (Kernig's positive). It is a feature of SAH but takes six hours to develop.

CONFUSA
Other differential diagnoses for stiff neck are—Shigella gastroenteritis and meningitis.
- Focal neurology (i.e. hemiplegia) in SAH may give diagnostic clues, e.g.
  - *Early development*—suggests intracerebral hematoma
  - *Late development*—suggests vasospasm and ischaemia

Investigation of choice
Early CT (shows subarachnoid or ventricular blood).

Immediate management
Immediate neurosurgical opinion if
- Consciousness decrease
- Progressive focal deficit
- Suspected cerebellar hematoma

Treatment of choice
Surgical clipping of aneurysms/guglielmi coils
 +
Control hypertension

79. A 74-year-old woman had a fall two weeks ago. She is brought into the A and E department with slowly increasing drowsiness. On examination you find mild hemiparesis and unequal pupils.

Diagnosis: Subdural hematoma.

Clinchers
- *74-year-old:* Bridging veins in the skull becomes more prone to rupture in old age. It is due to cortical atrophy producing gradual shrinkage of brain and thereby producing more traction on the veins.
- *Slowly increasing drowsiness:* It means that the hematoma which is now behaving like a SOL (space occupying lesion) is still expanding and there is danger if it is not evacuated urgently.
- *Two weeks ago:* Remember subdural hematomas are usually subdued in appearance, i.e. they can occur weeks to months after the initial injury (as the bleeding is from very small veins).
- *Mild hemiparesis and unequal pupils:* Ipsilateral pupillary dilatation is a lagte sign. Focal neurological signs are an indication for urgent intervention.

CONFUSA
Do not rely on absence of ipsilateral pupillary dilatation as it is a late sign. Alteration in the conscious level is the cardinal feature; lateralising signs may be absent or minimal.

Investigation of choice
CT scan is diagnostic, showing a collection with an inner concave border (extradural—binconvex).

Immediate management
Urgent neurological opinion.

Treatment of choice
Surgical evacuation of the hematoma.

Your notes:

80. A 73-year-old man presents with hemianopia, hemisensory loss, hemiparesis and aphasia of 16 hours duration.

Diagnosis: TIA involving the carotids.

Clinchers
- *73-year-old man:* Incidence of TIA increases with age. Most common cause is atherosclerosis.
- *Hemianopia:* Homonymous hemianopia is typical of a carotid territory ischaemia.
- *Hemisensory loss:* Contralateral weakness/numbness is present in *hemiparesis* carotid territory ischaemia.
- *Aphasia:* Dysphasia, aphasia and dysarthria are characteristic pointers for carotid territory ischaemia.
- *Of 16 hours duration:* The sudden onset of focal CNS signs or symptoms due to temporary occlusion, usually by emboli, of part of the cerebral circulation is termed a TIA if symptoms are present for less than 24 hours and fully resolve within this period.

CONFUSA
80% of the TIA are in the carotid territory. Suspect then whenever there is:
- Unilateral paresis
- Unilateral sensory loss
- Aphasia
- Monocular visual loss.

Investigation of choice
CT is usually not indicated in patients over 55 years. Do a routine screen (FBC, ESR, U and E, glucose, ECG, CXR).

Immediate management
Give O_2 + monitor vital signs.

Treatment of choice
Oral aspirin (300 mg) unless contraindicated thereafter 150 mg daily.

Your notes:

81. Immunization of health workers who are in contact with body fluid.

Diagnosis: Risk of hepatitis B

Clinchers
- *Health workers:* Health workers should be particularly immunised against hepatitis B vaccine as its seroconversion rate after accidental exposure are dangerously high (much more than HIV). Now the protocol is to immunise everyone (and not just health workers) for hepatitis B vaccine in UK. The past strategy of vaccinating at risk gropus—health workers, IV drug abusers, homosexual, hemodialysis patients have been unsuccessful here.
- *Who are in contact with body fluid:* Body fluid can transmit many infections of which hepatitis B, hepatitis C and HIV are of not. Of these hepatitis B has maximum potential of seroconversion but because of its effective screening and immunization, the incidence of hepatitis C is on the rise.

CONFUSA
Older age, smoking and male sex correlates to low antibody levels even after immunization against hepatitis B vaccine. So time boosters with serology. Often there are cases of nonresponders to the vaccine. If the the question is about social worker, then hepatitis A vaccine (Havrix Monodose) would have been the answer.

Investigation of choice
Anti HBs status (positive in vaccinated or after recovery).

Immediate management
Universal precautions.

Treatment of choice
Passive immunization (specific anti HBV immunoglobulin) may be given to nonimmune contacts after high risk exposure).

Your notes:

82. Immunization of hepatitis B, besides preventing hepatitis B also prevents.

Diagnosis: Reduction in risk of hepatocellular carcinoma.

Clinchers
- *Immunization of hepatitis B:* Hepatitis B vaccine (Engerix B) is given as a 1 mL dose into deltoid and is repeated at 1 and 6 months (child: 0.5 mL x 3 into anterolateral thigh). Now it is given to everyone in UK. The immunocompromised may need more boosters.
- *Besides preventing hepatitis B also prevents:* Since chronic viral hepatitis (HBV, HCV) also causes hepatocellular carcinoma in the long run, the hepatitis B vaccine is preventive against it also.

CONFUSA
Anti HBs serology advice in UK is different from rest of the world. Please note:

Anti HBs	Actions and comments
> 1000 IU/L	Retest in 4 years
100-1000 IU/L	Retest in 1 year
< 100 IU/L	Given booster and retest
< 10 IU/L	Non-responder, give booster and retest if still < 10, get consent to check hepatitis B status

Investigation of choice
Anti HBs serology.

Immediate management
See previous question.

Treatment of choice
See previous question.

Your notes:

83. Avoidance of alcohol for six months after hepatitis A.

Diagnosis: To decrease risk of cirrhosis.

Clinchers
A small proportion of patients with hepatitis A experience relapsing hepatitis weeks to months after apparent recovery from acute hepatitis. Relapses are characterised by recurrence of symptoms, aminotransferase elevations, occasionally jaundice and faecal excretion of HAV. Rarely, liver test abonormalities persits for many months, even upto a year. So it is advisable to avoid alcohol or drugs whose metabolism is primarily through liver (especially drugs which can precipitate cholestasis), because they can induce severe liver damage in this period which can lead to cirrhosis.

CONFUSA
Kumar and Clark's textbook of medicine says that there is no reason to stop alcohol consumption other than for the few weeks when the patient is ill (pg 304, 4th edn).

Investigation of choice
LET (to cheek resolution).

Immediate management
Symptomatic.

Treatment of choice
Avoidance of alcohol.

Your notes:

84. Counselling for intravenous (IV) drug users to use needle exchange facilities.

Diagnosis: To decrease risk of hepatitis B

Clinchers

IV drug user: They constitute a risk group of hepatitis B infection. Other risk groups are:
- Health workers
- Haemophiliacs
- Hemodialysis patients
- Sexually promiscuous
- Homosexual

It is endemic in:
- Far east
- Africa
- Mediterranean

Hepatitis B spread by:
- Direct contact—common in African children
- Vertical transmission—common in Asia

> **CONFUSA**
> IV drug users are also at risk for HIV and if would have been a better choice as an answer (if given in the list of options) since hepatitis B can be more effectively prevented by vaccination. Also there is controversy over the extent to which addicts should be supplied with clear needles.

Investigation of choice
Anti HBs (presence signifies vaccination).

Immediate management
Notify home office (required by law in UK).

Treatment of choice
Motivation for a proper deaddiction.

Your notes:

85. Immunization of sewage workers.

Diagnosis: To decrease risk of hepatitis A.

Clinchers
Hepatitis A spreads by faecal-oral route, so sewage workers are at special risk. Active immunization against hepatitis A is available and very effective. It is made from an inactivated protein derived from hepatitis A virus.

Dose: If > 16 years, 1 IM dose (1 mL to deltoid) gives immunity for 1 year (10 years if booster is given at 6 months).

Note: Trade name of hepatitis A vaccine in UK.
- Havrix monodose.
  Passive immunization is with normal human Ig. It gives less than 3 months immunity to those at acute risk, i.e.
- Travellers
- Household contacts

> **CONFUSA**
> Sewage workers are also at risk of leptospirosis as its spread is by contact with infected rat urine. But there is no effective vaccination against it.

Investigation of choice
IgG antibody (presence signifies previous infection).

Immediate management
Rule out recent exposure. If present give immunoglobulin.

Treatment of choice
Vaccination.

Your notes:

86. A 7-year-old boy has right sided earache and rhinorrhea. On examination his right sided tympanic membrane appears pink in colour.

Diagnosis: Acute suppurative otitis media (ASOM) (presuppurative stage)

Clinchers
- *7-year-old:* ASOM is more common in infants and children especially of lower socioeconomic group.
- *Right sided earache:* In presuppurative stage there is marked earache which may disturb sleep and is of throbbing nature.
- *Rhinorrhea:* Typically ASOM follows viral infection of upper respiratory tract (hence rhinorrhoea). Most common route of spread of infection is via eustachian tube.
- *Right sided tympanic membrane appears pink in colour:* Normal tympanic membrane should be pearly grey in colour. It is abnormal (i.e. inflamed) if it looks pink. In stage of presuppurative in ASOM, because of prolonged tubal occlusion, pyogenic organisms invade tympanic cavity causing hyperemia of its lining (hence pink colour). Tympanic membrane becomes congested.

CONFUSA
This condition may be confused with sphenoidal sinusitis, whose pain refers to retroauricular region and teeth (increase on walking). But in sinusitis there will be pyogenic discharge and facial tenderness.

Investigation of choice
Otoscopy/tympanometry.

Immediate management
Analgesia (Paracetamol).

Treatment of choice
Adults—IM benzylpenicillin
Less than 5 years—Amoxicillin
  If resistant strain: amoxicillin + clavulinic acid.

Your notes:

87. A 4-year-old with right sided earache is examined using otoscopy. This reveals a red bulging tympanic membrane

Diagnosis: Acute suppurative otitis media (ASOM) (suppurative stages).

Clinchers
- *4-year-old:* The most common infection causing ASOM in under 5 years age is *H. influenzae*.
- *Right sided earache:* In presuppurative stage the pain in ear becomes marked which may disturb sleep and is of throbbing nature. But in suppurative stage the pain becomes excruciating.
- *Red bulging tympanic membrane:* In suppurative stage the tympanic membrane appears red and bulging with loss of landmarks. Handle of malleus may be engulfed by the swollen and protruding tympanic membrane and may not be discernible. A yellow spot may be seen on the tympanic membrane which rupture is imminent.

CONFUSA
Pain is immediately relieved once the tympanic membrane ruptures to discharge its contents. In serous otitis media (Glue ear) the eardrum looks concave.

Investigation of choice
Otoscopy/tympanometry.

Immediate management
Analgesia (paracetamol).

Treatment of choice
Myringotomy—to evacuate pus
Indications of myringotomy in ASOM
1. Bulging drum and acute pain
2. Incomplete resolution despite antibiotics
3. Persistent effusion beyond 12 weeks.

Your notes:

88. An 8-year-old boy who has been playing outside now complains of right sided earache. On inspection a green bead is seen protruding into his ear canal. The walls of the canal are red.

Diagnosis: Foreign body in ear.

Clinchers
- *8-year-old boy:* Children are prone to put inanimate foreign bodies like beads in their ear.
- *Complains of right sided earache:* Foreign bodies in ear can cause conduction deafness, discomfort usually. If they cause pain then the ear canal must be inflamed.
- *A green bead is seen protruding into his ear canal:* Beads are smooth round foreign bodies which can easily slip deeper if their removal is attempted by a inexperienced person.
- *The walls of the canal are red:* This suggests inflammation secondary to impaction of the foreign body and hence the reason for pain (as the mucosa of ear canal swells up because of inflammation).

CONFUSA
Only things that a casuality SHO should attempt to remove are insects. They are drowned into olive oil and then syringed out. An expert should remove all other foreign bodies. Forceps should not be used for removal.

Investigation of choice
Otoscopy.

Immediate management
Pain relief.

Treatment of choice
- Hooks or suction (not forceps)
- GA is often needed especially when the child is uncooperative or if inflammation is present (as in this case).

Your notes:

---

89. A 9-year-old girl with a history of recurrent otitis media now complains of left sided earache. On examination the right sided tympanic membrane appears scarred. On examination of the left ear, pus is seen throughout the ear canal.

Diagnosis: Recurrent acute otitis media.

Clinchers
- *9-year-old girl:* It usually occurs in infants and children.
- *History of recurrent otitis media:* It may occur 4-5 times a year. The child remain free of symptoms between the episodes. Recurrent middle ear infections may sometimes be superimposed upon an existing otitis externa.
- *Complains of left sided earache:* It can be due to otitis externa or an acute episode of otitis media in this ear.
- *Right sided tympanic membrane appears scarred:* This signifies stigmata of previous episodes of otitis media in this ear.
- *Left ear, pus is seen thoughout the ear canal:* This pus can either be due to rupture of tympanic membrane (i.e. from middle ear) or due to otitis externa. But since the pain still present, we shall consider it to be from otitis externa.

CONFUSA
Chronic suppurative otitis media presents with discharge and hearing loss but no pain.

Investigation of choice
Otoscopy.

Immediate management
Ear toilet.

Treatment of choice
Amoxicillin + calvulinic acid (as recurrent infections are usually resistant)
+ medicated wicks (aluminium acetate or silver nitrate).

Your notes:

90. A 54-year-old female develops mild fever, malaise and ear pain. 3 days dilater she developed multiple painful vesicles over her early canal and external meatus.

Diagnosis: Herpes zoster

Clinchers
- *Mild fever, malaise, ear pain:* Fever, malaise signifies viral infection. Herpes zoster oticus is a viral infection involving geniculate ganglion of facial nerve. There may be anaesthesia of face, giddiness and hearing impairment due to involvement of V and VIII nerves.
- *Multiple painful vesicles;* Herpes zoster infection (oticus) is characterised by appearance of veiscles on the tympanic membrane, deep meatus, concha and reteroauticular sulcus. There may be a vesicular rash in the external auditory canal and pinna.

CONFUSA
Nose tip involvement is virtually diagnostic if present in a case of Herpes Zoster. It is known as Hutchinson's signs and means involvement of the nasociliary branch of the trigeminal nerve which also supplies the globe and makes it highly likely that the eye will be affected.

Investigation of choice
Fluoroscent antibody tests and Tzank smears (but both rarely needed as the diagnosis is clinically easy).

Immediate management
Keeping cool may reduce the number of lesions. Tell her to avoid scratching. Give adequate analgesia.

Treatment of choice
Aciclovir 800 mg
- five times a day
- for 7 days

Your Notes:

---

91. A fair 18-year-old girl has had dark black facial patches, one of which is now growing rapidly in size.

Diagnosis: Malignant melanoma (MM)—Superficial spreading type.

Clinchers
- *Fair:* It is seen in all racial types but is more common in fair-skinned caucasian types.
- *18-year-old girl:* Malignant melanoma is extremely rare before puberty but can occur at any age after that. The incidence is slightly more common in females.
- *Dark black facial patches:* Some 30% of lesions of MM develop from a pre-existing melanocytic naevus and other develop de novo on any part of skin surface. Benign moles may be very dark brown or black but are usually a uniform colour.
- *One of which is now growing rapidly in size:* Any change in the size, shape or colour of a pre-existing lesion should be suspected of being MM. Particular signs that are valuable in recognition of MM are irregularity in the margin, irregularity in the degree of pigmentation and erosion or cursting of skin surface.

CONFUSA
Acral lentiginous melanoma is more frequent in black skinned individuals and subjects of Japanese and Asian descent. It has particularly poor prognosis.

Investigation of choice
Clinical examination by a dermatologist.

Immediate management
Examine whole body to rule out other foci.

Treatment of choice
Excision biopsy with wide margin of normal skin and subsequent pathological examination.

Your Notes:

92. A 70-year-old bald gardener has had a brownish patch on his scalp which has been slowly growing for the last 30 years.

Diagnosis: Solar keratoses (actinic keratosis, senile keratosis).

Clinchers
- *70-year-old:* Usually found in elderly (hence the name senile keratosis) due to cumulative effect of sun exposure over the years.
- *Bald:* It means that his scalp is a perennially sun exposed area and hence a potential site for solar keratotis.
- *Gardener:* As he is a gardener, sun exposure is a professional hazard to him. Men seem to be at more risk than women.
- *Brownish patch on his scalp:* It appear as crumbly yellow-white crusts (may be brownish) in fair skinned people. It is a raised, scaling or warty hyperkeratotic plaque or papule.
- *Slowly growing for the last 30 years:* Solar keratoses are typically slow growing and any rapid growth in them should raise suspicious of a malignant change (SCC more common).

CONFUSA
Clinical diagnosis of solar keratosis may be quite difficult even for experienced clinicians. So a simple biopsy must be done.

Investigation of choice
Simple biopsy.

Immediate management
Avoid further sun exposure.

Treatment of choice
Cautery/cryotherapy/5-FU cream.

Your Notes:

93. A young HIV positive man develops raised patches in his skin and in his mouth.

Diagnosis: Kaposi's sarcoma (Idiopathic haemorrhagic sarcoma).

Clinchers
- *Young HIV positive man:* There are many cutaneous manifestations of HIV disease, due to both infectious and noninfectious conditions.
  - *Infections:* Oral candidiasis, molluscum contagiosum, HSV, varicella zoster, cryptococcosis (on face), scabies, oral hairy leukoplakia.
  - *Others:* Seborrhic dermatitis, psoriasis, eosinophilic folliculitis, drug reactions.
- *Develops raised patches in his skin and in his mouth:* Kaposi's sarcoma typically affects both skin and mucus membranes (especially oral mucosa). It presents as purpulish macules, papules, nodules and plaques affecting the feet, legs, face and oral mucosa (in fact before the advent of HIV, it was known to affect only mucosa surfaces).

CONFUSA
Lichen planus is another disease which presents as raised purple polygonal plaques on both skin and oral mucosa. However, it is not so typically associated with HIV, is itchy and characteristically differentiated by Wickham's striaes (whitish criss-cross lines). Another differential diagnosis is bacillary angiomatosis (Bartonella).

Investigation of choice
Biopsy.

Immediate management
Examine whole body as the disease is usually multifocal.

Treatment of choice
- Cryotherapy
- Intralesional vincristine
- Radiotherapy
- Treatment of HIV disease

Your Notes:

94. A builder has been exposed to sun for long periods of time develops an ulcerated lesion on his face.

Diagnosis: Squamous cell carcinoma (SCC).

Clinchers
- *Builder:* Sun exposure is a professional hazard for him.
- *Exposed to sun for long periods of time:* UV rays exposure is by far the most important causative factor of both actinic keratoses and SCC.
- *Develops an ulcerated lesion on his face:* SCC presents as a persistently ulcerated or crusted from irregular lesion. It is usually found on sun-exposed sites (face in this question). It may occur in pre-existing actinic keratoses which might be present because of his profession (builder).

CONFUSA
The main problem is to differentiate between a BCC and SCC.

BCC	SCC
Rolled margins	Everted margins
Pearly	Ulcerated
Usually on face	Ears, dorsa of hands, bald-scalp

Investigation of choice
Clinical evaluation by a dermatologist.

Immediate management
Clinical evaluation by a dermatologist.

Treatment of choice
- Excision
- Metastases are relatively uncommon but more frequent at certain sites, e.g. ears.

Your Notes:

95. An 18-year-old girl with moles on her back of different colour and sizes.

Diagnosis: Intradermal melanoma (Naevi).

Clinchers
- *18-year-old girl moles on her back:* Nearly everyone possesses one or more moles some have hundreds, although they may not become apparent until after puberty. Those moles that are entirely within the dermis remain benign, but a small percentage of the junctional naevi, so called because they are seen in the basal layer of the epidermis at its junction, with the dermis, may undergo malignant change.
- *Of different colour and sizes:* Intradermal melanoma is the most common variety of mole. The naevus may be light or dark in colour and may be flat or raised, hairy or hairless. A hairy mole is nearly always intradermal. They never undergo malignant change, and need no treatment unless the diagnosis is uncertain.

CONFUSA
Intradermal melanoma may be found in every situation except the palm of the hand, the sole of the foot or the scrotal skin.

Investigation of choice
Histology only on suspicious of a malignant change (excision biopsy).

Immediate management
Reassurance.

Treatment of choice
None required.

Your Notes:

96. A 70-year-old woman has taken 20 mg of temazepam at night for the last 30 years. She has begun to suffer with falls and has agreed that the temazepam might be contributing to the falls.

Diagnosis: Benzodiazepine addiction.

Clinchers
- *70-year-old:* A large number of older patients take benzodiazepines regularly, particularly temazepam and nitrazepam.
- *Falls:* There is good evidence in published trials that sedative medications increase the risk of falls and that sedative withdrawal reduces this risk.

CONFUSA
Benzodiazepine withdrawal symptoms are very common if the drug has been taken regularly for longer than six months (30 years in this case). But in this case the symptoms are due to sedative action and not due to withdrawal. Withdrawal is easier from long acting benzodiazepines, such as diazepam or chlordiazepoxide.

Investigation of choice
Neurological examination to rule out it as a cause for falls.

Immediate management
Counselling.

Treatment of choice
Patient converted to an equivalent dose of diazepam, which is then reduced by 3 mg every one or two weeks.

Your Notes:

97. A 26-year-old heroin addict is worried because her partner has been diagnosed as having HIV infection. She is HIV negative. She does not feel able to stop using heroin currently.

Clinchers
- *Heroin addict:* Heroin is usually taken IV by drug addicts.
- *Her partner has been diagnosed as having HIV infection:* This makes her very susceptible for HIV infection because they might be sharing needles.
- *Is HIV negative:* Usually HIV antibodies do not appear in blood till three months. A PCR antigen test is required to detect early infection after exposure. So HIV negative status is dependent on the type of test she has undergone. If it was ELISA then she need another testing after three months to completely rule out the infection.
- *She does not feel able to stop using heroin currently:* Its the duty of the doctor to counsel and convince her for deaddiction. But the first priority is to eurol her in a needle exchange programme to decrease her risk of exposure to HIV, hepatitis B and C.

CONFUSA
Narcotic withdrawal is dangerous in patients with heart disease, tuberculosis or other debilitating conditions.

Investigation of choice
ELISA for HIV after three months.

Immediate management
Counselling.

Treatment of choice
Enrolment in needle exchange programme.

Your Notes:

98. A 40-year-old man has become increasingly dependent on alcohol since his wife died last year. He admits that he has a problem and wishes to stop drinking. He does not with to take antidepressants.

Diagnosis: Alcohol dependence.

Clinchers
- *Since his wife died:* Alcohol dependence is often precipitated by breavment, in the false belief that it alleviates the symptoms of depression. But infact, alcohol does the opposite, as it a depressant and will exacerbate the problem.
- *Admits problem drinking and wishes to stop drinking:* Treatment of any dependency is only beneficial if the patient recognises the problem and wants to give up drinking. But even so, the relapse rates are very high. Supportive counselling and group psychotherapy (e.g. alcoholics anonymous) is of most benefit.
- *Does not wish to take antidepressants:* Since the patient is aware of the problem and has insight in it, antidepressants may not be needed (group psychotherapy alone can help). If he still experience difficulty abstaining, disulfiram may be used. It produces an unpleasant reaction (flushing and nausea) when taken with alcohol and will discourage a patient from drinking.

CONFUSA
Drugs which help in abstinence:
- Disulfiram—makes drinking unpleasant
- Naltrexone—takes pleasure out of drinking (halve the relapse rates)
- Acamprosate—mitigates anxiety, insomnia and craving.

Investigation of choice
Gamma GT (increased); LFTs to rule out liver damage.

Immediate management
Admit.

Treatment of choice
Group psychotherapy.

Your Notes:

99. A 63-year-old retired surgeon is admitted with a short history of bizarre behaviour. He claims that GMC are investigating him for murder and have hired a private detective to follow him. He has evidence of a coarse tremor, horizontal nystagmus and an ataxic gait. His wife says that the story about GMC is untrue but is worried about the amount of gin that her husband has drunk since retirement.

Diagnosis: Wernicke's encephalopathy + Korsakoff's psychosis.

Clinchers
- *Bizzare behaviour:* Due to dementia in Korsakoff's psychosis.
- *"GMC are investigating him for murder and have hired a private detective to follow him":* It is a delusion (a false, unshakeable belief). Delusions and paranoia are commonly features of Korsakoff's psychosis. Other features can be impairement of new learning and confabulations.
- *Coarse tremor, horizontal nystagmus and ataxic gait:* These are features of Wernicke's encephalopathy. It usually presents as a traid of nystagmus, ophthalmoplegia (commonly external recti) and ataxia. Other eye signs such as ptosis, abnormal pupillary reactions and altered consciousness may also occur. It may present with headache, anorexia, vomiting, and confusion.
- *Wife is worried about alcohol (gin) intake:* it substantiates our diagnostic suspicious of alcohol abuse.

CONFUSA
Wernicke's encephalopathy appears before Korsakoff's psychosis in patients of alcohol abuse. Wernicke's encephalopathy is a potentially reversible stage with thiamine treatment. Korsakoff's psychosis is irreversible.

Investigation of choice
Red cell transketolase (decrease).

Immediate management
IV thiamine amine urgently.

Treatment of choice
Thiamine 200-300 mg/24 h PO.
Note: Give Pabrinex (2-3 pairs of high potency ampoules every 8 hr IV over 10 min for $\leq$ 2 days) if—oral route is impossible.

100. A 37-year-old retired professional footballer admits of using cocaine and heroin for the last three years. He has recently signed a contract to present a sports show on television and wishes to 'clean his life up' first. His wife and family are very supportive of this.

Diagnosis: Narcotic drug abuse.

Clinchers

- *Cocaine and heroin addiction:* They are common drugs of abuse.
- *Wishes to clean his life up first:* i.e. he is willing to leave drug addiction. Any patient who is clearly willing to leave drug addiction should be provided proper medical deaddiction. Even those patient's who are not willing to leave should be counselled for enrolement in deaddiction programmes.
- *His wife and family are very supportive:* Since this patient had adequate social support, there is not reason for his receiving in patient treatment only. Drug dependency teams can arrange supported outpatient withdrawal programmes.

CONFUSA
Abuse of drugs is a criminal offence in UK, but still patient confidentiality does not allow you to inform the police. Although it is the duty of the doctor to make sure that the patient is registered as a drug addict in the confidential registers of the regional health authorities.

Investigation of choice
A complete health check up to ensure risk-free out patient treatment.

Immediate management
Outpatient referral to drug dependency team.

Treatment of choice
Drug withdrawal programme (outpatient).

Your Notes:

101. A middle-aged woman develops a purulent cough with some hemoptysis. A chest X-ray reveals right upper lobe consolidation.

Diagnosis: *Streptococcus pneumoniae.*

Clinchers
- *Middle-aged woman:* Streptococcal pneumonia affects all ages, but is more common in middle-aged and elderly.
- *Purulent cough:* Mycoplasma, *Legionella*, *Chlamydia* and *Pneumocystis carinii* characteristically presents with dry cough. Streptococcal and staphylococcal generally presents with purulent cough.
- *Some hemoptysis:* Acute bronchitis, pneumonia, neoplasm (primary) hemoptysis in the united kingdom. TB is common in third world countries.
- *Right upper lobe consolidation:* Lobar consolidation is sign of streptococcal pneumonia, more commonly on right side.

CONFUSA
When there is history of hemoptysis, always think of TB and malignancy first.

Investigation of choice
Chest X-ray.

Treatment of choice
Ampicillin or cefuroxime.

Your Notes:

CXR: Pneumonia

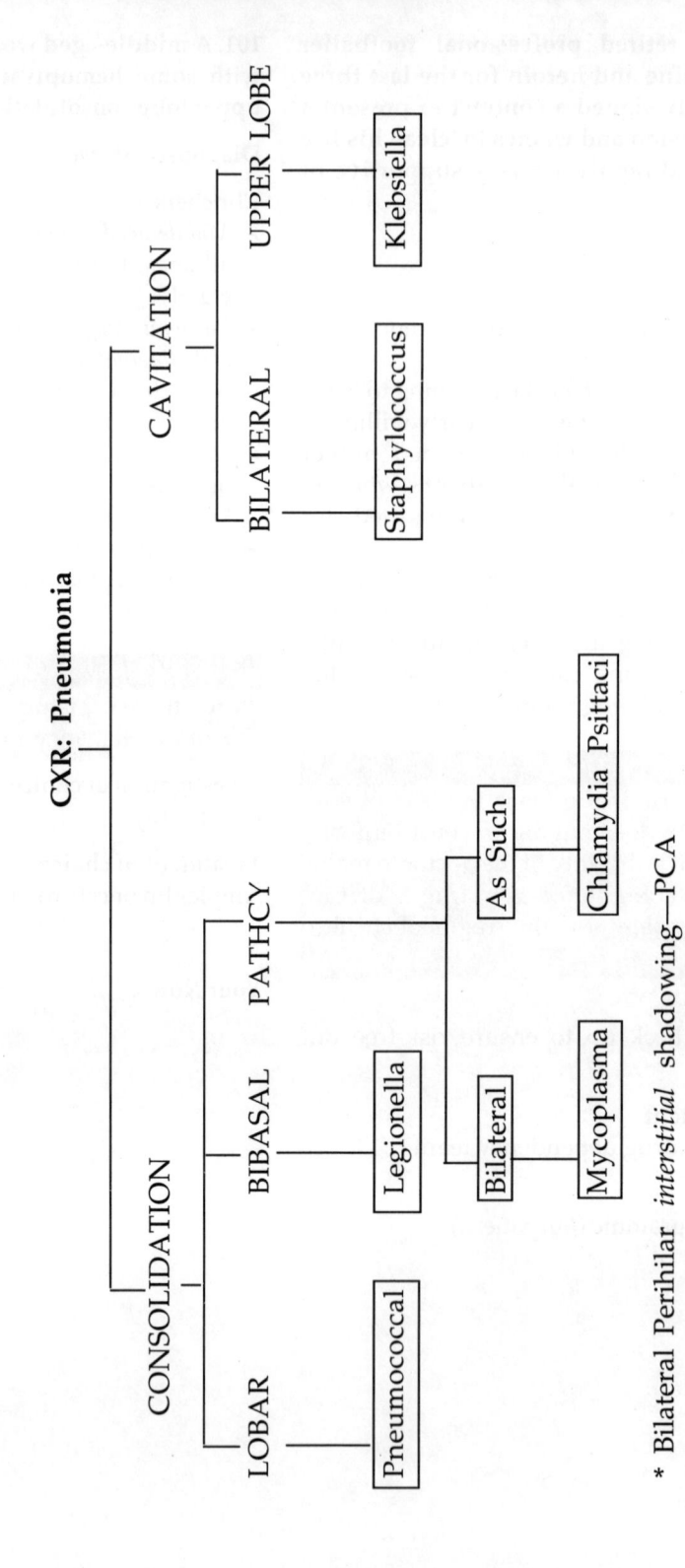

- CONSOLIDATION
  - LOBAR — Pneumococcal
  - BIBASAL — Legionella
  - PATCHY
    - Bilateral — Mycoplasma
    - As Such — Chlamydia Psittaci
- CAVITATION
  - BILATERAL — Staphylococcus
  - UPPER LOBE — Klebsiella

* Bilateral Perihilar *interstitial* shadowing—PCA

102. A young woman with no relevant medical history develops a severe purulent cough. A chest X-ray reveals multiple cavitating bilateral lung lesions.

Diagnosis: Staphylococcal pneumonia.

Clinchers
- *Young woman:* Staphylococcal pneumonia occurs in young and elderly patients.
- *No relevant medical history:* Helps rule out any chronic condition like tuberculosis, though not that significant.
- *Severe purulent cough:* History of severe purulent cough is common is staphylococcal pneunomia.
- *Multiple cavitating bilateral lung lesions:* Bilateral cavitating bronchopneunomia is characteristic of *Staphylococcal pneumonia*.

Investigation of choice
Chest X-ray.

Treatment of choice
Flucloxacillin.

Your Notes:

103. A young male prostitute develops a dry cough. A chest X-ray reveals bilateral interstitial infiltrates.

Diagnosis: *Pneumocystis carinii* pneumonia (PCP).

Clinchers
- *Young male prostitute:* Pneumocystis carinii causes pneumonia in the immunosuppressed (e.g. HIV).
- *Dry cough:* Pneumocystis carinii presents with fever, dry cough, exertional dyspnoea, and bilateral crepitation.
- *Bilateral interstitial infiltrates:* In PCP chest X-ray may be normal or bilateral interstial (perihilar) infiltration can be seen.

Investigation of choice
Chest X-ray.

Treatment of choice
High dose co-trimoxazole IV or pentamidine by slow IV for 2-3 weeks. In case of severe hypoxaemia, steroids can be added.

Your Notes:

104. A young man has recently suffers from a bout of influenza. He now develops a purulent cough.

Diagnosis: Staphylococcal pneumonia.

Clinchers
- *Young man:* Staphylococcal pneumonia occurs in young and elderly patients.
- *Recently suffers from a bout of influenza:* Staphylococcal pneumonia, very commonly present as a complication of influenza infection. More commonly seen in intravenous drug users or patients with underlying disease (e.g. leukemia, lymphoma, cystic fibrosis).
- *He now develops a purulent cough:* History of purulent cough supports the diagnosis of staphylococcal pneumonia.

CONFUSA
Though there should be no confusion in this question, but the diagnosis should be supported with chest X-ray findings. In staphylococcal pneumonia typical bilateral cavitating bronchopneumonia is seen.

Investigation of choice
Chest X-ray.

Treatment of choice
Flucloxacillin.

Your Notes:

---

105. Man comes back from a holiday in Malaysia and he develops malaise, fever and dry cough. Chest X-ray reveals bilateral consolidation.

Diagnosis: Legionella pneumophila.

Clinchers
- *Back from holiday to Malaysia:* Legionella pneumophila colonizes water tanks kept at < 60°C (e.g. hotel airconditioning and hot water system). Therefore this is a very good clincher in this question.
- *Fever, malaise, myalgia:* These flu like symptoms often precede dry cough and dyspnoea in Legionella pneumonia.
- *Bilateral basal consolidation:* Chest X-ray showing bilateral basal consolidation is feature of Legionella pneumonia.

CONFUSA
There should be no confusion in this question. This is very commonly asked in PLAB.

Investigation of choice
Chest X-ray and legionella serology.

Treatment of choice
High dose erythromycin.

Your Notes:

106. A businessperson has just returned from a business trip to Asia. He now develops copious watery and bloody diarrhea.

Diagnosis: Amoebic dysentery.

Clinchers

- *Business person:* Risk of amoebiasis in developed countries is more in travellers, recent immigrants and homosexual men.
- *Just returned from a business trip to Asia:* Highest incidence of amoebiasis is seen in developing countries in the topics, particularly Mexico, India, tropical Asia, central and south America and Africa.
- *Copious watery and bloody diarrhea:* In amoebiasis diarrhoea develops slowly, but becomes profuse and bloody.

> **CONFUSA**
> Bacillary dysentery often has sudden onset and may cause dehydration. Stools are more watery. Acute ulcerative colitis has more gradual onset and stools are very bloody.

Investigation of choice
Stool microscopy showing trophozoites, blood and pus cells.

Immediate management
Correct dehydration: Oral rehydration is more beneficial than IV rehydration. In severe dehydration give 0.9% saline + 20 mmol K^+/L IVI.

Treatment of choice
Metronidazole 800 mg/8h PO for 5 days then diloxanide furoate 500 mg/8h for 10 days to destroy gut cysts.

Your Notes:

---

107. A middle-aged man develops constipation with overflow diarrhea and bright red bleeding per rectum. A barium enema reveals an ulcerated stricture in the sigmoid colon.

Diagnosis: Sigmoid carcinoma.

Clinchers

- *Middle-aged man:* Carcinoma of colon usually occurs in patients over 50 years of age but it is not rare earlier in adult life.
- *Constipation with overflow diarrhea:* In the carcinoma of left side of colon (sigmoid), alteration of basal habit is seen. The episodes of constipation are followed by attacks of diarrhoea.
- *Bright red bleeding per rectum:* Low tumors may result in tenesmus accompanied by the passage of mucus and blood, especially in the early morning.
- *An ulcerated stricture in the sigmoid colon:* Ulcerated stricture is a sign of malignancy, but it may well be Crohn's involvement of the colon. Sigmoidoscopic examination becomes important here. Biopsy should be taken to ascertain the diagnosis.

> **CONFUSA**
> This question may be confused with Crohn's involvement of the colon. Sigmoidoscopy and biopsy should be performed.

Investigation of choice
- Sigmoidoscopy
- *Barium enema*: It shows 'apple core' appearance, i.e. a short, irregular stenosis with sharp shoulders at each end (look at Figure 57.43, page 1051, Bailey and Love, 23rd edn).

Treatment of choice
Preoperative treatment: Bowel is cleared by enemas and oral stimulant laxatives (e.g. picolax). Principle of operative treatment is wild resection of the growth together with a regional lymphatics.

In obstructed cases, where bowel preparation is contraindicated the primary goal is to relieve obstruction.

Your Notes:

108. A young man develops bloody diarrhea. A rigid sigmoidoscopy examination revealed granular ulceration in the sigmoid colon with proximal sparing.

Diagnosis: Crohn's involvement of the colon.

Clinchers
- *Young man:* Peak occurrance between 15 and 30 years of age and between 60 and 80 years of age, but onset may occur of any age.
- *Bloody diarrhea:* Though bloody diarrhoea is more commonly seen in ulcerative colitis, sometimes Crohn's disease may present with bloody diarrhoea. Moreover the options include ulcerative pancolitis and not ulcerative colitis, therefore since rectal involvement is not there we can safely exclude UC.
- *Granular ulceration in the sigmoid colon with proximal sparing:* Inflammation seen in UC is continuous (no skip areas), where as in Crohn's disease any part of GI involved, usually terminal ilium and/or colon, with linear ulcerations and submucosal thickening leading to cobblestone pattern, discontinuous skip areas are characteristic of Crohn's disease.

CONFUSA
There may be confusion with ulcerative collitis (UC) but in that case rectum involvement should be there. In UC rectal involvement is almost always seen.

Investigation of choice
Sigmoidoscopy.

Immediate management
Antidiarrhoeal agents, IV hydration and blood transfusion in severe cases.

Treatment of choice
5 ASA oral or enema, metronidazole and/or ciprofloxacin.

Your Notes:

109. A middle-aged woman has been on several antibiotic treatments recently because of a persistent pneumonia. She now develops a severe watery diarrhea. Colonoscopy reveals whitish plaques scattered throughout the colon.

Diagnosis: Pseudomembranous colitis.

Clinchers
- *On several antibiotic treatments recently:* Pseudomembranes colitis is caused by overgrowth of clostridium difficile, following any antibiotic therapy.
- *Severe watery diarrhoea:* Most often diarrhoea is profuse and watery, although bloody diarrhoea occurs in 5% cases.
- *Whitish plaques scattered thoughout the colon:* Characteristic multiple, discrete, yellowish plaques are seen on sigmoidoscopy which on biopsy shows features of acute inflammation and ulceration with a pseudomembrane of fibrin and necrotic material.

CONFUSA
Currently, strains of C. difficile that produce toxins detectable in the stool the only identified cause of colitis idncued by antibiotics, therefore there should be no confusion in this question.

Investigation of choice
Sigmoidoscopy occasionally colonoscopy may be required.

Immediate management
Should be initially directed in eradicating C. difficile from the stool.

Treatment of choice
Vancomycin 125 mg/6h PO or metronidazole 400 mg/8h PO.

Your Notes:

110. An elderly woman is found anemic. As part of her examination, she has a barium enema, which reveals a mass lesion in the ascending colon.

Diagnosis: Caecal carcinoma.

Clinchers

- *Elderly woman:* Caecal carcinoma presents in older age group with a long history.
- *Anaemia:* Carcinoma of caecum presents with anaemia diarrhoea weight loss, and sometimes as right iliac fossa mass. Anaemia occurs due to occult blood loss.
- *Mass in the ascending colon:* Barium enema showing mass in ascending colon confirms our diagnosis of caecal carcinoma.
- *Ascending colon:* Right sided colonic carcinoma typically presents with constipation with or without diarrhoea, whereas left sided colonic carcinoma presents with anorexia, weight loss and constipation.

CONFUSA
Young parents with diarrhoea and right iliac fossa a mass focus on Crohn's disease and there should be no confusion with an appendicular mass.

Investigation of choice
Barium enema and occult blood test.

Immediate management
Estimate hemoglobin.

Your Notes:

111. A middle-aged woman with a history of rheumatoid arthritis develops sudden swelling in One of her knees. This knee is swollen and hot to touch.

Diagnosis: Pseudogout.

Clinchers

- *Middle-aged:* Though pseudogout occurs more commonly in old age, no age after thirties is exempt from it.
- *Woman:* There is a slight preponderance of female incidence.
- *Sudden swelling in one of her knees:* Knee is the main joint to get involved in it. A minority will have involvement of multiple joints.
- *This knee is swollen and hot to touch:* involved joint is erythematous, swollen, warm and painful.
- *History of rheumatoid arthritis:* Any existing arthritis is a risk factor for pseudogout. Other risk factors are old age, dehydration, intercurrent illness, hyperparathyroidism, myxoedema, diabetes mellitus, phosphate decrease, magnesium deficiency, hemochromatosis, acromegaly, gout, ochronosis, surgery.

CONFUSA
Acute pseudogout is less severe and longer lasting than gout and affects different joints. Pseudogout can even be secondary to gout. It cannot be septic arthritis also as there is no preceding history of joint trauma of presence of fever.

Investigation of choice
- *Screening:* Wrist X-ray (calcium deposition in triangular ligament or chondrocalcinosis)
- *Definitive:* Joint fluid aspiration and microscopy (positively birefringent calcium pyrophosphate crystals in plane polarised light).

Immediate management
Analgesia.

Treatment of choice
NSAIDs ± intra-articular injection of glucocorticoids ± colchicine.

Your Notes:

112. An elderly man with recently diagnosed heart failure has been treated with diuretics. He now develops severe joint pain in his left ankle with swelling and redness.

Diagnosis: Gout (acute attack).

Clinchers
- *Diuretics:* Attacks of gout can be precipitated by:
  - Trauma
  - Surgery/some antibiotics
  - Starvation/purine rich foods (liver, offal, oily fish)
  - Infection
  - Diuretics
  - Alcohol
- *Severe joint pain in his left ankle:* Gout produces an acute inflammatory arthritis which is exquisitely painful monoarthritis (usually) but can be polyarticular also. It is often accompanied by fever. It usually affects the distal joints of the hands and feet and the knees. It particularly (and characteristically) affects the metatarso-phalangeal joints of the great toes.
- *Swelling and redness of ankle:* In acute attacks the affected joints, usually single, become severely painful, swollen, often red and impossible to move. This usually settles in less than three weeks.

> **CONFUSA**
> Gout is a chronic disease, but is characterised by acute attacks. Predisposing conditions to gout can be blood dyscrasias such as myeloid leukemia and polycythaemia. Most common extra-articular complication of gout is recurrent renal stones. Paradoxically renal failure can be a cause for gout.

Investigation of choice
Synovial fluid microscopy (urate crystals—negatively birefringent).

Immediate management
Pain relief by NSAID (Ibuprofen/Naproxen)
- If NSAID contraindicated—colchicine
- If cholchicine contraindicated—streroids

Treatment of choice
Allopurinol (but not until 3 weeks after an attack).

Note: Aspirin is absolutely contraindicated in gout.

Your Notes:

---

113. A 78-year-old woman complains of a stiff left hip joint after walking some distance. This is Most evident when she attempts to abduct the hip joint (limited abduction).

Diagnosis: Osteoarthritis (OA).

Clinchers
- *78-year-old woman:* The mean age of onset of OA is 5 years. OA is symptomatic three times more in women.
- *Shift hip joint after walking some distance:* Typically in OA, there is pain on movement. It is usually worse at end of day. There may be some background pain at rest.
- *Limited adduction of hip joint:* There can be stiffness of the joint which limits the movements (poor range of movements). There can be associated joint instability.

Joints affected in OA
- Most commonly: DIP joints, first MCP joint, cervical and lumbar spine
- Next most common: Hip joint
- Other most common: Knee joint.

> **CONFUSA**
> Lets have a good look at the differentiating features of osteoarthritis and rheumatoid arthritis, the two most common arthritis of elderly females
>
> | | OA | RA |
> |---|---|---|
> | Joint stiffness | Late evening | Early evening |
> | Palpable osteophytes | + | - |
> | Skin redness | +/- | + |
> | Swelling | +/- | + |
> | Ligaments stretch | - | + |
> | Age | Usually older | Usually adolescents |
> | Arthrodesis use | Good | Poor |
> | Fibrillation | + | - |
> | Pannus | - | + |
> | Bone arround joint | Sclerotic | Osteoporotic |
> | Joint deformity | Varus | Valgus |

Investigation of choice
Joint X-ray (findings: Loss of joint space, Subchondral sclerosis, Subchondral cysts, Marginal osteophytes).

Immediate management: Paracetamol for pain.

Treatment of choice
Reduce weight + walking aid
- Contralateral hand—for hip
- Ipsilateral hand—for knee
- Joint replacement is done for end stage disease.
- If PCM does not bring relief from pain, then give
  - Day pain—NSAID
  - Night pain—TCA in low doses (tricyclic antidepressant)

114. A 34-year-old woman complains of bilateral stiff and painful joints in her hands and feet.

Diagnosis: Rheumatoid arthritis (RA)

Clinchers
- *34-year-old woman:* Although the peak onset of RA is fifth decade, no age is exempt from it. The incidence of RA is three times more in women.
- *Bilateral:* RA is a symmetrical arthropathy, i.e. affect the same joints bilaterally.
- *Stiff and painful joints in her hands and feet:* RA presents typically with swollen, painful and stiff hands and feet, especially in the morning. This gradually gets and feet, especially in the morning. This gradually gets worse and large joints become involved

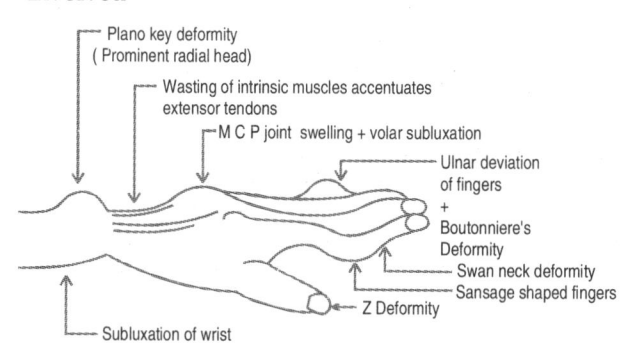

Labels on figure:
- Plano key deformity (Prominent radial head)
- Wasting of intrinsic muscles accentuates extensor tendons
- M C P joint swelling + volar subluxation
- Ulnar deviation of fingers + Boutonniere's Deformity
- Swan neck deformity
- Sansage shaped fingers
- Z Deformity
- Subluxation of wrist

Fig. "Handy" thesaurus for signs of RA

CONFUSA
In the PLAB exams, Felty's syndrome has been indirectly asked on at least a couple of occasions. So always keep an eye open for any mention of splenomegaly in a patient of RA.
(Felty's syndrome: RA + Splenomegaly + WCC ↓)

Investigation of choice
Rheumatoid factor often negative at start, but becomes positive in 80% over the time. But note that it may be false positive in several other chronic diseases.

Immediate management
Analgesia.

Treatment of choice
- Naproxen/Ibuprofen
- Disease modifying drugs if:
  - 12 week trial of 3 NSAIDs do not control pain.
  - Synovitis > 2 months.

Your Notes:

115. A 67-year-old woman complains of right hip pain. On examination the right hip is adducted, externally rotated and flexed.

Diagnosis: Fracture neck of femur.

Clinchers
- *67-year-old woman:* Osteoporosis is the main cause of spontaneous fractures of neck of femur in elderlies (as it is a weight bearing joint). Usually females are more prone to fracture neck of femur in old age.
- *Right hip pain:* There is pain in the hip, thigh or knee but may be little to see on local examination.
- *Right hip is adducted, externally rotated and flexed:* The affected leg may be shortened and externally rotated but this classical appearance is dependent on the grade of the fracture. A more valuable sign is pain on gental passive rotation of the extended leg. If the fracture has impacted, other movements may be good with minimal pain including even straight leg raising. Tenderness is most marked posteriorly.

CONFUSA
There are three circumstances in which fracture neck of femur occurs:
1. At any age: Associated with major voilence and multiple injuries
2. In the elderly: After a simple fall.
3. Spontaneously: As a result of osteoporosis or bony secondary deposits.

Investigation of choice
X-ray
- AP view of hips and pelvis
- Lateral view of affected hip.

Immediate management
A box splint to control leg movements + Analgesia.

Treatment of choice
Internal fixation or hemiarthroplasty is usually performed within 24 hours.

Your Notes:

116. A tall 34-year-old man develops severe central chest pain radiating to his back. He soon develops a dense hemiplegia.

Diagnosis: Dissecting aortic aneurysm (DAA)

Clinchers
- *Tall 34-year-old man:* Peak incidence of DAA occurs in sixth and seventh decade. Men are more commonly affected. DAA in young 34-year-old man (tall) may focus our attention towards Marfan's syndrome. Marfan's sydnrome is a dominent connective tissue disease with following criteria (diagnostic, e.g. > 2 criteria with positive family history)—lens dislocation, aortic dissection/dilatation, dural ectasia and skeletal features, e.g. arachnodactyly (long spidery fingers) armspan greater than height.
- *Severe central chest pain radiating to his back:* DAA presents with sudden onset, severe and tearing chest pain which may be localised to front or back. Other causes of chest pain are
  - *Cardiovascular:*
    - Angina
    - Myocardial infarction
    - Acute aortic dissection
    - Pericarditis.
  - *Gastrointestinal*
    - Oesophageal spasm
    - Reflux oesophagitis
    - Peptic ulcer disease
  - *Pulmonary*
    - Pneumonia
    - Pulmonary embolism
    - Pneumothroax
  - *Musculoskeletal*
    - Chest wall injuries
    - Costochondritis
    - Rib secondaries
    - Herpes zoster
  - *Emotional*
    - Depression
    - De Costa's syndrome
- *Develops dense hemiplegia:* Hemiplegia and hemianesthesia both are neurological findings in DAA due to carotid artery obstruction. It may also lead to spinal cord ischemia (paraplegia).

CONFUSA
Echocardiogram that shows no evidence of ischemia is helpful in distinguishing aortic dissection from myocardial infarction.

Investigation of choice
Chest X-ray/aortography or noninvasive techniques like two-dimentional echocardiography, CT scan or MRI (If haemodynamically compromised). MRI gives the best differentiation owing to high resolution.

Immediate management
Monitor hemodynamics and urine output. Unless hypotension is there, aim at reducing cardiac contractility and systemic arterial pressure.

Treatment of choice
For acute aortic dissection, beta-adrenergic blockers should be administered IV to achieve heart rate of about 60 beats/minute, followed by sodium nitroprusside infusion to lower systolic BP to 120 mmHg.

Long-term aim—control hypertension and reduce cardiac contractility.

Your Notes:

117. An elderly gentleman suffers a sudden severe crushing central chest pain radiating to his neck

Diagnosis: Myocardial infarction (MI).

Clinchers
- *Elderly gentleman:* Myocardial infarction (MI) occurs in elderly, more common in males. Other risk factors include family history of IHD, smoking, hypertension, diabetes, hyperlipidemia, obesity and sedentary lifestyle.
- *Sudden onset:* Chest pain in MI is of sudden onset, lasting >20 minutes which may be associated with nausea, sweatiness, dyspnoea, and palpitations.
- *Severe, central crushing chest pain radiating to neck:* Crushing, squeezing and heavy are some adjectives used by the patient to describe the pain in MI. The pain is severe involving central portion of chest and/or the epigastrium radiating to arms, back, lower jaw and neck.

CONFUSA
When the pain begins during a period of exertion, it does not usually subside with cessation of activity in contrast to angina pectoris.
Two out of three are essential for diagnosis of MI, A typical history ECG changes and cardiac enzyme rise.

Investigation of choice
- *Screening:* ECG changes—hyperacute T wave, ST elevation or new LBBB occur within hours of acute Q wave.
- *Definitive:* Cardiac enzymes↑ and troponin T increases.

Immediate management
- High flow O_2 by facemask
  ↓
- Aspirin 300 mg chewed (unless clear contraindication)
  ↓
- Morphine 5-10 mg IV + metoclopromide 10 mg IV
  ↓
- GTN sublingually 2 puff or 1 tablet as required
  ↓
  β-blockers
  ↓
  thrombolysis

Your Notes:

---

118. A middle-aged man has severe chest pain. Repeated St elevation patterns are seen and a Pericardial rub is heard.

Diagnosis: Pericarditis.

Clinchers
- *Severe chest pain:* The pain in pericarditis is often severe. It is characteristically reterosternal of left precordial, referred to the back and the trapezius. Pain gets worse on inspiration or lying flat, relieved by sitting up and learning forward.
- *Repeated ST elevation pattern:* ECG classically shows concave (saddle-shaped) ST segment elevation, but may be normal.
- *Pericardial rub:* This is the most important physical sign of pericarditis. It may have upto three components per cardiac cycle, heard most frequently during expiration with patient in sitting position.

CONFUSA
Myocardial infarction can be confused here as with acute pericarditis, serum transaminase and creatine kinase levels rise. However, these enzyme elevations in pericarditis are quite modest, given the extensive ECG. ST segment elevation in pericarditis.

Investigation of choice
ECG.

Immediate management
Observe for development of pericardial effusion, and if it is there watch for tamponade. If manifestations of tamponade appear pericardiocentesis must be carried out at once.

Your Notes:

119. A woman 10 days following hysterectomy complaints of severe left sided chest pain and breathlessness. Chest X-ray and ECG failed to relieve any abnormality.

Diagnosis: Pulmonary embolism.

Clinchers
- *10 days following hysterectomy:* Any cause of immobility or hypercoagulability, e.g. recent surgery (in this case hysterectomy), recent stroke or MI, disseminated malignancy, thrombophilia/antiphospholipid syndrome, prolonged bed-rest and pregnancy.
- *Severe left chest pain/breathlessness:* Symptoms of pulmonary embolism are—acute breathless, pleuritic chest pain, hemoptysis, dizziness and syncope.
- *Chest X-ray and ECG show no abnormality:* Chest X-ray and ECG is generally normal in pulmonary embolism.

Investigation of choice
- *Screening:* V/Q scan or spiral CT.
- *Definitive:* CT pulmonary angiography. This shows clots down to 5th order pulmonary arteries.

Immediate management
Screen for DVT.

Treatment of choice
Anticoagulation.

Your Notes:

120. A 52-year-old obese man has had episodic anterior chest pain, particularly at night, for three weeks. Chest X-ray and ECG are normal. (Question change in theme)

Diagnosis: Reflux oesophagitis.

Clinchers
- *Obesity:* A risk factor for reflux oesophagitis.
- *Episodic anterior chest pain:* Refer causes of chest pain in question 116. Episodic character of chest pain is more likely to be de to angina or reflux oesophagitis.
- *At night:* Burning, retrosternal discomfort related to meals, lying down, stooping and straining is likely to be due to refulx.
- *Chest X-ray and ECG are normal:* Rules out cardiovascular + pulmonary causes of chest pain.

CONFUSA
Oesophagitis (corrosive, NSAIDs), duodenal and gastric ulcer, infections (CMV, herpes, candida).

Investigation of choice
Investigation not required in isolated symptoms:
Tests—barium swallow (shows hiatus hernia).

Immediate management
Antacids, e.g. magnesium trisilicate mixture.

Treatment of choice
Change in lifestyle— ↓weight, stop smoking, ↓ alcohol inatke, raise bed head, take small regular meals, avoid hot drinks, eating < 3 hours before bed.
- Upper GI endoscopy
- H_2 antagonists (ranitidine)
- Proton pump inhibitor (lansoprazole)
- Prokinetic drugs (metoclopramide)

Your Notes:

121. A woman in the eight-week of her pregnancy develops bright red bleeding of four hours duration. On examination her cervical os is completely closed.

Diagnosis: Threatened abortion.

Clinchers

- *Eight-week of her pregnancy:* This can well be a case of first trimester abortion. Abortion is the loss of pregnancy before 24 week gestation.
- *Develops bright red bleeding;* In threatened abortion the bleeding is usually slight and bright red in colour.
- *Cervical OS is completely closed:* This is the most important point in this question. If the symptoms are mild and cervical os is closed, it is a threatened abortion.

In this case we go for ultrasonography. On USG a well-formed gestational ring and positive cardiac activity state 98% chance of continuation of pregnancy.

$$\text{USG} \begin{cases} \text{gestational ring} \\ + \\ \text{cardiac activity} \end{cases} 98\% \text{ chances of survival}$$

Investigation of choice
Ultrasonography (USG)

Immediate management
Rest (until bleeding stops)

Treatment of choice
Advice rest, 75% will settle. In others sedation and relief of pain may be ensured by phenobarbitone 30 mg or diazepam 5 mg twice daily.

Your Notes:

122. A woman in the twelfth week of her pregnancy develops bright red bleeding of four hours duration with large clots. On examination the cervical os is wide open.

Diagnosis: Inevitable abortion.

Clinchers

- *Twelfth week of pregnancy:* Abortion is loss of pregnancy before 24 weeks gestation.
- *Bright red bleeding with clots:* Increased vaginal bleeding with clots and increased pain that is colicky in nature is a sign of inevitable abortion.
- *Cervical OS is wide open:* This is again the most important point in this question, because internal examination revealing dilated internal os of the cervix through which the products of conception can be felt is diagnostic of inevitable abortion.

Diagnosis can be confirmed an ultrasonography. On USG if it is found that most of the products of conception have already been passed, it is incomplete abortion.

Investigation of choice
USG (ultrasonography).

Immediate management
If bleeding is profuse consider ergometrine 0.5 mg IM.

Treatment of choice
Take appropriate measures to look after general condition (e.g. bleeding, shock, etc). Accelerate the process of expulsion.

Your Notes:

123. A woman in the tenth week of her pregnancy develops bright red bleeding of one day duration. Her Gp organises an ultrasound examination which reveals heart contractions.

Diagnosis: Probable threatened abortion.

Clinchers
- *Tenth week:* After 24 weeks (and effectively after 20 weeks for the purpose of management in A and E department), vaginal bleeding is classed as an antepartum hemorrhage. Before this time it may be:
  - A threatened abortion
  - An incomplete abortion
  - A complete abortion
  - Other local causes
- *USG reveals heart contractions:* Formal scanning may detect a heart beat at 7 weeks gestation. A presence of contracting fetal heart rules out fetal loss. Other indications for fetal loss can be:
  - Significant pain and tenderness
  - Heavy of continuing bleeding
  - Passage of placental material in addition to blood clots.

CONFUSA
Vaginal bleeding occurs in upto one-fifth of all pregnant women but in over 50% of cases the pregnancy will continue successfully. A fresh bleed can due to local trauma to vaginal walls or cervix. So always rule it out by colposcopic examination.

Investigation of choice
Colposcopy to rule out local bleeding.

Immediate management
Early USG (aldready done in this case).

Treatment of choice
Patients with threatened abortion without symptoms or signs of fetal loss may be referred back to the GP for bed-rest at home.

Your Notes:

124. A 23-year-old woman has a history of a termination of pregancy at 12 weeks. She subsequently suffers a spontaneous miscarriage after 22 weeks of pregnancy. She has history of deep vein thrombosis (DVT).

Diagnosis: Antiphospholipid syndrome.

Clinchers
- *History of termination of pregnancy at 12 weeks and now suffer with miscarriage at 22 weeks:* Untreated < 20% of pregnancies proceed to live birth in antiphospholipid syndrome. This is due to:
  - First trimester loss
  - Placental thrombosis causing placental insufficiency leading to:
    - Intrauterine growth retardation and
    - Fetal death
- *History of DVT:* Apart from recurrent pregnancy loss history of arterial thrombosis/venous thrombosis supports the diagnosis of DVT.

Investigation of choice
Lupus plasma marker.

Treatment of choice
Careful regular fetal assessment (Doppler flow studies and ulstrasound for growth are required for 20 weeks). Treat affected woman from conception with aspirin 75 mg daily (heparin SC/12h until 34 weeks improves outcome). In this question since she has suffered from prior thrombosis, she should be given Warfarin (may cause abnormal fetal cartilage development) or heparin (causes maternal osteoporosis).
Some recommend
  Heparin—first trimester
  Warfarin—thereafter until time of delivery.
Use one of these postpartum as risk of thrombosis is high.

Your Notes:

125. A young lady had a miscarriage in her second trimester following which she bleed profusely, needing 6 units of blood and had to be taken for surgical evacuation of her uterus. She needed medical treatment as she had milk secretion for a few days, but since she has had no periods.

Diagnosis: Sheehan's syndrome (Simmonds disease).

Clinchers
- *She bleed profusely, needing 6 units of blood:* The most common cause of Sheehan's syndrome in females is severe obstetric hemorrhage causing necrosis of pituitary (due to ischaemia).
- *Milk secretion for a few days:* This is completely normal to occur for a few days after a second trimester abortion. But eventually there will be a failure to lactate because of panhypopituitarism of Sheehan's syndrome.
- *No periods:* Amenorrhoea sets in because of failure of pituitary to secrete gonadotrophins.

CONFUSA
Galactorrhoea is milk secretion unrelated to pregnancy or postpartum period. If present it suggests pituitary function (or hyperfunction exactly) and excludes a diagnosis of Sheehan's syndrome.

Investigation of choice
CT/MRI pituitary fossa.

Immediate management
Refer to endocrinologist.

Treatment of choice
Hormone therapy.

Your Notes:

---

126. This test of lung function is characteristically not involved in asthmatic patients.

Diagnosis: Asthma.

Clinchers
- Amongst all the options given in this question only vital capacity is not a criteria to assess an asthmatic patient. Vital capacity refers to the largest amount of air that can be expired after a maximal inspiratory effort. It is an index of pulmonary function. The fraction of vital capacity expired during the first second of a forced expiration (FEV_1, timed vital capacity) is reduced in diseaes like asthma, in which airway resistance is increased because of bronchial constriction, but the vital capacity remains unaffected.
- *Important tests in asthmatic patients:* Pulmonary expiratory flow rate (PEFR) monitoring (It correlates well with the forced expiratory volume in 1 sec, i.e. FEV_1 and used as an estimate of airway calibre).

CONFUSA
PEFR should be monitored regularly in asthmatics to monitor response to therapy and disease control. Spirometry: Obstructive defects ($\downarrow FEV_1/FVC, \uparrow$residual volume), *Aspergillus* serology, and hyperinflation on chest X-ray. In acute attack arterial blood gases analysis and blood culture may be helpful besides other regular tests.

Investigation of choice
Spirometry for obstructive defects ($FEV1$, FVC_1 and $\uparrow$ residual volume), PEFR.

Immediate management
In acute attack—Sit patient up and give O_2 (100% via non rebreathing bag) followed by salbutamol nebulization and hydrocortisone 200 mg IV/prednisolone 30 mg go for chest X-ray to exlclude pneumothorax.

Your Notes:

127. This substance is released by mast cells and causes flushing.

Diagnosis: Asthma

Clinchers
- Histamine, the richest source being the mast cells, released by degranulation of mast cells in response to variety of stimuli.
  Along with serotonin, histamine is available from preformed stores and is among the first mediators to be released during inflammation.
  In humans, histamine causes dilatation of the arterioles and increases vascular permeability of the venules (it, however, constricts large arteries) causing venular gaps and hence flushing.

CONFUSA
A direct question with no scope for any confusion.

Immediate management
Of asthma discussed in Question 126.

Your Notes:

128. This substance is characteristically found in the sputum of most asthma patients.

Diagnosis: Raised eosinophil count.

Clinchers
- Sputum examination of asthmatic patients reveals
  - Eosinophilia
  - Curschmann's spirals (costs of small airways)
  - Charcot-Layden crystals
  - Large number of neutrophils (suggesting bronchial infection)
- Complete blood count may also show eosinophilia.
- IgE may show mild elevations in blood. Marked elevation of IgE suggests evidence of allergic bronchopulmonary *Aspergillosis*.

CONFUSA
There is no question of confusion in this question. IgA is predominant class of immunoglobulin in secretions (tear, saliva, nasal secretions, GIT fluid and human milk) not to be confused with this question.

Immediate management
Of asthma is discussed in question 126.

Your Notes:

129. This test is done as a diagnostic test for asthma.

Diagnosis: Asthma

Clinchers
- The diagnosis of asthma is established by demonstrating reversible airway obstruction. Though there are various tests to diagnose asthma, traditionally 15% or greater improvement of FEV_1 following two puffs of keto adrenergic agonist is considered to be diagnostic of asthma.
- *Other tests for asthma:* Pulmonary expiratory flow rate (PEFR) monitoring (If correlates well with the forced expiratory volume in 1 sec, i.e. FEV_1 and used as an estimate of airway calibre).

CONFUSA
No confusion in this question.

Immediate management
Of asthma is discussed in question 126.

Your Notes:

130. Blocking of these can cause worsening of asthma.

Diagnosis: Asthma

Clinchers
- The walls of bronchi and bronchioles are innervated by the autonomic nervous system. There are abundant muscarinic receptors and cholinergic discharge causes bronchoconstriction. There are β_1 and β_2 adrenergic receptor in bronchial epithelium and smooth muscles. Some are located on cholinergic endings and ganglia where they inhibit acetylcholine release. In humans, β_2 receptors predominate. Therefore if β_2 receptors are blocked, there will be increased stimulation of cholinergic system which will lead to bronchoconstriction, worsening asthma.
- Here we can discuss role of β_2 agonists in asthma. β_2 agonists relax bronchial smooth muscle acting within minutes. Salbutamol is best given by inhalation, but can be given per oral or IV.

CONFUSA
No confusion in this question.

Immediate management
Given in question 126.

Your Notes:

131. An HIV patient develops a severe headache and confusion. She is discovered to have bilateral papillodema.

Diagnosis: Cerebral toxoplasmosis.

Clinchers
- *HIV patient:* The most common CNS infections in a HIV poistive patient are cerebral toxoplasmosis and cryptococcal meningitis.
- *Severe headache:* The clinical presentation of cerebral toxoplasmosis is of focal neurological features, convulsions, fever, headache and possible confusion.
- *Bilateral papilloedema:* It may be positive due to increased intracranial tensions as toxoplasmosis behave like a space occupying lesion.

CONFUSA

In addition to classic presentation as a CNS mass lesion, *T. gondii* has been reported to cause a variety of other clinical problems in HIV infected patients, including a CNS presentation more characteristic of herpes simplex with a negative CT scan, chorioretinitis, pneumonia, peritonitis with ascites, gastrointestinal tract involvement, cystitis and orchitis.

Investigation of choice
- *Screening:* CT scan—multiple ring enhancing lesions.
  Note:
  - A single lesion on CT may be found to be one of several on MRI
  - A solitary lesion on MRI mitigates against toxoplasmosis
- *Definitive:*
  Brain biopsy.

Immediate management
Medical management of raised ICT.

Treatment of choice
Pyrimethamine + Sulfadiazine
(side effects: Renal stones)

Your Notes:

132. An 8-year-old with acute leukemia is admitted in a comatose state. He is found to have lymphoblast depletion prevention of infectious diseases.

Diagnosis: Tumor lysis syndrome.

Clinchers
- *8-year-old:* Leukemias are the most common type of childhood malignancies are over 95% of cases are of acute variety. In the acute series ALL accounts for 70-80% cases. The peak age of onset of ALL is 3-7 years.
- *Acute leukemia:* As his diagnosis is known he must be on some treatment. Usually chemotherapy is given for ALL.
- *Lymphoblast depletion:* Since lymphoblasts rapidly proliferate in ALL, their depletion should raise a suspicion of any treatment with chemotherapeutic drugs. Tumor lysis syndrome is due to rapid cell death on starting chemotherapy for rapidly proliferating tumors like ALL. It results in rise in serum urate, potassium and phosphate, precipitating renal failure, which can lead to comatose condition if not treated urgently.

CONFUSA

Coma can also occurs in ALL as leukemic blast cells can infiltrate brain to produce leukemic meningitis.

Investigation of choice
Serum urate level (increased).

Immediate management
Immediate hydration.

Treatment of choice
Haemodialysis.

Your Notes:

133. A 14-year-old boy presents with drowsiness and generalised headache. He is recovering from a bilateral parotitits. His CT scan is normal.

Diagnosis: Viral meningitis (aseptic meningitis)

Clinchers

- *14-year-old boy:* Mumps is generally a childhood disease caused by RNA paramyoxovirus. Incidence of meningitis in males is three times more after mumps.
- *Drowsiness and generalised headache:* There are cardinal symptoms of increased ICP. Other symptoms can be:
  - Irritability
  - Vomiting
  - Fits
  - Bradycardia
  - BP increase
  - Impaired consciouness (confusion)
  - Coma
  - Irregular respiration
  - papilloedema (late sign)
- *Recovering from bilateral parotitis:* Meningitis secondary to mumps usually occur in convalescent phase. Mumps is characterised by painful swelling of the parotids, unilaterally at first, becoming bilateral in 70%.
- *CT scan is normal:* Rules out any space occupying lesion in the brain or ventricular dilatation, both of which are contraindication to lumbar puncture.

CONFUSA
In aseptic meningitis, CSF has cells but is Gram stain negative and no bacteria can be cultured on standard media. Mumps infection confers life-long immunity, so a documented history of previous infection excludes this diagnosis.

Investigation of choice
- *Screening:* Lumbar puncture, will show a picture of aseptic meningitis
- *Definitive:* Isolation of virus from CSF.

Immediate management
Symptomatic (hospital admission usually not required).

Treatment of choice
Bed-rest in a quiet and dark room.

Your Notes:

134. An intravenous drug abuser presents with suspected meningitis. The organism is confirmed in the CSF by India ink preparation.

Diagnosis: Cryptococcal meningitis.

Clinchers

- *IV drug abuser:* He must be having an undiagnosed HIV infection resulting in immunodeficient state. Cryptococcal meningitis does not occur in immunocompetent people.
- *Suspected meningitis:* CNS infections in HIV positive people are usually by toxoplasmosis, CMV and *Cryptococcus*. Toxoplasmosis causes a SOL and CMV causes encephalitis. *Cryptococcus* is associated with meningitis usually.
- *Organism confirmed in CSF in India Ink preparation:* This is characteristic of *Cryptococcus neoformans* (a fungi) whose thick capsule resist staining and can only be demonstrated as translucencies against black background in India ink preparations.

CONFUSA
Cryptococcal meningitis have an insidious onset and is often without neck stiffness. The etiology of neck stiffness is inflammation and it is often absent in immunodeficients and neonates. Conditions (other than meningitis) which can produce neck stiffness are *Shigella* gastroenteritis and subarachnoid hemorrhage.

Investigation of choice
India ink staining of CSF.
or
Detection of cryptococcal antigen in blood/CSF.

Immediate management
Transfer to ITU.

Treatment of choice
Amphotericin/fluocytosine IV
Fluconazole can be given in milder cases (better tolerated).

Your Notes:

135. An anxious mother called you to say that her son's best friend in school has caught meningitis.

Diagnosis: Immediate 'contact' of meningitis.

Clinchers
Meningitis prophylaxis:
Talk to your consultant in community disease control. Offer prophylaxis is:
- Household/nurser contacts (i.e. within droplet range)
- Those who have kissed the patient's mouth.

> **CONFUSA**
> If the student suffering from meningitis is just a classmate and the best friend of her son, then there is no need of any chemoprophylaxis.

Investigation of choice
None required except screening the skin for any nonblanching petechiae.

Immediate management
Reassure mother

Treatment of choice
Rifampicin prophylaxis
- 600 mg/12 h PO for 2 days
- Children   > 1 yr 10 mg/kg/12 h
                < 1 yr 10 mg/kg/12 h

or
Ciprofloxacin
- 500 mg PO, 1 dose, adult only

Your Notes:

---

136. Cimetidine.

Diagnosis: Impotence

Clinchers
As it is a direct question, lets discuss cimetidine in particular,
- It is a H_2 blocker
- Cimetidine crosses placenta and reaches milk, but penetration in brain is poor.
- Well-tolerated by most patients: adverse effects occur in 5% people. Main side effects is evident in males because of:
  - *Antiandrogenic action*
    It displaces dihydrotestosterone from its cystoplasmic receptor.
  - *Increases plasma prolactin*
  - *Inhibits degradation of estradiol by liver*

So, high doses of cimetidine for long periods have produce.
- Gynaecomastia
- Loss of libido
- Impotence
- Temporary decrease in sperm count

> **CONFUSA**
> This antiandrogenic profile of side effects of cimetidien is not shared by any other H_2 blocker.

Investigation of choice
Serum estradiol.

Immediate management
Reassure.

Treatment of choice
Discontinue cimetidine.

Your Notes:

137. Cyclophosphamide.

Diagnosis: Haemorrhagic cystitis.

Clinchers
Hemorrhagic cystitis can develop in patients receiving cyclophosphamide or ifosphamide. Both these drugs are metabolized to acrolein (a strong chemical irritant) excreted in urine. Prolonged contact or high concentrations may lead to bladder irritation and hemorrhage.

Other side effects of cyclophosphamide:
- Bone marrow suppression
- Bladder carcinoma
- Gonadal suppression
- GI intolerance
- Hypogammaglobulinemia
- Pulmonary fibrosis
- Myelodysplasia
- Oncogenesis

Immediate management
In hemorrhagic cystitis, the maintenance of a high urine flow may be sufficient supportive care.

Treatment of choice
Conservative management. If it fails irrigation of the bladder with 0.37 to 0.74 percent formalin solution for 10 min stops bleeding in most cases.

In extreme cases, cystectomy may be necessary.

Your Notes:

138. Diamorphine.

Diagnosis: Constipation.

Clinchers
Opioid analgesia is a leading cause of constipation in herpitalized patients. It is aggravated by low fluid fibres intake. Diamorphine is a semisynthetic opiate. It is 3 times more potent than morphine. It is considered to be more euphorient and highly addicting. This drug is favoured in illcit drug trafficking. This drug has been banned in most countries except UK.

Constipation is a prominent side effec of diamorphine.

CONFUSA
Drugs that lead to constipation are:
- Opiate analgesics (e.g. morphine, diamorphine, codiene)
- Anticholinergics (tricyclics, phenothiazines)
- Iron

Immediate management
Laxative.

Treatment of choice
Treat the cause. Advice high fibre diet with adequate fluid intake (unless cause is GI obstruction, megacolon or colonic hypotonia). Encourage exercise

Drugs used rarely
- Bulking agents (ispaghula husk)
- Stool softners (arachis oil enema)
- Osmotic laxative
- Stimulated laxatives.

Your Notes:

139. Amoxycillin.

Diagnosis: Stevens-Johnson syndrome

Clinchers
Drugs like amoxycillin (penicillins), sulfonamides and sedatives, may induce a systemic illness with fever, arthralgia, myalgia ± pneumonitis and conjunctivitis. The skin develops typical target lesions of erythema multiforme often on plams.

Other causes of Stevens-Johnson syndrome include viruses or other infection (e.g. of herpes simplex) and neoplasm.

Treatment of choice
Calamine lotion for the skin, steroids (systemic and eye-drops) were once used, but ask a dermatologist and ophthalmologist.

Your Notes:

140. Oral contraceptive pill.

Diagnosis: Deep vein thrombosis.

Clinchers
The older preparations of oral contraceptives increased the incidence of venous thromboembolism, but this is found to be only marginal with the newer reduced steroid content pills. However, even these phase significant risk in woman > 35 years age diabetics, hypertensives and those who smoke.

The most common symptoms of DVT are of pain in the calf, with varying degree of redness and swelling.

Investigation of choice
Venography, or Doppler ultrasound. Venography is invasive technique. Colour Doppler ultrasound is now preferred first line method of investigating suspected DVT.

Immediate management
In any women with suspicion of DVT, heparin or low molecular weight heparin should be given in treatmet doses, until the diagnosis is confirmed or refuted.

Your Notes:

141. Middle-aged man with hematuria and colicky left loin pain.

Diagnosis: Renal colic.

Clinchers

- *Middle-aged man:* Fifty percent of patients of renal colic present between the ages of 30 until and 50 years. The male:female ratio is 4:3.
- *Hematuria:* Hematuria is sometimes a leading symptom of stone disease and occasionally the only one. As a rule the amount of feeding is small. Other causes of hematuria are:
  - Kidney
    - Glomerular diseases
    - Polycystic kidney
    - Carcinoma
    - Stone
    - Trauma (including renal biopsy)
    - Vacuolar malformation
    - Embolism
    - Renal vein thrombosis
  - Ureter
    - Stone
    - Neoplasm
  - Bladder
    - Carcinoma
    - Stone
    - Trauma
    - Inflammatory, e.g. TB, cystitis, schistosomiasis
  - Prostate
    - Benign prostatic hypertrophy
    - Carcinoma
  - Urethra
    - Trauma
    - Stone
    - Urethritis
    - Neoplasm
  - General
    - Anticoagulant therapy
    - Thrombocytopenia
    - Haemophilia
    - Sickle cell disease
    - Malaria
    - Exercise (heavy)
  - Red urine
    - Haemoglobinuria
    - Myoglobinuria
    - Acute intermittent prophyria
    - Beet root
    - Senna
    - Phenolphthalein
    - Rifampicin

- *Colicky left loin pain:* Ureteric colic is an agonising pain passing from loin to groin. It starts suddenly and may be associated with strangury (painful passage of few drops of urine). Colic pain is the result of smooth muscle contraction against a resistance. Common causes of colicky pain are
  - Biliary tract
    - Stone in Hartmann's pouch
    - Stone in cystic duct
    - Stone in ampula of vater
  - Renal tract
    - Ureteric colic due to stone, blood clot or tumor
  - Intestinal tract
    - Mechanical obstruction
    - Appendicular colic as appendix lumen occludes
  - Uterus
    - Parturition
    - Menstruation
    - Ectopic pregnancy in fallopian tube

Investigation of choice

Radiography (plain films of kidneys, ureter and bladder) [KUB film]. Following radiography, excretion urography may be done to confirm calculus and its location. USG scanning can be performed in locating stones.

Your Notes:

142. An elderly gentleman with left iliac fossa pain and tenderness and rectal bleeding.

Diagnosis: Diverticulitis.

Clinchers
- *Elderly gentleman:* Diverticulitis is unusual before 40 years. Sex distribution is roughly equal.
- *Left iliac fossa pain:* Acute diverticulitis is well nicknamed left-sided appendicitis. Here abdominal pain shifts to left iliac fossa (LIF) accompanied by fever, vomiting, local tenderness and guarding.
- *Rectal bleeding:* In chronic cases passage of mucosa or bright red blood per rectum or malaena or occult bleeding is present. There may be diarrhoea alternating with constipation.

Bleeding from a diverticulum is the most likely cause of a sudden perfuse, bright red bleed in an elderly, often hypertensive patient.

Diverticulitis may lead to
- Perforation
- Chronic infection
- Haemorrhage.

CONFUSA
The symptoms and presentation in this question may very much be confused from neoplasm of the colon. It is imposible to be certain of this differentiation clinically or even on special investigations, unless positive biopsy is obtained by flexible sigmoidoscopy or colonoscopy.

Investigation of choice
Sigmoidoscopy (fibre optic-flexible)—can be performed to visualize colonic diverticula and to take a biopsy. This is an investigation of choice. Barium enema should not be performed in the acute phase to prevent iatrogenic perforation of friable and inflamed bowel, rather in acute cases CT scan may be useful to exclude other causes of lower abdominal pain.

Treatment of choice
This case should be managed conservatively. Perform flexible sigmoidoscopy and place the patient on fluid diet and antibiotics. In chronic cases bowels are regulated by means of lubricant laxative (e.g. Milpar) and prescribe high roughage diet (fruit, vegetables, whole meal bread and barley).

Your Notes:

143. A middle-aged woman with recurrent right upper abdominal pain radiating to the right shoulder. She is tender in this region.

Diagnosis: Cholelithiasis.

Clinchers
- *Middle-aged woman:* Always remember the five F's of cholelithiasis: fair, fat, fertile, female of fourty (40). But this is just an approximation to the truth. The incidence of cholelethiasis is higher in overweight, middle-aged women.
- *Recurrent right upper abdominal pain:* Recurrent bouts of pain occur due to mild cholecystitis, which may or may not be accompanied by fever. In acute cases upper abdomen is extremely tender and often a palpable mass develops in the region of the gall-bladder.

Though stones may be absent from the duct system, a tinge of jaundice may be produced due to pressing of common bile duct by sudden gallbladder.

Fatty meals cause discomfort, as they stimulate release of cholecystokinin which causes the gallbladder to contract onto stones.

CONFUSA
Differentiate it from pancreatitis, chronic dyspepsia, including peptic ulceration and hiatus hernia. So for serum amylase to exclude pancreatitis, and chest X-ray to rule out pneumonia.

Investigation of choice
Ultrasonography—show presence of stones in inflamed gallbladder with edema around the gallbladder wall.

Immediate management
Conservative management.

Treatment of choice
Conservative treatment followed by cholecystectomy.

Your Notes:

144. Middle-aged chronic alcoholic presents with severe pain in upper abdomen, radiating to the back.

Diagnosis: Pancreatitis

Clinchers

- *Middle-aged chronic alcoholic:* Pancreatitis is more commonly seen in obese and middle-aged or elderly, women being affected more than male.
  Alcoholism is the main cause of chronic pancreatitis. Acute cases are associated with either gallstones or alcohol.
- *Severe pain (upper abdomen) radiating to back:* In pancreatitis the pain severe, constant, usually epigastric and often radiates to back. Pain is sometime relieved on bending forward. Abdomen is tender with positive guarding.
  To diagnose pancreatitis go for serum amylase. Amylase is liberated into circulation by damaged pancreas. Amylase may be raised in variety of other conditions like—renal failure, salivary gland diseases (like parotitis) severe diabetic ketoacidosis, morphine administration (causing sphincter of Oddi spasm), perforated' peptic ulcer, acute cholecystitis, intestinal obstruction and many more.

Investigation of choice
Serum amylase.

Immediate management
Conservative consists of analgesia with pethidine (avoid morphine, which may produce sphincter spasm) and fluid replacement.

Treatment of choice
In acute cases, conservative management is done. Surgery is indicated if diagnosis is not certain, but should be avoided. In chronic pancreatitis—analgesia and diet control is advised. Surgery if very frequent attacks or severe pain—partial pancreatectomy or pancreaticojejunostomy.

Your Notes:

145. A fit 17-year-old man present with a 12 hour history of central abdominal pain localising to his right iliac fossa. He is pyrexical with tenderness, guarding and rebound tenderness in the right iliac fossa.

Diagnosis: Acute appendicitis

Clinchers

- *17-year-old man:* Acute appendicitis may occur at any age but is most common between the ages of 15 and 30 years and is uncommon under the age of 2 years.
- *12 hour history of central abdominal pain localising to his right iliac fossa:* The pain in appendicitis is initially periumbilical or epigastric, later radiating to right iliac fossa.
- *Pyrexical with tenderness, guarding and rebound tenderness in RIF:* Right iliac fossa is usually most tender and guarded part of the abdoman in appendicitis. Rebound tenderness points towards peritonitis. Pyrexia and tachycardia are usual.

CONFUSA
Differentiate it from other causes of acute abdomen. Refer page 196, lecture notes on general surgery, 9th edn.

Investigation of choice
Diagnostic laparoscopy. This is the best answer amongst all the options given. Though it is important to note that the diagnosis of acute appendicitis is made on the basis of history and examination. No special investigation is indicated unless alternative diagnosis is being considered.

Immediate management
The treatment of acute appendicitis is appendicectomy, except in following conditions
- Patient is morifund with advanced peritonitis
- Attack has already resolved, in such a case appendicectomy can be adviced as an elective procedure.

Your Notes:

146. A 35-year-old female with a high blood glucose level is noted to be obese and has abdominal striae.

Diagnosis: Determination of diurnal steroid level pattern.

Clinchers
- *35-year-old female:* Cushings disease is more common in women with peak age between 30-50 years.
- *High blood glucose level:* One of the secondary causes of diabetes include Cushing's disease (Other endocrine diseases associated are acromegaly, pheochromocytoma, thyrotoxicosis).
- *Obese with abdominal striae:* Weight gain, menstrual irregularities, amenorrhoea, hirsutism, impotence, depression, muscle weakness are the symptoms of Cushing's disease.
  Important signs include—tissue wasting, thin skin, puple abdominal striae, buffalow hump, osteoporosis water retention, etc.

Investigation of choice
Determination of diurnal steroid level pattern.

Immediate management
Monitor blood and urine glucose and adopt treatment accordingly.

Treatment of choice
Manage high sugar levels and investigate for Cushing's disease. For Cushing's disease selective removal of pituitary adenoma via a transsphenoidal and rarely transfrontal approach is done. Bilateral adrenalectomy is done if source cannot be located.

Your Notes:

147. An elderly gentleman with frequency is found to have a raised random blood glucose level.

Diagnosis: Diabetes mellitus.

Clinchers
- *Elderly gentleman with frequency:* Signs and symptoms attributable to an osmotic diuresis (polyuria, polydipsia) supported with hyperglycemia makes the diagnosis of diabetes mellitus unequivocal.
- *Raised random blood glucose level:* If the random blood glucose level is raised, we go for fasting venous palsma glucose. Fasting plasma glucose level ≥ 7 mmol/L is diagnostic. A glucose of 6-7 mmol/L implies impaired fasting glucose. If there is any doubt, the 2 hour value in oral glucose tolerance test (OGTT) should be used (diagnostic if levels >11.1 mmol/L).

Investigation of choice
Fasting glucose level (diagnostic if ≥ 7 mmol/L)

Immediate management
Monitor blood and urine glucose and adopt treatment accordingly.

Your Notes:

DIABETES—treatment
(NIDDM)

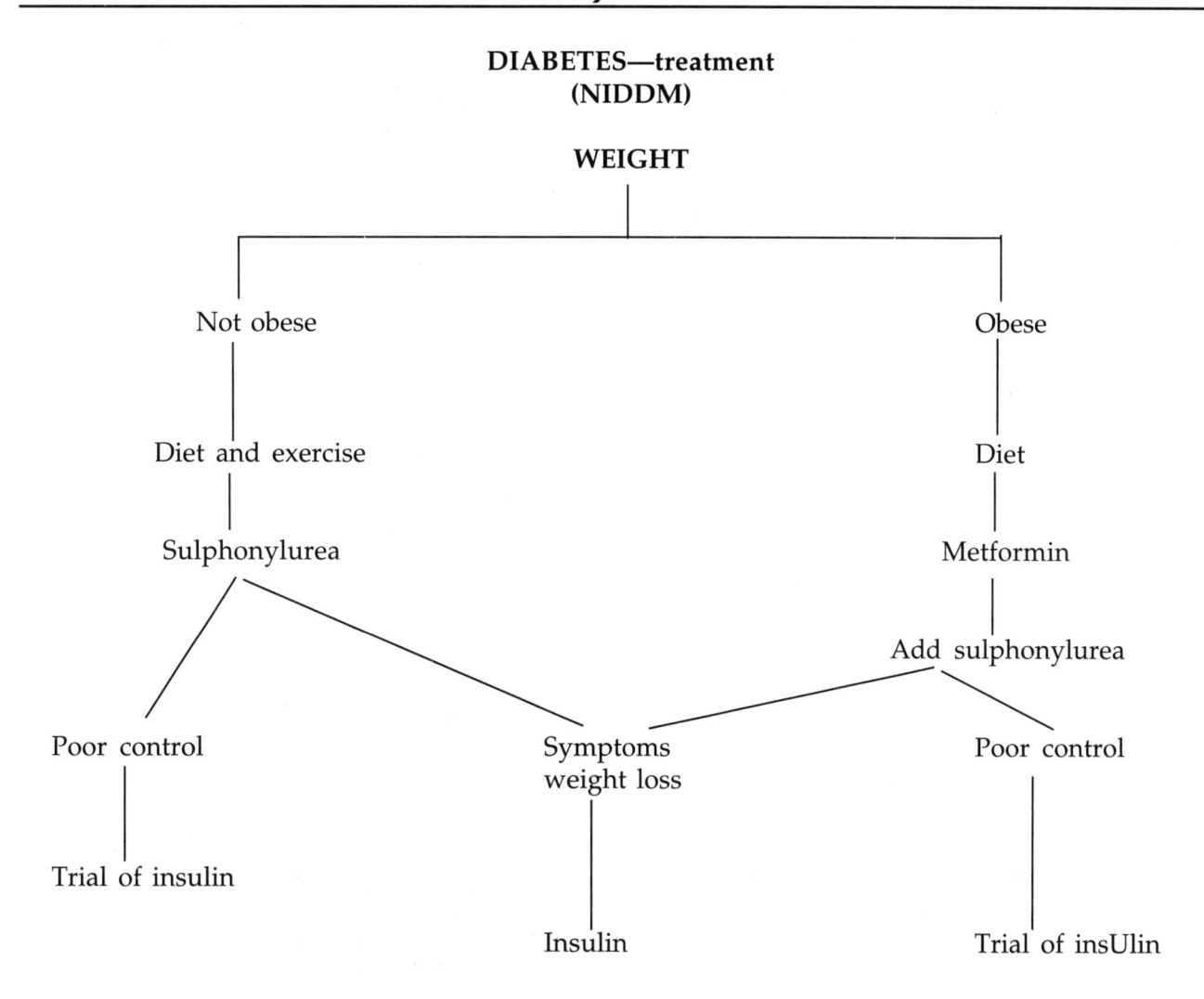

WEIGHT

```
                    WEIGHT
                      │
        ┌─────────────┴─────────────┐
    Not obese                     Obese
        │                           │
  Diet and exercise               Diet
        │                           │
   Sulphonylurea                Metformin
        │                           │
        │                    Add sulphonylurea
        │                           │
   ┌────┴────────┐           ┌──────┴──────┐
Poor control   Symptoms              Poor control
               weight loss
   │              │                     │
Trial of       Insulin            Trial of insUlin
insulin
```

148. An elderly gentleman with polyuria is found to have a raised fasting blood glucose level.

Diagnosis: Diabetes mellitus.

Clinchers

➢ *Elderly gentleman with polyuria:* Though this question directly points towards diabetes mellitus, let us familiarise ourselves with *causes of polyuria*.

Diuretics
- Therapeutic
  - Frusemide
  - Amiloride
  - Bendrofluazide
- Osmotic
  - Hyperglycaemia
  - Mannitol
  - Hypercalcaemia
  - Urea

Diabetes insipidus
- Cranial
  - Idiopathic deficiency of ADH production
  - Inherited (dominant or recessive)
  - Head injuries
  - Neurosurgery
  - Brain tumors
  - Opiates
- Nephrogenic
  - Drugs
    - Lithium
    - Demechocycline
  - Inherited (X-linked)
  - Chronic hypercalcaemia
  - Hypokalaemia
  - Chronic tubulointestinal nephritis
- Excessive fluid intake
  - Psychogenic
  - Drug induced thirst—anticholinergics
  - Hypothalamic disease

➢ *Raised fasting glucose level:* As already discussed in previous question fasting glucose (plasma) level of ≥ 7 mmol/L is diagnostic and glucose of 6-7 mmol/L implies impaired fasting glucose. We should never go for a single glucose value. In case of any doubel 2 hour value in oral glucose tolerance test (OGTT) should be used (diagnostic if value ≥ 11.1 mmol/L).

Method for performing OGTT:
- Fast overnight and give 75 gm of glucose in 300 ml under to drink.
- Venous palsma glucose before and 2 hours after drink.

Investigation of choice: Glucose tolerance test.

Immediate management: Go for OGTT.

149. A known diabetic on treatment has several episodes of hypoglycemia.

Diagnosis: Improper treatment.

Clinchers

➢ *Known diabetic on treatment:* In hospital settings drugs are the most common cause of hypoglycaemia, the three drugs most frequently implicated being
- Insulin
- Sulphonylurea
- Alcohol

➢ Here in this question we can assess glycaemic control from glycosylated hemoglobin (HbA_{1c}), the levels 8 weeks (i.e. RBC half-life). The target HbA_{1c} should be set individually. Complications increase in frequency with increasing HbA_{1c}.

In conditions interfering with HbA_{1c} measurements (e.g. some hemoglobinopathies), fructosamine (glycated plasma protein) levels can be assessed, this related to control over previous 1-3 weeks.

➢ Plasma HbA_{1c} values—if >7%. DM is likely and risk of microvascular complications occurs.

Investigation of choice
Hemoglobin A_{1c} (glycosylated hemoglobin).

Immediate management
Monitor blood and urine glucose levels and adjust the treatment accordingly.

Treatment of choice
Educate patient—recognition and treatment of hypoglycaemia (e.g. sweets/sugar) is essential
- Regular exersise and healthy eating habits ($\downarrow$ sugar, $\downarrow$ saturated fat, starch-carbohydrate $\uparrow$)

Your Notes:

150. A 27-year-old woman was found to have glycosuria at a routine antenatal clinic visit. A glucose tolerance test confirmed the diagnosis of gestational diabetes. What will be your like of action.

Diagnosis: Gestational diabetes.

Clinchers
- *Gestational diabetes:* Diabetes arising for the first-time in pregnancy, is often treated with diet alone. The patient requires good education and must be encouraged to monitor blood glucose at home. A very few cases may require insulin to achieve glycaemic control. Oral hypoglycaemia should not be used in pregnancy.
- *Glycosuria:* Is common in pregnancy due to lowering of renal threshold. If glycosuria persistently present, a glucose tolerance test is performed. Some women with gestational diabetes either remain diabetic or subsequently develop diabetes.

CONFUSA
Only minority will require insulin to achieve glycaemic control.

Investigation of choice
GTT.

Immediate management
Dietary adjustment + monitor.

Your Notes:

151. A female lawyer is becoming anxious when she has to speak in front of people. This is affecting her work as she needs to speak out in court

Diagnosis: Anxiety.

Clinchers
- *Becoming anxious when she has to speak in front of people:* It is a type of performance anxiety and has a recognised anxiety provoking stimulus.
- *Affecting her work:* Anxiety is acceptable and require no treatment until and unless it becomes symptomatic, i.e.
  - Affect work/social life
  - Somatization symptoms

CONFUSA
If not treated, she may become less efficient because of her constant performance anxiety. This might lead to more interference with her work more and hence may be predisposed to develop anxiety neurosis.

Investigation of choice
A detailed psychiatric history.

Immediate management
Reassurance.

Treatment of choice
Desensitization, i.e. a graded exposure to the anxiety provoking stimulus (behaviour therapy). Anxiolytics may be needed to enable effective work to be done with the patient.

Your Notes:

152. A student approaching her secondary level exams is becoming increasingly anxious a few days ahead of her exam.

Diagnosis: Anxiety.

Clinchers

> *Approaching her secondary level exams:* This is an anxiety provoking stimulus in this patient. Usually sterss and life events precipitate anxiety which can be exaggerated in some individuals, thus producing symptoms.
> *Becoming increasingly anxious:* Since the condition is progressive, she need treatment. This will also ensure that the anxiety will not hamper her preparation and performance in the exams.

CONFUSA
Desensitization cannot work in this patient as the anxiety provoking stimulus is an isolated event in future and not something she has to cope up with every day.

Investigation of choice
Detailed psychiatric history.

Immediate management
Anxiolytics indicated if the condition is hampering her studies.

Treatment of choice
Progressive relaxation training (the patient is taught to tense and relax groups of muscles in an orderly way—e.g. starting with the toes and working up the body. By concentrating on this, anxiety and muscle tone are reduced).

Your Notes:

153. A 20-year-old woman attends A and E complaining of sudden breathlessness and anxiety. She describes palpitations and paraesthesiae of her hands, feet and lips. ECG shows sinus tachycardia and O_2 saturation is normal.

Diagnosis: Panic attacks.

Clinchers

> *20-year-old female:* young females are most prone to have panic attacks.
> *Sudden breathlessness and anxiety:* Classically the symptoms begin unexpectedly or 'out-of-the-blue'. Usually there is no apparent precipitating factor. The patient becomes increasingly frightened by an apparent inability to breath adequately. Attempts to breadth rapidly results in dizziness and further anxiety.
> *Palpitations:* It is due to sympathetic overactivity. Other symptoms attributed to sympathetic stimulation are—tachycardia, sweating, flushes, dyspnoea, hyperventilation, dry mouth, frequency and hesitancy of micturition, dizziness, diarrhoea, mydriasis.
> *Paraesthesiae of her hands, feet and lips:* Tachypnoea blows off CO_2 and the resultant respiratory alkalosis causes a fall in ionised calcium. This hypocalcaemia manifest as paraesthesiae in the fingers and perioral area.
> *Sinus tachcycardia:* Due to sympathetic stimulation.
> O_2 *saturation is increased:* due to hyperventilation.

CONFUSA
The most important differential diagnosis in a female is from MVPS (mitral valve prolapse syndrome). This syndrome, more commonly seen in young females (like panic disorder), presents with classical symptoms of panic disorder occurring in episodes. It is caused by prolapse, usually congenital, of the mitral valve into the atrium during ventricular systole. On auscultation, a mid systolic click and a systolic murmur can be heard sometimes. The clininical differentiation between MVPS and panic disorder is difficult. The diagnosis is usually established on echocardiography.

Investigation of choice
To rule out organic respiratory problems (ECG, CXR, ABG).

Immediate management
Confirmation of normality with warm reassurance to the patient.

Treatment of choice
Re-breathing into a closed bag and mask system without oxygen.

154. This treatment is very effective in endogenous anxiety and phobias.

Diagnosis: Panick attacks associated with phobias.

Clinchers

The drug of choice of panic attacks associated with phobias is MAO inhibitor.

MAO inhibitors act on mono amine oxidase which is responsible for the degradation of catecholamines after reuptake. Their final effects is the same as tricyclic antidepressants, i.e. functional increase in the NE and/or 5HT levels at the receptor site. The increase in brain amine levels is probably responsible for their action.

CONFUSA

It takes 5-10 days before a MAO inhibitor has any evident action. Therefore it is useless to give it on a SOS basis. They must be administered regularly in sufficient doses to achieve desired effect.

Investigation of choice
A detailed psychiatric history.

Immediate management
Lorazepam if immediate agitation is present.

Treatment of choice
MAO inhibitors (phenelzine).

Your Notes:

155. A 25-year-old woman finds it difficult to leave her house. She becomes very agitated in supermarkes and describes palpitations and difficult breathing when in crowds.

Diagnosis: Agoraphobia.

Clinchers

➢ *25-year-old woman:* All phobic disorders are more common in females.
➢ *Difficult to leave her house:* This is fear of open places, public places, crowded places, any other place from where there is not easy escape to a safe place (safe place is usually home according to the patients).
➢ *Becomes very agitated in super and describes palpitations and difficult breathing when in crowds:* If patient of agoraphobia finds herself/himself in a crowded place like supermarkets, he/she will suddenly develop incapaciating symptoms of palpitations or a full blown panic attack, which can lead to agitation. Difficulty breathing leading to hyperventilation is a typical symptoms of panic attacks.

CONFUSA

As the agoraphobia increases in severity, there is a gradual restriction in normal day to day activities. The activity may become so severely restricted that the person becomes self-imprisoned at home. One or two persons (usually close relations) may be relied upon, with whom the patient can leave home. Claustrophobia is just the opposite—fear of closed spaces from where there is no easy escape to a safe place.

Investigation of choice
Detailed psychiatric history.

Immediate management
Rebreathing into a bag if panic attack is present.

Treatment of choice
Behaviour therapy

Your Notes:

156. A pregnant woman has a vaginal discharge. The pH is 2 and mycelia are seen.

Diagnosis: Candidiasis.

Clinchers
- *Pregnant woman has vaginal discharge:* Pregnancy favrous candidial infection becomes of increased vaginal acidity and high glycogen content. Other risk factors for candidial infections are:
  - Hormonal contraceptive pills
  - Diabetes
  - Immunodeficiencies
  - Antibiotics
  - Steroids
- *pH is 2:* Gram-positive fungus 'Candida albicans' flourishes in an acid medium with an abundant supply or carbohydrates.
- *Mycelia are seen:* In candidial infection, microscopy reveals strings of mycelium or typical oval spores. Culture or Sabouraud's medium.

CONFUSA
If still any confusion, the diagnosis of thrush (candia albicans) can be established by following features
- Candidial discharge is classically white curds
- Vulva and vagina may be red, fissured and rose.

Investigation of choice
Microscopy + culture

Treatment of choice
A single imidazole pessary, e.g. clotrimazole 500 mg. For further treatment you may refer page 48 (OHCS), 5th edn.

Your Notes:

---

157. A woman has a vaginal discharge. The pH is 8 and clue cells are seen.

Diagnosis: Bacterial vaginosis.

Clinchers
- *Vaginal discharge:* The character of discharge is not specified, so let us have an idea of type, of vaginal discharges:
  - White curdy discharge—Thrush (*Candida albicans*)
  - Thin, bubbly, fishy smelling discharge—*Trichomonas vaginalis*
  - Offensive discharge with fishy odour—bacterial vaginosis.
- *pH is 8:* Vaginal pH > 5.5 is seen in bacterial vaginosis, candidiasis occurs in acidic vaginal pH.
- *Clue cells:* Stippled vaginal epithelia 'clue cells' seen on met microscopy supports the diagnosis of bacterial vaginosis.

CONFUSA
Though the diagnosis is settled for bacterial vaginosis, the nature of vaginal discharge should have been mentioned. In bacterial vaginosis offensive discharge with fishy odour occurs.

Investigation of choice
Wet microscopy and culture.

Treatment of choice
Metronidazole 2 g PO once or clindamycin 2% vaginal cream. If recurrent treat the partner also. And in pregnant females use metronidazole alone 200 mg/8 hr PO for 7 days.

Your Notes:

158. A woman has severe right sided abdominal pain and fever. She has a foul smelling vaginal discharge. She has a palpable right sided firmness.

Diagnosis: Pelvic inflammatory disease (PID).

Clinchers
- *Right sided abdominal pain and fever:* PID presents with pain which is usually bilateral but may be localized to one side, with fever. Most of the cases are because of *Chlamydia* but rarely gonococcus and *Streptococcus* may be the culprits.
- *Foul smelling vaginal discharge:* Along with pain and fever PID presents with cervicals with profuse purulent or blood vaginal discharge.
- *Palpable right sided firmness:* In chronic cases inflammation leads to fibrosis, so adhesions may develop between pelvic organs. The tubes may get distended with pus (pyosalpinx) or fluids (hydrosalpinx).

> **CONFUSA**
> In endometeriosis, pelvic pain is the most common symptom (classically cyclical during periods), but foul smelling vaginal discharge is not seen. Here secondary dysmenorrhoea and deep dyspareuria are common.

Investigation of choice
Endocervical and urethral swabs if practicable. Check for *Chlamydia*. Later we can go for blood culture if fever is present.

Immediate management
Admit for blood culture and IV antibiotics if very unwell.

Treatment of choice
Refer page 50 (OHCS) 5th end.

Your Notes:

---

159. A woman on the contraceptive pill for several years has a slight whitish vaginal discharge. On inspection she is found to have a pinkish coloration of the outer cervix.

Diagnosis: Cervical erosion (cervical ectropion).

Clinchers
- *On contraceptive pills:* Ectropions extend temporarily under the influence of hormones in following conditions:
  - During puberty
  - With the combined pill and during pregnancy
- In this case endocervical epithelium extends its territory over paler epithelium of ectocervix. Endocervical canal is lined by mucus columnar epithelium and vaginal cervix with squamous epithelium, therefore columnar epithelium in ectocervix giving if pinkish colouration.
  Columnar epithelium is soft and glandular therefore ectropion is prone to bleeding and there is excess mucus production, and hence they are also prone to infection.

> **CONFUSA**
> History of women being an contraceptive pills with vaginal discharge may point towards thrush (*Candida albicans*), but the discharge of thrush is white curdy. In candidiasis microscopy will reveal stringe of mycelium.

Treatment of choice
Generally no treatment is required. But in case it creates nuisance, cautery can be done.

Your Notes:

160. A middle-aged woman with a vaginal discharge is found to have several ulcers at the vaginal introitus.

Diagnosis: Herpes simplex.

Clinchers
- *Vaginal discharge:* Vaginal discharge occurs in herpes due to exudation from the lesion in the cervix and vagina.
- *Several ulcers at vaginal introitus:* In herpes simplex the vulva is ulcerated and exquisitely painful. Herpes type II is sexually acquired, this classically causes genital infections. This may be caused by type I transferred from cold sores. Several ulcers at vaginal introitus are characteristically seen in herpes.

Immediate management
If painful give strong analgesia.

Treatment of choice
Analgesia, lidocaine gel 2%, salt baths (and micturating in the bath) help. Aciclovir topically and 200 mg 5 times daily PO for 5 days shortens symptoms and infectivity.

Reassure the patient that subsequent attacks are shorter and less painful.

Your Notes:

161. Man involved in road traffic accident is found to have comminuted fractures of the tibia and fibula. He develops rapid swelling of the lower limb below the knee. Arterial pulses are absent below the knee.

Diagnosis: Compartment syndrome.

Clinchers
- *Comminuted fractures of tibia and fibula:* A comminuted fracture will cause much more swelling and local inflammation than a simple fracture. Also polytrauma usually causes obstructed venous outflow from a compartment.
- *Rapid swelling of the lower limb below the knee:* Swelling of the leg in any compartment of the leg produces the pressure to rise gradually within the compartment. The situation is compounded by an obstructed venous outflow from the compartment due to trauma. When the pressure reaches a critical level any nerves passing through the compartment cease to function, causing paraesthesiae intially, followed by loss of sensation in the area supplied by nerve. As the pressure continues to rise, tissue perfusion may cease, particularly in the muscles, and rarely a point can be reached when the pressure rises above arterial level and all structures within the compartment rises above arterial level and all structures within the compartment becomes ischaemic.

CONFUSA
Since the fractures involve both tibial compartment and fibular compartment, there will be no arterial pulses on either side. Otherwise the findings are limited to the affected compartment only.

Investigation of choice
Measure intracompartmental pressures using a simple manometer (pressure higher than 30 mmHg are an indication for urgent decompression).

Immediate management
Orthopaedics referral.

Treatment of choice
Immediate decompression by fasciotomy to prevent impending muscle necrosis and to save the leg (since evn arterial pulses are blocked, the intracompartmental pressure must be much higher than 30 mmHg).

Your Notes:

162. An elderly male develops pain in his thigh and leg when walking for approximately 20 metres. This pain resolves with rest. He is a long time smoker. In examination his dorsalis pedis pulse on the affected side is absent.

Diagnosis: Buerger's disease (thromboangiitis obliterans).

Clinchers

- *Elderly:* The disorder develos most frequently in men under 40. The prevalence is higher in Asians and individual of eastern european descent.
- *Pain in his thigh and leg when walking for approximately 20 meters:* This is claudication and 20 meters is the claudication distance. Buerger's disease presents as a triad of claudication of the affected extremity, Raynaud's phenomenon, and migratory superficial vein thrombophlebitis. Claudication is usually confined to the lower calves and feet or the forearms and hands, because this disorder primarily affects distal vessels.
- *Pain resolves with rest:* A hallmark of caludication.
- *Long-time smokers:* While the cause of Buerger's disease is unknown there is a definite relationship to cigarette smoking and an increased incidence of HLA-B5 and A9 antigens in patients with this disorder.
- *Dorsalis pedis pulse absent:* The physical examination shows normal branchial and popliteal pulses but reduced or absent radial, ulnar, and/or tibial and dorsalis pedis pulses.

CONFUSA
Buerger's disease can be clinically indistinguishable from atheromatous peripheral vascular disease.

Investigation of choice
- *Screening:* Arteriography
- *Definitive:* Biopsy

Immediate management
Local debridement if gangrene is present.

Treatment of choice
Advise stop smoking and exercise. The prognosis is worst in patients who continue to smoke.

Your Notes:

163. A 70-year-old with known atrial fibrillation on treatment dvelops a sudden cold leg. Pulses are absent in the level at and below the knee.

Diagnosis: Femoral artery emboli.

Clinchers

- *Known atrial fibrillation:* Emboli commonly arise from the heart secondary to atrial fibrillation and infarcts.
- *Develops a sudden cold leg:* Sings or symptoms of acute leg ischaemia due to emboli are described by six Ps—the part is pale, pulseness, painful, paralysed, paraesthetic and perishing with cold. All these symptoms can be explained by occlusion of the arterial supply.
- *Pulses are absent in the levell at and below the knee:* it indicates that the site of occlusion by emboli is above popliteal artery, i.e. in superficial femoral artery.

CONFUSA
The other common source of leg emboli an aneurysm (aorta, femoral or popliteal). So perform an extensive clinical examination to rule it out.

Investigation of choice
Urgent arteriography (only if diagnosis in doubt).

Immediate management
Urgent surgical referral.

Treatment of choice
Femoral embolectomy (Fogarty catheter)
or
Local thrombolysis (t-PA)

Your Notes:

164. A 67-year-old male with a history of peripheral vascular disease develops sever ulceration and cellulitis in his left foot and extending up his left leg above the left ankle. The popliteal pulse is absent on that side. He has a history of ulceration on the contralateral side which resolved following a bypass graft operation on that side.

Diagnosis: Peripheral vascular disease (PVD) with gangrene.

Clinchers
- *67-year-old male:* It chiefly occurs over the age of 50 years, chiefly in men.
- *Severe ulceration and cellulitis in his left foot and extending up his left leg above the left ankle:* Ulceration and gangrene of the affected limb is prsent in severe disease. It usually start at the toes.
- *Popliteal pulse absent:* There are diminished or absent pulses to diseased areas. The limb is cold with dry skin and lack of hair due to chronic ischaemia.
- *History of ucleration on contralateral side which resolved following a bypass graft operation:* Aortoiliac bypass grafts give good results in PVD. Aslo PVD is usually bilateral.

> **CONFUSA**
> Atherosclerotic PVD can be easily confused clinically with Buerger's diseases, but in Buerger's disease, the popliteal pulse is almost always present. Also patients with atherosclerotic PVD usually have symptomatic ischaemic heart disease.

Investigation of choice
Arteriography.

Immediate management
Urgent surgical referral.

Treatment of choice
Amputation is necessary for severely ischaemic limbs, usually those with gangrene (as in this case).

Note: Bypass operations are not done till 3 months after an acute attack (to let a collateral circulation develop).

Your Notes:

---

165. A 55-year-old man complains of intermittent pain in his toe on walking. He says that in addition it looks 'white'.

Diagnosis: Peripheral vascular disease (PVD).

Clinchers
- *55-year-old:* Patients with arterial disease tend to be elderly and have generalised atherosclerosis.
- *Intermittent pain on walking:* This is intermittent claudication, the hallmark of PVD. It is typically relieved by rest (except in severe disease, where it may be present at rest).
- *Toe looks 'white':* It is due to arterial narrowing and decreased perfusion of the toe.

> **CONFUSA**
> Arterial diseases produces white toes or feet, while venous disease will produce blue extremities (cyanosis). Arterial diseases, when minimal can be demonstrated by mild exercise. Exercise produces vasodilatation below the obstructing lesion and the arterial, inflow, reduced by the lesion, cannot keep pace with the increasing vascular shape, arterial pressure falls and the pulse disappears producing the white limb or toe.
> Some important points in PVD differential diagnosis:
> - PVD symptoms in young females—suspect Raynaud's disease
> - PVD symptoms in young males—suspect Buerger's disease
> - PVD symptoms in migraine patient—suspect ergotamine overdose
> - PVD symptoms in TIA patient—suspect atherosclerosis

Investigation of choice
- *Screening:* Ankle branchial pressure index (ABPI)
  - Resting value is 1.0
  - < 0.9 signify some degree of arterial obstruction
  - < 0.5 signify severe ischaemia
  - < 0.3 signify imminent necrosis
- *Definitive:* Arteriography.

Immediate management
Detailed work up to rule out diabetes and coronary artery disease.

Treatment of choice
If claudication is a significant handicap to the patient, the possibility of reconstructive surgery or angiographic intervention should be considered.

166. A 33-year-old boxer who complains of left sided weakness 24 hours after a boxing match.

Diagnosis: Subdural hematoma.

Clinchers
- *Boxer:* Bridging veins in the cranium weakens in boxers because they sustain regular blows to the head. This increases the risk of their rupture and hence the formation of a subdural hematoma.
- *24 hours after a boxing match:* Subdural hematomas usually have an insiduous and delayed presenation (subdural is subdned) because the bleeding is venous and through very small vessels. They can present even weeks or months later.
- *Left sided weakness:* Focal neurological signs appear once the hematoma short behaving like a space occupying lesion in brain.

CONFUSA
Other risk groups for subdural hematoma are:
- Alcoholics (due to recurrent falls)
- Elderly (due to cortical shrinkage)

Investigation of choice
CT skull ("concave inside" lesion).

Immediate management
A complete neurological assessment + decrease ICT.

Treatment of choice
Evacuation (sugical) of hematoma.

Your Notes:

167. An 18-year-old man who has sustained stab wounds to his abdomen and trunk. His respiratory rate is 23 breaths/min, his breath sounds appear normal but his pulse is 142/min and his BP is only 80/40 mm Hg.

Diagnosis: Hypovolemic shock.

Clinchers
- *Stab wounds in abdomen and trunk:* Hemothorax and hemoperitoneum are the two conditions producing hypovolemic shock by internal bleeding. This person is at risk of both.
- *Respiratory rate is 23 breaths/min:* Tachypnoea is an early feature of hypovolemic shock.
- *Breath sounds normal:* This rules out haemothorax which can lead to absence of breath sounds on affected side.
- *Pulse rate is 142/min:* Tachycardia is also a characteristic feature of circulatory failure due to shock.
- *BP is only 80/40 mm Hg:* This signifies that the blood loss is significant and requires urgent resuscitation.

CONFUSA
It is very important to remember that in a young and fit person (like this man of 18 years age), BP can remain stable even upto loss of 30% of circulating blood volume (though the pulse pressure will fall).

Investigation of choice
Ultrasound (abdomen)
Note: Peritoneal lavage is often indicated in older textbooks but rarely indicated.

Immediate management
Colloid infusion followed by infusion of crossmatched blood (or "O-ve" blood in emergency).

Treatment of choice
Urgent explorative laparotomy.

Your Notes:

168. A 48-year-old woman complains of left shoulder and neck pain after having fallen off her bicycle. She has a graze on her forehead and also complains of tingling in her left ring and little fingers [digits IV and V].

Diagnosis: Cervical spine injury.

Clinchers
- *Fallen off her bicycle:* Cervical spine injury is more likely if the mobile head hits a fixed object (deceleration accleration) tha if a mobile object hits the fixed head (assault).
- *Left shoulder and neck pain:* It might be due to soft tissue injury she had sustained during the fall. Neck pain as such after trauma always require cervical spine injury to be excluded.
- *Graze on her forehead:* If it is anterior, suspect cervical joint dislocation/instability. If it is near the top of skull, suspect axial compression injury.
- *Tingling in her left ring and little fingers:* These indicated a lesion in the domain of ulnar nerve. Either an imminent cervical cord compression or injury to posterior root of ulnar nerve might be responsible.

CONFUSA
A normal neurological examination does not exclude cervical spine injury. Moreover, conscious patients with other painful injuries may not always complain of neck discomfort. So neck injury must be assumed to have occurred in all patients who have sustained polytrauma until clinical examination and good quality radiographs prove otherwise. So in a major trauma the first X-ray to be performed after resuscitation is a cross-table lateral of the cervical spine. All seven cervical vertebrae, including C8-T1 junction, must be seen.

Investigation of choice
Cervical spine X-ray
There are three standard views of the cervical spine in UK practice:
- Lateral view (90% sensitivity)
- Upper AP (open mouth or peg) view
- Lower AP view

Supplementation oblique views are used to visualize the apophyseal joints, looking for facet joint dislocation.

Immediate management
Neck immobilization immediately with a well-fitting hard collar and a purpose-build head holder (except in situations where the patient struggles violently—a collar above will do here).

Treatment of choice
Skull traction × 6 weeks.

169. A 28-year-old motorcyclist has been involved in an accident and complains of loss of sensation below the umbilicus and paralysis of both legs. His BP is 80/50 mm Hg with a pulse rate of 72/min.

Diagnosis: Neurogenic shock (spinal shock)

Clinchers
- *Motor cyclist:* Most serious injuries in RTAs are sustained by motrocyclists. Injuries of head, thorax and legs are more frequent in them.
- *Loss of sensation below the umbilicus and paralysis of both legs:* This suggest cord compression at T_{10} level (as umbilicus is supplied by T_{10} dermatome). There is complete anaesthesia and flaccid paralysis of all segments and muscles innervated below the level affected. Tendon reflexes are absent and there is retention of urine.
- *BP is 80/150 mmHg:* Hypotension in neurogenic shock is not due to hypovolemia but due to sympathetic interruption below the lesion.
- *Pulse rate at 72/min:* Pulse rate is always normal in neurogenic shock.

CONFUSA
Neurogenic shock is the only "shock" in which tachycardia is absent. The thoracic spine lesions are more likely to be complete than cervical and lumbar lesions because of least free space between cord and canal. Also it has the poorest blood supply. Ischaemic injury often spreads below the level of mechanical injury.

Investigation of choice
MRI spine (around T_{10} level)

Immediate management
Arrange early and expert transfer to a spinal injuries unit after proper immobilization (in semiprone position).

Treatment of choice
Surgical decompression
+
Methylprednisolone
(started within 8 hours of trauma).

Your Notes:

170. A 55-year-old roofer complains of lower back pain radiating into the right leg having fallen from a scaffold. He has no loss of power or sensation when examined.

Diagnosis: Lumbar fracture

Clinchers

- *55-year-old:* Elderlies can have osteoporotic bones which can fracture on slightest trauma or spontaneously. Spine, especially lumbar region, is most prone to sustain on osteoporotic fracture.
- *Lower back pain radiating into right leg:* Trapped nerve roots of lumbar plexus can lead to pain in right leg. Lower back pain is directly attributable to the presence of fracture in that region.
- *Having fallen from a scaffold:* This is the reason for his lumbar fracture. He is entitled to compensation under UK laws as this injury qualifies as a professional hazard.
- *No loss of power or sensation:* Lumbar fractures are not usually associated with paraplegia, but they are variably unstable, so neurological deficits can be a complication anytimy.

CONFUSA

In the absence of any neurological deficit a plain X-ray should be the first investigation. Subsquently a CT scan or MRI can be done to assess the stability of the injured vertebra and integrity of the spinal canal.

Investigation of choice
X-ray lumbar spine.

Immediate management
Orthopaedics (spinal injury unit) referral.

Treatment of choice
If there is no paraplegia, external support with a moulded polythene or plaster jacket until union occurs is adequate.

Your Notes:

171. A couple aged 25 years have been trying for a baby for six months.

Diagnosis: Normal

Clinchers

- *Trying for a baby for six months:* Infertility cannot be a diagnosis before one year of unprotected intercourse in healthy couples of child-bearing age. Usually 80% couples achieve a pregnancy after 12 months and 90% after two years (in young couples it is 90% within one year).
- *25 years age:* Infertility decreases with age, but this is a young couple and this age factor is ruled out. They must be given more time to try for a baby.

CONFUSA

Infertility is a symptom and not a diagnosis. High fertility in one partner can compensate low fertility in the other. Investigations of infertility can be a tremendous strain on patients. So, sympathetic management is crucial.

Investigation of choice
Infertility investigations are not initiated before one year.

Immediate management
Reassurance.

Treatment of choice
None.

Your Notes:

172. Useful in determining ovulation.

Diagnosis: Day 21 progesterone.

Clinchers
Tests for ovulation are often asked in the themes on investigation of infertility. So lets discuss them.
> *Indication:* Infertility with regular menstrual cycles.
  Eamples:
  - *USG:* Visualization of follicle development or change to secretory endometrium
  - *Midcycle mucus test:* Ovulatory mucus is like raw egg white.
  - *Clear plan kit:* detects LH surge
  - *21 day progesterone test:* detect a luteal rise in progesterone to >30 nmol/L 7 days before the onset of menstruation at 21st day.
  - *BBT:* Detecting a rise in basal body temperature at midcycle.

CONFUSA
The only proof of ovulation is pregnancy. It is possible for a follicle to luteinize without rupturing, so tests may be positive in the absence of an ovum. Negative results imply failure to ovulate.

Investigation of choice
Day 21 progesterone test is the best test.

Your Notes:

173. An essential investigation for all heterosexual infertile couples.

Diagnosis: Semen analysis.

Clinchers
Semen analysis is an essential investigation and can be perforemd in a primary care setting.

Requirements:
- 3 days abstinence
- Two samples at one month interval

Normal values in semen analysis:
- Volume—mean 2.75 ml
- Count > 20 million sperm/mL
- Mortility > 40% motile
- Form > 60% normal morphology

Impaired sperm production can be a side effect of:
- Psychotropic drugs
- Antiepileptics
- Antihypertensive
- Chemotherapy

CONFUSA
A satisfactory postcoital test can obviate the need for a semen analysis, so it should be done first.
Interesting fact: Mean sperm count is 66 million/mL and this is falling at a rate of 100 sperms/mL/hour worldwide.

Immediate management
Reduced counts require specialist referral.

Your Notes:

May—2002

174. This investigation is of little value in infertility.

Diagnosis: Bacteriological examination of urine.

Clinchers
It is a non-specific question, so let us see the role of pelvic inflammatory diseases and venereal diseases in causing infertility.

Tubal dysfunction: If affects the normal transport of oocyte and embryo. PID is a major cause of tubal infertility. Sexually transmitted diseases with chlamydia-trachomatis, gonococci and other microorganisms may lead to tubal damage (*Chlamydia* is most common). Tuberculosis is a leading cause of tubal damage in developing countries.

CONFUSA
Either acute or chronic urinary tract infections rarely produce infertility. Bacteriological examination of urine can tell about any UTI but signify almost nothing about a possible cause of infertility.

Your Notes:

175. It is an essential investigation of the female partner.

Diagnosis: Tubal patency test.

Clinchers
It is an essential investigation as it is important to exclude tubal causes which account to 14% cases of infertility. It interfers with meeting of sperm and ova and assisted reproductive technique may required to help in conception. Main tests of tubal patency are:
1. Laproscopy with dye
2. Hysterosalpingogram (constant X-ray)
3. High contrast ultrasonography (HyCoSy)

Note:
- HyCoSy is a modern, ultrasound based investigation using a negative (normal saline) and positive (Echovist) contrast media to outline the uterine cavity and fallopian tubes, tubal patency and avoid exposure to X-rays.
- Hysterosalpingogram is done within first ten days of menstruation in order to avoid inadvertent exposure of the early embryo to X-rays.

CONFUSA
Tubal patency tests are same of the few investigations in context of infertility that yield a definitive result and are potentially remediable. That makes them essential to either exclude or treat.

Investigation of choice
HyCoSy.

Immediate management
Reassurance.

Treatment of choice
Tubal problems may be remedied by surgery but the results are poor. So in-vitro fertilization (IVF) is a better option.

Note: Gamete intrafallopian transfer (GIFT) can be used only when tubes are potent.

Your Notes:

176. A 23-year-old woman develops an acute pain in her right chest radiating to her right shoulder associated with a fever. She is vomiting and has mild yellowing of her skin.

Diagnosis: Acute cholecystitis

Clinchers

- *23-year-old woman:* Female sex is a definitive risk factor for gallstones. Acute cholecystitis follows stone impaction in the neck of gallbladder.
- *Acute pain:* The pain may begin suddenly but is then constant and very severe.
- *Pain in right chest radiating to her right shoulder:* There is constant right upper quadrant pain referred to back and shoulder.
- *Fever:* Pyrexia and malaise are commonly part of the presentation.
- *Vomiting:* Nausea and vomiting are almost always present.
- *Mid yellowing of skin:* Obstructive jaundice may be present as the common causes of acute cholecystitis in a female are biliary calculi.

CONFUSA
Acute pancreatitis usually do not occur as commonly in young females. Pyrexia is uncommon in it. It is more characterised by tachycardia and cyanosis due to hypovolemic shock (third space sequestration of fluids).

Investigation of choice
Early USG

Immediate management
Analgesia and admission.

Treatment of choice
Cefuroxime 1.5 g/8 h IV.

In suitable cases, do cholecystectomy within 48 hours (laparoscopic if no question of GB perforation). Otherwise operate after 3 months.

Your Notes:

---

177. A tall young man developed sharp chest pain on his right, following a road traffic accident. On palpation, this area is tender. A chest X-ray shows his lungs are not injured.

Diagnosis: Fracture rib.

Clinchers

- *Tall young man:* Nothing of much significance in this question.
- *RTA:* Fracture ribs result from direct blows or falls an are a common component of polytrauma in RTAs.
- *Tender on palpation:* It is present in the area of fracture and is inevitable. Moreover there is pain on inspiration and coughing along with considerable difficulty with trunk movements.
- *Lungs are not injured (on CXR):* The chest should be examined thoroughly to exclude underlying pneumo/haemothorax and contusion in any case of rib fracture. A clear CXR rules out these

CONFUSA
A chest X-ray (CXR) is mandatory in the presence of dyspnoea or past history of respiratory problems. There are usually more tibs fractured than you can easily see on the X-ray. Multiple rib fractures on an adults CXR usually indicate past episodes of alcohol abuse; in case of a child—nonaccidental injury should be considered.

Investigation of choice
Chest X-ray.

Immediate management
Analgesia.

Treatment of choice
> 3 ribs fractured:
- High concentration O_2 by mask
- Monitor SaO_2, BP, ECG, respiratory rate and blood gases
- Request anaesthetic opinion for intensive care

< 3 ribs fractured: Exclude underlying problems and respiratory difficulties and discharge with adequate analgesia.

Your Notes:

178. A 23-year-old male prostitute develops severe chest pain. This area of chest pain corresponds to an area with an erythematous rash.

Diagnosis: Herpes Zoster (shingles)

Clinchers

- *Male prostitute:* Undiagnosed HIV infection may be present (acquired as a professional hazard) which has caused reactivation of the Herpes virus lying dormant in ganglion cells. The etiology of the primary herpes infection can also be similar.
- *Severe chest pain:* Pain heralds infection and may precede the development of vesicles by 48-72 hrs. It is severe and burning in character. Thoracic dermatomes and ophthalmic division of trigeminal are most vulnerable.
- *Pain corresponds to an area with an erythematous rash:* Herpes zoster is characterised by a unilateral vesicular eruption within a dermatome accompanied by severe local pain. Vesicles start as erythematous maculopapules.

CONFUSA
Motor nerves are rarely affected in shingles and almost all the symptoms are sensory. Other high risk group for shingles are elderly people.

Investigation of choice
- Rarely necessary for shingles
- HIV seropositivity tests (after consent)

Immediate management
Aciclovir (start as early as possible) + refer to pain clinic.

Treatment of choice
- Pain—oral analgesic or low dose amitryptiline
- Virus—Aciclovir
- Post herpetic neuralgia prophylaxis—4 week course of prednisolone.

Your Notes:

---

179. A 69-year-old man develops crushing chest pain associated with nausea and profuse sweating radiating to the neck. By the time he gets to the hospital [quarter of an hour later] the pain is gone.

Diagnosis: Angina pectoris

Clinchers
Angina pectoris, the most common clinical manifestation of coronary artery disease, results from an imbalance between myocardial O_2 supply and demand, most commonly resulting from atherosclerotic coronary artery aneurysm.

- *69-year-old man:* Angina, like other common heart ailments, increase in incidence with age.
- *Crushing chest pain:* It may present variably as a central chest tightness or heaviness, crushing chest (more like MI). Usually it is precipitated by exertion and relieved by rest.
- *Nausea and profuse sweating:* Associated symptoms of an acute attack are: dyspnoea, nausea, vomiting, sweatiness, faintness.
- *Radiating to neck:* The pain may radiate to
  - One/both arms
  - Neck
  - Jaw
  - Teeth

CONFUSA
The main clinical criterion to differentiate between severe episode of angina and MI (myocardial infarction) is the duration of pain. If the pain is for more than 20 minutes (OHCM, 104) it qualifies as MI. All other characteristics and associations of the pain are same in both conditions.

Investigation of choice
- ECG (usually normal, may show ST depression)
- If resting ECG normal—do exercise ECG

Immediate management
GTN spray/sublingual tablet for an acute attack.

Treatment of choice
Aspirin (75-150 mg/24 h)
+
According to angina guidelines in UK.

Your Notes:

180. Minutes after upper GI endoscopy a 57-year-old man develops chest pain. When you examine him, he has a crackling feeling under the skin around his upper chest and neck.

Diagnosis: Ruptured oesophagus

Clinchers
- *Minutes after upper GI endoscopy:* Oesophageal injury is a well recognised complication of upper GI endoscopy. The most common site of perforation is the level of cricopharyngeus.
- *57-year-old man:* Elderly people have a lax musculature of oesophagus which is more prone to perforation by instrumentation or rupture by repeated vomiting against a closed glottis (Boerhaave's syndrome).
- *Chest pain:* After instrumentation, perforation is suspected if the patient complains of pain in the neck, chest or upper abdomen. Pyrexia and dysphagia are also present. Consider oesophageal perforation if there is:
  - Inexplicable shock after trunk injury
  - Left pneumothorax without rib fracture
  - Gastric contents in a chest drain
- *Crackling feeling under the skin around his upper chest and neck:* This is subcutaneous emphysema and its location (i.e. supraclavicular) is pathognomic of oesophageal rupture. It is due to the gas escaping into the mediastinum.

CONFUSA
Since the site of pain in this patient is chest, this is most probably a thoracic rupture (usually instrumentation produce perforation in the neck). It is important to differentiate a thoracic rupture from a rupture in neck as the latter can be conservatively managed.

Investigation of choice
- *Screening:* Chest X-ray (mediastinal gas)
- *Definitive:* Gastrograffin swallow (a water soluble contrast fluid) will confirm the perforation and define its position.

Immediate management
Crossmatch 10 units blood and inform surgeons.

Treatment of choice
Thoractomy and suturing of oesophagus (or resection if a carcinoma is instrumentally perforated).

Your Notes:

181. A 35-year-old woman complains of abdominal discomfort relieved by passing flatus or- defecation. Over the last 6 months she has had episodes of diarrhoea and constipation, but denied she had lost weight. Her mother died of bowel carcinoma.

Diagnosis: Irritable bowel syndrome (IBS).

Clinchers
- *35-year-old woman:* Patients of IBS are usually between 20-40 years and females are more frequently affected.
- *Abdominal discomfort relieved by flatus or defecation:* This is a very important point. This supports the diagnosis of IBS. Other important history is the sensation of incomplete evacuation and the passage of mucus.
- *Episode of diarrhoea and constipation:* Altered bowel habits (constipation alternating with diarrhoea) present in IBS.
- *Since last 6 months:* These symptoms must be present for atleast 3 months, before the diagnose of IBS could be established.
- *No history of weight loss:* Helps to exclude carcinoma.

Investigation of choice
Flexible sigmoidscopy: In over 48 years to exclude colonic neoplasm. In younger patients exclude inflammatory bowel disease.

Treatment of choice
Though there is no treatment for IBS, focus on dietary modification with fiber supplements. Treatment should be directed to the predominant symptom.

Your Notes:

182. A 37-year-old woman presents with a sudden onset of severe left iliac fossa pain. On vaginal USG, 2 cm echogenic masses are seen in the broad ligament. She says this pain seems to come every month.

Diagnosis: Endometriosis

Clinchers

- *37-year-old woman:* Endometriosis is typically seen in those with postmenstrual exposure, common in fourth decade of life.
- *Severe left iliac fossa pain (comes every month):* Pelvic pain classically cyclical at the time if periods is the most common symptoms. Periods are usually heavy and frequent.
- *On USG, 2 cm echogenic masses seen in broad ligament:* Foci if endometrial tissue may be found on an ovary, rectovaginal pouch, uterosacral ligaments, surface if pelvic peritoneum, broad ligament and sometimes in distant organs like lungs.
- *On vaginal examination*
  - Fixed retroverted uterus
  - Nodules in uterosacral ligament
  - General tenderness.

Investigation of choice
Laproscopy shows
- Types cysts
- Peritoneal deposits

Treatment of choice
- Danazol 400-800 mg OD
- Gestrinone 2.5-5 mg PO twice weekly
- Buserelin/goserelin (LHRH analyses)

Surgical local exicision or diathermy of endometriotic tissue or hysterectomy may depend upon site of lesion and women's with for future fertility.

Your Notes:

183. A 23-year-old woman just had an intrauterine device fitted. She complains of a watery brown vaginal discharge and abdominal pain.

Diagnosis: Pelvic inflammatory disease (PID).

Clinchers

- *Intrauterine device fitted:* 10% of cases of PID follow childbirth or instrumentation (insertion of IUCD, TOP) though 90% are sexually acquired (mostly due to *Chlamydia*).
- *Watery brown vaginal discharge:* PID present with abdominal pain and vaginal discharge. Discharge is come times profuse and purulent, or it may be bloody. These is spasm of lower abdominal muscles.
  In chronic cases abdominal mass may also be palpated because the inflammation leads to fibrosis, so adhesions develop between pelvic organs.

Investigation of choice
Endocervical and urethral swabs if practicable. Always check for chlamydia. Go for blood culture if febrile.

Immediate management
Admit for blood culture and IV antibiotics if very unwell.

Treatment of choice
Page 50 (OHCS), 5th edn.

Your Notes:

184. An 18 weeks pregnant female presents with lower abdominal pain and tenderness, with offensive vaginal discharge. She has high grade fever since last two days.

Diagnosis: Septic abortion

Clinchers
- *Lower abdominal pain:* In this question this pain may be due to pelvic infection.
- *Offensive vaginal discharge with high grade fever:* This point towards the infection (probably uterus). To support the diagnosis of septic abortion, fever more than 38°C for more than 24 hours (with or withour chills and rigors) should be present. Offensive and purulent vaginal discharge support the diagnosis of infection.
Majority of infection occurs following illegal induced abortion (rare in UK) in developing countries.
Any abortion associated with clinical evidence of infection of the uterus and it content is called septic abortion.

Investigation of choice
Cervical or high vaginal swab for culture. Ultrasonography.

Treatment of choice
Hospitalization. Aim at
- To control sepsis
- Remove source of infection
- Supportive therapy

Go for analgesia, sedatives and antibiotics.

Your Notes:

185. A 32-year-old who conscientiously uses the oral contraceptive pill, has experienced monthly vaginal bleeding. On abdominal examination she is comfortable. Her temperature is 37°C. She is otherwise healthy.

Diagnosis: Break through bleeding.

Clinchers
- *Conscientiously uses—OCP:* It means she is a regular in taking the pills.
- *Monthly vaginal bleeding:* Menstruation is initiated by the withdrawal of oestrogen and progesterone. Such as effect is produced in women receiving oestrogens and progestogens in the form of the combined contraceptive pill or hormone replcement therapy—withdrawal bleeding on completion of a pack.
- *On abdominal examination she is comfortable:* This rules out any pelvic inflammatory disease. Otherwise also OCP use decreases the risk of PID. The only infection whose incidence is increased by using OCP is monoilial vaginitis (candidiasis).

CONFUSA
Intermenstrual spotting is common in the first three months of the start of the pills, but it gradaully disappears. Heavy spotting can be stopped by increasing the dose for a few months.

Investigation of choice
None required.

Immediate management
Reassurance.

Treatment of choice
None required.

Your Notes:

186. A patient in her third pregnancy presents to her GP at 12 weeks gestation. She was mildly hypertensive in both of her previous pregnancies. Her BP is 150/100 mm Hg. Two weeks later at the hospital antenatal clinic her BP is 150/95 mm Hg.

Diagnosis: Essential hypertension (EH)

Clinchers

> *Third pregnancy:* EH is common in older multiparas, and present before pregnancy or in first trimester (in this case 12 weeks).
> *Mildly hypertensive in both of her previous pregnancies:* Those with EH are five times more likely to develop pre-eclampsia. Also increased BP is a positive risk factor for PIH.
> *BP is 150/100 mmHg, two weeks later 150/95 mmHg:* Isolated BP measurements are never reliable in pregnancy. So BP has to be recorded on at least two occasions (at least >4 hrs apart) to make a diagnosis. In this case the BP is more of less the smae on two occasions (two weeks apart). Also the diastolic BP is > 90 mmHg on both occasions.

CONFUSA
If the symptoms are episodic, think of phaeochromocytoma. PIH by definition does not present before 20 weeks for the first-time.

Investigation of choice
24 hours urinary proteins (to screen for pre-eclampsia).

Immediate management
BP monitoring (biweekly).

Treatment of choice
Oral antihypertensive (as BP should be kept < 140/90 mmHg).

Your Notes:

---

187. A 22-year-old Nigerian woman has an uneventful first pregnancy to 30 weeks. She is then admitted as an emergency with epigastric pain. During the first two hours her BP rises from 150/105 to 170/120 mmHg. On dipstick test she is found to have 3+ proteinuria. The fetal cardiotocogram (CTG) is normal.

Diagnosis: Fulminating PIH.

Clinchers

> *First pregnancy:* 70% cases of pre-eclampsia occur in primigravidas. A recurrence rate of 20% is present for multigravidas (with same partner). With a new partner the incidence of recurrence increases.
> *30 weeks:* By definition PIH present for the first-time after 20 weeks.
> *Epigastric pain:* It is due to stretching of liver capsule.
> *PB rises from 150/105 to 170/120 mmHg in two hours:* A rapid rise in BP is a characteristic feature of fulminant PIH and require immediate IV antihypertensives.
> *3+ proteinuria:* It signifies significant proteinuria and hence qualifies for the diagnosis of fulminant PIH.
> *CTG is normal:* Abnormal CTG signifies fetal distress and warrants an immediate caesarean section. In this case it is not required as CTG is normal. Still regular CTG monitoring (1 to 2 per day of one hour each) must be done.

CONFUSA
In severe (fulminating) PIH, delivery is the only definitive treatment (Note: PIH regress by delivery of placenta and not only fetus). The delivery is often vaginal, except in conditions given below where a caesarian section is preferred (A B C D E)
  A—Abruption
  B—BP unctrollable; breech
  C—Cervix unfavourable
  D—Distress of fetus
  E—Error in induction of delivery (failed induction)
Note: Delivery criteria in PIH
  Mild PIH—can continue till 40 weeks
  Moderate PIH—can continue till 37 weeks
  Severe PIH—as soon as possible
  and eclampsia

Investigation of choice
CTG (already done in this case).

Immediate management
IV hydralazine/Labetalol.

Treatment of choice
Intravenous antihypertensive (hydralazine/labetalol) immediately + Regular monitoring

188. At an antenatal clinic visit at 38 weeks gestation, a 36-year-old multiparous woman has a BP of 140/90 mmHg. She has no proteinuria and is otherwise well.

Diagnosis: Normal.

Clinchers
- *38 weeks gestation:* PIH usually present in the second trimester and not this late.
- *36-year-old:* Age > 35 years (or < 20 years) is a positive risk factor for PIH/eclampsia.
- *Multiparous:* Usually multiparous females are not affected by PIH if there is no history of it in the previous pregnancies.
- *BP 140/90 mmHg:* By definition the diastolic BP has to cross 90 to qualify for a diagnosis of PIH. The classification criteria of PIH are given in next question (Q 189). This BP does not classify as a criteria for diagnosis.
- *No proteinuria:* Excludes pre-eclampsia/severe PIH.
- *Otherwise well:* Excludes other medical disorders.

CONFUSA
In cases of PIH (pregnancy induced hypertension), admit if
- BP rises by >30/20 mmHg over booking BP
- BP reaches
  - 160/100 without proteinuria
  - 140/90 with proteinuria

PIH can be diagnosed only with BP elevation above in criteria on at least 2 occasions (> 4 hours apart).

Investigation of choice
Biweekly BP monitoring.

Immediate management
Take second BP measurement after four hours.

Treatment of choice
A period of observation for blood pressure.

Your Notes:

---

189. At 32 weeks, a 22-year-old primigravida is found to have a BP of 145/100 mmHg. She has no proteinuria but is found to have edema of her knees.

Diagnosis: Pregnancy induced hypertension (PIH).

Clinchers
- *32 weeks:* By definition PIH called so only if it appears for first-time after 20 weeks. Hypertension occurring before is usually due to an existing and non-pregnancy induced condition.
- *Primigravida:* PIH is an almost exclusive disease of primigravidas.
- *BP of 145/100 mmHg with no proteinuria:* PIH is classified according to BP and proteinuria.
  Mild PIH—BP upto 140/100 without proteinuria
  Moderate PIH—BP upto 160/110 without proteinuria
  Severe PIH—BP more than 160/110 with proteinuria
  (Proteinuria is > 300 mg excretion of proteins in urine in 24 hours).
- *Oedema of her knees:* Peripheral edema in pregnancy has little significance if it occurs as an isolated finding. But it signifies severe PIH if it occurs along with hypertension and proteinuria.

CONFUSA
PIH is almost exclusively seen in primigravidas. But in multiparous women its risk is increased if the existing pregnancy is with a new partner. Other risk factors for PIH in multigravidas are: history of first pregnancy, H. mole, multiple pregnancy, gestational diabetes mellitus.

Investigation of choice
Fetal USG.

Immediate management
Admit in first instance for assessment and monitoring.

Treatment of choice
Since the disease in question is a moderate PIH, its management is:
- Care in day assessment until/hospital
- Oral antihypertensives if—BP > 160/100 (sustained)
  Note: It is > 170/110 according to OHCS.
- Can continue upto 37 weeks with regular monitoring of:
  Daily—urinary proteins
  Bi-weekly—LFT
  Weekly—Plasma U and E, plasma urate, total urinary proteins.

Indications of delivery in moderate disease
- Progression to pre-eclampsia
- Declining maternal renal function
- Fetal distress
  - Abnormal CTG (cardiotocogram)
  - Absence of end diastolic flow in doppler of umbilical circulation
- Placental abruption.

Your Notes:

190. At 34 weeks, an 86 kg woman complains of persistent headaches and 'flashing lights'. There is no hyperreflexia and her BP is 150/100 mmHg. Urinalysis is negative but she has finger edema.

Diagnosis: Pre-eclampsia

Clinchers

Preclampsia is a syndrome of sings and when the symptoms occurs, it is usually too late.

➢ *34 weeks:* It develops after 20 weeks and usually resolves within 10 days of delivery.

➢ *86 kg woman:* Predisposing factors of pre-eclampsia are

Maternal	Fetal
• Primiparity • History of severe pre-eclampsia • Positive family history • Height <155 cm • Overweight • Age < 20 or > 35 yrs • Pre-existing migraine • BP ↑ or renal disease	• H mole • Multiple pregnancy • Placental hydrops (e.g. Rh disease)

➢ *Persisting headaches:* Frontal>occipital, reason is cerebral edema. It is of dragging/throbbing type
  - Worsen on
    - Supine position
    - Morning
  - Resolves on—mobility

➢ *Flashing lights:* Visual symptoms are common in pre-eclampsia. They are due to edema of neural layer in retina.
  The most common visual symptoms are
  - Black holes
  - Double vision
  - Flashing lights

➢ *No hyperreflexia:* Hyperreflexia is said to be present when a reflex can be obtained away from the tendon that usually causes it, e.g. knee reflex by tapping anterior surface of tibia (rather than the tendon). It is an important sign of impending eclampsia.

➢ *BP is 150/100:* A diastolic BP exceeding 90 mmHg on at least two occasions in the second half of pregnancy, where the blood pressure was previously normal, accompanied by significant proteinuria (> 300 mg/24 h) qualifies for a diagnosis of pre-eclampsia.

➢ *Urinalysis negative:* It means no proteinuria. Proteinuria is the last feature of pre-eclampsia to appear. It may be trace or at times coupious. There may be few hyaline casts, epithelial cells or even few red cells. It is considered significant only when >300 mg/24 h.

Proteinuria may also be missed in an isolated urinary examination, so do a 24 hours total urinary protein excretion measurement to rule it out.
- *Finger oedema:* Traditionally the presence of peripheral oedema has been included in the definition, however, this is a common finding in otherwise normal pregnancy and its absence does not preclude the diagnosis (nor does its presence makes the diagnosis). However, tightness of the ring on the finger (finger oedema) is an early manifestation of pre-eclampsia oedema. Gradually the swelling may extend to face, abdominal wall, vulva and even the whole body.

CONFUSA
In the UK, high quality antenatal care has reduced the problems of pre-eclamptic toxaemia to such an extent that 75% of cases of eclampsia now occur in the post-partum period and a similar proportion occur without pre-existing hypertension.

Investigation of choice
24 hours urinary protein.

Immediate management
BP control by IB hydralazine/Labetalol if there is an acute or progressive increase in BP.

Treatment of choice
Oral antihypertensive are given in case of sustained rise of BP till > 160/100 mmHg or at lower levels if cerebral edema is present (i.e. in this case). Antihypertensives that can be uses are;
- Methyldopa—contraindicated in liver disease
- Labetalol—contraindicated in asthma
- Magnesium sulfate—(preferred drug in USA)

Your Notes:

191. A 35-year-old man presents with pain in the right eye, vomiting and loss of vision.

Diagnosis: Acute glaucoma

Clinchers
- *Painful loss of vision:* In this question the presentation seems to be acute. Let us see the causes of sudden painful loss of vision.
  - Acute congenital glaucoma
  - Acute iridocyclitis
  - Chemical/mechanical injuries to the eyeball
- *Vomiting:* Severe pain in eye with loss of vision associated is the typical attack of acute congestive glaucoma.

CONFUSA
In iridocyclitis there is painful deterioration of vision, along with circumcorneal congestion. The onset is usually gradual. Moreover history of coloured haloes is present in glaucoma and not in iridocyclitis.

Immediate management
Injectable analgesics (pethidine) to releive pain. Systemic hyperosmotics (mannitol IV) given initially to lower IOP.

Treatment of choice
It is essential surgical. However, medical therapy is instituted as an emergency and temporary measure before the eye is ready for operation.
Surgical treatment may consists of either
- peripheral iridectomy
- filtration surgery.

Your Notes:

192. A 55-year-old known diabetic and hypertensive wakes up in the morning with diminished vision.

Diagnosis: Retinal detachment (RD)

Clinchers

- *55-year-old:* RD is most common in 40-60 years of age.
- *Diabetic:* Diabetes induces a high retinal blood flow—microangiopathy in capillary, precapillary arterioles and venules—occlusion and leakage—ischaemia—new vessel formation in retina (proliferative retinopathy)—new vessels carry along them fibrous tissue—increased traction—seperation of neurosensory retina proper from pigment epithelium (as there are loosely attached)—retinal detachment.
- *Hypertensive:* It predisposes to accumulation of fluid beneath retina and a hypertensive retinopathy, both of which can potentially produce RD.
- *Wakes up in morning with diminished vision:* RD usually present as a sudden painless loss of vision.

CONFUSA

Only 50% of patients developing detachment have premonitary symptoms—flashing lights or the sensation of spots before the eyes as the retina has been abnormally stimulated prior to detachment. Detachment of lower half of the retina tends not to pull of the macula, whereas upper half detachments do (if the macula becomes detached, central vision is lost and does not recover completely even if the retina is successfully replaced). RD is sometimes described as a curtain falling over the vision.

Investigation of choice
Retinoscopy (grey opalescent retina, ballooning forward).

Immediate management
Urgent ophthalmology referral.

Treatment of choice
Scleral silicone implants, cryotherapy, pneumatic retinopathy or argon or laser coagulation.

Your Notes:

193. A 25-year-old man present to the accident and emergency department with pain in the right eye associated with backache.

Diagnosis: Uveitits.

Clinchers

- *25-year-old man:* Ankylosing spondylitis is more common in men, in second and third decades of life.
- *Pain in right eye with backache:* In ankylosing spondylitis patient (young man) typically presents with morning stiffness, backache, sacroiliac pain, progressive loss of spinal movement. Other features are uveitis, carditis, thoracic excursion ↓, chest pain, plantar fascitis, lung fibrosis, etc.
  Diagnosis is clinically supported by radiological findings. Though the clinical findings in this question are hard to find, but then this is what PLAB is all about.

Investigation of choice
Radiology.

Treatment of choice
Exercise not rest, for backache. NSAIDs may releive pain and stiffness. Rarely spinal osteotomy is useful.

Your Notes:

194. An elderly woman presents with a history of visual loss and scalp soreness.

Diagnosis: Cranial arteritis.

Clinchers
- Elderly woman: Cranial arteritis is rare under 55 years,
- History of visual loss and scalp soreness: Typical symptom of giant cell (cranial/temporal) arteritis are:
  - Headahe
  - Scalp tenderness (e.g. on combing hair)
  - Jaw claudication
  - Sudden blindness in one eye

Tests: ESR ↑, CRP ↑, platelets, alkaline phosphatase ↑ and Hb is decreased.

Investigation of choice
Erythrocyte sedimentation rate.

Immediate management
Start prednisolone 40-60 mg/24 hr PO immediately.

Treatment of choice
Reduce prednisolone after 5-7 days in light of symptoms and ESR.

Your Notes:

195. An elderly man who is an inpatient (for hypertension) wakes in the morning note that he cannot see his breakfast. He has no other complaints. He has a carotid bruit.

Diagnosis: Occipital lobe infarct.

Clinchers
- In patient (for hypertension): Elderly hypertensive is a risk factor for occipital lobe infant/stroke and myocardial incarction
  - Contralateral visual field defects (homonymous hemianopia) occur in occipital lesions.
- Carotid bruit: May signify stenosis (>30%) often near the internal carotid origin. Usual cause: arthroma.
- Cannot see his breakfast: Hypertensive patient with carotid bruit cannot see his breakfast in the morning as majority of the attacks occurs in early morning and on waking up.

Investigation of choice
Carotid Doppler.

Treatment of choice
If stenosis (carotid) is > 80%, go for surgery.

Your Notes:

196. A six-year-old boy complains of intermittent hip pain for several months. Hematological investigations are normal. X-rays show flattening of the femoral head.

Diagnosis: Perthes' disease (Legg-Calve-Perthes disease).

Clinchers

- *Six-year-old boy:* Perthes' disease is commonly present in the 3-11 years age group though the usual presentation is at age 4-7 years.

  It is more common in boys and about 15% cases are bilateral. There is a definite familiar tendency and the condition has been described in identical twins.
- *Intermittent hip pain for several months:* In the initial stages, the symptoms tend to be relatively minor. Pain and a limp are usual presenting features. Pain is often slight and may have been present over several weeks or months.
- *Hematological investigations are normal:* Since the disease is secondary to epiphyseal ischaemia and infarction and not due to inflammation, the hematological investigations are usually normal.
- *X-rays show flattening of the femoral head:* This specific feature is caused by localized osteonecrosis. The X-ray changes are characteristic and it is often obvious that the condition has been present for time prior to presentation.

Radiological progression of perthes disease:

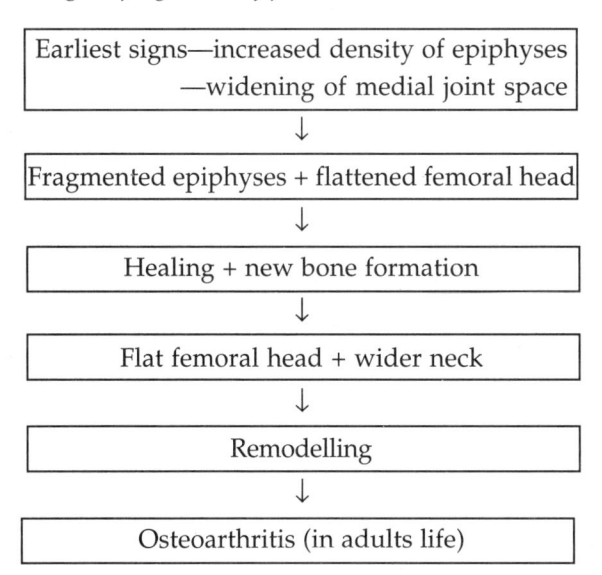

```
Earliest signs—increased density of epiphyses
              —widening of medial joint space
                        ↓
Fragmented epiphyses + flattened femoral head
                        ↓
            Healing + new bone formation
                        ↓
            Flat femoral head + wider neck
                        ↓
                    Remodelling
                        ↓
            Osteoarthritis (in adults life)
```

CONFUSA
The prognosis is better in
- Younger child
- Partial involvement of head of femur
- Boys.

Investigation of choice
Early X-rays (lateral view)

Immediate management
Admission for observation and rest

Treatment of choice
Depends upon femoral head involvement:
- *<½ of femoral head affected + joint space depth well preserved*—bed rest until pain subsides, followed by X-ray surveillance.
- *>½ of femoral head affected + narrowing of total joint space*—surgery may be considered.

Your Notes:

197. A two-year-old girl with one day history of increasing hip pain has become unable to weight bear. Her WCC is 21/fl, with an ESR of 89 mm/hr and a CRP of 300 mg/l. A radiograph of the hip shows a widened joint space.

Diagnosis: Septic arthritis.

Clinchers
- *Two-year-old girl:* It occurs most commonly below the age of four years. When it occurs in neonates it is known as Smith's arthritis.
- *One day history of increasing hip pain:* In older child it usually presents as an acute fever with extensive pain and spasm in the joint. It is rapid in onset (difference from Perthes' disease).
- *Unable to weight bear:* Child is unable to walk in septic arthritis because of pain (difference from Perthes' disease in which child can walk but with a limb).
- *WCC 21/fl, ESR 89 mm/hr, CRP 300 IU/l:* Normal WCC is 4-11/fl, ESR < 20 mm/hr and CRP < 10 IU/L. Any increase in these inflammatory markers denotes a sepsis somewhere in the body.
- *Radiograph of the hip shows a widened joint space:* Fluid in joint makes the joint space look wide on radiographs. An aspiration will confirm the presence of fluid.

CONFUSA
Differential diagnosis of septic arthritis is from 'irritable hip' and acute onset of Perthes' disease. Rheumatic fever and Still's disease occasionally present initially as a monoarthritis.

Investigation of choice
Diagnostic aspiration and culture of joint.

Immediate management
Joint aspiration, as it releives pain also + Analgesia.

Treatment of choice
Open surgical drainage and appropriate antibiotics.

Your Notes:

---

198. A 12-year-old boy with left groin pain for 6 weeks is noticed to stand with the left leg externally rotated. Examination reveals negligible internal rotation of the hip.

Diagnosis: Slipped upper femoral epiphyses (SUFE).

Clinchers
- *12-year-old boy:* SUFE is found in older children. The child is frequently overweight and may have delayed sexual development
- *Boys > girls:* It is a bilateral in 24% of patients.
- *Left groin pain for 6 weeks:* Classically symptoms are insiduous in onset, as the displacement is gradual. It is often associated with a limp (like Perthes' disease).
- *Stand with the left leg externally rotated:* External rotation of the limb at rest is pathognomic. Also the limb may be slightly short.
- *Negligible internal rotation of the hip:* Passive internal rotation is characteristically diminished in SUFE.

CONFUSA
The condition may not be apparent in early stages on an AP X-ray, but is detectable on a lateral film. A line drawn through the centre of the femoral neck in any X-ray projection should pass through the centre of the head. If it does not then some displacement has occurred.

Investigation of choice
Special lateral X-ray view
(Findings: Posterior displacement of the upper femoral epiphysis)

Immediate management
Orthopaedics referral.

Treatment of choice
- *Acute symptoms*
  - Traction in internal rotation
  - Alternatively manipulation under GA
- *Chronic symptoms*
  - Pinning
  - If not possible—osteotomy.

Your Notes:

199. A four-year-old boy complains of right hip pain a few days following an upper respiratory tract infection. Blood tests are as follows: WCC 12/fl, ESR 10 mm/hr and CRP 2 mg/l.

Diagnosis: Irritable hip syndrome (transient synovitis).

Clinchers
- *Four-year-old boy:* It is essentially a disease of childhood.
- *Right hip pain:* It is because of a sterile effusion in the hip (as it is a type of reactive arthritis).
- *A few days following an upper respiratory tract infection:* It often follows an upper respiratory tract infection.
- *WCC 12/fl, ESR 10 mm/hr and CRP 2 mg/l:* Blood tests are usually normal in irritable hip syndrome. Moreover the children are not systemically ill. Also there are no X-ray changes.

CONFUSA
When there has been unilateral limitation of all hip movements but a spontaneous recovery after bed-rest in the presence of normal X-rays, a retrospective diagnosis of transient synovitis is made. If other joints are involved, consider the diagnosis of juvenile rheumatoid arthritis. Rarely in irritable hip, an X-ray taken several weeks later may show the early changees of Perthes' disease.

Investigation of choice
Microscopy of hip joint aspirate.
(Typical findings: fluid containing WBC but no organisms).

Immediate management
Aspiration of the hip joint (as it reduces pain).

Treatment of choice
Bed-rest + observation.

Your Notes:

200. A five-year-old girl complains of progressively increasing severe pain in her left hip and upper leg for 6 days. She is able to walk but limps visibly. Blood tests are as follows: WCC 19/fl, ESR 72 mm/hr and CRP 94 mg/l. X rays and ultrasound scans of the hip are normal.

Diagnosis: Osteomyelitis (acute).

Clinchers
- *Five-year-old girl:* Acute osteomyelitis occur mainly in children. Poor lining conditions predispose to it, and there may be an obvious primary focus of infection such as a boil, sore throat, etc.
- *Progressively increasing severe pain in her left hip and upper leg for 6 days:* Pain is usually localized to the metaphyseal region of the bone.
- *Able to walk but limps visibly:* There is an unwillingness to move because of pain. There may be a visible limp if area of hip and femur and involved.
- *WCC 19/fl, ESR 72 mm/hr and CRP 94 mg/l:* All the inflammatory markers rise as it is as infective condition.
- *X-rays and ultrasound scans of the hip are normal:* X-ray changes are not apparent for few days but then shows haziness and loss of density of affected bone—subperiosteal reaction—sequestrum and involucrum.

CONFUSA
Osteomyelitis can be difficult to differentiate clinically from septic arthritis. But a typical difference between the two is in walking. In osteomyelitis the child may still be able to walk which is not the case with septic arthritis. Also the pain in osteomyelitis is more chronic in onset and less severe than septic arthritis.

Investigation of choice
MRI.

Immediate management
Send blood culture (positive in 60%).

Treatment of choice
Flucloxacillin 250-500 mg/6hr IVI or IM till sequesterum culture reports are known.
Open surgery to drain abscess and remove sequestera.

Your Notes:

March—2002

RxPG Analysis

Total themes:	**40**
Repeat themes:	**4**
Repeat themes with a different header:	**9**

March—2002

THEME 1: DIAGNOSIS OF HEARING LOSS

OPTIONS
a. Acoustic neuroma
b. Blast injury
c. petrous temporal bone fracture
d. wax impaction
e. Acute otitis media
f. Ototoxicity
g. Fracture base of skull
h. CSOM
i. Glue ear
j. Herpes zoster
k. Foreign body

*For each presentation below, choose the **most likely** diagnosis from the above list of options. Each option may be used once, more than once, or not at all.*

QUESTIONS

1. Man treated with gentamicin for peritonitis for 10 days presents with deafness.

2. Man with poor physical hygiene presents with pain and deafness after taking a shower.

3. Woman presents with deafness and corneal anaesthesia. On MRI, a widened internal auditory meatus is seen.

4. Male, 20 years, with history of head injury, bruising on the side of head complains of hearing loss.

5. A 54-year-old female develops mild fever, malaise and ear pain. 3 days dilater she developed multiple painful vesicles over her ear canal and external auditory meatus.

THEME 2: DIAGNOSIS OF EPISTAXIS

OPTIONS
a. Nasopharyngeal angiofibroma
b. Carcinoma maxillary antrum
c. Nasal polyposis
d. ORF
e. Septal perforation
f. Coagulopathy
g. Anticoagulant overdose
h. Sarcoidosis
i. Trauma
j. HTN

*For each presentation below, choose the **single most likely** diagnosis from the above list of options. Each option may be used once, more than once, or not at all.*

QUESTIONS

6. A sheep farmer with a bleeding polyp on anterior part of nasal septum.

7. Man working in a chrome factory presents with whistling sound on talking

8. Man with prosthetic heart valve presents with epistaxis.

9. Man who is involved in furniture making presents with recurrent epistaxis and anaesthesia of right cheek.

10. An 80-year-old man with history of epistaxis since 2 hours.

THEME 3: MECHANISM OF ACTION OF DRUGS

OPTIONS
a. Ipratropium
b. Amoxycillin
c. Salbutamol
d. Doxapram
e. Theophylline
f. Trimethoprim

*For each presentation below, choose the **correct answer** from the above list of options. Each option may be used once, more than once, or not at all.*

QUESTIONS

11. β_2 agonist

12. Antimuscarinic

13. Interferes with cell wall synthesis

14. Increases the activity of respiratory muscles

15. Urinary antiseptic

THEME 4: DRUGS USED IN MANAGEMENT OF ASTHMA

OPTIONS
a. Nebulised β_2 agonist
b. Inhaled short acting β_2
c. Inhaled long acting β_2
d. Oral short acting β_2
e. Oral long acting β_2
f. Leukotriene antagonist
g. Na cromoglycate
h. Oral theophylline
i. Paracetamol
j. β-blocker
k. carcinoma channel antagonists

*For each presentation below, choose the **correct answer** from the above list of options. Each option may be used once, more than once, or not at all.*

QUESTIONS

16. First line drug used in treating mild asthma.

17. Not given in a chronic asthmatic after a myocardial infarction.

18. Used to control acute severe asthma in a 15-year old with severe breathlessness in A and E.

19. Used to control intermittent night wheeze in a person using inhaled high dose steroids presently.

20. A nine-year-old boy has a mild cough and wheeze after playing football in the cold weather.

THEME 5: DIAGNOSIS OF ELECTROLYTE DISTURBANCES

OPTIONS
a. Metabolic acidosis
b. Metabolic alkalosis
c. Renal failure
d. Fluid overload
e. Hypokalemia
f. Respiratory acidosis
g. Hyperkalemia

*For each presentation below, choose the **most likely** diagnosis from the above list of options. Each option may be used once, more than once, or not at all.*

QUESTIONS

21. Man with pyloric stenosis, profuse vomiting, hypokalaemia and increased bicarbonate.

22. Man who is not able to pass urine, tired, complains of hiccups.

23. Man with villous adenoma, profuse diarrhoea.

24. Female, 24 hours after hysterectomy complains of breathlessness, increased JVP.

25. A patient in severe renal failure has potassium level of 2.5 mmol/L.

THEME 6: DIAGNOSIS OF UNCONSCIOUS PATIENTS

OPTIONS
a. Subdural hematoma
b. Extradural hematoma
c. Mild injury
d. Moderate injury
e. Fracture base of skull
f. Fracture cervical spine
g. Meningitis

*For each presentation below, choose the **most likely** diagnosis from the above list of options. Each option may be used once, more than once, or not at all.*

QUESTIONS

26. A chroni alcoholic with history of recurrent falls comes to A and E with complaint of ataxia. Blood glucose is 7.

27. A 17-year-old rugby player becomes unconscious after a fall. After sometime, he recovers, gives his name and address to the people in the ambulance. Later condition deteriorates.

28. A child becomes unconscious after falling off his bicycle, later he is better and active. Only complaint is headache.

29. Man with head trauma—GCS found to be 12.

30. Man with GCS=5, hemotympanum.

THEME 7: INVESTIGATION OF UNCONSCIOUS PATIENTS

OPTIONS
a. CT skull
b. Blood glucose
c. Lumbar puncture
d. Full blood count
e. Serum urea electrolytes
f. MRI Scan
g. Toxicology screen
h. X-ray skull
i. Blood alcohol
j. Plasma osmolarity
k. Arterial blood gases

*For each presentation below, choose the **most appropriate answer** from the above list of options. Each option may be used once, more than once, or not at all.*

QUESTIONS

31. A 10-year-old girl, unconscious, brought to A and E. She is found to be dehydrated on examination and respiratory rate is 40/min.

32. A young boy is brought to A and E by his grandparents. He is unconscious with a bruise on the temporal area.

33. A 10-year-old boy is drowsy, febrile with a rash.

34. A old lady fell and broke her hand one week back. After that slowly increasing confusion. Today her relatives could not wake her up from sleep.

35. A 21-year-old female found unconscious next to her 22-year-old husband, who was found dead. Her ECG shows evidence of acute MI.

THEME 8: MANAGEMENT OF BURNS

OPTIONS
a. Referral to burns unit
b. IV opioid
c. Dressing
d. Escharotomy + referral to burns unit
e. Anaesthesia and intubation
f. IV fluids in A and E before discharge
g. Reassure
h. Deroof blisters
i. Aspirate blisters
j. Antibiotics
k. Fasciotomy
l. IV fluids + referral for admission to burns unit

*For each presentation below, choose the **most appropriate management** from the above list of options. Each option may be used once, more than once, or not at all.*

QUESTIONS

36. Man rescued from burning building. Burns on face and anterior chest, soot in pharynx and singed nasal hair, asking about his family members.

37. Baby with less than 3 percent burns on chest and shoulders[scald due to tea falling on him] is irritable, crying, not allowing examination.

38. Man was electrocuted. Full thickness burn on fingers complaining of pain.

39. Man with 40 percent burns over trunk an limbs.

40. Man, slept while sunbathing comes with redness, pain all over his body. otherwise well.

THEME 9: VACCINES

OPTIONS
a. Delay by 2 weeks
b. Omit pertussis and meningitis
c. Give vaccine in hospital
d. Continue as per schedule
e. Give inactivated vaccines
f. Omit pertussis, Hib, measles
g. Do not give any vaccines
h. Omit pertussis only
i. Omit meningitis only
j. Omit measles only
k. Delay by 2 months

*For each presentation below, choose the **correct answer** from the above list of options. Each option may be used once, more than once, or not at all.*

QUESTIONS
41. Child who is HIV+ is due for MMR.
42. Child due for Hib, DPT, etc suffering from acute febrile illness.
43. Child cried for 2 hours after Hib, DPT, etc.
44. Family history of egg allergy. Child due for MMR.
45. History of convulsions. Child due for HiB, DPT, etc.

THEME 10: INVESTIGATIONS IN POSTOPERATIVE PATIENTS

OPTIONS
a. Pulse oximetry
b. Wound swab
c. V/Q scan
d. ECG
e. Ultrasound abdomen + pelvis
f. Coronary angiogram
g. Serum urea, electrolytes
h. Blood culture
i. MSU
j. Chest X-ray

*For each presentation below, choose the **correct answer** from the above list of options. Each option may be used once, more than once, or not at all.*

QUESTIONS
46. Woman after open cholecystectomy presents with fever, redness, tenderness of wound.
47. Chronic smoker 1 day after splenectomy presents with chest pain and dyspnea.
48. Female after anterior resection of rectum complains of anterior chest pain radiating to her left arm.
49. Man with COPD presents with central cyanosis.
50. Man after appendicectomy presents with spiking fever with rigors, tenesmus, diarrhoea.

THEME 11: CONTRACEPTION

OPTIONS
a. Condoms
b. COCP
c. POPs
d. OCPs + condom
e. Depovera
f. Mirena coil
g. Diaphragm
h. IUCD
i. Abstinence

*For each presentation below, choose the **best answer** from the above list of options. Each option may be used once, more than once, or not at all.*

QUESTIONS
51. A 14-year-old girl has just started having sexual relationship with her boyfriend of 2 months.
52. A 35-year-old female after her third child wants reliable contraception. She is a smoker and does not want to gain weight.
53. An 18-year-old girl has been on OCP's since 2 years, has to have rifampicin prophylaxis since her roommate has meningitis.
54. Girl with learning disorder begins to find males attractive. Her parents and teachers are worried.
55. Female after her first-child wants reliable contraception but wants no chemicals in her body, complains of heavy periods and dysmenorrhoea, husband does not want to use condoms.

THEME 12: DEMENTIA DIAGNOSIS

OPTIONS
a. Alzheimer's
b. Multi infarct
c. Lewy body
d. Pseudodementia
e. Frontal dementia
f. CJD
g. Alcoholic dementia

*For each presentation below, choose the **single most likely diagnosis** from the above list of options. Each option may be used once, more than once, or not at all.*

QUESTIONS
56. Most common form of dementia in the UK.
57. Characterised by neurofibrillary tangles and senile plaques.
58. May respond to antidepressants.
59. Increased disinhibition, preservation of intellect
60. An elderly hypertensive with recurrent faints presents with deteriorating mental functions.

THEME 13: SIDE EFFECTS OF ANTIPSYCHOTIC DRUGS

OPTIONS
a. Chlorpromazine
b. Phenelezine
c. Lithium
d. Fluoxetine
e. Haloperidol
f. Amitryptiline
g. Clozapine

*For each presentation below, choose the **correct answer** from the above list of options. Each option may be used once, more than once, or not at all.*

QUESTIONS

61. A schizophrenic on long-term treatment complains of impotence, has high prolactin levels, extrapyramidal side effects.

62. Drug with anticholinergic side effects, dry mouth, blurred vision, tremor.

63. Patient on treatment for bipolar disorder, hypothyroidism features.

64. Schizophrenic patient under treatment presents with sore throat, decreased WBC, agranulocytosis.

65. Schizophrenic patient under treatment presents with fever, increased WBC, increased muscle creatinine kinase levels.

THEME 14: DEMENTIA DIAGNOSIS

OPTIONS
a. Alzheimer's
b. Delirium
c. Depression
d. Late onset schizophrenia
e. Frontal dementia
f. Chronic anxiety state
g. Vascular dementia

*For each presentation below, choose the **most likely diagnosis** from the above list of options. Each option may be used once, more than once, or not at all.*

QUESTIONS

66. Man living in a hostel, brought to hospital after he collapsed. On the 3rd day, he points out things other people cannot see, disorientation in time and place.

67. An 80-year-old female is on no medication. Cause of concern is that she was trying to get into a shop at 6:00 AM. Neighbours say she is ok except her memory is not as good as it used to be since 2 years. She is otherwise well.

68. Female brings her husband to A and E, says he talks about their sex life in public. There is loss of inhibition, (intellect normal) in him.

69. Man has cough and fever since 2 days. Wife notices he has disorientation in time and place, decreased concentration and confused. He was ok mentally 1 day before.

70. A 70-year-old man says his life is not worth living, his existence is a waste, he performs all his work very slowly, he has lost weight.

THEME 15: DIAGNOSIS IN TRAUMA PATIENTS

OPTIONS
a. Aortic rupture
b. Splenic rupture
c. Diaphragmatic rupture
d. Cardiac tamponade
e. Renal contusion
f. Renal pedicle avulsion
g. Bladder rupture
h. Pancreatic rupture
i. Tension pneumothorax

*For each presentation below, choose the **most likely** **diagnosis** from the above list of options. Each option may be used once, more than once, or not at all.*

QUESTIONS

71. Boy was riding his bicycle when he was hit by a car. After examination in A and E, he was found to have left upper quadrant tenderness. He is pale.

72. Man fell off a ladder, has diffuse pain on right side of the trunk. IVU shows no excretion on right side.

73. Man was stabbed with a 10 cm knife in the left upper quadrant, stable for 20 min after which BP falls to 90/60 mmHg. On ultrasound, no free fluid seen in abdomen.

74. Known asthmatic patient involved in road traffic accident (RTA). Has a right-sided chest pain. On auscultation right side is hyper-resonant. Trachea is deviated to the left.

75. A 19-year-old girl has fallen off her horse. Neck is immobilised + 100% oxygen. Has left upper abdominal pain, is pale and tachycardiac.

THEME 16: CRANIAL NERVE PALSIES

OPTIONS
a. I cranial nerve
b. II cranial nerve
c. III cranial nerve
d. IV cranial nerve
e. V cranial nerve
f. VI cranial nerve
g. VII cranial nerve
h. VIII cranial nerve
i. IX cranial nerve
j. X cranial nerve
k. XI cranial nerve
l. XII cranial nerve

*For each presentation below, choose the **correct answer** from the above list of options. Each option may be used once, more than once, or not at all.*

QUESTIONS

76. Fracture of anterior cranial fossa, rhinorrhoea, anosmia.

77. Cavernous sinus affected, pupil not responding to light and accommodation, ptosis present.

78. After head trauma, patient cannot shrug his shoulder.

79. Forehead sparing, lower face no voluntary movements. Involuntary movements possible.

80. Fracture of base of skull, loss of taste in anterior two-thirds of tongue, deviation of angle of mouth.

THEME 17: MANAGEMENT OF FRACTURES

OPTIONS
a. Strapping and discharge
b. Strapping and review in hospital
c. Urgent orthopaedic referral
d. X-ray wrist including oblique scaphoid view
e. Isotope scan of the wrist

*For each presentation below, choose the **most appropriate step in management** from the above list of options. Each option may be used once, more than once, or not at all.*

QUESTIONS

81. A 16-year-old boy falls from a tree. Complains of pain in left anatomical fossa. X-rays are normal.

82. Man falls on hand. X-ray shows perilunate dislocation.

83. A 43-year-old man after a fall, pain in anatomical snuff box and X-ray shows impacted distal radius fracture.

84. Man falls on hand, pain in anatomical fossa.

85. Young girl tripped while holding mother's hand. Now cannot use arm at all.

THEME 18: CHILD CARE

OPTIONS
a. Child protection conference
b. Nutritional assessment
c. CT skull
d. Skeletal survey
e. Coagulation profile
f. Continue regular health care
g. Examine under anaesthesia
h. High vaginal swab
i. Gluten free diet

*For each presentation below, choose the **correct answer** from the above list of options. Each option may be used once, more than once, or not at all.*

QUESTIONS

86. A 12-month-old child of unemployed parents, did not gain weight from 6 months.

87. Child brought to AandE, age 6 months, swollen thigh, X-ray shows transverse fracture of shaft of femur.

88. A nine-year-old female child with itching, sore vagina, perineum is red and excoriated.

89. An 18-year-old female brings her baby unconscious to A and E, cyanosed, dilated fixed left pupil.

90. Child with forearm bruise, brought by teacher, Mom says she held her to prevent her from running across the road.

THEME 19: DIAGNOSIS OF CONFUSION

OPTIONS
a. Schizophrenia
b. Substance abuse
c. Opiate abuse
d. Opiate withdrawal
e. Generalized tonic clonic seizure
f. Panic attack

*For each presentation below, choose the **single most likely diagnosis** from the above list of options. Each option may be used once, more than once, or not at all.*

QUESTIONS

91. A 40-year-old lady stops talking suddenly, says someone took away her thoughts.

92. A 17-year-old girl comes anxious and tearful to A and E. She is unkempt and dishevelled, says she lost her medication, says she aches all over and demand immediate pain relief.

93. Unconscious boy with pin point pupils, respiratory rate 4/min.

94. Boy brought by his friend to the A and E. History of suddenly falling to the ground, jerky movements, urine incontinence. He is confused now but neurological examination is normal.

95. A 20-year-old woman attends A and E complaining of sudden breathlessness and anxiety. She describes palpitations and paresthesiae of her hands, feet and lips. ECG shows sinus tachycardia and O_2 saturation is normal.

THEME 20: MANAGEMENT OF ECZEMA

OPTIONS
a. Emollient with 1percent hydrocortisone
b. Emollient with 3 percent beclomethasone
c. Admit in hospital
d. Oral antihistamine
e. Desensitisation
f. Oral prednisolone
g. Steroids and flucloxacillin
h. Breastfeeding
i. Emollient with 2.5% hydrocortisone
j. Psychiatric referral
k. None required

*For each presentation below, choose the **most appropriate management** from the above list of options. Each option may be used once, more than once, or not at all.*

QUESTIONS

96. A bottle-fed baby has developed flexural eczema. His brother has the same history. Family history of asthma. Mom is presently avoiding using soap.

97. Young girl with eczema, treated with emollient and topical hydrocortisone, did not get better.

98. Young girl with severe eczema, weeping vesicles, skin swab was taken, topical steroids did not work.

99. A 49-year-old woman complains of itchy blisters, which are occurring in groups on her knees and elbows. The itch is becoming unbearable and she is contemplating suicide. She responds to 180 mg of dapsone within 48 hours of treatment.

100. An 18-month-old baby, red swollen lips after eating egg. Presently under treatment with emollients and topical hydrocortisone three times a day.

THEME 21: INVESTIGATIONS OF INFECTIOUS DISEASES

OPTIONS
a. Lyme disease serology
b. Leptospirosis serology
c. Viral serology
d. Wound swab
e. Lumbar puncture
f. MSU
g. LFT's [liver function tests]
h. Serum urea and electrolytes
i. Well-felix test
j. Ultrasound abdomen
k. Blood culture

*For each presentation below, choose the **most appropriate investigation** from the above list of options. Each option may be used once, more than once, or not at all.*

QUESTIONS
101. Girl goes into a forest, remembers getting bitten by a tick, redness near the bite is slowly increasing in size.
102. A policeman bit on his hand by a heroin addict while arresting him. He comes to the A and E, on examination, a deep wound seen on his hand.
103. An 18-month-old baby, drowsy, febrile, headache, CT normal.
104. A chronic alcoholic presents with flapping tremors and confusion.
105. A 70-year-old woman, confusion, constipation, frequency of urine.

THEME 22: MECHANISMS OF HYPERTENSION

OPTIONS
a. Renal artery stenosis
b. Conn's syndrome
c. Cushing's syndrome
d. Chronic pyelonephritis
e. Phaeochromocytoma
f. Glomerulonephritis
g. Polycystic kidney disease
h. Acromegaly
i. Coarctation of aorta
j. Systemic sclerosis
k. Diabetic neuropathy

*For each presentation below, choose the **most likely cause of hypertension** from the above list of options. Each option may be used once, more than once, or not at all.*

QUESTIONS
106. Due to increased catecholamines.
107. Autosomal dominant.
108. Increased production of aldosterone.
109. Deposition of immune complexes on basement membrane.
110. A 17-year-old girl with hypertension of 160/100 is found to have a femoral pulse delay.

THEME 23: DIFFERENTIAL DIAGNOSIS OF HEMOPTYSIS

OPTIONS
a. Bronchiectasis
b. TB (tuberculosis)
c. Inhaled foreign body
d. Pneumonia
e. Pulmonary embolism
f. Pulmonary oedema
g. Goodpasture's syndrome
h. Wegener's granulomatosis
i. Mitral stenosis
j. Hereditary haemorrhagic telengiectasia
k. Coagulation disorders
l. Carcinoma of lung

*For each presentation below, choose the **most likely cause of haemoptysis** from the above list of options. Each option may be used once, more than once, or not at all.*

QUESTIONS

111. A 40-year-old man underwent removal of tooth under anaesthesia, presents after one month with coughing up of blood.

112. Female with cough, copious blood tinged sputum for more than a month. She is from south-east Asia.

113. Female presents with acute pleuritic chest pain, hemoptysis after undergoing hysterectomy.

114. A middle-aged women develops a purulent cough with some haemoptysis. A chest X-ray reveals right upper lobe shadows.

115. A patient with an area of consolidation and fever on his chest X-ray is treated with antibiotics. His fever resolves but four weeks later he still has a large area of consolidation.

THEME 24: COMPLICATIONS OF MYOCARDIAL INFARCTION

OPTIONS
a. Papillary muscle rupture
b. Acute pericarditis
c. PE
d. Acute atrial fibrillation
e. Ventricular fibrillation
f. Congestive cardiac failure
g. Complete heart block
h. Ventricular free wall rupture
i. Ventricular aneurysm
j. Cardiac tamponade
k. Dressler's syndrome

*For each presentation below, choose the **most likely complication** from the above list of options. Each option may be used once, more than once, or not at all.*

QUESTIONS

116. Patient, 12 hours after MI presents with recurrent chest pain, breathlessness, heart rate—40/min.

117. Patient with pulmonary edema features presents with irregular pulse, heart rate—140/bpm.

118. A woman 10 days following hysterectomy complaints of severe left sided chest pain and breathlessness. Chest X-ray and ECG failed to relieve any abnormality.

119. 10 days after MI, female presents with chest pain on inspiration, persistently elevated ST segment on ECG.

120. Patient after MI found to have a harsh pansystolic murmur at the apex.

THEME 25: INVESTIGATIONS OF NEUROLOGICAL COMPLAINTS

OPTIONS
a. Carotid Doppler
b. MRI temporal lobe
c. MRI occipital lobe
d. CT scan
e. ESR
f. Echocardiography
g. MRI pituitary fossa
h. Skull X-ray
i. MRI cervical spine
j. MRI lumbar spine
k. Tensilon test

*For each presentation below, choose the **most appropriate** investigation from the above list of options. Each option may be used once, more than once, or not at all.*

QUESTIONS

121. Man with recurrent amaurosis fugax of right eye.

122. An elderly female with scalp tenderness on both sides of the head, complains of headache, sudden loss of vision in one eye.

123. A 40-year-old female comes with complaints of headache, bitemporal hemianopia, increase in shoe size.

124. Patient with attacks of numbness in left hand and right sided headache.

125. Patient gets diplopia when he works very hard.

THEME 26: INVESTIGATION OF COMPLICATIONS OF PROSTATIC CARCINOMA

OPTIONS
a. PSA
b. Serum acid phosphatase
c. Serum alkaline phosphatase
d. Transrectal ultrasound
e. Abdominal ultrasound
f. Serum calcium
g. Gallium scan
h. Technitium scan
i. Thallium scan
j. Transrectal biopsy
k. HLA status
l. Urodynamic studies

*For each presentation below, choose the **most appropriate** investigation from the above list of options. Each option may be used once, more than once, or not at all.*

QUESTIONS

126. 80-year-old with prostatic carcinoma comes with 4 month history of low backache.

127. Patient with prostatic cancer has been treated, now complains of confusion, thirst, bodyaches, constipation.

128. Man on GnRH's for prostate cancer comes after 2 months for a follow up.

129. Man with prostate carcinoma which has extended outside the capsule presenting with features of renal failure.

130. A man having adenocarcinoma prostate which has already spread to pelvic side walls has to be given chemotherapy.

THEME 27: DIAGNOSIS OF ALTERED BOWEL HABIT

OPTIONS
a. Irritable bowel syndrome
b. Inflammatory bowel disease
c. Acute gastroenteritis
d. Faecal impaction
e. Carcinoma colon
f. Diverticular disease
g. Diverticulitis

*For each presentation below, choose the **most likely diagnosis** from the above list of options. Each option may be used once, more than once, or not at all.*

QUESTIONS

131. An elderly female has history of uncontrollable loose stools many times a day. On examination, packed solid faeces in rectum.

132. A 30-year-old female has history of alternating constipation and diarrhoea for 7 months. She told that she is passing hard pellet like stools.

133. Female, 22-year-old, with bleeding and mucus per rectum, fever, loss of weight, has never been abroad.

134. An 80-year-old woman, fever 39 degrees centigrade, acute generalized abdominal pain, diarrhoea and vomiting, slightly dehydrated.

135. A 55-year-old man, history of altered bowel habit from 2 months, anemia, loss of weight.

THEME 28: MANAGEMENT OF EPILEPSY

OPTIONS
a. EEG
b. CT skull
c. Add 2nd drug
d. Check drug levels
e. IV lorazepam
f. Give rectal diazepam to parents and teach them how to use it
g. Evaluate dose of drug

*For each presentation below, choose the **most appropriate management** from the above list of options. Each option may be used once, more than once, or not at all.*

QUESTIONS

136. A 4-year-old boy has fever since 2 days, presents with convulsions since 5 min, still convulsing in the ambulance, IV line has been established.

137. A 2-year-old boy with past and family history of febrile convulsions. He is ok now.

138. Young girl on Na valproate, parents come with complaints of increased seizure frequency and frequent absences from school. On examination, she is mildly obese.

139. A 12-year-old girl, one episode of grandmal seizure of 3 min duration in her sleep.

140. A 14-year-old girl has had been academically brilliant, lately has had difficult with her schoolwork. She has been caught day dreaming in class on a number of occasions.

THEME 29: DIAGNOSIS OF GYNAECOLOGICAL CONDITIONS

OPTIONS
a. Endometrial carcinoma
b. Cervical ectropion
c. Polycystic ovarian disease
d. Cervical carcinoma
e. Pregnancy
f. Hypothalamus related disorder
g. Trauma

*For each presentation below, choose the **most likely diagnosis** from the above list of options. Each option may be used once, more than once, or not at all.*

QUESTIONS

141. A 55-year-old lady with history of intermittent postmenopausal bleeding. Vaginal and speulum examinations are normal.

142. Young girl has put on weight, hirsutism, oligomenorrhoea

143. Female on OCP's complains of postcoital bleeding.

144. An 18-year-old university student with history of 3 months of amenorrhoea and starvation.

145. A woman on the contraceptive pill for several years has a slight whitish vaginal discharge. On inspection she is found to have a pinkish coloration of the outer cervix.

THEME 30: FEEDING

OPTIONS
a. PEG feeding (gastrostomy)
b. Nasogastric tube feeding
c. Parenteral feeding
d. Gluten free diet
e. Low protein diet
f. Low calorie diet
g. Lactose free diet

*For each presentation below, choose the **most appropriate feeding modality** from the above list of options. Each option may be used once, more than once, or not at all.*

QUESTIONS

146. Patient with long-standing Parkinson's disease with intractable dysphagia.

147. Patient after a stroke, 5 days later, fluids still being aspirated from stomach.

148. Man after large bowel resection and ileostomy is septicaemic.

149. Man with jaundice and ascites suddenly deteriorates.

150. Girl with diarrhoea and jejunal villous atrophy.

THEME 31: PAIN RELIEF

OPTIONS
a. NSAIDs
b. Methotrexate
c. Home exercises
d. Local steroid injection
e. Splinting
f. IV biphosphonates
g. Oral steroids
h. Physiotherapy
i. Exercise training

*For each presentation below, choose the **most appropriate way of pain relief** from the above list of options. Each option may be used once, more than once, or not at all.*

QUESTIONS

151. An elderly busy man with indigestion, acute pain lateral side of hip.

152. Patient with symmetrical polyarthritis, pain does not decrease with simple analgesia.

153. Patient with hot swollen MT joint, pain does not decrease with paracetamol.

154. Pregnant woman with numbness, tingling on lateral side of hand.

155. A 35-year-old woman treated one year ago for a breast cancer with 12/20 nodes positive, presents with a two days history of increasing confusion, She is drowsy and disoriented. Her husband reports that she has been complaining of severe thirst for the past week.

THEME 32: PALLIATIVE CARE

OPTIONS
a. Cyclizine
b. Haloperidal
c. Hyoscine
d. Oral dexamethasone
e. Oral beclamethasone
f. Per rectal predisolone
g. Metronidazole gel
h. Long-term catheterisation
i. Intermittent self-catheterisation

*For each presentation below, choose the **most appropriate palliative method** from the above list of options. Each option may be used once, more than once, or not at all.*

QUESTIONS

156. Patient with intractable hiccups.

157. Patient cannot cough up bronchial secretions. Noise is distressing to attendants.

158. Patient after radiotherapy for bowel adenocarcinoma comes with bright red rectal bleeding.

159. Patient with superior vena cava obstruction after radiotherapy.

160. Female with fungating breast carcinoma with a bad adour.

March—2002

THEME 33: ANAEMIA INVESTIGATIONS

OPTIONS
a. Blood film for parasites
b. Serum B12
c. Schilling test
d. Bone marrow biopsy
e. Serum/gel electrophoresis
f. Mesenteric angiogram

*For each presentation below, choose the **most appropriate** investigation from the above list of options. Each option may be used once, more than once, or not at all.*

QUESTIONS

161. A middle-aged man with hepatosplenomegaly, fatigue, immature cells seen in blood film.

162. Man returns from Ghana presents with fever with rigors.

163. A 60-year-old man presents with fatigue and backache with localised tenderness. He also have decreased visual acuity.

164. Old lady with Hb is 3g/dl, MCV is 120fl, family history presents with fatigue, lethargy.

165. An eldelry female with past history of rectal bleeding, normal on endoscopy and enema studies done previously presents with profuse fresh rectal bleeding.

THEME 34: MANAGEMENT OF GYNAECOLOGY CONDITIONS

OPTIONS
a. Vaginal estrogens
b. Infection control
c. Prophylactic antibiotic treatment
d. Ring pessary
e. High fibre diet
f. Surgery

*For each presentation below, choose the **most appropriate** step in management from the above list of options. Each option may be used once, more than once, or not at all.*

QUESTIONS

166. 85-year-old with 14 children, severe heart failure, complains of dysuria, feeling of pressure in lower abdomen.

167. Female with well-controlled diabetes mellitus type 2 with recurrent UTI.

168. A young female with long-standing irregular bowel habit and persistent UTI.

169. An 80-year-old sexually active woman with dyspareunia and recurrent dysuria.

170. A middle-aged woman with a vaginal discharge is found to have several ulcers at the vaginal introitus.

THEME 35: MANAGEMENT OF VARICOSE VEINS

OPTIONS
a. Injection sclerotherapy
b. Graded compression stockings
c. Operation for varicose veins
d. Reduce weight
e. Prophylactic anticoagulation

For each presentation below, choose the most appropriate management from the above list of options. Each option may be used once, more than once, or not at all.

QUESTIONS
171. Female with bilateral varicose veins, lipodermatosclerosis. She is using compression stockings. Despite that increase in itching and eczema. BMI is 27.

172. 75-year-old, underwent 2 operations for varicose veins, presents with painful legs, has history of heart failure. On examination bilateral gross varicose veins, lipodermatosclerosis, no ulcers.

173. Female with BMI 33, comes with complaints of varicose veins and eczema.

174. Man with varicose veins has to fly for 20 hours. His father has a history of pulmonary embolism after flying.

175. A patient presents with a shallow ulcer, with no inrolled edges, situated over the medical malleolus. It has been reducing in size with compression bandaging. There is some evidence of lipodermatosclerosis and varicose veins in the distribution of the greater saphenous veins.

THEME 36: INVESTIGATIONS IN JAUNDICE

OPTIONS
a. Liver biopsy
b. Liver ultrasound
c. Oral cholecystography
d. Viral serology
e. ERCP
f. Percutaneous transhepatic cholangiography
g. Serum AMAs

*For each presentation below, choose the **most appropriate investigation** from the above list of options. Each option may be used once, more than once, or not at all.*

QUESTIONS
176. Man returned from trip to Asia, complains of anorexia, malaise, dark urine, pale stools.

177. An 80-year-old man has never been out of UK, one month history of epigastric pain, dark urine, pale stools, jaundice.

178. Female with fever, rigors, right upper quadrant pain, jaundice, ultrasound is normal.

179. Female, 50-year-old, 5 years history of mild pruritus. History of pale stools, dark urine, jaundice.

180. Man with history of hemochromatosis and alcohol addiction presents with jaundice, ascites, variceal bleed. USG is unequivocal, high ferritin level.

THEME 37: INVESTIGATION OF SCROTAL PAIN

OPTIONS
a. MSU
b. Urethral swab
c. Urgent surgical exploration
d. IVU
e. Ultrasound
f. Syphilis serology
g. Three glass test
h. CT scan
i. Laparoscopy
j. Testicular biopsy
k. None required

*For each presentation below, choose the **most appropriate investigation** from the above list of options. Each option may be used once, more than once, or not at all.*

QUESTIONS

181. Man after trip to Asia presents with red, swollen scrotum.

182. Man with painful red scrotum and vomiting.

183. Man with painless testicular swelling since 2 months.

184. Man with a swelling of scrotum since 3 years.

185. Man with no history of unsafe sex presents with dysuria and urinary frequency.

THEME 38: DIAGNOSIS OF ABDOMINAL CONDITIONS

OPTIONS
a. Acute pancreatitis
b. Chronic pancreatitis
c. *H. pylori* infection
d. Pernicious anemia
e. Barrett's esophagus
f. Prostatic carcinoma
g. Acute cholecystitis
h. Hepatitis
i. Chronic cholecystitis
j. Duodenal ulcer
k. Aplastic anemia

*For each presentation below, choose the **most likely diagnosis** from the above list of options. Each option may be used once, more than once, or not at all.*

QUESTIONS

186. Condition that can cause necrosis, formation of fluid-filled spaces that can get infected.

187. Condition associated with gastroesophageal reflux, epithelial metaplasia, increased risk of carcinoma.

188. Condition associated with epigastric pain radiating to the back, pale loose stools, associated with alcohol consumption.

189. Condition associated with persistent inflammation, can cause lymphoma.

190. Condition associated with megaloblastic anemia, increased risk of carcinoma.

THEME 39: DIFFERENTIAL DIAGNOSIS OF THYROID DISORDERS

OPTIONS
a. Anaplastic carcinoma
b. Follicular carcinoma
c. Papillary carcinoma
d. Hashimoto's thyroiditis
e. Thyrotoxic goitre
f. Autoimmune hypothyroidism
g. Drug induced thyrotoxicosis
h. Graves' disease
i. Riedel's thyroiditis
j. De Quervian thyroiditis
k. Small bowel lymphoma

*For each presentation below, choose the **most likely diagnosis** from the above list of options. Each option may be used once, more than once, or not at all.*

QUESTIONS
191. Female, 41-year-old, presents with hard, irregular fixed swelling, stridor, dysphagia since 3 months.
192. Old lady with smooth neck swelling, bradycardia, spare coarse hair, macrocytic anemia.
193. Female on treatment for supraventricular tachycardia complains of seeing dots and glare on driving at night, exophthalmos, no goitre.
194. Female, swelling in the neck, tremor irritability, diarrhoea, bruit.
195. A 35-year-old woman who was diagnosed as having coelic disease at the age of 12 years has had good control of her abdominal symptoms for a number of years. She presents with a recent history of weight loss, tiredness, diarrhoea and abdominal pain.

THEME 40: COMPLICATIONS OF BREAST CARCINOMA

OPTIONS
a. Pathological fracture
b. Cerebral metastases
c. Hypocalcemia
d. Lymphedema
e. Spinal cord compression
f. Hypercalcemia
g. Hyperparathyroidism

*For each presentation below, choose the **most common complication** from the above list of options. Each option may be used once, more than once, or not at all.*

QUESTIONS
196. Female with breast carcinoma 3 years back, was treated with mastectomy and lymph node clearance on the left side, presents with a swollen limb and decreased hand movements.
197. Presents with thirst, confusion, constipation.
198. Presents with weakness of both legs, difficulty walking, urine retention.
199. Presents with headache, confusion. On examination, papilledema present.
200. Presents with features of fracture femur.

March—2002

General Medical Council PLAB Test Part 1

Full Name
Test Centre/Date

- Use pencil only   • Make heavy makrs that fill the lozenge completely
- Write your candidate number in the top row of the box to the right **AND** fill in the appropriate lozenge below each number
- Give **ONE** answer only for each question

Specimen

DO NOT WRITE IN THIS SPACE

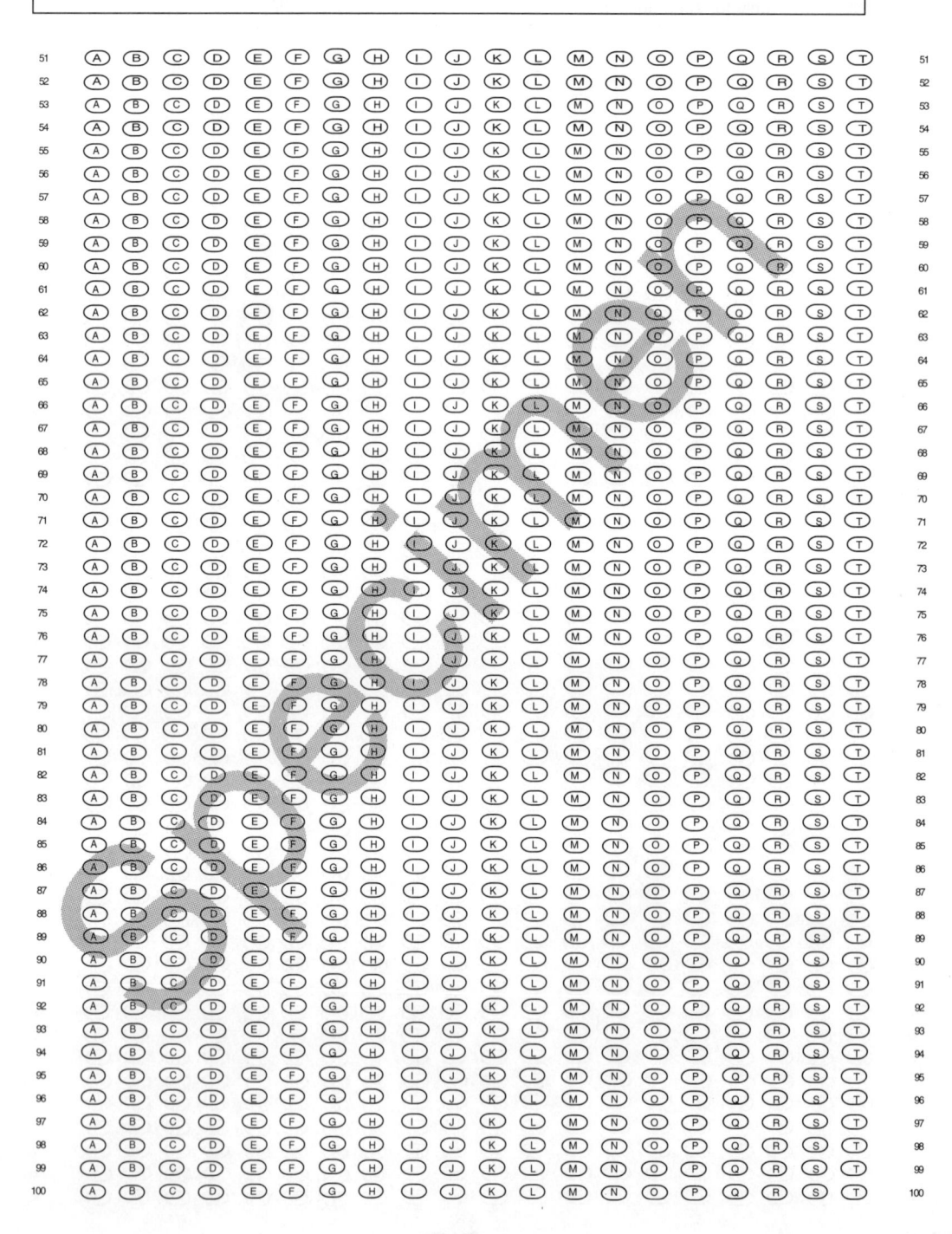

March—2002

DO NOT WRITE IN THIS SPACE

DO NOT WRITE IN THIS SPACE

Answers

March—2002

#		
1	f	Ototoxicity
2	d	Wax impaction
3	a	Acoustic neuroma
4	c	Petrous temporal bone fracture
5	j	Herpes zoster
6	d	Orf
7	e	Nasal perforation
8	g	Anticoagulant overdose
9	b	Carcinoma of maxillary antrum
10	j	Hypertension
11	c	Salbutamol
12	a	Impratropium bromide
13	b	Amoxycillin
14	d	Doxapram
15	f	Trimethoprim
16	b	Inhaled short acting β_2-agonist
17	j	Beta-blockers
18	a	Nabulized β_2-agonist
19	c	Inhaled long-acting β_2-agonist
20	g	Na cromoglycate
21	b	Metabolic alkalosis
22	c	Renal failure
23	e	Hypokalaemia
24	d	Fluid over load
25	e	Hypokalaemia
26	a	Subdural hematoma
27	b	Extradural hematoma
28	c	Mild injury
29	d	Moderate injury
30	e	Fracture base of skull

#		
31	b	Blood glucose
32	a	CT skull
33	c	Lumber puncture
34	a	CT skull
35	g	Toxicology screen
36	e	Anaesthesia and intubation
37	b	IVopioid
38	d	Escharotomy
39	l	IV fluids + referral for admission to burns unit
40	g	Reassure
41	d	Continue as her schedule
42	a	Delay by 2 weeks
43	d	Continue as per schedule
44	d	Continue as per schedule
45	d	Continue as per schedule
46	b	Wound swab
47	a/j	Chest X-ray/pulse oximetry
48	d	ECG
49	a	Pulse oximetry
50	e	USG abdomen + pelvis
51	d	OCP + Condom
52	h	IUCD
53	d	OCP+Condom
54	e	Depovera
55	f	Mirena coil
56	a	Alzheimer's
57	a	Alzheimer's
58	d	Pseudodementia
59	e	Frontal dementia
60	b	Multi infarct

61	a	Chlorpromazine		93	c	Opiate abuse
62	f	Amitriptyline		94	e	GTCS
63	c	Lithium		95	f	Panic attack
64	g	Clozapine		96	a	Emollient with 1% hydrocortisone
65	e	Haloperidol		97	i	Emollient with 25% hydrocortisone
66	b	Delirium		98	g	Steroids and flucloxacillin
67	a	Alzheimer's		99	j	Psychiatric referral
68	e	Frontal dementia		100	c	Admit in hospital
69	b	Delirium		101	a	Lyme disease serology
70	c	Depression		102	d	Wound swab
71	b	Splenic rupture		103	e	Lumbar puncture
72	f	Renal pedicle avulsion		104	g	LFT
73	d	Cardiac tamponade		105	f	MSU
74	i	Tension pneumothorax		106	e	Phaeochromocytoma
75	b	Splenic rupture		107	g	Polycystic kidney disease
76	a	I cranial nerve		108	b	Conn's syndrome
77	c	III cranial nerve		109	f	Glomerulonephritis
78	k	XI cranial nerve		110	i	Coarctation of aorta
79	g	VII cranial nerve		111	c	Inhaled foreign body
80	g	VII cranial nerve		112	b	TB
81	e	Isotope scan		113	e	Pulmonary embolism
82	c	Urgent ortho referral		114	b	TB
83	c	Urgent ortho referral		115	l	Carcinoma
84	d	X-ray wrist including oblique view of scaphoid		116	g	Complete heart block
85	c	Urgent ortho referral		117	d	Acute AF
86	b	Nutritional assessment		118	c	PE
87	d	Skeletal surgery		119	b	Acute pericarditis
88	g	Examine under anaesthesia		120	a	Papillary muscle rupture
89	c	CT skull		121	a	Carotid doppler
90	e	Coagulation profile		122	e	ESR
91	a	Schizophrenia		123	g	MRI pituitary fossa
92	d	Opiate withdrawl		124	d	CT scan

125	k	Tensilon test
126	h	Technitium scan
127	f	Serum calcium
128	a	PSA
129	l	Urodynamic studies
130	d	Trans rectal USG
131	d	Faecal impaction
132	a	IBS
133	b	IBD
134	c	Acute gastroenteritis
135	e	Carcinoma colon
136	e	IV lorazepam
137	f	Give rectal
138	d	Check dry levels
139	a	EEG
140	a	EEG
141	a	Endemetrial carcinoma
142	c	Polycystic ovarian disease
143	b	Cervical ectropion
144	f	Hypothalamus related disorders
145	b	Cervical ectropion
146	a	PEG feeding
147	c	Parenteral feeding
148	c	Parenteral feeding
149	e	Low protein diet
150	d	Gluten free diet
151	d	Local steroid
152	a	NSAID
153	a	NSAID
154	e	Splinting
155	f	IV bisphosphonates
156	b	Haloperidol

157	c	Hyoscine
158	f	Per rectal diazepam
159	d	Oral dexamethasone
160	g	Metronidazole gel
161	d	Bone marrow biopsy
162	a	Blood film for parasites
163	e	Serum/gel electrophoresis
164	c	Schilling test
165	f	Mesenteric angiogram
166	d	Ring pessary
167	b	Infection control
168	f	Surgery
169	a	Vaginal estrogens
170	b	Infection control
171	d	Reduce weight
172	b	Graded compression stockings
173	d	Reduce weight
174	b	Graded compression stockings
175	a	Injection sclerotherapy
176	d	Viral serology
177	e	ERCP
178	c	Oral cholecystography
179	a	Liver biopsy
180	a	Liver biopsy
181	b	Urethral swab
182	c	Urgent surgical exploration
183	e	USG
184	k	None required
185	a	MSU
186	a	Acute pancreatitis
187	e	Barget's oesophagus
188	b	Chronic pancreatitis

189	c	H pylori infection
190	d	Pernicious anaemia
191	a	Anaplastic carcinoma
192	d	Hashimotos's thyroiditis
193	g	Dry induced thyrotoxiosis
194	h	Graves' disease

195	k	Small bowel lymphoma
196	d	Lymphoedema
197	f	Hypercalcaemia
198	e	Spinal cord compression
199	b	Cerebral metastases
200	a	Pathological fracture

March—2002

EXPLANATIONS

1. Man treated with gentamicin for peritonitis for 10 days presents with deafness.

Diagnosis: Ototoxicity.

Clinchers

Various drugs and chemicals can damage the inner ear and cause sensorineural deafness and tinnitus.

Symptoms of ototoxicity are—hearing loss, tinnitus, and/or giddiness, may manifest during treatment or after completion of treatment.

Ototoxic drugs: *Aminoglycoside antibiotics*: Gentamicin is the most important of all. Other includes—streptomycin, tobramycin, neomycin, etc.
- *Diuretics*: Furosemide, ethacrinic, etc.
- *Antimalarials*: Quinine, chloroquine.
- *Cytotoxic drugs*: Nitrogen, mustard, cisplatin
- *Analgesics*: Salicylates, indomethacin, ibuprofen.
- *Chemicals*: Alcohol, tobacco, marijuana, carbon monoxide poisoning.

Investigation of choice

Rinne test (positive), i.e. air conduction < bone conduction.

Immediate management

Weber lateralised to better ear.

Treatment of choice

Stop gentamicin at once.

Your Notes:

2. Man with poor physical hygiene presents with pain and deafness after taking a shower.

Diagnosis: Wax impaction.

Clinchers

- *Man with poor physical hygiene*: Wax impaction is common in people with poor hygiene.
- *Pain and deafness after shower*: During bathing and swimming if water enters the ear, it may swell the wax and this will give rise to sudden pain, sense of blocked ear and/or hearing loss.

Tinnitus and giddiness may result from impaction of wax against the drum head. Patient may also complain of reflux cough, due to stimulation of auricular branch of vagus.

Wax or cerumen is secreted by ceruminous glands (modified sweat glands) situated in cartilaginous part of meatus.

Treatment of choice

Treatment consists of its removal by syringing or instrumental manipulation. Hard impacted mass may sometimes require prior softening with wax solvents.

Your Notes:

3. Woman presents with deafness and corneal anaesthesia. On MRI, a widened internal auditory meatus is seen.

Diagnosis: Acoustic neuroma.

Clinchers
- *Woman:* No significance. Acoustic neuroma is present equally in both the sexes. It is mostly seen in age group of 40-60 years.
- *Deafness:* Progressive unilateral sensorineural hearing loss often accompanied by tinnitus is the presenting symptom of acoustic neuroma.
- *Corneal anaesthesia:* Acoustic neuroma may uninvolve V, IX, X and XI cranial nerve as it grows. The earliest cranial nerve to be involved is V cranial nerve, presenting with reduced corneal sensitivity, numbness or paraesthesia of face.
- *Widened internal auditory meatus:* Acoustic neuroma, a benign, slow growing tumor of 8th nerve expands and causes widening and erosion of the internal auditory meatus.

CONFUSA
Acoustic neuroma should be differentiated from the cochlear pathology (i.e. Meniere's disease) and other cerebellopontine angle tumours, e.g. meningioma, primary cholesteatoma and arachnoidal cyst.

Treatment of choice
Surgical removal.

Your Notes:

4. Male, 20 years, with history of head injury, bruising on the side of head complains of hearing loss.

Diagnosis: Petrous temporal bone fracture.

Clinchers
- *Head injury:* Head injury can cause hearing loss due to:
  - Ossicular disruption
  - Haemotypmpanum
  - CSF otorrhoea
  - VIII cranial nerve palsy

All these can occur in fracture of petrous temporal bone which houses of the middle ear and VIII nerve.
- *Bruising on side of head:* This almost confimrs our suspicion of pterous temporal bone.

CONFUSA
A complaint of reduced hearing in one ear after trauma points to a haemotypanum most commonly. Blood in the external auditory meatus after trauma is usually caused by basal fracture but is rarely secondary to temporomandibular joint injury. In such cases direct auroscopic examination of the canal should be avoided as it may introduce infection via torn meninges.

Investigation of choice
Skull X-rays (special views).

Immediate management
GCS + admit

Treatment of choice
Usually conservative. For hearing loss discuss with an ENT surgeon.

Your Notes:

5. A 54-year-old female develops mild fever, malaise and ear pain. 3 days later she developed multiple painful vesicles over her ear canal and external meatus.

Diagnosis: Herpes zoster

Clinchers

- *Mild fever, malaise, ear pain:* Fever, malaise signifies viral infection. Herpes zoster oticus is a viral infection involving geniculate ganglion of facial nerve. There may be anaesthesia of face, giddiness and hearing impairment due to involvement of V and VIII nerves.
- *Multiple painful vesicles;* Herpes zoster infection (oticus) is characterised by appearance of vesicles on the tympanic membrane, deep meatus, concha and reteroauricular sulcus. There may be a vesicular rash in the external auditory canal and pinna.

CONFUSA
Nose tip involvement is virtually diagnostic if present in a case of Herpes zoster. It is known as Hutchinsons signs and means involvement of the nasociliary branch of the trigeminal nerve which also supplies the globe and makes it highly likely that the eye will be affected.

Investigation of choice
Fluoroscent antibody tests and Tzank smears (but both rarely needed as the diagnosis is clinically easy).

Immediate management
Keeping cool may reduce the number of lesions. Tell her to avoid scratching. Give adequate analgesia.

Treatment of choice
Aciclovir 800 mg
- five times a day
- for 7 days.

Your Notes:

6. A sheep farmer with a bleeding polyp on anterior part of nasal septum.

Diagnosis: Orf

Clinchers

- *Sheep farmer:* Certain pox viruses can cause localized vesicular lesions when humans come into direct contact with infected animals. *Orf virus* is one such virus, which is known as contagious pustular dermatitis virus, caught from sheep.
- *Bleeding polyp on anterior part of nasal septum:* People who come into contact with the affected fluid from animal lesions (especially from young lambs) may develop lesions on the hands and the body parts they touch (especially face and nose).

CONFUSA
Occasionally Orf infection is transmitted from goats.

Investigation of choice
None

Immediate management
Tell him not to touch vesicles

Treatment of choice
Lesions resolve spontaneously after 4-6 weeks and immunity lasts life-long.

Your Notes:

7. Man working in a chrome factory presents with whistling sound on talking.

Diagnosis: Nasal perforation.

Clinchers
- *Working in chrome factory:* Inhalation of chrome salts is an important cause of septal perforation.
- *Whistling sound:* Signifies perforation.
- *Causes of septal perforation*
  - Inhalation of chrome salts
  - Postseptal surgery
  - Trauma/nose picking
  - Sniffing cocaine
  - Rodent ulcer
  - Malignancy
  - Granuloma
  - Infections (TB, syphilis)
  - Perforations irritable, crust and bleed.

Immediate management
Symptomatic.

Treatment of choice
Symptomatic (closure of perforation is difficult).

Your Notes:

8. Man with prosthetic heart valve presents with epistaxis.

Diagnosis: Anticoagulant overdose.

Clinchers
- *Prosthetic heart valve:* Patients with prosthetic heart valves are treated with anticoagulants, indefinitely.
- *Epistaxis:* Littles area is very prone to bleeding. Here there is convergence of the anterior ethmoidal artery, the septal branches of the sphenopalatine and the superior labial arteries and greater palatine. Anticoagulant overdose is an important cause of bleeding tendency (e.g. Warfarin anticoagulation) Other causes of epistaxis are degenerative arterial disease and hypertension in older people, and local causes are atrophic rhinitis, hereditary telangiectasia and tumors of the nose of sinuses.

Investigation of choice
INR.

Immediate management
Treat shock and replace blood if necessary.

Treatment of choice
Titrate the dose of anticoagulant for prosthetic heart valve. For epistaxis:
- Apply firm uninterrupted pressure of nostrils f/w finger and thumb for 10 minutes, possibly with ice pack over bridge of nose.
- If still bleeding spray—2.5-10% cocaine solution over mucosa. This will anaesthetize the mucosa and reduce bleeding by constricting vessels. Cauterize any bleeding points.
- Pack the nose.
- If bleeding recurs, further packs.
- Rarely arterial ligation.
- In severe, resistant bleeds, consider embolization of the feeding vessel.

Your Notes:

9. Man who is involved in furniture making presents with recurrent epistaxis and anaesthesia of right cheek.

Diagnosis: Carcinoma of maxillary antrum.

Clinchers
> *Involved in furniture making:* People working in hardwood furniture industry, nickel refining, leather work and manufacture of mustard gas has shown higher incidence of sinunasal cancer.
> Maxillary carcinoma is common in Bantus of South Africa. They use locally made snuff, rich in nickel and chromium.
> *Recurrent epistaxis and anaesthesia of maxillary antrum:* These are the early features of maxillary antrum. Other features are nasal stiffness, blood stained discharge, facial paraesthesia or pain and epiphora.

CONFUSA
Workers of furniture industry develop adenocarcinoma of the ethmoids and upper nasal cavity, while those engaged in nickel refining get squamous cell and anaplastic carcinoma.

Investigation of choice
Radiograph of sinuses. CT scan helps in staging the disease. Biopsy confirm the suspicion of malignancy.

Immediate management
Embolization of feeding vessel as epistaxis of malignancy is not remediable by simple measures.

Treatment of choice
Investigate as above for malignancy. If malignancy proved, histological nature of malignancy is important in deciding the line of treatment, e.g. in squamous cell carcinoma, combination of radiotherapy and surgery gives better result then either alone.

Your Notes:

10. An 80-year-old man with history of epistaxis since 2 hours.

Diagnosis: Hypertension.

Clinchers
> *An 80-year-old man:* Since only age is specified in this question, and no other relevant history is given, we can think of only two important factor, that relate age to epistaxis. They are:
> - Hypertension and
> - Degenerative arterial disease.
> *Since 2 hours:* This further supports our diagnosis of hypertension. Since local causes of epistaxis (atrophic rhinitis, hereditary telangectasia and tumor of nose and sinuses) can be excluded.

Immediate management
Immediate lowering of BP.

Treatment of choice
- For epistaxis refer Q-8 (March 2002)
- For hypertension—hypertension is a major risk factor for stroke and myocardial infarction. Out aim should be for BP < 140/85, but in 130/80 in patients with diabetes.

Your Notes:

11. β₂ agonist.

Diagnosis: Salbutamol.

Clinchers
Salbutamol is a sedative β₂ adrenergic receptor agonist (other example: terbutaline).

β₂ receptors are present in brochi, blood vessels, uterus, GIT, urinary tract, eye.

β₂ stimulation causes—bronchodilatation, vasodilatation and uterine relaxation, without producing significant cardiac stimulation.

Salbutamol is primarily and in bronchial asthma. Other uses are:
- Uterine relaxant: to delay premature labour
- In hyperkalemic familial periodic, paralysis—cause increased uptake of K⁺ by muscles.

Side effects
Most important side effects is muscle tremor. Tachycardia and arrhythmias are less likely.

Your Notes:

12. Antimuscarinic

Diagnosis: Ipratropium bromide.

Clinchers
Ipratropium bromide is a semisynthetic anticholinergic drug. It blocks the action of acetylcholine on autonomic effectors and in the CNS exerted through muscarinic receptor.

Ipratropium bromide 40-80 µg by inhalation, acts selectively on bronchial muscles without altering volume on consistency of respiratory secretions.

It is suitable for regular prophylactic use rather than rapid symptomatic relief during an attack, because of gradual onset and late peak (at 60-90 min) of bronchodilator effect in comparison to inhaled sympathomimetics.

Ipratropium bromide is more effective in COPD (chronic obstructive pulmonary disease), since parasympathetic tone is the major reversible factor here.

CONFUSA
Atropine is highly selective for musurinic receptors, the synthetic derivatives do passes significant nicotinic blocking property in addition.

Your Notes:

13. Interferes with cell wall synthesis.

Diagnosis: Beta-lactum antibiotics.

Clinchers

- Amoxicillin is a semisynthetic penicillin, with extended spectrum of activity, containing a beta-lactum ring.
  All the beta-lactum antibiotics interfere with the synthesis of bacterial cell wall.
  Beta-lactum antibiotics inhibit the transpeptidase so that cross linking (which maintains the does knit structure of the cell wall) does not take place.
- *Mechanism of action:* When bacteria divide in the pressure of a beta-lactum antibiotic, cell wall deficient (CWD) forms are produced. Because the interior of the bacterium is hyperosmotic, CWD forms smell and burst—bacteriolysis.

CONFUSA
Drugs that inhibit cell wall synthesis are: penicillin, cephalosporins, cycloserine, vancomycin, bacitracin.

Your Notes:

14. Increases the activity of respiratory muscles.

Diagnosis: Analeptics.

Clinchers

- *Doxapram:* At low doses it is more selective for the respiratory centre than other analeptics. It stimulates respiration through carotid and arotic body chemoreceptors as well.
  Its role in therapeutics is very narrow, with narrow safety margin. Mechanical support to respiration and other measures to improve circulation are more effective.
- *Mechanism of action:* Doxapram acts by promoting excitation of central neurons, thus stimulating respiration.
- *Other analeptics:* Ethyl and propyl butamide, Nikethamide.

Your Notes:

15. Urinary antiseptic.

Answer: Trimethoprim

Clinchers

Trimethoprim is a diaminopyrimidine, a structural analogue of pteridine moiety of folic acid. It is a competitive inhibitor of dihyrofolate reductase, the enzyme responsible for reduction of dihydrofolic acid to tetrahydrofolic acid, the essential final component in the folic acid synthesis pathway that is necessary for all one-carbon transfer reactions like the sulfonamides, timethoprim is bactericidal in the absence of thymine but is only bacteriostatic when this pyrimidine is present in high concentration. The selective antibacterial activitiy of trimethoprim is based on the extreme sensitivity of bacterial dihydrofolate reductase to inhibition by this drug in comparison with the mammalian enzyme. The bacterial enzyme is approximately 50,000 times more sensitive to such inhibition.

CONFUSA

Trimethoprim is used for treatment of UTI, i.e. for acute cases, suppressive treatment of chronic and recurrent cases—specially in females

Your Notes:

16. First line drug used in treating mild asthma.

Diagnosis: Asthma

Clinchers

Guidelines laid by the British Thoracic Society should be followed here.

In mild asthma, first line of drugs used is short acting inhaled β_2-agonists (as and when required for symptom relief). But this should be used only once daily. If used more than once daily add standard dose inhaled steroid, beclometasone or budesonide. Cromoglycate or nedocromil can be tried but if they do not control symptoms change to inhaled steroids.

β_2 adrenoreceptor agonists relax bronchial smooth muscle, acting within minutes. Salbutamol is best given by inhalation, but can be given PO or IV (do not use regular short acting β-agonists as maintenance).

CONFUSA

Since British Thoracic Society has laid down strict guidelines, there should be no confusion in this question. For guidelines refer page 172 (OHCM), 5th edn.

Immediate management (in acute severe asthma)
- Sit patient up and give high dose O_2
- Salbutamol 5 mg/terbutaline 10 mg nebulized with O_2
- Hydrocortisone 200 mg IV or prednisolone 30 mg PO (if very ill)
- Exclude pneumothorax (CXR).

Your Notes:

17. Not given in a chronic asthmatic after a myocardial infarction.

Diagnosis: Myocardial infarction in chronic asthmatic.

Clinchers
β-adrenergic blockers reduce myocardial O_2 consumption, limit infarct size, and reduce mortality. But is contraindicated in asthmatic patient.

$β_2$-receptors induces peripheral vasoconstriction and bronchoconstriction.

Important contraindications of β-blockers are:
- Asthma/COPD
- Peripheral vascular disease
- Heart failure/heart block.

Immediate management
Aspirin 300 mg PO. Analgesia, e.g. morphine 5-10 mg IV + metoclopromide 10 mg IV

Treatment of choice
Stop smoking and avoid precipitants. Follow British Thoracic Society guidelines refer page 172 (OHCM), 5th edn for chronic asthma. For management of MI refer page 781 (OHCM), 5th edn.

Your Notes:

18. Used to control acute severe asthma in a 15-year-old with severe breathlessness in A and E.

Diagnosis: Acute severe asthma.

Clinchers
➢ *Control acute severe asthma:* Acute severe asthma is a medical emergency, presented with acute breathlessness and wheeze. The first step in management is to sit patient up and give high-dose O_2.
Nabulised $β_2$ agonist (salbutamol or terbutaline) nebulised with O_2 is the fastest acting bronchodilator, therefore used to control acute severe asthma.

➢ *15-year-old:* 15-year-old can receive a full dose of $β_2$ agonists (i.e. salbutamol 5 mg or terbutalin 10 mg). Half dose is given in very young children.

In very young children add ipratrapium 0.25 mg to nabulized beta-agonist.

> **CONFUSA**
> Hydrocortisone 200 mg IV or prednisolone 30 mg PO are both added if the patient is very ill, but they are no substitute to nabulised beta-agonists.
> In life-threatening conditions nabulised ipratropium and IV aminophylline can be added.

Investigation of choice
In acute asthma PEFR, sputum culture, U and E, blood culture and ABG. In chronic cases look for obstructive defects ($↓FEV_1/FVC$, ↑residual volume).

Your Notes:

19. Used to control intermittent night wheeze in a person using inhaled high dose steroids presently.

Diagnosis: Asthma.

Clinchers
- *Control intermittent night wheeze:* Salmeterol is a long acting inhaled β_2-agonist that can help nocturnal symptoms and reduce morning dips.
- *Inhaled high dose steroids presently:* Long acting inhaled β_2-agonists (salmetrol) is an alternative to ↓ steroid dose when symptoms are uncontrolled (rinse mouth after inhaled steroid to prevent and candidiasis).

Therefore intermittent night wheeze in a person using inhaled high dose steroids presently can be controlled by long acting (inhaled) β_2-agonists like salmetrol.

Do refer to the British Thoracic Society guidelines for control of asthma in page 172 (OHCM), 5th edn.

CONFUSA
Aminophylline may be tried as prophylaxis, at night PO, to prevent morning dipping, but not in this question.

Immediate management
Long acting inhaled β_2-agonists (salmetrol).

Your Notes:

20. A nine-year-old boy has a mild cough and wheeze after playing football in the cold weather.

Diagnosis: Exercise induced asthma

Clinchers
- *Nine year old boy:* Exercise induced asthma is most commonly present in childhood.
- *Mild cough and wheeze:* These are the diagnostic symptoms of asthma.
- *After playing football in cold weather:* Cold weather and exercise are both precipitants of asthma. Exercise is one of the most common precipitants of acute episodes of asthma. Exercise probably provokes bronchospasm to some extent in every asthmatic patients, and in some it is the only trigger that produces symptoms. There is a significant interaction between the ventilation produced by exercise, the temperature, and the water content of the inspired air and the magnitude of the postexertional obstruction.

CONFUSA
Cromoglycate is used prophylaxis is mild and exercised asthma (always inhaled), especially in children. Note that it may precipitate asthma. Exercise induction differs from other naturally occurring provocations of asthma, such as antigens or viral infections, in that it does not evoke any long term sequelae nor does it change airway reactivity.

Investigation of choice
PEFR

Immediate management
Nebulisation

Treatment of choice
Prophylactic inhaled sodium cromoglycate.

Your Notes:

21. Man with pyloric stenosis, profuse vomiting, hypokalemia and increased bicarbonate.

Diagnosis: Metabolic alkalosis.

Clinchers

- *Pyloric stenosis:* Presents with vomiting of large amounts of food some hours after meal. Metabolic alkalosis develops as a result of net gain of (HCO_3^-) or loss of nonvotile acid (usually HCl by vomiting) from extracellular flush.
- *Profuse vomiting:* Which is a sign of pyloric stenosis will lead to loss of acid (HCl). Vomiting/pyloric stenosis is an important cause of hypokalaemia..

The combination of hypokalemia and alkalosis in a normotensive, nonedematous patient can be due to Bartter's syndrome, magnesium deficiency, vomiting, evogenosis alkali or diuretic ingestion.

Gastrointestinal loss of H^+ results in retention of HCO_3^-. Increased H^+ loss through gastric secretions can be caused by vomiting, gastric aspiration, or gastric fistula. This loss of fluid and NaCl in vomitus, results in contraction of extracellular fluid volume (ECFV) and increased in secretion of renin and aldosterone. Volume contraction causes a reduction in GFR and an enhanced capacity of the renal tubule to reabsorb HCO_3^-. Thus during active vomiting, there is continued addition of HCO_3^- to plasma in exchange for Cl^-.

CONFUSA
Presence of hypertension and hypokalemia in an alkalotic patient suggests either mineralocorticoid excess or a hypertensive patient receiving diuretics.

Investigation of choice
ABG and serum electrolytes (already done in the patient).

Immediate management
Correct contracted extracellular fluid volume (ECFV) with NaCl, along with K^+ supplements.

Your Notes:

22. Man who is not able to pass urine, tired, complains of hiccups.

Diagnosis: Renal failure.

Clinchers

- *Not able to pass urine:* Oliguria (urine output < 400 mL/d) is a frequent but not invariable feature of acute renal failure.
- *Complains of hiccups:* Hiccups occur when there is increased retention of nitrogenous waste products. In renal failure, there is increase in plasma urea and creatine concentration.

Features suggestive of chronic renal failure include anaemia, neuropathy, radiological evidence of renal osteodystrophy or small scared kidney.

CONFUSA
Renal failure may cause high anion gap acidosis, poor filtration and reabsorption of organic onions contribute to the pathogenesis. In this question the answer could have been metabolic acidosis, if renal failure was not amongst the options.

Investigation of choice
- Blood urea and S creatinine
- Arterial blood gas (ABG) analysis
- S electrolyte

Immediate management
In case of acidosis, replace alkali ($NaHCO_3$), to maintain (CHO_3^-) between 20 and 24 mmol/L.

Treatment of choice
- Identify the cause of ARF
- Eliminate triggering insult (e.g. nephrotoxin) and/or institute disease specific therapy.
- Prevent and manage uremic complications
- Metabolic acidosis is not treated unless, serum bicarbonate concentration falls below 15 mmol/L or arterial pH falls below 7.2.

Your Notes:

23. Man with villous adenoma, profuse diarrhoea.

Diagnosis: Hypokalemia.

Clinchers
Diarrhoea may be associated with villous adenoma (usually with large tumors, more than 3-4 cm in diameter). Here hypokalemia due to potassium loss is common.

Acute diarrhoea is generally infectious. Chronic diarrhoea can be inflammatory, osmotic (malabsorption) or secretory due to intestinal dysmotility.

In cases of villous adenoma, diarrhoea is secretory in nature, caused by abnormal fluid and electrolyte transport not necessarily related to ingestion of food.

Vomiting, diarrhoea, villous adenoma rectum, pyloric stenosis, diuretics, Cushing's syndrome, alkalosis, all are important causes of hypokalaemia. Normal potassium levels in serum: 3.5-5 mmol/L.

> **CONFUSA**
> Metabolic alkalosis has been described in cases of villous adenoma, but this is most likely the result of potassium depletion.

Investigation of choice
Serum electrolytes.

Immediate management
In mild cases (>2.5 mmol/L, no symptoms) give oral K^+ supplement. If no thiazide diuretic, hypokalaemia > 3.0 mmol/L rarely needs treating. In severe cases (< 2.5 mmol/L, dangerous symptoms) give IV potassium cautiously, not more that 20 mmol/h, and not more concentrated than 40 mmol/L. Do not give K^+ if oliguric.

Your Notes:

24. Female, 24 hours after hysterectomy complains of breathlessness, increased JVP.

Diagnosis: Fluid overload.

Clinchers
- *24 hours after hysterectomy:* Intravenous fluid and blood components that may have been transfused to this female in this whole process of hysterectomy, may have lead to these signs of fluid overload (breathlessness and increased JVP).

  Blood components are excellent volume expanders and transfusion may quickly lead to volume overload.
- *Breathlessness and increased JVP:* JVP is best indicator of estimating the central venous pressure (CVP), which is no doubt raised in fluid overload. Fluid overload will lead to elevated pulmonary capillary pressure, which may be due to left ventricular dysfunction. This elevation of hydrostatic pressure in the pulmonary vascular bed leads to dyspnoea by multiple mechanisms like pulmonary edema.

Investigation of choice
Central line to measure CVP.

Immediate management
Treatment is aimed by reducing extracellular fluid volume by lowering total body Na^+ stores by following mechanisms:
- Reducing dietary intake of Na^+
- Increasing its urinary excretion with the aid of diuretics

Treatment of choice
Monitoring the rate and volume of transfusion, along with the use of a diuretic, can minimise this problem of fluid overload.

Your Notes:

25. A patient in severe renal failure has potassium level of 2.5 mmol/L.

Diagnosis: Hypokalemia (Answer: frusemide)

Clinchers
- *Severe renal failure:* May be due to glomerulonephritis, pyelonephritis, interstitial nephritis, DM, hypertension, cystic diseases, etc. In CRF there is usually, irreversible and long-standing loss of renal function. In CRF treatment is aimed at treating reversible causes (relieve obstruction, stop nephrotoxic drugs, treat hypercalcemia). High does of loop diuretics (furosemide) are used to treat edema.
- *Potassium level of 2.5:* Normal range of potassium is 3.5-5 mmol/L. Hypokalaemia is the most significant problem with high ceiling diuretics (frusemide) and thiazides. Usual manifestations of hypokalemia are weakness, fatigue, muscle cramps and cardiac arrhythmias.

CONFUSA
Hypokalemia is less common with standard doses of high ceiling diuretics (frusemide), than with thiazides, possibly because of shorter duration of action of the former which permits intermittent operation of compensatory reflection mechanism.

Investigation of choice
- Blood: FBC, ESR, U and E, Creatinine, S calcium
- Urine: Microscopy, creatinine clearance
- Renal ultrasound

Immediate management
Change furosemid with potassium sparing Diuretics

Treatment of choice
For hypokalaemia: Attempt to maintain serum K^+ at or above 3.5 mEq/L, by:
- High dietary K^+ intake
- Supplements of KCl (24-72 mEq/day) or
- Concurrent use of K^+ sparing diuretics

Your Notes:

26. A chronic alcoholic with history of recurrent falls comes to A and E with complains of ataxia. Blood glucose is 7.

Diagnosis: Subdural hematoma.

Clinchers
- *Chronic alcoholic:* Chronic alcoholics are more prone for subdural hematomas because of recurrent falls weakens the bridging veins.
- *No recurrent falls:* This substantiates the above argument.
- *Complains of ataxia:* Unsteadiness, sleepiness, headache and personality changes are frequent symptoms in an evolving subdural hematoma.
- *Blood glucose is 7:* This rules out hypoglycemia to be a cause for all of the above symptoms.

CONFUSA
Drunkenness increases the risk of sustaining a head injury and of that injury causing brain damage. Nevertheless, changes in conscious level must not be attributed to alcohol or other drugs except by exclusion and in retrospect. The plasma osmolality may be a useful investigation in this circumstance.

Investigation of choice
CT skull.

Immediate management
ICP lowering.

Treatment of choice
Evacuation of hematoma via surgery or burr holes.

Your Notes:

27. A 17-year-old rugby player becomes unconscious after a fall. After sometime, he recovers, gives his name and address to the people in the ambulance. Later condition deteriorates.

Diagnosis: Extradural hematoma.

Clinchers
- *Becomes unconscious after a fall:* Initial loss of consciousness is due to cerebral contusion (because of the severity of attack). It resolves in sometime usually.
- *He recovers, gives his name and address to the people in the ambulance:* This is the characteristic lucid interval, between initial trauma and onset or return of depressed consciousness. It is typical for extradural hematoma.
- *Later condition deteriorates:* Now, the impairment is due to local pressure effects and increasing ICP.

CONFUSA
The lucid interval is said to be characteristic for extradural haematoma but is by no means inevitable. Extradural collections are typically seen on CT scanning as binconvex, whereas subdural collections have inner concave borders. The classical unilateral, fixed, dilated, pupil is a very late sign in extradural bleeds (it occurs as a result of a ipsilateral third nerve palsy which is caused by cerebral herniation). An impaired level of consciousness is the first feature. Limb weakness, from direct pressure on the motor cortex, is usually found on the contralateral side. Lateralizing signs may be preterminal.

Investigation of choice
CT skull.

Immediate management
ICP lowering.

Treatment of choice
Surgical evacuation or multiple burr holes.

Your Notes:

28. A child becomes unconscious after falling off his bicycle, later he is better and active. Only complaint is headache.

Diagnosis: Mild injury.

Clinchers
- *Unconscious:* This is due to cerebral contusion that can produce unconsciousness immediately after injury.
- *Better and acting now:* This rules out any immediate neurological impairment or injury. However, a watch should be kept as extradural hematoma can still develop.
- *Only complaint in headache:* It is due to local pain and resolving cerebral contusion.

CONFUSA
An extradural hematoma cannot be ruled out till it develops. But among the given options, mild injury is the most suitable answer. However, a more correct and definitive criterion of mild head injury is GCS 13-15.

Investigation of choice
X-ray skull (to rule out any fracture).

Immediate management
A complete neurological evaluation.

Treatment of choice
Discharge with written advise (only if some responsible adult is accompanying him) and analgesia.

Your Notes:

March—2002

29. Man with head trauma—GCS found to be 12.

Diagnosis: Moderate injury

Clinchers
- *Glasgow Coma Scale (GCS)*
  - Maximum possible score = 15 (not necessarily equivalent to alert and oriented)
  - Minimum possible score = 3 (even if dead)
  - Coma = GCS $\leq$ 8
  - Minor/mild injury = GSS 13-15
  - Mild injury = GCS 9-12
  - Severe injury = GCS $\leq$ 8
- *TIP:* Mnemonic to remember best motor response scoring in GCS

See = C	obeys Commands	6
Low = Lo	Localises pain	5
Wit	Withdraws from pain	4
Flex Fl	abnormal flexion	3
ex	extension to pain	2
None	None	1

> **CONFUSA**
> Some centre in UK score GCS and of 14, not 15, omitting 'withdrawal to pain' in the best motor response category.

Investigation of choice
Skull X-ray.

Immediate management
Rule out cervical spine injury.

Treatment of choice
Monitoring for any complication or neurological impairment.

Your Notes:

30. Man with GCS=5, haemotympanum.

Diagnosis: Fracture base of skull.

Clinchers
- *GCS 5:* The implies a severe brain injury as GCS $\leq$ 8 is coma.
- *Haemotympanum:* It is a characteristic finding after fracture base of skull. It may produce reduced hearing so a complaint of reduced hearing in one ear after head injury moments an urgent otoscopy. Other pointers for fracture base of skull are:
  - Bleeding from ear canal
  - Bleeding from nose in absence of direct injury
  - Nasopharyngeal bleeding (this may be torsential and even severe enough to compromise the airway)
  - Cerebrospinal fluid leakage from the nose or ear
  - Subconjunctival haemorrhage without a posterior edge
  - Retro-orbital haematoma
  - Bilateral periorbital haematomas (*racoon or panda eyes*)
  - Bruising around the mastoid area (*Battle's sign*)

> **CONFUSA**
> Blood in the external auditory meatus after trauma is usually caused by basal fracture but is rarely secondary to temporomandibular joint injury. Deep auroscopic examination of the canal should be avoided as it may introduce infection via torn meninges. These are usually no radiographic signs of a basal skull fracture. However, there may be:
> - Blood in the sphenoid sinus (look for a fluid level)
> - A fracture line which appears to continue towards the base of the skull

Investigation of choice
- *Screening:* Skull X-ray.
- *Definitive:* CT scan.

Immediate management
Admission for observation for 48 hours + get neurosurgeon's opinion.

Treatment of choice
Surgical repair if appropriate, otherwise symptomatic.

Your Notes:

31. A 10-year-old girl, unconscious, brought to A and E. She is found to be dehydrated on examination and respiratory rate is 40/min.

Diagnosis: Salicylate poisoning

Clinchers
- *10-year-old girl:* Children can accidentally consume household drugs, often in large amounts. Salicylates are a common drug to be taken in this way as they are easily available in almost every household.
- *Unconscious:* In severe poisoning, convulsions and coma may occur.
- *Dehydrated:* It is a marked and potentially fatal symptom of salicylates poisoning. It also differentiate if from paracetamol poisoning.
- *Respiratory rate is 40/min:* Hyperventilation is due to direct stimulation of the central respiratory centres and produce respiratory alkalosis initially in salicylate poisoning. It also differentiate the clinical condition from that of paracetamol poisoning.

CONFUSA
In salicylate poisoning, initial stimulation of the respiratory centre causes a respiratory alkalosis. As more of the drug is absorbed a metabolic acidosis supervenes. In between there two phases there may be a transitory period with a relatively normal blood gas picture.

Investigation of choice
Blood glucose immediately (plasma salicylates concentration measured usually 4 hours after ingestion).

Immediate management
Toxicology screen + Correct dehydration

Treatment of choice
Gastric lavage—if present with 1 hr
+ Activated charcoal
+ Intensive monitoring
+ Dialysis if plasma level > 700 mg/L
  or forced alkaline diuresis if > 300 mg/L (500 mg/L for adults).

Your Notes:

32. A young boy is brought to A and E by his grandparents. He is unconscious with a bruise on the temporal area.

Diagnosis: Nonaccidental injury (probably).

Clinchers
- *Brought by grandparents:* Always suspect a nonaccidental injury whenever the accompanying adult to a suspiciously injured child is not an immediate parent.
- *Unconscious:* Due to head injury, most probably cerebral contusion in this case. But injury to temporal area is a risk factor for massive extradural hematomas (due to rupture of lateral sinus).
- *Bruise on temporal area:* This necessiaties a radiological investigation, CT-skull in this case as he is unconscious. Otherwise a skull X-ray would have sufficed.

CONFUSA
Diagnosis of child abuse is a complex problem. False accusations may produce great distress. In suspicious circumstances, experienced advice should be obtained before a full examination is undertaken.

Investigation of choice
CT skull.

Immediate management
Admit to hospital. Refer to neurosurgery if CT is abnormal. Look for the child name on the child protection register.

Treatment of choice
As per the CT findings. If normal, admit for 24 hours and if nonaccidental injury is proven, inform social services.

Your Notes:

33. A 10-year-old boy is drowsy, febrile with a rash.

Diagnosis: Meningococcal meningitis.

Clinchers
- *10-year-old boy:* It is an increase in UK and is most most common seen in young children. It is also the commonest cause of death from infectious disease in UK. In recent years, there has been a marked rise in incidence in young people aged 15 to 24 and the case fatality in this age group is twice as high as that in children under five.
- *Drowsy:* In meningococcal meningitis photophobia and neck stiffness are relatively unusual features; the most common symptoms are fever, malaise and drowsiness. Although meningism, if present, is associated with a worse prognosis.
- *Febrile:* It is due to bacteremia and is a very common symptom.
- *Rash:* The characteristic purpuric skin rash can be found in over 70% of cases of meningococcal septicaemia if a careful examination is made.

CONFUSA
The rash may not be purpuric in the early stages of the disease (it may be macular initially). A rapid increase in the distribution of the purpura is often associated with circulatory failure. In children, always screen for ICP increase. If raised, do not do a lumbar puncture. All children with raised ICP with require intubation and ventilation to control the $PaCO_2$.

Investigation of choice
Lumbar puncture (after a preliminary CT to rule out ICP↑).

Immediate management
Benzyl penicillin IM (as soon as possible—before everything).

Treatment of choice
Benzyl penicillin slow IV
Dexamethasone and mannitol if raised ICP.

Your Notes:

34. A old lady fell and broke her hand one week back. After that slowly increasing confusion. Today her relatives could not wake her up from sleep.

Diagnosis: Subdural hematoma.

Clinchers
- *Broke her hand one week back:* Since she fall and the injury was severe enough to break hand, she might have suthered head injury also (common in injuries due to fall). At that time it might have been ignored because of masking by severe pain in the hand.
- *Slowly increasing confusion since one week:* Development of subdural haemorrhage may be insidious and fluctuating level of consciousness if often present as a preceding symptom.
- *Today her relatives could not wake her up from sleep:* It could be because of unconscious produced by increased ICP and local pressure effects of the subdural hematoma.

CONFUSA
The elderly are more susceptible to subdural hematoma formation after trivial injuries, as brain shrinkage makes bridging veins more vulnerable. Other at risk are those prone to falls (epileptics, alcoholics) and those on long-term anticoagulation. Midline shift is often visible on CT scan except in bilateral isodense clots.

Investigation of choice
CT skull (Clot ± midline shift)

Immediate management
ICP lowering.

Treatment of choice
Evacuation of hematoma via surgery/burr holes.

Your Notes:

35. A 21-year-old female found unconscious next to her 22-year-old husband, who was bound dead. Her ECG shows evidence of acute MI.

Diagnosis: Cocaine abuse

Clinchers
- *21-year-old female and 22-year-old husband:* The experimentation with recreational drugs of abuse is highest amongst young persons. Also it is very rare to have a MI at this young age.
- *Husband dead:* It is most probably due to drug overdose. This couple might be the first times on drugs and most probably did not know how much is enough for them.
- *Female—ECG shows acute MI + is unconscious:* MI per se do not produce unconsciousness. She might be unconscious due to the effect of drug. As cocaine is a potent vasoconstrictor, it can cause MI by inducing coronary artery spasm.

CONFUSA

Cocaine is rarely used for homicide or suicide. Accidental cases occur from addiction, hypodermic injection and from urethral, vesical and rectal injection. It is believed to be an aphrodisiac and to increase the duration of sexual act by paralysing sensory nerves of glans penis. Sudden death by cocaine is due to cardiac arrhythmias due to direct action on myocardium and cardiopulmonary arrest.

Investigation of choice
Toxicology screen

Immediate management
Airway and circulatory stabilization.

Treatment of choice
Amyl nitrate is an antidote and is given by inhalation.

Your Notes:

36. Man rescued from burning building. Burns on face and anterior chest, soot in pharynx and singed nasal hair, asking about his family members.

Diagnosis: Inhalation injury.

Clinchers
- *Rescued from burning building:* Inhalation of hot smoke and fumes is common in patients exposed to house fires.
- *Burns on face and anterior chest:* Burns around the lips, mouth, throat or nose suggest high likely hood of inhalation injury.
- *Soot in pharynx:* Soot in pharynx and production of carboniferous (black) sputum is virtually diagnostic o inhalation injury.
- *Signed nasal hair:* It should always arouse the suspicious of inhalation injury. One should always check a burns patient for singeing of nasal vibrissae to rule out inhalation injury.
- *Asking about his family members:* This rules out impaired consciousness or confusion which is a common complication after inhalation injury. It is caused by a combination of hypoxia, carbon monoxide poisoning and hydrogen cyanide poisoning.

CONFUSA

Fumes may contain gases which impair surfactant activity and irritate the respiratory mucosa. Early bronchospasm may occur but there may be no obvious evidence of damage until pulmonary oedema develops some hours later. Airway obstruction may also rapidly result from delayed sloughing of tracheal or bronchial mucosa.

Beware of conventional blood gas analyser readings in patients who may have high carboxy- or methaemoglobin levels. The oxygen electrode measure oxygen dissolve in plasma only and oxygen saturation in then calculated assuming all hemoglobin to be normal. PaO_2 and oxygen saturation may thus appear to be satisfactory despite very low total blood oxygen content.

Investigation of choice
Fibreoptic bronchoscopy + ABG + COHb

Immediate management
- High concentration O_2
- Ask for senior anaesthetic advice about intubation

Treatment of choice
Early intubation (late intubation is difficult because of oedema).

Note: Endotracheal tubes should be left long and uncut to allow for swelling.

37. Baby with less than 3 percent burns on chest and shoulders [scald due to tea falling on him] is irritable, crying, not allowing examination.

Diagnosis: Superficial small burns.

Clinchers
- *Less than 3 percent burns:* This patient does not require a referral for admission to burns unit. The criteria for admission are:
  - Children and elderly—>10% burns
  - Adults—>15% burns
  - Other—facial, hand, perineal burns.
- *Scald due to tea falling on him:* A scald from hot fluid with produce a cascade effect, with streaks of burnt skin following the path of the falling fluid, possibly with increasing depth of injury where its flow has been held up by constricting clothes such as waistbands or socks.
- *Irritable, crying:* That means the burn is painful. This is significant as full thickness burns are painless because of destruction of nerve endings.
- *Not allowing examination:* To perform examination, analgesia need to be given.

CONFUSA
Simple erythema is extremely painful. Even patients expected to go home after treatment may need parenteral analgesia. A scald with a glove or stocking distribution is unusual and suggests abuse (non-accidental injury) in children.

Investigation of choice
Determination of depth of burn.

Immediate management
IV opioid (analgesia must be given as soon as possible, especially to children. The beneficial effects of morphine is small children greatly outweigh any haemodynamic side effects).

Treatment of choice
Dressing with medication and discharge with follow up instructions.

Your Notes:

38. Man was electrocuted. Full thickness burn on fingers complainting of pain.

Diagnosis: Electric burns.

Clinchers
- *Electrocuted:* Electric burns are of two types:
  1. *High voltage injury:* Produce ECG changes (RBBB and/or ST changes ± SVT) and are usually fatal. The causes include lightning.
  2. *Low voltage injury:* These are usually sustained from the domestic electricity supply and usually localised without cardiac complications. The case described in question is most probably of this type.
- *Full thickness burns on fingers with pain:* Local burns even in low voltage injury are almost always full-thickness and much deeper than it appears. Pain may be present in adjoining ischaemic area which usually also necrose within few days.

CONFUSA
The fingers quickly stiffen up and conventional bandages become very dirty, with an increased risk of infection. These complications are avoided if plastic gloves are used initially instead of standard dressings. Silver sulphadiazine cream is applied and a loosely fitting examination glove is fitted in place with tape around the wrist. The gloves tend to burst, so patients must be given a supply to apply themselves.

Investigation of choice
ECG.

Immediate management
Escharotomy.

Treatment of choice
Early excision and grafting.

Your Notes:

39. Man with 40 percent burns over trunk and limbs.

Diagnosis: Burns requiring admission to burns unit.

Clinchers
- *40% burns:* The criteria for admissions are:
  - Adults—>15% burns
  - Child (<10 yrs)—>10% burns
  - Elderly (>70 yrs)—>10% burns

  The admission is required as these patients require IV fluid resuscitation to correct haemodynamic changes.
- *Over trunk and limbs:* This rules out inhalation injury (but sill check ABG and nasal vibrissae singeing).

CONFUSA
Fluid replacement must be calculated from the time of burns and not from the time of admission. This is so because exudative fluid loss start immediately after burns. Fluid given in the first time band has to be given at a faster rate if there is a delay between time of burns and time of arrival at hospital.

Investigation of choice
U and E.

Immediate management
IV fluids + referral for admission to burns unit.

Treatment of choice
Monitoring + care in specialist burns care unit ± skin grafting later on.

Your Notes:

40. Man, slept while sunbathing comes with redness, and pain all over his body. Otherwise well.

Diagnosis: Sunburns.

Clinchers
- *Sunbathing:* It can cause sunburns if prolonged, but these are usually not serious.
- *Redness:* It is superficial erythema and is never taken into accounting when calculating the area of burn.
- *Pain:* Simple erythema is extremely painful. Even patients expected to go home after treatment may need parenteral analgesia.
- *Other wise well:* This rules out any other injury or fluid compromise. Since simple erythema do not require active treatment, he can be safely discharged home.

CONFUSA
Unprotected exposure to UV radiation can cause extremely painful, blistering, oedematous skin. In general the treatment is as for any other burn.

Investigation of choice
None required.

Immediate management
Oral analgesia if required.

Treatment of choice
Reassure and discharge
+
Regular application of hydrocortisone 1% cream.

Your Notes:

41. Child who is HIV positive is due for MMR.

Diagnosis: Balanced risk.

Clinchers
- *MMR vaccines:* Those age 18 months to 5 years who have not had the vaccine (even if they have had single measles vaccine) may have MMR with the preschool of DPT. There is no upper age limit.
- As per the UK schedule, first dose of MMR (0.5 mL SC) is given between 12-18 months.
- *HIV positive:* Immunodeficiencies are a contraindication for MMR vaccination but these include only primary immunodeficiencies and not HIV or AIDS (208, OHCS, 5th edn).

CONFUSA
Contraindications for MMR vaccination

Condition	Delay for
Fever	till fever resolves
Pregnancy	till one month postpartum
Previous line vaccine	till 3 weeks
Previous Ig	till 3 months
Primary immunodeficiencies (except HIV and AIDS)	not given
Steroid therapy	till 3 months after discontinuation
Leukemia	not given
Lymphoma	not given
Recent radiotherapy	till 6 months to one year
Anaphylaxis history by • egg • neomycin • kanamycin	not given

- Steroid therapy implies prednisolone ≥ 2 mg/kg/day from > 1 week (or equivalent doses)
- Neomycin or kanamycin are the vaccine preservatives
- The vaccine is chick embryo based, so a history of anaphylaxis by egg protein (and not egg allergy) is a contraindication

Investigation of choice
None required.

Immediate management
None required.

Treatment of choice
Continue as per schedule.

Your Notes:

42. Child due for HiB, DPT, etc. suffering from acute febrile illness.

Diagnosis: Risk of febrile convulsions.

Clinchers
Note: An acute febrile illness is a contraindication for any vaccine.
- *HiB vaccine:* It is a bacterial polysaccharide protein conjugate vaccine for hemophilus influenza type V strain. It has a few insignificant local effects and no serious reactions.
- *DPT vaccination:* It is a combination vaccine against diphtheria, pertussis and tetanus. In them diphtheria and tetanus are toxoids and pertussis is an acellular vaccine. According to UK schedule the first dose is given at 2 months of age (in preterm babies—2 month postnatally).
- *Acute febrile illness:* It is a contraindication for DPT vaccination (not so for H:B) as the pertussis component in it produces a post vaccination fever of >39.5°C within 48 hours. Since the child is already febrile, it can compound the problem and can lead to febrile convulsions. Its better to delay the vaccine till the fever resolves or at least 2 weeks.

CONFUSA
The only other contraindication for pertussis vaccination is a past severe reaction to pertussis vaccine—i.e. indurated redness most of the way around the arm, or over most of the anterolateral thigh (depending on the site of injection) or a generalised reaction.
Note: According to BNF (British National Formulary) website, evolving neurological problems are also a contraindication untill the condition is stable.

Investigation of choice
Fever workup.

Immediate management
Paracetamol ± tepid sponging.

Treatment of choice
Delay by 2 weeks.

Your Notes:

43. Child cried for 2 hours after Hib, DPT, etc.

Diagnosis: No risk from further vaccination.

Clinchers
- *Cried for 2 hours after Hib, DPT:* Persistent, inconsolable crying lasting ≥ 3 hours within 48 hours after DPT vaccination is a valid *precaution* for further vaccination. Since this child does not meet this criteria, the rest of the immunisation schedule can be safely continued.

CONFUSA
Since the above criterion is only a precaution and not a contraindication, it warrants further vaccination after careful review. The benefits and risk of administering a specific vaccine to an individual under the circumstances are considered. It benefits outweigh the risk, e.g. during on outbreak or foreign travel, the vaccine should be administered.

Investigation of choice
A complete work up to find the cause of inconsolable crying.

Immediate management
A complete work up to find the cause of inconsolable crying.

Treatment of choice
Continue as per schedule.

Your Notes:

44. Family history of egg allergy. Child due for MMR.

Diagnosis: Insignificant risk of anaphylaxis.

Clinchers
- *Family history of egg allergy:* The only contraindication for MMR (a chick embryo based vaccine) is previous history of anaphylaxis by egg intake. History of other egg allergies in the subject to be vaccinated or in his family is a contraindication.

Note: Other vaccine which can produce complications in previous history of egg allergy is Hib vaccine.

CONFUSA
Persons with a history of anaphylactic reactions (and not just history of egg allergy in himself or in family) following egg ingestion be vaccinated only with caution. Protocols have been developed for vaccinating such persons and should be consulted.

Investigation of choice
None.

Immediate management
Cautions vaccination and monitoring thereafter.

Treatment of choice
Continue as per schedule.

Your Notes:

March—2002

45. History of convulsions. Child due for HiB, DPT, etc.

Diagnosis: Insignificant risk of febrile convulsions.

Clinchers
➢ *History of convulsions:* The parents of children with a tendency to have convulsions should be counselled on the management of any fever developing after immunization. Febrile convulsions may occur 5-10 days after measles vaccination (or MMR) whereas they may take place in the first 72 hours after pertussis immunization. Suggestion may include paracetamol, sponge with tepid water, give extra fluids, dress in thin clothing and place in a cool room. In high-risk children, an antipyretic drug may be suggested routinely for the first 72 hours after immunization. Where the tendency is severe, the parents may be instructed on rectal diazepam administration (source: BNF website).
➢ *HiB, DPT*—Only the pertussis component is known to produce a febrile syndrome postvaccination (Hence increase the risk of febrile convulsions)

CONFUSA
Presence of history of convulsions (personal/family) is a special consideration (i.e. require individual care review) and not a contraindication for vaccination. Most children with idiopathic epilepsy, or a family history of epilepsy (sibling or parent) should be vaccinated. If in doubt, seek expert advice rather than withholding the vaccine. Those with special CNS conditions (e.g. cerebral palsy, spina bifida) are *especially recommended* for vaccination.

Investigation of choice
None required.

Immediate management
Counsel and teach the parents about the prevention and management of febrile convulsions.

Treatment of choice
Continue as per schedule.

Your Notes:

46. Woman after open cholecystectomy presents with fever, redness and tenderness of wound.

Diagnosis: Wound infection.

Clinchers
➢ *Open cholecystectomy:* Wound infections are especially common when the alimentary, biliary or urinary tract is opened during surgery, allowing bacterial contamination to occur.
➢ *Fever with redness and tenderness of wound:* The onset of would infection is usually a few days after operations; this may be delayed still further, even upto weeks, if antimicrobial chemotherapy has been employed. The patient complaints of
- pain and swelling in the wound
- general effects of infection, e.g.
  - malaise
  - anorexia
  - vomiting
- runs a swinging, pyrexia.

The wound is red, swollen, hot and tender.

CONFUSA
The principal causes of wound infection are the penicillin resistant *Staphylococcus aureus*, together with *Streptococcus faecalis*, *Pseudomonas*, coliform bacilli and other bowel bacteria including bacteroides. With continued use of antibiotics, mothicillin resistant *Staphylococcus aureus* (MRSA) and the vancomycin resistant enterococcus (VRE) becoming more common.

Investigation of choice
Wound swab.

Immediate management
Removal of sutures of probing of the wound to release the contained pus.

Treatment of choice
Established infection is treated by drainage. Antibiotics are given, if there is, in addition, a spreading cellulitis.

Your Notes:

47. Chronic smoker 1 day after splenectomy presents with chest pain and dyspnea.

Diagnosis: Pulmonary collapse.

Clinchers
- *Chronic smoker:* Smokers are at particular risk, with increased secretions and ineffective cilia.
- *Splenectomy:* Some degree of pulmonary collapse occurs after almost every abdominal or transthoracic procedure.
  Mechanism: Mucus is retained in the bronchial tree
  ↓
  blocks smaller bronchi
  ↓
  alveolar air is then absorbed
  ↓
  collapse of the supplied lung segments (usually the basal lobes)
  ↓
  Collapsed lung continued to be perfused and acts as a shunt
  ↓
  this reduced oxygenation
  ↓
  secondary infection of collapsed segment
  ↓
  abscess formation
- *1 day after:* Pulmonary collapse occurs within the first post-operative 48 hours. Also this excludes other conditions which occurs:
  - Pulmonary embolism—10th postoperative day
  - Infection—5th postoperative day
- *Chest pain and dyspnoea:* The patient is dyspnoeic with a rapid pulse and elevated temperature. There may be cyanosis. The patient attempt to cough, but this is painful.

CONFUSA
To relieve chest pain or abdominal pain (of operative scar), intercostal nerve blocks and epidural anaesthesia are preferred over opiate analgesia as the latter causes respiratory depression and worsens the already reduced O_2 saturation.

Fruity cough is typical pulmonary collapse and results from the sound of the bronchial secretions rattling within the chest (A good clinicians should be able to make the diagnosis while skill several yards away from the patient)

Investigation of choice
CXR (mediastinal shift + opacity of involved segment—usually basal or mid zone)
+
Pulse oximetry (reduced saturation)

Immediate management
Referral to a physiotherapist

Treatment of choice
Symptomatic + breathing exercises.

Your Notes:

March—2002

48. Female after anterior resection of rectum complains of anterior chest pain radiating to her left arm.

Diagnosis: Myocardial infarction (probably).

Clinchers
- *Anterior resection of rectum:* It suggest that a rectal tumor has been resected. In any pelvic surgery there is an increased incidence of arterial or venous embolisation postoperatively which can lead to coronary artery thrombosis or pulmonary embolism.
- *Anterior chest pain radiating to left arm:* This is a typical pain presentation it is MI as angina usually require also some precipitant (e.g. exertion) and patient also give a previous history most of the times.

CONFUSA
Although pain from pulmonary embolism can present in the same way as that of MI, it is highly unlikely as a answer in this question as the presentation is not cliched. Usually GMC do not ask for such "far-sighted" diagnoses.

Investigation of choice
12 lead ECG

Immediate management
High flow O_2 by facemask.

Treatment of choice
See MI protocol on pg 781, OHCM, 5th edn.

Your Notes:

---

49. Man with COPD presents with central cyanosis postoperatively.

Diagnosis: Pulmonary collapse.

Clinchers
- *COPD:* Pre-existing chronic pulmonary disease like emphysema or COPD is a risk factor for complicated pulmonary collapse after surgery.
- *Central cyanosis:* Cyanosis may or may not be present depending upon the severity of pulmonary collapse. In pre-existing diseases it tends to be severe enough to produce cyanosis.

Risk factors for pulmonary collapse
- Preoperative
  - Pre-existing acute or chronic pulmonary infection
  - Smokers
  - Chronic inflammatory diseases
  - Chest wall diseases, e.g. ankylosing spondylitis
- Operative
  - Anaesthetic drugs
  - Atropine
- Postoperative
  - Pain

Investigation of choice
Pulse oximetry (as cyanosis is the main feature; if dyspnoea is the main feature; CXR will be done first).

Immediate management
Referral to a physiotherapist.

Treatment of choice
See Q 47.

Your Notes:

50. Man after appendicectomy presents with spiking fever with rigors, tenesmus, diarrhoea.

Diagnosis: Pelvic abscess.

Clinchers
- *Appendicectomy:* Pelvic abscess formation is an occasional complication of appendicitis and can occur irrespective of the position of the appendix within the peritoneal cavity.
- *Spiking fever with rigors:* The most common presentation is a spiking pyrexia several days following appendicitis (the patient may have been discharged from hospital).
- *Tenesmus and diarrhoea:* Pelvic pressure or discomfort associated with loose stool or tenesmus is common.

CONFUSA
A pelvic abscess may follow any general peritonitis, but it is particularly common after acute appendicitis (75%), or after gynaecological infections. In the male the abscess lies between the bladder and the rectum, in the female between the uterus and posterior fornix of the vagina anteriorly, and the rectum posteriorly (pouch of Douglas). Left untreated the abscess may burst into the rectum or vagina or may discharge onto the abdominal wall, particularly if there has been previous abdominal laparotomy incision at the time of the original episode of peritonitis (as in this case).

Investigation of choice
- *Screening:* Per rectal examination (foggy mass in pelvis, anterior to rectum, at the level of peritoneal reflection).
- *Definitive:* Pelvic USG/CT scan.

Immediate management
Antipyretics + short course chemotherapy.

Treatment of choice
Transrectal drainage under GA.

Note: Very often even this is not required, as firm pressure by the finger in the rectum may be followed by rupture of the abscess through the rectal wall.

Your Notes:

51. A 14-year-old girl has just started having sexual relationship with her boyfriend of 2 months.

Best option: OCPs + condom

Clinchers
- *14-year-old girl:* OCP's are not preferral over 35 years of age, as it increases the risk of thromboembolism (more common if they smoke). Smokers: stop pill at 30 years.
- *With her boyfriend:* In steady relationships only OCPs would be the fine, but here to reduced risk of transmission of most STDs, condom together with OCP would help.

When prescribing OCPs tell her about the risks. Look for any contraindications.

Contraindications to OPCs

Absolute contraindications
A. Circulatory diseases (past/present)
  - Arterial or venous thrombosis
  - Severe hypertension
  - Angina/valvular heart disease/ischaemic heart diseases
  - Migraine
  - Hyperlipidemia
B. Diseases of liver
  - Active liver disease
  - Liver adenoma, carcinoma
  - History of cholestatic, jaundice in pregnancy
C. Others
  - Pregnancy
  - Breast cancer (estrogen dependent neoplasms)
  - Undiagnosed genital tract bleeding

Relations contraindications
- Obesity
- Epilepsy
- Age over 35 years
- Varicosities
- Bronchial asthma
- Smoking

CONFUSA
Condoms would not only prevent pregnancy, but will also give protection against STDs.

Your Notes:

52. 35-year-old female after her third child wants reliable contraception. She is a smoker and does not want to gain weight.

Best option: IUCD.

Clinchers

- Death due to the pill in 35-year-old is 8 times more common if they smoke. At 30 years either stop smoking or stop the pills.
- *35-year-old female:* A relative contraindications for OCPs. For other contraceptives refer previous question.
- *She is a smoker:* Smoking is contraindication for OCPs. Increases the risk of thromboembolism.
- *Does not want to gain weight:* Weight gain is an adverse effect of OCPs. The progestin have got an anabolic effect due its chemical relation to testosterone which results in a positive nitrogen balance and fat deposition.

CONFUSA

Sterilization would have been a better option, since she already has three children. If this female is quite sure that she does not want further children, then sterilization is the most effective form of contraception for this female.

IUCD is the best form of contraception after sterilization for older women.

Side effects of OCPs
- Nausea, vomiting, headache
- Mastalgia
- Weight gain
- Chloasma and acne
- Menstrual abnormalities
- Libido may be diminished

Major complications are:
- Depression
- Hypertension
- Thromboembolism/coronary thrombosis
- Cholestatic jaundice.

Your Notes:

53. An 18-year-old girl has been on OCPs since 2 years ,has to have rifampicin prophylaxis since her roommate has meningitis.

Best option: OCPs + condom.

Clinchers

- *Rifampicin prophylaxis:* Liver enzyme inducers, e.g. rifampicin, anticonvulsants and griseofulvin reduce the efficacy of oral contraceptives by decreasing circulating, oestrogen. For rifampicin take precaution besides OCPs whilst use and four weeks after. Best alternatives would be to change the contraceptives method if on long-term rifampicin.

  Barrier method along with OCPs can be used here. With long-term use of these drugs consider using 50 Hg estrogen pills with higher doses of progesterone, e.g. Norinyl-I.

Your Notes:

54. Girl with learning disorder begins to find males attractive. Her parents and teachers are worried.

Best option: Depovera.

Clinchers

Depovera 150 mg given deep IM is given 12 weekly, started during the first 5 days of a cycle. It is medroxyprogesterone acetate, simple, safe and very effective.

Since it is given once in 12 weeks it has following advantages.
- Secret
- No compliance problems
- No estrogen content
- Reduced for menstrual syndrome
- Suppresses ovulation.

Therefore in a girl with learning disorder depovera is the best option.

Your Notes:

55. Female after her first-child wants reliable contraception but wants no chemicals in her body, complains of heavy periods and dysmenorrhoea, husband does not want to use condoms.

Best option: Mirena coil.

Clinchers
- Mirena coil (carries levonorgesterol) is an IUCD carrying hormone. It has been shown to be *helpful in dysmenorrhoea*. Local effects make implantation less likely, and *periods lighter*. It lasts 3 years. There may be less risk of ectopic pregnancy.
- *Heavy periods and dysmenorrhoea:* Mirena coil is beneficial in both of these conditions.

CONFUSA
Diaphragm (intravaginal device made of rubber), could have been the answer, but it is not a popular method. Complaints of dysmenorrhoea favours mirena coil.

Your Notes:

March—2002

56. Most common form of dementia in the UK.

Diagnosis Alzheimer's disease (AD)

Clinchers
About 25% of the elderly population suffer from a psychiatric disability, mainly anxiety and depression. However, dementia affects about 10% of those aged over 65 years and 20% of those over 80 years of age a total of 650 thousand people in England and Wales. Seventy percent are due to Alzheimer's disease.

CONFUSA
Neurotransmitter changes with disease
- Depression—decreased NE and 5-HT
- Alzheimer's—decreased Ach
- Huntingtons's disease—decreased GABA and ACh
- Schizophrenia—increased dopamine
- Parkinsonism—decreased dopamine

Investigation of choice
AD is a diagnosis of exclusion
- MRI or CT—exclude
  - Multi infarct dementia
  - Subdural hemorrhage
  - Abscess
  - Tumor

Immediate management
Usually none required, otherwise symptomatic.

Treatment of choice
Donepezil

Your Notes:

57. Characterised by neurofibrillary tangles and senile plaques.

Diagnosis: Alzheimer's disease (AD)

Clinchers
- *Neurofibrillary tangles and senile plaques:* Neuropathological changes include neuronal reduction, neurofibrillary tangles, senile neuritic plaques and a variable amyloid angiopathy. These changes are particularly seen in the hippocampus, substantia innominate, locus cenuleus and the tempoparietal and frontal cortices.
- *TIP:* 6 A's of dementia
  - Aphasia
  - Apraxia
  - Agnosia
  - Amnesia
  - Abstract thought
  - Agitation

CONFUSA
Usually pathophysiology questions are not asked in PLAB exam, but there may be a couple of questions or whole theme on these features. So do not skip these topics during your first reading.

Investigation of choice
See previous question.

Immediate management
See previous question.

Treatment of choice
See previous question.

Your Notes:

58. May respond to antidepressants.

Diagnosis: Pseudodementia.

Clinchers
Depression can produce cognitive impairment, called pseudodementia contributed to by lack of motivation, concentration and self-confidence.

CONFUSA
Pseudodementia must be differentiated from dementia, as the foramen can respond to antidepressants. Two questions can help in distinguishing them:
- Did low mood or poor memory come first?
- Is the failure to answer questions due to lack of ability or lack of motivation?

Note that dementia and depression can also occur together.

Investigation of choice
Clinical diagnosis.

Immediate management
Rule out delirium by checking level of consciousness.

Treatment of choice
Antidepressants.

Your Notes:

59. Increased disinhibition, preservation of intellect

Diagnosis: Frontal dementia.

Clinchers
- *Increased disinhibition:* Frontal lobe lesions produces personality changes and disinhibition increases, i.e. the patient becomes
  - Indecent
  - Indolent
  - Indiscreet
- *Preservation of intellect:* There is no intellectual impairment in frontal lobe dementia. Psychosis is never present in frontal lobe dementia.

CONFUSA
Intellectual deterioration is a hallmark of corpus callosum lesions. Also do not confuse increased disinhibition with hypersexuality which is a feature of temporal lobe lesions.

Investigation of choice
CT/MRI.

Immediate management
Nose required.

Treatment of choice
- Conservative and symptomatic
- Surgery if SOL present.

Your Notes:

60. An elderly hypertensive with recurrent faints presents with deteriorating mental functions.

Diagnosis: Multiinfarct dementia (MID)

Clinchers
- *Hypertensive:* Hypertension is a risk factor for CVA which in turn is a cause for MID.
- *Recurrent faints:* There is usually a history of transient ischaemic attacks with brief impairment of consciousness, fleeting pareses or visual loss. The dementia may follow a succession of acute CVA or less commonly, a single major stroke. Vessel occlusion is the most common cause of vascular dementia, and this may produce a variety of cognitive defects depending on the site of the ischaemic damage.

Note: MID results from involvement of several vessels supplying the cerebral cortex and subcortical structures and is typically associated with signs of cortical dysfunction.

CONFUSA
MID is the second most common cause of dementia in UK and is distinguished from Alzheimer's disease by its history of onset, clinical features and subsequent course. MID is also known as vascular dementia, so do not get confused between them!

Investigation of choice
CT/MRI.

Immediate management
Usually none required.

Treatment of choice
Symptomatic.

Your Notes:

61. A schizophrenic on long-term treatment complains of impotence, has high prolactin levels, extrapyramidal side effects (EPS).

Diagnosis: Side effects (Chlorpromazine)

Clinchers
- *Schizophrenic on long-term treatment:* After a single episode of schizophrenia, medication is continued for 12-24 months. If the person remains week it should be tailed off because there is little evidence that further medication is beneficial and because of the risk of tardive dyskinesia. Patients who have had multiple episodes or persistent symptoms usually remain on medication for many years, though the need for it should remain under regular review.
- *Impotence:* Inhibition of ejaculation is more common with low potency phenothiazines and is due to α-adrenergic blockade.
- *High prolactic levels:* It occurs infrequently after prolonged use and is associated with low levels of gonadotrophins which may also be responsible for impotence. It is due to blockade of hypothalamic dopamine receptors.
- *Extrapyramidal side effects:* These are the major dose limiting side effects—more prominent with high potency drugs.

CONFUSA
Akathisia is an EPS which can be mistaken for exacerbation of psychosis—differentiation may be helped by an IM injection of benzotropin (2 mg): akathesia will respond but not exacerbation of psychosis. Parkinsonism is another EPS that can be mistaken for depression or for negative symptoms in schizophrenia.

Investigation of choice
Serum prolactin (already done in this case).

Immediate management
Reduce dose of antipsychotics.

Treatment of choice
Symptomatic:
- Acute dystonia—IM/IV anticholinergics
- Parkinsonism—reduce dose or add anticholinergic
- Alkathesia—reduce dose + propranolol
- Tardine dyskinesia—reduce! stop drug
- Impotence—α agonist

Your Notes:

62. Drug with anticholinergic side effects, dry mouth, blurred vision, tremor.

Diagnosis: Side effects of tricyclics.

Clinchers
- Anticholinergic side effects: These can be
  - Dry mouth
  - Bad taste
  - Constipation
  - Epigastric distress
  - Urinary retention/heritancy (especially in males with enlarged prostate)
  - Blurred vision
  - Palpitation

CONFUSA
Though anticholinergic side effects can also occurs with antipsychotics, they are more characteristic and common with tricyclics. Amitriptyline especially produce sedation, mental confusion and weakness in addition.

Investigation of choice
None required.

Immediate management
Reduce dose.

Treatment of choice
Stop or change dry if troublesome.

Your Notes:

63. Patient on treatment for bipolar disorder, now present with weight gain and loss of appetite.

Diagnosis: Lithium side effects.

Clinchers
- *Bipolar disorder treatment:* Its first line prophylactic treatment is lithium. Majority of patients stabilizes on lithium and usually do not need alternative or second line drugs.
- *Weight gain and loss of appetite:* This suggests hypothyroidism which is infact a prominent yet rare side effects of lithium. It is due to interference with iodination of tyrosine—decreased thyroxine synthesis.

CONFUSA
Lithium induced hypothyroidism is seen in 20% women. In men it is rare. Other main side effect of lithium on long-term usage is renal diabetes insipidus. Lithium induces granulocytosis and infact sometimes used to treat agranulocytosis (e.g. chemotherapy induced leukopenia and agranulocytosis).

Investigation of choice
TSH.

Immediate management
Rule out primary thyroid disease.

Treatment of choice
Thyroxine administration.

Your Notes:

March—2002

64. Schizophrenic patient under treatment presents with sore throat, decreased WBC, agranulocytosis.

Diagnosis: Clozapine side effects.

Clinchers

- *Schizophrenic patient:* Clozapine is an atypical antipsychotic and is pharmacologically distinct from other in that it has only weak D_2 blocking action and produces few extrapyramidal symptoms; tardive dyskinesia is also rare with it. It suppresses both positive and negative symptoms of schizophrenia and many patients refractory to typical neuroleptics respond.
- *Sore throat:* It is due to infections secondary to agranulocytosis.
- *Decreased WBC and agranulocytosis:* The major limitation of clozapine is higher incidence of agranulocytosis and other blood dyscrasias.

CONFUSA
Clozapine is used only as a reserve drug in resistant schizophrenia (who have not responded to, or are intolerant of, two other antipsychotics). In UK it is given on a named patient basis and weekly white cell counts are mandatory. It is very expensive (~£3000 per year in UK)—though cost benefit analyses are favourable as in-patient care is reduced.

Investigation of choice
Weekly white cell counts.

Immediate management
Stop drug.

Treatment of choice
Change clozapine with new antipsychotics, i.e. risperidone, olanzapine and questiapine which do not have EPS like clozapine but do not need blood tests.

Your Notes:

---

65. Schizophrenic patient under treatment presents with fever, increased WCC, increased muscle creatinine kinase levels.

Diagnosis: Neuroleptic malignant syndrome (NMS).

Clinchers

- *Schizophrenic patient under treatment:* Most probably he is taking some high potency antipsychotics with whom this syndrome is common.
- *Fever:* Pyrexia is pathognomonic of this condition.
- *Increased WCC:* Investigations invariably show increased WCC.
- *Increased muscle creatinine kinase levels:* Increased creatinine phosphokinase and myoglobin may be present in blood. It lasts 5-10 days after drug withdrawal and may be fatal.

CONFUSA
NMS occurs in 0.2% of patients on antipsychotics (particularly with high potency drugs i.e. Haloperidol). Its symptoms appear a few days to a few weeks after initiation of therapy. Its main presenting symptoms are:
- Hyperthermia
- Muscle rigidity
- Autonomic instability (tachycardia, labila BP, pallor)
- Fluctuating level of consciousness.

Investigation of choice
CPK (↑); WCC (↑); LFT (deranged)

Immediate management
Stop drug immediately and give symptomatic treatment (e.g. temperature reduction)

Treatment of choice
Bromocriptine (to enhance dopaminergic activity)
+
Dantrolene (to reduce muscle tone)

Your Notes:

66. Man living in a hostel, brought to hospital after he collapsed. On the 3rd day, he points out things other people cannot see, disorientation in time and place.

Diagnosis: Delirium tremens (DT).

Clinchers
- *Living in a hostel:* Alcoholism or binges drinking is more prevalent in hostels and young people. Often they do not drink in moderation resulting in withdrawal symptoms.
- *Brought to hospital after he collapsed:* He must have collapsed because of a heavy prolonged drinking session (alcohol intoxication)
- *On 3rd day:* Onset of DT is typically 24-72 hours after prolonged drinking.
- *Points out things other people cannot see:* Visual hallucinations are characteristic (e.g. pink elephants) in DT.
- *Disorientation in time and place:* Clouding of consciousness and disorientation is a feature of DT.

CONFUSA
In alcoholic hallucinosis, heavy drinker experiences recurrent auditory hallucinations, usually of threatening or derogatory nature. In contract to delirium tremens, the hallucinations typically occur in clear consciousness.

Investigation of choice
The diagnosis is purely clinical.

Immediate management
Adequate sedation + intensive monitoring.

Treatment of choice
Supportive therapy.

Your Notes:

67. An 80-year-old female is on no medication. Cause of concern is that she was trying to get into a shop at 6:00am. Neighbours say she is ok except her memory is not as good as it used to be since 2 years. She is otherwise well.

Diagnosis: Alzheimer's dementia (AD).

Clinchers
- *An 80-year-old:* The onset of AD can be in middle adult life or even earlier (of pre-senile onset) but the incidence is higher in later life. It is the most common cause of dementia in elderly. The frequency of AD increases with each decade of adult life to reach 20 to 40% of population over the age of 85.
- *Female:* Female gender may also be a risk factor independent of the greater longevity of women. Unconfirmed studies have suggested that postmenopausal estrogen use is associated with a decreased frequency of AD.
- *She was trying to get into a shop at 6:00 AM:* AD produced cognitive problems which interfere with daily activities, such as keeping track of finances, following instructions on the job, driving, shopping and house keeping. In this case the patient seem to have completely lost sense of judgement and forgot the opening time of the shop.
- *Memory is not as good as it used to be:* Failing memory is the most common presenting feature of AD.
- *Otherwise well:* This rules out any acute cause for confusional state.

CONFUSA
Rarely AD patients may have a form of cortical blindness in which they deny their inability to see. In AD, social graces, routine behaviour and superficial conversation may be surprisingly retained. Patients at risk of developing AD are with:
- Family history
- Down's syndrome
- ALL
- Head injury.

Investigation of choice
Neuroimaging (rule out frontal lobe dementia, Lewy body dementia and Pick's disease).

Immediate management
Usually none required, otherwise symptomatic.

Treatment of choice
Donepezil.

68. Female brings her husband to A and E, says he talks about their sex life in public. There is loss of inhibition (intellect normal) in him.

Diagnosis: Frontal lobe dementia (FLD).

Clinchers
- *Talks about sex life in public:* In FLD, the patient typically have loss of inhibitions (indiscreet, indolent, indecent). In fact this feature differentiates FLD from other dementias.
- *Normal intellect:* FLD patients may do better than those with Alzheimer's dementia on construction and calculation tasks.

CONFUSA
FLD is not a specific entity (not even regarded as such by some authors) and the designation usually includes Pick's disease. In FLD, in addition to progressive memory loss and confusion, the patients are often irritable.

Investigation of choice
Neuroimaging (atrophy confined to frontal or frontal and temporal lobes)

Immediate management
Counselling of the wife on how to take care of him.

Treatment of choice
Symptomatic.

Your Notes:

---

69. Man has cough and fever since 2 days. Wife notices he has disorientation in time and place, decreased concentration and confused. He was ok mentally 1 day back.

Diagnosis: Delirium.

Clinchers
- *Cough and fever since 2 days:* Medical conditions which can cause delirium are:
  - Febrile illness
  - Septicaemia
  - Organ failure (cardiac, renal, hepatic)
  - Hypoglycemia
  - Postoperative hypoxia

  Or it can occur because of prescribed drugs in illness, i.e.
  - Any drug with anticholinergic properties (highly likely in this case)
  - Sedatives including opiates
  - Digoxin
  - Diuretics
  - Lithium
  - Steroids
- *Disorientation in time and place:* This is typical of delirium. Orientation in "person" is usually normal.
- *Decreased concentration and confused:* Impaired concentration and memory is a feature of delirium. Confusion is so prominent that delirium is also known as acute confusional state.
- *Mentally OK 1 day back:* It proves that the condition is acute in onset. Note that delirium is always acute in onset.

CONFUSA
In delirium there is usually no disorientation in "person" element, only disorientation in time and place are found. Clouding of consciousness is the most important diagnostic sign. It is manifested as drowsiness, decreased awareness of surroundings, disorientation and distractibility. At its most severe the patient may be unresponsive, but more commonly the impaired consciousness is quite subtle. Often the first clue to the presence of delirium is one of its features other than delirium.

Investigation of choice
Neuroimaging to rule out SOL or encephalitis.

Immediate management
Take psychiatric opinion.

Treatment of choice
Symptomatic + treat the cause.

70. A 70-year-old man says his life is not worth living, his existence is a waste, he performs all his work very slowly, he has lost weight.

Diagnosis: Depression.

Clinchers
- *70-year-old man:* The incidence of depression increases with age; the disorder is approximately twice as prevalent in women as in men, regardless of age.
- *Say his life is not worthlining, his existence is a waste:* In depression thoughts are negative and pessimistic, centring upon unpleasant memories, past failings and a bleak future. Hopelessness, helplessness and worthlessness readily supervene, not only reinforcing the depressed mood but leading to suicidal thoughts. Mood is infact a criterion to differentiate minor (transiently low mood) and major (persistently low mood) depression.
- *Performs all his work very slowly:* This is *psychomotor retardation* a typical feature of depression.
- *Lost weight:* Loss of appetite in depression leads to loss of weight. Rarely some patients have increased appetite leading to weight gain.

CONFUSA
Many depressed patients do not complain of or admit to, low mood, but present because of the associated cognitive, behaviourly or somatic symptoms. Somatic presentations of depression are particularly common in Asian cultures. In depression, pcyhomotor retardation can increase to the point where the person sits motionless and mute—depressive stupor. This used to end in death from dehyhdration; it now calls for emergency ECT.

Investigation of choice
A detailed psychiatric history.

Immediate management
Exclude suicidal ideation.

Treatment of choice
Fluoxetine.

Your Notes:

71. Boy was riding his bicycle when he was hit by a car. After examination in A and E, he was found to have left upper quadrant tenderness. He is pale.

Diagnosis: Probable splenic rupture.

Clinchers
- *Riding bicycle when he was hit by a car:* Road traffic accidents (RTA) are the most common cause of traumatic splenic rupture. Usually the patient has sustained a blunt trauma to the abdomen.
- *Left upper quadrant pain:* This is the anatomical site of spleen. Always rule out splenic rupture by USG in RTA with LUQ pain.
- *Tenderness:* Most probably due to associated rib fractures.
- *Pale:* If a patient is abnormally pale following an injury always suspect splenic rupture if no other bleeding sites or cause of blood loss is evident.

CONFUSA
There is an increasing trend to preserve the spleen after rupture, if its salvageable, in children. It is so because of the risk of sudden, overwhelming sepsis which can occur at any time of lift after splenectomy.

Investigation of choice
USG (early).

Immediate management
Resuscitation + crossmatch blood.

Treatment of choice
Urgent laparotomy.

Your Notes:

March—2002

72. Man fell off a ladder, has diffuse pain on right side of the trunk. IVU shows no excretion on right side.

Diagnosis: Avulsion of renal pedicle.

Clinchers

- *Fell of a ladder*: Injuries to the loins are common after all and assault.
- *Diffuse pain on right side of trunk*: Local pain and tenderness are invariably present in renal injury. Hematuria is characteristically absent in complete avulsion of renal pedicle.
- *IVU shows no excretion on right side*: This is characteristic of pedicle avulsion (see confusa below). It may also suggest absence of kidney on right side due to previous nephrectomy. In that case a history will exclude this diagnosis. Absence of one kidney may be due to congenital aplasia which can be confirmed by USG. Also in this case the other kidney will be hypertrophied. An absent or grossly atrophic kidney is found in about 1:1400 individuals.

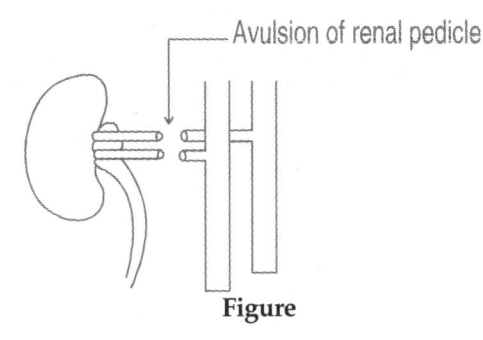

Figure — Avulsion of renal pedicle

CONFUSA

Superficial soft tissue bruising may testify to the severity of the blow but is often absent. The main differential diagnosis is from renal contusion but an IVU will differentiate that. In contusion injuries there is at least some uptake of the contrast and there may be extravasation of contrast media outside the renal outline. Hematuria is the main symptom in renal contusion which will be completely absent in avulsion of renal pedicle. In avulsion injuries, the detachment may be partial or complete. There may be complete detachment of a pole of kidney.

Investigation of choice
USG to confirm the existence of kidney.

Immediate management
Fluid resuscitation and crossmatch.

Treatment of choice
Urgent nephrectomy is the only course of treatment.

73. Man was stabbed with a 10 cm knife in the left upper quadrant, stable for 20 min after which BP falls to 90/60 mmHg. On USG, no free fluid seen in abdomen.

Diagnosis: Cardiac tamponade.

Clinchers

- *Stabled with 10 cm knife*: A long blade is invariably required to produce cardiac lacerations. A shorter knife may only result in open haemopneumothorax.
- *LUQ*: That is the anatomical site of the heart.
- *Stable for 20 min*: A small laceration to the heart will be asymptomatic till the leak fills up the pericardial cavity.
- *BP falls to 90/60 mmHg*: Cardiac tamponade is characterised by a rise in venous pressure and fall in arterial pressure. Overall BP falls due to blood loss and restricted heart function.
- *No free fluid in abdomen*: This rules out splenic rupture, which is also common cause of hypotension after LUQ injury.

CONFUSA

The main differential diagnosis in this case is from tension pneumothorax which can also result in cardiac tamponade. But in that case the patient will present with acute breathlessness and there will be a suckling wound. A haemopneumothorax (not necessarily tension) invariably will be present with such injuries.

Investigation of choice
CXR (enlarged cardiac shadow)

Immediate management
Crossmatch blood + careful fluid resuscitation.

Treatment of choice
Pericardiotomy (urgent)
↓
evacuation of blood
↓
Suturing of cardiac laceration

Your Notes:

74. Known asthmatic patient involved in road traffic accident (RTA). Has a right-sided chest pain. On auscultation, right side is hyper-resonant. Trachea is deviated to the left.

Diagnosis: Tension pneumothorax (right side).

Clinchers
- *Asthmatic patient:* In patients over 40 years of age, COPD most commonly predisposes to pneumothorax. Rarer causes include bronchial asthma, carcinoma, a lung abscess breaking down and leading to bronchopulmonary fistula and severe pulmonary fibrosis with cyst formation.
- *RTA:* A simple pneumothorax in a patient of trauma may develop into a tension pneumothorax—particularly when the patient receives IPPV.
- *Right sided chest pain:* This is pleuritic pain which is variably in intensity.
- *Hyperresonance on same side:* This rules out cardiac tamponade and confirms pneumothorax.
- *Trachea is deviated to left:* Signs of tension pneumothorax are:
  - Hypotension
  - Distended neck veins
  - Trachea deviated away from the side of pneumothorax
  - Severe respiratory distress.

CONFUSA
A CXR should not be performed if a tension pneumothorax is suspected as it will delay immediate necessary treatment. The clinical picture of tension pneumothorax may be mistaken for that of a cardiac tamponade. However, tension pneumothorax is more common and may be differentiated by the hyper-resonance over the affected side.

Investigation of choice
CXR but only after needle thoracocentesis.

Immediate management
Needle thoracocentesis urgently.

Treatment of choice
Chest drain (always required in a traumatic pneumothorax irrespective of its size).

Your Notes:

75. A 19-year-old girl has fallen off her horse. Neck is immobilised + 100% oxygen. Has left upper abdominal pain, is pale and tachycardiac.

Diagnosis: Splenic rupture (hypotensive shock).

Clinchers
- *19-year-old has fallen off her house:* Falls in a young person usually produce polytrauma and blunt injuries.
- *Neck is immobilized + 100% O_2:* This means that the airway and breathing in primary survey is taken care of. Now there is a need to assess the circulation (ABC approach).
- *Left upper abdominal pain:* This could be due to rib fracture or blunt impact over this area. Such a finding should make one strongly suspicious of splenic rupture.
- *Pale and tachycardiac:* This suggest that patient is in hypotensive shock (most probably due to massive blood loss into peritoneum after splenic rupture).

CONFUSA
In hypotensive shock after massive blood loss, give colloid (Haemaccel) fast IV until BP ↑, pulse ↓, urine flows (> 30 mL/h) and crossmatched blood arrives.

Investigation of choice
USG/peritoneal lavage.

Immediate management
Crossmatch blood and inform surgeons after starting IV fluids.

Treatment of choice
Immediate laparotomy.

Your Notes:

76. Fracture of anterior cranial fossa, rhinorrhoea, anosmia.

Diagnosis: Olfactory (I cranial nerve)

Clinchers

- *Fracture of anterior cranial fossa:* Palsy of first cranial nerve is often followed by head trauma especially the fracture of anterior cranial fossa due to local trauma to the nerve.
- *Rhinorrhoea:* This must be CSF leakage from the fracture of cribriform plate of ethmoid. It must be confirmed to be CSF by glucose dipstick testing.
- *Anosmia:* Sense of olfaction is definitely lost. To examine occlude each nostril sequentially. Use a mild test stimulus such as soap, toothpaste, coffee or lemon oil. With the eyes closed, the patient sniffs and try to identify the stimulus.

CONFUSA
Anosmia may also be produced by
- tumors of the olfactory groove
  - meningioma
  - frontal glioma
- meningitis

The sense of smell is often lost, sometimes permanently, after upper respiratory viral infections. It is diminished in nasal obstruction.

Investigation of choice
Glucose dipstick test for CSF rhinorrhoea.

Immediate management
Neurosurgery opinion.

Treatment of choice
Conservative/surgical repair.

Your Notes:

77. Cavernous sinus affected, pupil not responding to light and accommodation, ptosis present.

Diagnosis: Oculomotor (III cranial nerve)

Clinchers

- *Cavernous sinus affected:* Cavernous sinus carries in its lateral wall the third and fourth cranial nerves and the ophthalmic and maxillary divisions of the fifth nerve. Hence in its pathology, any of these can be affected.
- *Pupil not responding to light:* A fixed and dilated pupil is characteristics of III nerve palsy and signify a complete palsy.
- *Ptosis present:* Total palsy of the oculomotor nerve lesions causes:
  - Ptosis (as it supplies, levator palpebrae superioris), which is unilateral and complete
  - The eye facing down and out
  - A fixed and dilated pupil.

An early or partial oculomotor palsy can present in any combination of the above features.

CONFUSA
Early dilatation of pupil implies a compressive lesion. Third nerve palsies without a dilated pupil are due to:
- diabetes mellitus
- other vascular causes (aneurysm)

Sparing of the pupil means that parasympathetic fibres which run in a discrete busidle on the superior surface of the nerve remain undamaged, and so the pupil is of normal size and reacts normally.

Investigation of choice
IV antibiotics.

Immediate management
Thrombolysis (as cavernous sinus thrombosis is the most usual pathology).

Treatment of choice
IV antibiotics.

Your Notes:

78. After head trauma, patient cannot shrug his shoulder.

Diagnosis: Spinal accessory (XI cranial nerve)

Clinchers
- *Head trauma:* This motor nerve to the trapezius and sternomastoid muscles arises in the medulla and leaves the skull through the jugular foramen with the ninth and tenth nerves. It is commonly injured in fracture base of skull.
- *Cannot string his shoulder:* A lesion of the eleventh nerve causes:
  - Weakness of the sternomastoid—rotation of the head and neck of the opposite side.
  - Weakness of trapezium—should shrugging lost.

CONFUSA
Causes of XI cranial nerve palsies are:
- Polio
- Syringomyelia
- Tumors near jugular foramen
- Stroke
- Bulbar palsy
- Trauma
- TB

Over all XI nerve palsy is a rare occurrence.

Investigation of choice
CT skull.

Immediate management
Refer to neurosurgery unit.

Treatment of choice
Conservative ± surgical repair of fracture base of skull.

Your Notes:

79. Forehead sparing, lower face no voluntary movements. Involuntary movements possible.

Diagnosis: Facial nerve palsy (VII cranial nerve)—UMN type.

Clinchers
- *Forehead sparing:* This is characteristic of facial nerve palsy of upper motor neurone (UMN) origin. The frontalis muscle is spared; the normal furrowing of the brow is preserved, and eye closure and blinking are not affect.
- *Lowerface—no voluntary movements:* UMN lesions cause weakness of the lower part only of the face on the side opposite the lesion. The earliest sign is simply slowing of one side of the face, for example on baring the teeth. Later on, voluntary movement is preserved.
- *Involuntary movement possible:* In UMN lesions, there is sometimes relative preservation of spontaneous emotion movement (e.g. similing) compared with voluntary movement.

CONFUSA
Differences between

	LMN	UMN
Weakness	All muscle of face	Forehead sparing
Eye closure	Weakness	Normal
Frontalis	Involved	Spared
Side of lesion	Same	Opposite

Investigation of choice
CT skull/MRI (cerebral infarction or tumor).

Immediate management
Admit and take neurosurgical opinion.

Treatment of choice
Conservative if stroke; surgery if SOL.

Your Notes:

80. Fracture of base of skull, loss of taste in anterior two-thirds of tongue, deviation of angle of mouth.

Diagnosis: Facial nerve (VII cranial nerve)—LMN type.

Clinchers
- *Fracture base of skull:* Facial nerve leaves skull through the stylomastoid foramen and can be injured here in head trauma such as fracture base of skull. This will be a lower motor neurone (LMN) lesion then.
- *Loss of taste in anterior two-thirds of tongue:* Facial nerve carries taste fibres from the anterior two-thirds of the tongue via the chorda-tympani, hence this finding confirms the suspicion of a facial nerve LMN palsy.
- *Deviation of angle of mouth:* The face, especially the angle of the mouth, falls, and dribbling occurs from the corner of the mouth.

CONFUSA
Lesions of the facial nerve within the petrous temporal bone cause the combination of:
- Loss of taste on the anterior two-third of the tongue
- Hyperacusis (unpleasantly loud distortion of noise) owing to paralysis of stapedius muscle

Investigation of choice
CT scan

Immediate management
Admit and urgent neurosurgery referral.

Treatment of choice
Surgical decompression (urgent).

Your Notes:

81. A 16-year-old boy falls from a tree. Complains of pain in left anatomical fossa. X-rays are normal.

Diagnosis: Fracture scaphoid (left hand).

Clinchers
- *16-year-old:* The relative compressibility of the bone in children makes scaphoid fracture uncommon under the age of 14 years. It is most common in men between the ages of 20 and 50 years.
- *Falls from a tree:* It is often sustained in falls when the impact is beared by hand.
- *Pain in left anatomical fossa:* Tenderness is typically found in the anatomical snuff box between the long and short extensors of the thumb and also on the dorsal and volar aspects of the scaphoid bone.
- *X-rays are normal:* Structures it is merely a crack fracture of scaphoid and not visible on initial X-rays until bone resorption at 10-14 days have widened the fracture line. Ultrasound and bone scan have been associated in such cases.

CONFUSA
A missed scaphoid fracture may cause more long-term morbidity than many major trunk injuries. In fracture scaphoid, swelling is usually minimal. Movements may be good, but forced thumb adduction and extension are usually painful. Unfortunately, many injuries to the soft-tissues may present a similar picture. Avascular necrosis may fellow a scaphoid fracture.

Investigation of choice
Isotope scan

Immediate management
Plaster cast is applied extending from the thumb interphalangeal joint to the elbow in all cases of suspected fracture scaphoid.

Treatment of choice
Plaster cast for 3 months in confirmed scaphoid fracture.

Your Notes:

First Aid for the PLAB

82. Man falls on hand. X-ray shows perilunate dislocation.

Diagnosis: Peri-lunate dislocation.

Clinchers
- *Falls on hand:* This is a common mode of injury in lunate or perilunate dislocations.
- *Perilunate dislocations:* In this dislocation, the lunate remains in position and the rest of the carpal bones dislocate dorsally.

CONFUSA
Perilunate and lunate dislocations are rare injuries of the wrist. In lunate dislocation the lunate dislocates anteriorly but the rest of the carpals remain in position. In both types severe loss of wrist movements is inevitable. Avascular necrosis of the lunate is a common complication.

Investigation of choice
Wrist X-ray.

Immediate management
Urgent orthopaedics referral.

Treatment of choice
Open reduction.

Your Notes:

83. A 43-year-old man after a fall, pain in anatomical snuff-box and X-ray shows impacted distal radius fracture.

Diagnosis: Colle's fracture.

Clinchers
- *43-year-old man:* It is the most common fracture in people above 40 years of age and is particularly common in women because of postmenopausal osteoporosis. It is much less common in young adults.
- *Fall:* A Colle's fracture is almost always produced by a fall on an outstretched hand.
- *Pain in anatomical snuff box:* The patient usually presents with pain, swelling and deformity of the wrist. On examination, tenderness and irregularity of the lower end of the radius is found which can be felt in anatomical snuff box.
- *X-ray shows impacted distal radius fracture:* Colle's fracture mean a fracture within 2-3 cm of the lower end of the radius with backward tilt, backward displacement and, often impaction of the distal fragment producing shortening of the radius and radial deviation of the wrist. The fracture may be comminuted. The styloid process of the ulnar is often avulsed by the triangular articular disc. So that the inferior radio-ulnar joint is disrupted.

CONFUSA
If Colle's fracture is only minimally displaced reduction is not necessary. A useful way of assessing the need for reduction is to draw a line between the two lips of the articular surface of the radius on the lateral film.

Reduction	drawn line relative to line of radial shaft
• not necessary	at right angle slight forward tilt
• necessary	any backward tilt

Investigation of choice
Lateral and anteroposterior X-ray wrist.

Immediate management
Urgent ortho referral.

Treatment of choice
- *Undisplaced fracture:* below elbow plaster cast for 6 weeks.
- *Displaced fracture:* manipulative reduction followed by immobilization in Colle's cast.

84. Man falls on hand, pain in anatomical fossa.

Diagnosis: Fracture scaphoid (probably).

Clinchers (Note: See question 81 in his theme also)
- *Fall on hand:* A common mode of injury for scaphoid fracture.
- *Pain in anatomical fossa:* Pain in this area with no obvious deformity or swelling following a fall on the outstretched hand, in an adult, should make one suspect strongly about the possibility of a scaphoid fracture.

Note: A force transmitted along the axis of second metacarpal may produce pain the region of the scaphoid bone.

CONFUSA
A scaphoid fracture is more common in young adults. It is rare in children and elderly. Commonly fracture occurs through the waist of the scaphoid. Rarely, it occurs through the tuberosity. It may be either a crack fracture or a displaced fracture

Investigation of choice
X-ray wrist including oblique view of scaphoid.

Immediate management
A scaphoid cast for at least 2 weeks in all suspected cases (irrespective of whether they are visible or not on X-ray—if invisible do a repeat X-ray after 2 weeks).

Treatment of choice
Scaphoid cast for 3 months in a confirmed scaphoid fracture.

Your Notes:

85. Young girl tripped while holding mother's hand. Now cannot use arm at all.

Diagnosis: Pulled elbow.

Clinchers
- *Young girl:* This condition occurs in children between 1-4 years of age.
- *Tripped while holding mother's hand:* It occurs when pulled up by the arms, while being lifted in play. The head of the radius is pulled partly out of the annular ligament when a child is lifted by the wrist.
- *Now cannot use arm at all:* The child starts crying and is unable to move the affected limb. The forearm lies in an attitude of pronation. There may be mild swelling at the elbow.

CONFUSA
It is not possible to see the subluxated head on an X-ray because it is still cartilagineous. X-rays are taken only to rule out any other bony injury. Do not attempt to reduce a pulled elbow if there is any doubt about the diagnosis.

Investigation of choice
Entirely clinical diagnosis.

Immediate management
Refer to orthopaedics.

Treatment of choice
Elbow rotation (forced supination with a thumb over the radial head). A click will be heard on reduction. Final reassurance for the doctor, and doubting parents, is obtained by letting the child play and watching normal movements return. This may take sometime.

Your Notes:

86. A 12-month-old child of unemployed parents, did not gain weight from 6 months.

Diagnosis: Failure to thrive

Clinchers
- *12-month-old:* Failure to thrive means poor weight gain in infancy. In 95% cases this is due to not enough food being offered, or not enough food being taken.
- *Unemployed parents:* This titles the suspicion more towards not enough food being offered.
- *Did not gain weight from 6 months:* This is a serious finding as infants usually gain 2-3 kg during this period.

CONFUSA
Failure to thrive is mainly because of poverty in developing countries. In UK it is
- Difficulty at home
- Emotional deprivation
- Unskilled feeding techniques

While investigating, focus on there points:
- Signs of abuse
- Family finances
- Chart family heights
- Feeding patterns
- Dysmorphic face
- Parenteral illness
- Activity level; behaviour
- General health and happiness

Investigation of choice
Nutrition assessment

Immediate management
Rule out any malabsorption disease.

Treatment of choice
Correct nutritional deficiencies in diet.

Your Notes:

---

87. Child brought to A and E, age 6 months, swollen thigh, X-ray shows transverse fracture of shaft of femur.

Diagnosis: Non-accidental injury (NAI) probable.

Clinchers
- *Age 6 months:* One-third of NAI occurs under 6 months of age (other one-third between 6 months—3 yrs and next one-third after that). It is due to stress of looking after young children.
- *Transverse fracture of femoral shaft:* Any fracture in a child under 12-year-old should raised suspicious of NAI until prove otherwise.

CONFUSA
A skeletal survey—to look for occult injuries—is usually only indicated in children under 2 years of age.
Osteogenesis imperfecta can also clinically present in this way but it would have been diagnosed on the X-ray (already done in this child) because of its typical radiological characteristics:
- translucent bone
- trefoil pelvis
- wormian bones (irregular patches of ossification)

Investigation of choice
Skeletal survey (to find out other old injuries)

Immediate management
Look for child's name on child protection register.

Treatment of choice
Follow local protocol.

Your Notes:

88. A 9-year-old female child with itching, sore vagina, perineum is red and excoriated.

Diagnosis: Sexual abuse

Clinchers
- *9-year-old:* In UK, before the age of 16, at least one in 10 girls and one in 15 boys will have been sexually assaulted. The peak incidence of first assault is at about 8-year-old.
- *Itching and sore vagina, perineum is red and excoriated:* Most probably there are symptoms of venereal disease. Presence of venereal disease in a prepubertal, child should always be considered as sexual abuse until proven otherwise.

CONFUSA
Sexual abuse of children can occur in all socio-economic, cultural and religion groups and is associated with:
- Acute perineal injury
- Chronic perineal damage
- Genitourinary infection
- Sexually precocious behaviour
- Sexualized drawings and play
- Regressive patterns of behaviour
- Eating and sleep disorders
- Psychosomatic symptoms
- Withdrawal and depression
- Self harm
- Promiscuity
- Running away from home

Investigation of choice
Examine under anaesthesia.

Immediate management
Referred for consideration of the need for child protection.

Treatment of choice
Follow local protocol after informing social services.

Your Notes:

89. 18-year-old female brings her baby unconscious to A and E, cyanosed, dilated fixed left pupil.

Diagnosis: Head injury

Clinchers
- *18-year-old female:* Child abuse causing NAI is more common in babies of teenaged mother as they are more prove to breakdown under stress of looking after the child. Suspect this always in an unexplained head injury. Also note that child abuse is the most common cause of a skull fracture in an infant.
- *Unconscious; cyanosed, dilated fixed pupil:* All these features point to a unilateral intracranial hematoma.

CONFUSA
Children are unique in invariably having a carer with them. This means that most can go home with their parents and a set of head injury instructions. They often sleep after trauma and should not be kept awake. Instead, they should be examined by their parents two or three times during the night. Parents are much better judges of their children's night-time behaviour than hospital doctors or nurses.

Investigation of choice
CT skull.

Immediate management
Immediately neurosurgery referral.

Treatment of choice
Surgical evacuation of hematoma.

Your Notes:

90. Child with forearm bruise, brought by teacher, Mom says she held her to prevent her from running across the road.

Diagnosis: Non-accidental injury (NAI) (probably)

Clinchers
- *Forearm bruise:* It is a common site of bruising by holding or bondage. They can occur by light grasp because of a pre-existing coagulopathy (haemophilia) or tight and violent grasp or bondage in NAI.
- *Brought by teacher:* Always suspect NAI when the accompanying adult is not one of the immediate parent.
- *Mom say she held her to prevent her from running across the road:* It can be a true explanation if the child have a coagulopathy. But then the mother would herself be bothered enough to bring her to medical attention. But since it did not happen, a NAI becomes a more probable diagnosis.

CONFUSA
Confirm the doubts of NAI by excluding coagulopathy definitely through laboratory tests. Most common coagulopathy is hemophilia.

Investigation of choice
Coagulation profile.

Immediate management
Informal social services if NAI is confirmed.

Treatment of choice
Depends on investigation report. Follow local protocol if NAI.

Your Notes:

91. 40-year-old lady stops talking suddenly, says someone took away her thoughts.

Diagnosis: Schizophrenia

Clinchers
- *40-year-old lady:* As compared to males, the onset of schizophrenia is usually late in females and often runs a more benign course.
- *Stops talking suddenly:* Thought blocking is a characteristic feature of schizophrenia. There is a sudden interruption of stream of speech before the thought is completed. After a pause, the subject cannot recall what she had meant to say.
- *Say someone took away her thoughts:* Thoughts blocking is characteristically associated with thoughts withdrawn in schizophrenia. This is perception of removal of thoughts by an external force. This is a diagnostic first rank symptom of schizophrenia.

CONFUSA
Thought blocking can also be seen in complex partial seizures (temporal lobe epilepsy; absence seizures). But they are more commonly seen in children and extremely unusual to present at this age. In temporal lobe epilepsy, the subject continues to speak after a pause, from where he/she have left but not in schizophrenia.

Investigation of choice
Schizophrenia is a clinical diagnosis. Physical investigations are mainly used to rule out the organic disorders. Brain imaging is considered if there are neurological symptoms or signs.

Immediate management
Admission: The mental health act may be needed, since patients are at risk from neglect or dangerous acts.

Treatment of choice
After a single episode of schizophrenia continue treatment for 12-24 months with antipsychotic drugs (lozapine/risperidone).

Your Notes:

92. A 17-year-old girl comes anxious and tearful to A and E. She is unkempt and dishevelled, says she lost her medication, says she aches all over and demand immediate pain relief.

Diagnosis: Opioid withdrawal.

Clinchers
- *17-year-old girl:* Substance misuse is more prevalent in teens and twenties.
- *Anxious and tearful:* Opioid withdrawal leads to an extremely unpleasant withdrawal syndrome (cold turkey) involving:
  - Craving (presents in this case)
  - Myalgia
  - Restlessness and insomnia
  - Sweating
  - Abdominal pain, vomiting, diarrhoea
  - Dilated pupils, running nose and eyes
  - Tachycardia
  - Yawning and
  - Goose bumps
- *Unkempt and dishevelled:* A typical condition of a drug addict.
- *Says she lost her medication:* The unbearable withdrawal syndrome forces the patient to steal, lie or do almost anything in order to get the drug. However, if you question her about the medication or the disease she is suffering from, she will have no answer and may respond with agitation.
- *Demand immediate pain relief:* This confirms that the substance being misused is opioid. It is so as its withdrawal produces pain to myalgia or the patients having knowledge of opioids being used in hospital for pain relief.

Investigation of choice
Toxicology screen—because she might have consumed large doses of analgesics in order to get pain relief.

Immediate management
Admission

Treatment of choice
Counselling to get enrolled in systematic withdrawal programme. If not agreeing, enrol in harm reduction and maintenance therapy. Report all patients for registration in confidential register of NHS.

Your Notes:

93. Unconscious boy with pin point pupils, respiratory rate—4/min.

Diagnosis: Opiate overdose

Clinchers
- *Unconscious:* Delayed reflexes, thready pulse and coma may occur in case of a large overdose.
- *Pinpoint pupil:* It is characteristic of opioid overdose. Other conditions in which pin point pupils can be seen are:
  - Positive hemorrhage
  - Heat stroke
- *Respiratory rate is 4/min:* Respiratory depression is the main fatal complication of opioid overdose as it suppresses the respiratory centres [tip: k (*k*appa) receptors are involved in "*k*ick" effects and µ (*m*u) receptors are involved in *m*edical effects like respiratory depression].

CONFUSA
In severe intoxication, mydriasis (instead of miosis) may occur due to hypoxia. Tolerance to all opioids rapidly develops (except to constipation and miotic effects). Because of this (and because of batch-to-batch variation in purity), overdose is common and frequently fatal due to respiratory depression. On the other hand, opioid withdrawal is rarely life-threatening although the symptoms are severe.

Investigation of choice
Urinary opioids test (but treatment is the first priority, testing follow it).

Immediate management
Ventilatory support.

Treatment of choice
Naloxane 0.8-2 mg IV
Repeat every 2 min until breathing adequate.

Your Notes:

94.
Boy brought by his friend to the A and E. History of suddenly falling to the ground, jerky movements, urine incontinence. He is confused now but neurological examination is normal.

Diagnosis: Generalised tonic clonic seizure (GTCS)

Clinchers
- *Brought by his friend:* Since after a GTCS, the patient is in postictal confusion, he is incapable of reporting himself to hospital. Usually such patients are accompanied by someone who has witnessed the seizure.
- *Suddenly falling to ground; jerky movements and urine incontinence:* A typical description of GTCS is following a vague warning, the tonic phase of the seizure commences. The body becomes rigid, for upto a minute. The patient utters a cry and falls, sometimes suffering injury. The tongue is usually bitten. There may be incontinence of urine or faeces.
- *Confused now but neurological examination is normal:* After a generalised seizure the patient may feel awful with headache, myalgia, confusion and a sore tongue. This postictal confusion is characteristic and differentiates from other causes of loss of consciousness (e.g. vagovagal). It may lost upto 24 hours.

CONFUSA
A GTCS can be mistakenly referred to a psychiatrist if nobody has witnessed the seizure and the person is found wandering in a postictal delirium GTCS is a classical grand mal seizure. An atypical generalized seizure is myoclonic jerk in which also the patient falls to the ground because of violently disobedient lower limb.
Note: TV-induced seizures are almost always generalised.

Investigation of choice
EEG (a normal EEG between seizures does not exclude epilepsy).

Immediate management
Admission for 24 hours for investigations and observations.

Treatment of choice
Sodium valproate (but may be unacceptable in prepubertal child because of facial coarsening effects—replace with carbamazepine then).

Your Notes:

95.
A 20-year-old woman attends A and E complaining of sudden breathlessness and anxiety. She describes palpitations and paresthesiae of her hands, feet and lips. ECG shows sinus tachycardia and O_2 saturation is normal.

Diagnosis: Panic attacks.

Clinchers
- *20-year-old female:* young females are most prone to have panic attacks.
- *Sudden breathlessness and anxiety:* Classically the symptoms begin unexpectedly or 'out-of-the-blue'. Usually there is no apparent precipitating factor. The patient becomes increasingly frightened by an apparent inability to breath adequately. Attempts to breadth rapidly results in dizziness and further anxiety.
- *Palpitations:* It is due to sympathetic overactivity. Other symptoms attributed to sympathetic stimulation are—tachycardia, sweating, flushes, dyspnoea, hyperventilation, dry mouth, frequency and hesitancy of micturition, dizziness, diarrhoea, mydriasis.
- *Paraesthesiae of her hands, feet and lips:* Tachypnoea blows off CO_2 and the resultant respiratory alkalosis causes a fall in ionised calcium. This hypocalcaemia manifest as paraesthesiae in the fingers and perioral area.
- *Sinus tachcycardia:* Due to sympathetic stimulation.
- *O_2 saturation is increased:* due to hyperventilation.

CONFUSA
The most important differential diagnosis in a female is from MVPS (mitral valve prolapse syndrome). This syndrome, more commonly seen in young females (like panic disorder), presents with classical symptoms of panic disorder occurring in episodes. It is caused by prolapse, usually congenital, of the mitral valve into the atrium during ventricular systole. On auscultation, a mid systolic click and a systolic murmur can be heard sometimes. The clininical differentiation between MVPS and panic disorder is difficult. The diagnosis is usually established on echocardiography.

Investigation of choice
To rule out organic respiratory problems (ECG, CXR, ABG).

Immediate management
Confirmation of normality with warm reassurance to the patient.

Treatment of choice
Re-breathing into a closed bag and mask system without oxygen.

96. A bottle-fed baby has developed flexural eczema. His brother has the same history. Family history of asthma. Mom is presently avoiding using soap.

Diagnosis: Atopic infantile eczema.

Clinchers
- *Bottle-fed baby develops flexural eczema:* Infantile eczema is common (most children will grow out of it before the teenage years). Breastfeeding is protective.
- *Brother has same history + family history of asthma:* There is a strong genetic component often with a positive family history of atopy. IL-4 receptor mutation has been found in atopic families.
- *Mom is presently avoiding using soap:* It deinforces the finding of family history of atopy in this case (This is irritant dermatitis). If one parent has atopic disease the risk for a child of developing eczema is about 20-30%. If both parents have atopic eczema the risk is greater than 50%.

CONFUSA
Animal dander often aggravates eczema and elevated IgE RAST is typical. A proportion of atopic children have significant hood allergies, e.g. egg, fish which can exacerbate eczema. Infantile eczema gets better with time although asthma is often the next events along the line.

Immediate management
Encourage the mother to breastfeed.

Treatment of choice
- Hydrocortisone cream for acute flare ups (1% hydrocortisone)
- Trimeprazine for sleep, deprivation due to itching.

Your Notes:

97. Young girl with eczema, treated with emollient and topical hydrocortisone, did not get better.

Diagnosis: Eczema not responding to first line drug.

Clinchers
- *Young girls:* Young children should be treated with mild and moderately patent steroids on the body.
- *Treated with emollient and topical hydrocortisone, did not get better:* Hydrocortisone is a mild steroid. Since it is not improving the condition, a trial with a higher dose is needed before changing the drug (a high potency steroid) or treatment modality.

CONFUSA

Classification of topical steroids by potency	
Very potent	Choketasol
	Diflucortolone
Potent	Betamethasone
	Fluocinolone
Moderately potent	Clobetasone
	Aldometrasone
Mild	Hydrocortisone

Investigation of choice
Usually none required.

Immediate management
Reassurance (as it can precipitate depression especially, in young girls)

Treatment of choice
2.5% hydrocortisone topically.

Your Notes:

98. Young girl with severe eczema, weeping vesicles, skin swab was taken, topical steroids didn't work.

Diagnosis: Severe non-responsive eczema

Clinchers
- *Young girl:* A failure to treatment can produce anxiety or depression especially in a young girl.
- *Severe eczema, weeping vesicles:* It signify a severe acute attack of eczema and should be treated on an urgent basis. Bacterial infections often exacerbate eczema to this extent.
- *Skin swab taken: Staph aureus* commonly colonies lesions and staph endotoxin is known to act as super antigen. Its elimination is a prerequisite for definitive treatment.
- *Topical steroids did not work:* It means that oral steroids will have to be given a trial.

CONFUSA
If the skin infection is by *Streptococcus*, give penicillin V (500 mg QID). Erythromycin (500 mg QID) is useful if there is already to penicillin.

Investigation of choice
Skin swab (already taken)

Immediate management
Topical antiseptics

Treatment of choice
Steroids + flucloxacillin.

Your Notes:

99. A 49-year-old woman complains of itchy blisters, which are occurring in groups on her knees and elbows. The itch is becoming unbearable and she is contemplating suicide. She responds to 180 mg of Dapsone within 48 hours of treatment.

Diagnosis: Coeliac disease (Gluten sensitive enteropathy).

Clinchers
- *49-year-old female:* It can present at any age. The peak incidence in adults is in the third and fourth decades with a females preponderance.
- *Itchy blisters which are occurring in group on her knees and elbows:* This is an uncommon blistering subepidermal eruption of the skin associated with gluten sensitive enteropathy. The clinical term for it is gluten sensitive enteropathy.
- *Itch is becoming unbearable and she is contemplating suicide:* This disease can produce severe depression in females and can lead to suicide.
- *Responds to 180 mg of dapsone within 48 hours of treatment:* This confirms our diagnosis.

CONFUSA
The skin condition (dermatitis herpetiformis) responds to dapsone but both the gut and the skin will improve only on a gluten free diet in this disease.

Investigation of choice
Endomysial antibodies (IgA).

Immediate management
Psychiatric referral (as she is contemplating suicide)

Treatment of choice
Gluten free diet
+
Dapsone

Your Notes:

100. 18-month-old baby, red swollen lips after eating egg. Presently under treatment with emollients and topical hydrocortisone three times a day.

Diagnosis: Food allergy (egg)

Clinchers
- *18-month-old baby, red swollen lips after eating egg:* A proportion of topic children have significant food allergies, e.g. egg, fish, etc.
- *Presently under treatment with emollients and topical hydrocortisone:* Any episode of food allergy in eczema typically worsens it. So use high dose (2.5%) hydrocortisone for a few days as a prophylactic measure.

CONFUSA
Red swollen lips suggests anaphylaxis and require prompt treatment with IM epinephrine and enough interventions to prevent laryngeal oedema from developing.

Investigation of choice
None.

Immediate management
Follow anaphylaxis protocol

Treatment of choice
Admission to hospital.

Your Notes:

101. Girl goes into a forest, remembers getting bitten by a tick, redness near the bite is slowly increasing in size.

Diagnosis: Erythema chronicum migraines (Lyme disease).

Clinchers
- *Forest:* Lymes disease spreading ticks (on deer and sheep) are widespread in the UK, particularly in the forests and woodlands.
- *Bitten by tick:* Although not every person remember getting bitten by a tick, any history of tick bite in a forest should arouse suspicion of Lyme disease. It is transmitted by ixodes dammini or related ixodid ticks (Iodes ricinus in Europe).
- *Redness near the bite is slowly increasing in size:* Erythema chronicum migraine is the rash of Lyme disease, and typically manifests as singular or multiple annular plaques. It presents as an annular rash with central clearing. It gradually increases in size with central clearing. Untreated rash usually fade within 3 months but may recur. May be multiple.

CONFUSA
Lympes disease was originally described in Lyme, connecticut, but is now known to occur in many parts of USA, Europe and in Australia. Differential features from other erythemas is as follows:
- Erythema nodosum—painful, red, raised
- Erythema marginatum—pink coalescent rings
- Erythema multiforme—target lesions.

Investigation of choice
Serology (if negative, do PCR).

Immediate management
Advice regarding protection from ticks.

Treatment of choice
Doxycycline 100 mg/12 hr PO her for 10-21 days (Amoxicillin or penicillin V if < 12 years).

Your Notes:

102.
A policeman bite on his hand by a heroin addict while arresting him. He comes to the A and E, on examination, a deep wound seen on his hand.

Diagnosis: Human bite

Clinchers
- *Bite by heroin addict:* As the most common mode of taking heroin is intravenous, he is most probably an IV drug abuser. Such person carry highest risk for hepatitis B or HIV because of needle sharing.
- *Deep wound on hand:* A deep wound is more dangerous as infection can reach the deep space of the hand, including the bone, joint and tendons. Moreover lacerations to hand tendons can also be present which can produce functional deficits.

CONFUSA
HIV and hepatitis B virus have both been reported to be transmitted by human bite, but these instances appear to be quite rare (837, Harrisons, 14th edn). HIV serology can be done if suspicion is there (as in this case) but wound culture and Gram staining is absolutely essential in every case. Suspicious human bite wounds should provoke careful questioning regarding domestic or child abuse. Human bite infections are usually more dangerous than other animal bites (because of diverse flora or human mouth) and upto 50% infecting organisms in human bite produces β-lactamares.

Investigation of choice
Wound swab ± hepatitis B serology ± HIV serology

Immediate management
Bite injuries to the hand warrant consultation with a hand surgeon for the assessment of tendon, nerve and muscular damage. So get its opinion.
+
Ensure tetanus prophylaxis

Treatment of choice
Amoxicillin
+
Clavulinic acid

Your Notes:

103.
A 18-month-old baby, drowsy, febrile, headache, CT normal.

Diagnosis: Meningitis

Clinchers
- *18-month-old:* This age has a significance in meningitis as neck stiffness (inability to kiss knees) is often absent if < 18-month-old.
- *Drowsy:* It is a sing of increased intracranial pressure and if found in meningitis. Other signs of increased ICP are:
  - Irritability
  - Vomiting
  - Tense fontanelle
  - Preherniation
- *Febrile:* It is a "septic sign" of meningitis and signifies bacteremia. Other septic signs can be:
  - Arthritis
  - Odd behaviour
  - Rashes
  - Cyanosis
  - DIC
  - Pulse increased
  - BP decreased
  - Tachypnoea
  - WCC increased
- *Headache:* Can be due to both ICP and ↑ meningitis per se.

CONFUSA
Do not expect only petechiae in meningococcal disease as it can present with any rash. Rash or skin lesions in meningococcal infection signifies a bacteremia which may well be absent sometimes. Always do a CT exam to rule out inappropriately raised ICP (evident by ventriculomegaly) or a space occupying lesion first. Only then proceed to do lumbar puncture (LP). If LP carries a risk of inadvertent herniation of brain if done in setting of severely increased ICP. (But in neonates preliminary CT is incapable of showing that LP would be safe). If LP is contraindicated (i.e. focal neurological signs, DIC, increase ICP) and you are suspecting meningococcal disease (i.e. purpura is present), blood culture would be a better option.

Investigation of choice
Lumbar puncture

Immediate management
Give penicillin 50 mg/kg at once before anything.

Treatment of choice
Start a broad spectrum antibiotic (i.e. cefotaxime) if CSF is cloudy. Change according to CSF culture and sensitivity report.
- Meningococcus—Benzyl penicillin
- Pneumococcus—Cefotaxime
- Hemophilus—Cefotaxime/chloramphenicol.

Your Notes:

104. A chronic alcoholic presents with flapping tremors and confusion.

Diagnosis: Alcoholic liver disease.

Clinchers
- *Chronic alcoholic:* Alcohol and chronic HBV or HCV infections are the most common causes of cirrhosis.
- *Flapping tremors:* This is a coarse irregular tremor of outstretched hands better known as asterixis. It is pathognomic of chronic liver disease.
- *Confusion:* Confusion is presence hepatic disease signifies grade II of hepatic encephalopathy
  - Grade I—altered mood or behaviour
  - Grade II—increasing drowsiness, confusion, slurred speech
  - Grade III—stupor, incoherence, restlessness, significant confusion
  - Grade IV—coma.

CONFUSA
Flapping tremor can be present in
- Wilson's disease
- Haemochromatosis

Encephalopathy is suspected chronic liver disease suggests acute on chronic hepatic failure.

Investigation of choice
- *Screening:* LFT (↑ bilirubin, AST > ALT-although both rise)
- *Definitive:* Liver biopsy

Immediate management
Nurse with a 20° head up tilt in ITU

Treatment of choice
Supportive
- 20% mannitol, slow infusion for ↑ ICP
- 10% dextrose infusion for hypoglycemia
- Potassium and calcium supplements
- IV vitamin K for coagulopathy

Your Notes:

105. A 70-year-old woman, confusion, constipation, frequency of urine.

Diagnosis: Urinary tract infection (UTI)

Clinchers
- *70-year-old:* UTI's are more common in the elderly, in whom impaired bladder emptying due to prostatic disease in males and neuropathic bladder—especially common in females—is frequently found.
- *Woman:* Impaired bladder emptying due to neuropathic bladder is common in elderly females and produce urinary stasis which can than lead to UTI especially proteus infections.
- *Confusion:* May be due to dementia of elderly or due to severe debilitating illness. Or it may be due to secondary bacteremia from UTI.
- *Constipation:* Quite common in elderly due to impaired mobility or poor nutrition. Note that constipation produces urinary incontinence in elderly.
- *Frequency of urine:* Incontinence, nocturia, smelly urine or vague changes in well-being are often the only symptoms of UTI in an elderly patient.

CONFUSA
This is a question from GMC PLAB booklet. Repition of this question in the actual exam shows that GMC has a very limited question bank.

Investigation of choice
MSU

Immediate management
Consider a PR examination to rule out fecal impaction.

Treatment of choice
Systemic treatment of UTI in elderly is required if bacteremia is present. Otherwise focus on local hygiene.

Your Notes:

106. Due to increased catecholamines.

Diagnosis: Phaeochromocytoma

Clinchers
- *Increased catecholamines:* Phaeochromocytoma is a rare catecholamine producing tumor and its clinical features are those of catecholamine excess and are frequently, but not necessarily intermittent.

Note: These tumors are not innervated and catecholamine release dose not result from neural stimulation.

Most common neurotransmitter secreted by:
- Most phaeochromocytoma—both norepinephrine and epinephrine (in ratio 80:20)
- Most extra-adrenal pheochromocytoma—only norepinephrine
- Malignant pheochromocytoma—Dopamine and homovanillic acid

CONFUSA
Phaeochromocytoma produce some paradoxical clinical features and these should be noted, i.e. it can cause both hypertensive and hypotensive episodes (postural BP drop). Similarly it can produce both pallor and flushing. Phaeochromocytomas presents with vague episodic symptoms that the patient might be diagnosed as being depressed. This will further aggravate their problems as the tricyclic antidepressants can precipitate hypertensive episodes in them. Other precipitating factors can be
- Stretching
- Sneezing
- Stress
- Sex
- Smoking
- Surgery
- Parturition
- Cheese
- Alcohol

Investigation of choice
- *Screening:* 24 hour urine for HMMA, VMA
- *Definitive:* MIBG scan/clonidine suppression test

Immediate management
Consult specialist centre for full investigations.

Treatment of choice
Surgery after BP control

107. Autosomal dominant.

Diagnosis: Polycystic kidney disease (PKD)

Clinchers

Adult polycystic kidney disease is an autosomal dominant disease characterised by multiple expanding cysts of both kidneys that ultimately destroy the renal parenchyma and cause renal failure. It is a common condition affecting roughly 1 out of every 400 to 1000 live births an accounting for about 10% of cases of chronic renal failure requiring transplantation or dialysis. The pattern of inheritance is autosomal dominant with high penetrance. The disease is universally bilateral, reported unilateral cases probably represent multicystic dysplasia.

- *Clinical features*
  - Episodic flank pain
  - Hematuria (often gross)
  - Hypertension
  - Urinary infection in third or fourth decade
- *Associations*
  - Hepatic cysts
  - Intracranial berry aneurysms
- *Genes of chromosome*
  - 16 (PKD 1)
  - 4 (PKD 2)

CONFUSA
The cysts intially involve only portions of the nephrons, so that the renal function is retained until about the fourth or fifth decade of life. The likelihood of developing renal failure is less than 2% in affected individuals younger than 40 years but rises to 25% by age 50 years, 40% by 60 years, and 75% by age 70 to 75 years.

Investigation of choice
USG

Immediate management
Monitor BP and U and E

Treatment of choice
- Treat infections
- Dialysis/transplantation for end stage renal failure

Your Notes:

108. Increased production of aldosterone.

Diagnosis: Conn's syndrome

Clinchers

Conn's syndrome is unilateral adrenocortical adenoma and is responsible for more than 50% cases of primary hyperaldosteronism. It causes excess production of aldosterone, independent of renin-angiotensin system.

Clinical features:
- Hypertension
- Hypokalemia   in someone not on diuretics
- Alkalosis

CONFUSA
Posture test helps in differential diagnosis of primary hyperaldosteronism. It involves measuring the effect of posture on renin, aldosterone and cortisol (measure of 9 AM lying, and at noon standing).
Interpretation

On standing	Cortisol	Aldosterone
Conn's/GRA	↓	↓
Adrenal hyperplasia	↓	↑

Investigation of choice
- *Screening:* Posture test for renin, aldosterone and cortisol
- *Definitive:* Abdominal CT/MRI

Immediate management
Treat hypokalemia and alkalosis

Treatment of choice
Surgical excision after spironolactone upto 300 mg/24 h PO for 4 weeks.

Your Notes:

109. Deposition of immune complexes on basement membrane.

Diagnosis: Glomerulonephritis

Clinchers
Renal disease is the most common secondary cause of hypertension. 3/4 cases are from intrinsic renal disease of which glomerulonephritis is the most common. In glomerulonephritis, IgA; nephropathy is the most common one worldwide and is characterised by deposition of immune complexes on the basement membranes.

CONFUSA
The cardinal feature of glomerulonephritis is hematuria (which may be microscopic), with red cells casts in urine.

Investigation of choice
- *Screening:* Urine analysis and microscopy (red cell casts ± dysmorphic red cells)
- *Definitive:* Biopsy and immunofluorescence

Immediate management
Refer to a nephrologist for management
Keep BP $\leq 130/80$.

Treatment of choice
Depends upon underlying condition.

Your Notes:

110. A 17-year-old girl with hypertension of 160/100 is found to have a femoral pulse delay.

Diagnosis: Coarctation of aorta (CoA)

Clinchers
- *17-year-old:* The condition often remain asymptomatic for many years. Headache, epistaxis, cold extremities, and claudication with exercise may occur, and attention is usually directed to the cardiovascular system when a heart murmur or hypertension in the upper extremities and absence, marked diminution, or delayed pulsations in the femoral arteries are detected incidentally on physical examination.
- *Girl:* Although CoA is twice as common in males as in females, it association with Turner's syndrome accounts for majority of its incidence in females.
- *Hypertension of 160/110:* Blood pressure in upper limbs remains elevated in CoA. BP measurement in lower limbs should be done in order to get an idea.
- *Femoral pulse delay:* Radiofemoral delay is characteristic of the condition.

CONFUSA
When surgery for CoA is performed in childhood, hypertension usually resolves completely. However, when the operation is performed on adults the hypertension persists in 70% because of previous renal damage.

Investigation of choice
- *Screening:* CXR ("Figure of 3" appearance)
- *Definitive:* MRI/aortography/digital vascular imaging).

Immediate management
Screen for Turner's syndrome.

Treatment of choice
Surgery/balloon dilatation.

Your Notes:

111. A 40-year-old man underwent removal of tooth under anaesthesia, presents after one month with coughing up of blood.

Diagnosis: Inhaled foreign body

Clinchers
- *Removal of tooth under anaesthesia:* Tooth removal may have a complication of aspiration of a piece of tooth, especially when it is done under anaesthesia.
- *Coughing up of blood after one month:* The foreign body may lodge in the right main bronchus or upper basal lobe (most common sites because approach to them is wider, straighter and almost in line with the trachea). Inside the lung it can trigger a granulomatous reaction or infection which can then lead to hemoptysis and other symptoms.

CONFUSA
If the hemoptysis in this case is due to infection by foreign body, it would have presented much earlier (i.e. within a week) and the predominant symptom would have been of a swinging pyrexia. The given presentation is thus more indicative of a granulomatous reaction which will present usually after one month and with hemoptysis mainly.

Investigation of choice
Chest X-ray.

Immediate management
Contact dental surgeon who has operated upon him for a detailed history.

Treatment of choice
Removal (endoscopic).

Your Notes:

---

112. Female with cough, copious blood tinged sputum for more than a month. She is from south-east Asia.

Diagnosis: Pulmonary tuberculosis.

Clinchers
- *Cough:* Pulmonary TB may be silent but it causes cough more commonly.
- *Coupious blood tinged sputum:* Coupious sputum is a typical feature of tuberculosis. It may be blood tinged or associated with frank hemoptysis. Other associated presenting features can be:
  - Pneumonia
  - Pleurisy
  - Pleural effusion
- *South-east Asia:* Tuberculosis is most prevent in Indian subcontinent and is mostly seen in UK among immigrants from there (Pakistan, India, Bangladesh).

CONFUSA
Primary TB is usually asymptomatic, but there may be fever, lassitude, sweats, anorexia, cough, sputum, erythema nodosum or phlyctenular conjunctivitis. The most common nonpulmonary infection is GI, most commonly affecting the ileocaecal junction and associated lymph nodes.

Investigation of choice
- *Screening:* CXR (consolidation, cavitation, fibrosis, calcification)
- *Definitive:* Sputum culture.

Immediate management
Trace family contacts for prophylaxis

Treatment of choice
Directly observed therapy (DOT) with rifampicin, isoniazid, pyrazinamide ± ethambutol x 2 months, and then only with rifampicin and isoniazid for next for months.

Your Notes:

113. Female presents with acute pleuritic chest pain, haemoptysis after undergoing hysterectomy.

Diagnosis: Pulmonary embolism.

Clinchers
- *Acute pleuritic chest pain:* It is the usual presenting feature of pulmonary embolism. Other common associated presenting features can be:
  - Acute breathlessness
  - Haemoptysis
  - Dizziness
  - Syncope
- *Haemoptysis:* Haemoptysis occurs in 30%, often three or more days after the initial event.
- *After undergoing hysterectomy:* Any cause of immobility, i.e. postoperative immobility can increase the risk of pulmonary embolism. This risk is much more in middle-aged females on oral contraceptive pills (it induces hypercoagulability).

CONFUSA
Peluritic chest pain is common with small or medium sized pulmonary embolism. A massive pulmonary embolism give rise to severe central pain because of cardiac ischaemia due to lack of coronary blood flow.

Investigation of choice
- *Screening*
  - If patient stable = V/Q scan
  - If unable to undergo the above test = spiral CT
- *Definitive:* Pulmonary angiogram.

Immediate management
Anticoagulation with LMW heparin

Treatment of choice
Oral warfarin 10 mg PO x 3 months.

Your Notes:

---

114. A middle-aged woman develops a purulent cough with some haemoptysis. A chest X-ray reveals right upper lobe shadows.

Diagnosis: Pulmonary tuberculosis (PTB)

Clinchers
- *Middle-aged women:* Usually symptomatic primary tuberculosis develops due to reactivation of a primary complex years after the exposure.
- *Purulent cough with some hemoptysis:* Sputum in PTB may be mucoid, purulent or blood-stained.
- *CXR reveals right upper lobe shadows:* The CXR typically shows patchy or nodular shadows in the upper zones, loss of volume, and fibrosis with or without cavitation.

CONFUSA
Reactivation of tuberculosis is usually due to:
- DM
- Malnutrition
- Immunosuppression
- Drugs
  - Cytotoxins
  - Steroids
- Lymphoma
- AIDS

Investigation of choice
- *Screening:* CXR
- *Definitive:* Sputum culture and microscopy.

Immediate management
Find out cause of reactivation (often none found).

Treatment of choice
Directly observed therapy (DOT) x 6 months

Your Notes:

115. A 58-year-old man with fever and an area of consolidation on his chest X-ray is treated with antibiotics. His fever resolves but four weeks later but he still has a large area of consolidation.

Diagnosis: Bronchial carcinoma.

Clinchers
- *58-year-old man:* Elderly males with lung symptoms should be investigated to rule out lung cancer especially if they have history of smoking.
- *Fever:* This is because of the secondary pneumonia. Carcinoma causing partial obstruction of a bronchus interrupts the mucociliary escalator, and bacteria are retained within affected lobe.
- *An area of consolidation on his chest X-ray:* Secondary pneumonia due to above described mechanism appears as a lobar consolidation on CXR.
- *Is treated with antibiotics:* Treatment with antibiotics usually clears the pneumonia and resolves the fever within few days.
- *His fever resolves but four weeks later:* Any opacity secondary to inflammation should have been resolved in four weeks.
- *He still has a large area of consolidation:* Any opacity persisting beyound this time should make one strongly suspicious of a neoplastic lesion in this age group.

CONFUSA
The only confusion in this question can exist if one overlook the age of the patient and remain focussed only on the complications of pneumonia.

Investigation of choice
- *Screening:* CXR (already done in this case)
- *Definitive:* Bronchoscopy with biopsy.

Immediate management
Assess operability.

Treatment of choice
- Non-small cell tumors: Surgery (avoided in > 65 yrs with metastatic disease as rate of mortality is more than expected five-year survival)
- Radiotherapy: For bronchial obstruction (as in this case).

Your Notes:

116. Patient, 12 hours after MI presents with recurrent chest pain, breathlessness, heart rate—40/min.

Diagnosis: Heart block with haemodynamic compromise

Clinchers
- *12 hours after MI:* It means that it must be an acute complication of MI. Complication of MI in acute phase (i.e. within first two or three days following MI are—cardiac arrhythmia, cardiac failure and pericarditis. Late complications of MI are post-myocardial infarction syndrome (Dressler's syndrome), ventricular aneurysm, and recurrent cardiac arrhythmias.
- *Recurrent chest pain and breathlessness:* These are the symptomatologies of the associated haemodynamic compromise.
- *Heart rate—40/min:* It is low as bradycardia is present.

CONFUSA
Condition of heart block in this patient may require pace maker insertion. But it may not be necessary after inferior MI if:
- QRS is narrow and reasonably stable
- And pulse ≥ 40-50 (as in this patient).

A more detailed evaluation is required to consider pacemaker insertion in this patient.

Investigation of choice
ECG monitoring

Immediate management
Atropine IV (0.5 mg initial, upto 2.0 mg total)

Treatment of choice
Persistent bradycardia (<40 bpm) despite atropine is treated with electrical pacing.

Your Notes:

117. Patient with pulmonary edema features presents with irregular pulse, heart rate—140 bpm.

Diagnosis: Acute atrial fibrillation (AF)

Clinchers
- *Pulmonary oedema:* It is indicative of heart failure. Heart failure usually precipitates AF due to atrial irritation.
- *Irregular pulse:* The pulse in AF is characteristically irregularly irregular, the apical pulse rate is greater than radial rate and the first heart sound is of variable intensity.
- *Heart rate—140/bpm:* AF is a chaotic, irregular atrial rhythm at 300-600 bpm. But radial pulse is always lesser. It is so as the AV node responds intermittently producing an irregular ventricular rate.

CONFUSA
Atrial fibrillation is an early complication of myocardial infarction, occurring in about 10% patients. Apart from heart failure, other precipitants of AF can be
- Pericarditis
- Acute ischaemia or infarction

Investigation of choice
ECG (absent P waves; irregular QRS complexes)

Immediate management
IV digoxin or IV amiodarone

Treatment of choice
Treatment of underlying pathology (in this case, heart failure).

Your Notes:

118. A woman 10 days following hysterectomy complaints of severe left sided chest pain and breathlessness. Chest X-ray and ECG failed to relieve any abnormality.

Diagnosis: Pulmonary embolism.

Clinchers
- *10 days following hysterectomy:* Any cause of immobility or hypercoagulability, e.g. recent surgery (in this case hysterectomy), recent stroke or MI, disseminated malignancy, thrombophilia/antiphospholipid syndrome, prolonged bed-rest and pregnancy.
- *Severe left chest pain/breathlessness:* Symptoms of pulmonary embolism are—acute breathless, pleuritic chest pain, hemoptysis, dizziness and syncope.
- *Chest X-ray and ECG show no abnormality:* Chest X-ray and ECG is generally normal in pulmonary embolism.

Investigation of choice
- *Screening:* V/Q scan or spiral CT.
- *Definitive:* CT pulmonary angiography. This shows clots down to 5th order pulmonary arteries.

Immediate management
Screen for DVT.

Treatment of choice
Anticoagulation.

Your Notes:

119. 10 days after MI, female presents with chest pain on inspiration, persistently elevated ST segment on ECG.

Diagnosis: Acute pericarditis

Clinchers
- *10 days after MI:* Acute pericarditis is common in the first few days after MI, particularly in anterior wall infarction.
- *Chest pain on inspiration:* It is characterised by sharp chest pain, aggravated by
  - Movement
  - Respiration
  - Lying down (characteristic)
- *Persistently elevated ST segment:* ECG in acute pericarditis shows generalised ST segment elevation (concave upward) with upright, peaked T waves.

CONFUSA
Sequence of ECG changes in MI are:
1. Normal ECG
2. ST elevation
3. Appearance of Q waves
4. Normalization of ST segments
5. Inversion of T waves

So ST elevation is a normal feature in MI. However, if it remains persistently elevated, always suspect pericarditis, especially with saddle-shaped ST elevation.
Note:
- In pericarditis after MI, anticoagulation is avoided.
- In case of recurrent pericarditis, suspect Dressler's syndrome.

Investigation of choice
ECG (already done in this patient).
Each to check effusions.

Immediate management
Stop anticoagulation if continuing after MI.

Treatment of choice
NSAIDs.

Your Notes:

120. Patient after MI found to have a harsh pansystolic murmur at the apex.

Diagnosis: Papillary muscle rupture.

Clinchers
- *After MI:* Mitral valve papillary muscle rupture is common complication of MI.
- *Harsh pansystolic murmur at apex:* It is due to mitral regurgitation. It can also be a finding in ventricular septal perforation, more common than papillary muscle rupture, after MI. A systolic thrill may be found in both the cases.

CONFUSA
The cardiac rupture syndrome results from the mechanical weakening that occurs in necrotic and subsequently inflamed myocardium and includes:
1. *Rupture of ventricular free wall* (***most common***)—with haemopericardium and cardiac tamponade and usually fatal.
2. *Rupture of ventricular septum (less commonly)*—leading to a left to right shunt.
3. *Papillary muscle rupture (least common)*—resulting in acute onset of severe mitral regurgitation.

Note:
- Pansystolic murmur can be heard in (2) and (3).
- ECG is usually normal in cardiac rupture.

Investigation of choice
Echocardiography (colour flow doppler)

Immediate management
Lowering aortic systolic pressure
- Intraortic balloon counter pulsation
- Nitroglycerin/Nitroprusside

Treatment of choice
Surgical repair/mitral valve repalcement.

Your Notes:

121. Man with recurrent amaurosis fugax of right eye.

Diagnosis: Carotid artery stenosis.

Clinchers

> *Man:* The incidence of artherosclerosis, which is the causative factor of carotid artery stenosis is more in males.
> *Recurrent amaurosis fugax:* Amaurosis fugax is sudden transient loss of vision in one eye. A TIA causing an episode of amaurosis fugax is often the first clinical evidence of internal carotid artery stenosis, which may herald a hemiparesis. A recurrent event points more towards this pathology.

CONFUSA

Amaurosis fugax occurs as a benign event in migraine, but in that case recurrent unilateral headache will be a more predominant symptom. Vertebrobasilar insufficiency or emboli can be confused with amaurosis fugax, because many patients mistakenly ascribe symptoms to their left or right eye, when in fact they are occurring in the left or right hemifield of both eyes. In amaurosis fugax, the patient typically describes the blindness as a "sudden falling of a curtain in front of the eye". The other conditions with such a description is retinal detachment, but that is usually precede by a prodrome of photopsia and is differentiable on retinoscopy.

Other common cause for sudden uniocular blindness is multiple sclerosis but that will not be painless, (as in above two conditions) as retrobulbar pain is frequently present, and the patient will give a typical history of multiple sclerosis.

Common causes of amaurosis fugax
- Carotid TIA
- Embolization of retinal circulation
- Papilloedema
- Giant cell arteritis
- Raynaud's disease
- Hypertensive retinopathy
- Migraine
- Venous stasis retinopathy
- As a prodromal symptom of:
  - Central retinal artery occlusion
  - Carotid artery occlusion.

Investigation of choice
- *Screening:* Carotid artery doppler.
- *Definitive:* Carotid angiography.

Immediate management
Aspirin 75 mg pO/d.

Treatment of choice
Carotid endarterectomy (if the patient is good operative risk).

Your Notes:

122. An elderly female with scalp tenderness on both sides of the head, complains of headache, sudden loss of vision in one eye.

Diagnosis: Giant cell arteritis (GCA)

Clinchers
- *Elderly females:* Common in elderly (rare under 55 years). More incidence in females.
- *Scalp tenderness:* Pain is felt over the inflamed superficial, temporal or occipital arteries. Touching the skin over the inflamed vessel (e.g. combing the hair) causes pain. Arterial pulsation is soon lost and the artery becomes hard, tortuous and thickened. The skin over the vessels may become red. Rarely, gangrenous patches appear on the scalp.
- *Headache:* Invariably present in GCA because of arteritis.
- *Sudden loss of vision in one eye:* Visual loss owing to inflammation and occlusion of the ciliary and/or central retinal artery occurs in 25% of cases of untreated GCA. The patient complains of sudden uniocular visual loss, either partial or complete, which is painless. Amaurosis fugax may precede total visual loss, which is usually permanent, if the transient loss of vision lasts more than an hour.

CONFUSA
Do not think that GCA is only confined to arteries of the scalp. There is always associated inflammation of other branches of the external carotid (i.e. facial, maxillary and lingual) and their involvement produces clinically important features, e.g. jaw claudication (pain worse or eating), painful opening of mouth, painful movements of tongue, etc.

Investigation of choice
- *Screening:* ESR
- *Definitive:* Temporal artery biopsy

Immediate management
IV steroid (since visual symptoms are present)

Treatment of choice
Prednisolone 60-100 mg (i.e. high dose) for 2 years

Note: Headache subsides within hours of the first large dose of steroid.

Your Notes:

123. A 40-year-old female comes with complaints of headache, bitemporal hemianopia, increase in shoe size.

Diagnosis: Acromegaly

Clinchers
- *40-year-old female:* It typically presents between the ages of 30 and 50 years. It is equally prevalent in men and women.
- *Headache and bitemporal hemianopia:* Because of the pituitary tumor (responsible for growth hormone hypersecretion). Bitemporal hemianopia is characteristic of compression of optic chiasm (most common cause of it—pituitary tumor).
- *Increase in shoe size:* GH excess results in bony and soft tissue overgrowth. The features are insidious, chronic and debilitating, i.e.
  - Increased teeth spacing
  - Increased shoe size
  - Thick spade like hands
  - Large tongue
  - Prominent supraorbital ridge
  - Prognathism.

CONFUSA
Acromegalics are said to look more like each other than their family members. Presence of bitemporal hemianopia in it clinically corroborates the presence of a pituitary tumor and that acromegaly is not due to some ectopic secretion of growth hormone.

Ectopic (other than pituitary) tumors causing acromegaly
- GnRH secreting tumors
  - Bronchial carcinoids
  - Pancreatic islet cell tumors
  - Hypothalamic gangliocytomas
  - Harmatoma
  - Gliomas
- GH secreting tumors
  - Pancreatic islet cell tumor

Investigation of choice
MRI pituitary fossa.

Immediate management
Obtain old photographs for comparison.

Your Notes:

124. Patient with attacks of numbness in left hand and right-sided headache.

Diagnosis: Space occupying lesion (SOL)

Clinchers
- *Attacks of numbness in left hand:* This suggests an evolving focal neurology. Usually focal neurology depends upon site of the tumor but the information provided in the question is insufficient to diagnose the site of SOL. Most probably it is a parietal lobe tumor (Hemisonsory loss, decreased two-point discrimination).
- *Right-sided headache:* It is a sign of increased ICP signs to space occupying property of the tumor. Other signs of ↑ ICP can be:
  - Vomiting
  - Papilloedema (only in 50% of tumors)
  - Altered consciousness.

CONFUSA
Evolving focal neurology must be differentiated from false localising signs which are produced by raised ICP. VI nerve palsy is the most common due to its long intracranial course.

Investigation of choice
CT (MRI is good for posterior fossa tumors).

Immediate management
Refer to neurology.

Treatment of choice
Complete removal if possible.

Your Notes:

125. Patient gets diplopia when he works very hard.

Diagnosis: Myasthenia gravis (MG)

Clinchers
- *Gets diplopia when he works very hard:* Fatiguability is the single most important feature of MG. Muscles are not commonly affected in the early stages:
  - Proximal limb muscles
  - Extraocular muscles
  - Muscles of mastication, speech and facial expression.

Complex extraocular palsies, ptosis and a typical fluctuating proximal weakness are found.

CONFUSA
The reflexes are initially preserved in MG but may be fatiguable. Muscle wasting is sometimes seen late in the disease. The clinical picture of fluctuating weakness may be diagnostic. Early symptoms of weakness and fatigue are frequently dismissed by attending doctors.

Investigation of choice
Tensilon test (only do if resuscitation facilities available)

Immediate management
Rule out
- Thymic tumor
- Hyperthyroidism
- Rheumatoid arthritis
- SLE

Treatment of choice
Pyridostigmine + prednisolone.

Your Notes:

126. 80-year-old with prostatic carcinoma comes with 4 month history of low backache.

Diagnosis: Metastatic disease.

Clinchers
- *Carcinoma prostate:* Carcinoma of prostate is more usually discovered at a stage when it has already spread beyond its capsule and may have invaded pelvic cellular tissues, bladder base and bone.
- *Low backache for 4 months:* Once the diagnosis of prostate carcinoma has been established, it would be normal to perform a bone scan as part of the staging procedure if the PSA is >20 nmol/mL. If the PSA is < 29 nmol/mL than a bone scan would only be performed on clinical indications (like low backache). So a bone scan is must in this case.

CONFUSA
The bone scan is performed by the injection of technetium-99m, which is then monitored using a gamma camera. It is more sensitive in the diagnosis of metastases than a skeletal survey, but false positives occur in areas of arthritis, osteomyelitis or a healing fracture.

Investigation of choice
Tc^{99} bone scan.

Immediate management
TNM staging of tumor.

Treatment of choice
The main stay of treatment of metastatic prostatic carcinoma is androgen suppression or the use of specific androgen antagonists, which produce symptomatic relief in 75% cases.

Your Notes:

127. Patient with prostatic cancer has been treated, now complains of confusion, thirst, body aches, constipation.

Diagnosis: Hypercalcemia

Clinchers
- *Prostate carcinoma:* It produces osteoblastic metastases to the bone.
- *Has been treated:* The patient might have been operated upon to remove the local disease. The metastases to bone would either have been missed then or have now presented as a recurrence.
- *Confusion, thirst, body aches, constipation:* These all are symptoms of hypercalcemia. Other symptoms and signs can be:
  - Lethargy
  - Anorexia
  - Nausea
  - Polydipsia
  - polyuria
  - Dehydration
  - Weakness.

CONFUSA
Hypercalcemia is produced by following cancers:
- Myeloma (40% cases of hypercalcemia in malignancy)
- Breast
- Prostate
- Bronchus
- Kidney
- Thyroid

Investigation of choice
Serum calcium.

Immediate management
Rehydrate (3-4 litres of 0.9% saline IV over 24 hours)

Treatment of choice
Bisphosphonate IV
- Best treatment is control of underlying malignancy
- Resistant hypercalcemia—calcitonin

Your Notes:

128. Man on GnRH's for prostate cancer comes after 2 months for a follow up.

Diagnosis: Follow-up case of hormone therapy for prostate carcinoma.

Clinchers
- *GnRH for prostate cancer:* GnRH agonists, e.g. buserilin and goserilin, which inhibit the release of luteinizing hormone (LH) from the anterior pituitary, with consequent reduction of testicular production of testosterone. The exact mechanism is

GnRH agonists
↓
Initially stimulate hypothalamic GnRH receptors
↓
Later down regulation of hypothalamic GnRH receptors
↓
Cessation of pituitary LH production
↓
Decrease in testosterone production to levels akin to castration levels

- *Comes after 2 months for a follow up:* GnRH agonists are usually given in 2-3 month depot injection so the patient has to come every 2 months for follow up. PSA (prostate specific antigen) is the best way to follow the response after hormone therapy.

CONFUSA
Though transrectal USG can also be used for follow up and to measures response to treatment, PSA is the accurate and best way. Transrectal USG will also be used, but as an additional investigation to measure the size and regression.

Investigation of choice
PSA

Immediate management
Check for gynaecomastia or other such side effects of GnRH therapy.

Treatment of choice
Give second depot injection of GnRH agonist.

Your Notes:

129. Man with prostate Ca which has extended outside the capsule presenting with features of renal failure.

Diagnosis: Bladder outflow obstruction (BOO).

Clinchers
- *Prostate carcinoma which has extended outside capsule:* It means that it is a locally advanced disease. Bladder base is a frequent site of prostatic metastases. Otherwise also, prostatic enlargement due to carcinomatous growth can produce BOO.
- *Features of renal failure:* The obstruction to outflow of the bladder may result in renal failure with drowsiness, headache and impairment of intellect due to uraemia.

CONFUSA
Pain is not a symptom of BOO and its presence should prompt the exclusion of acute retention, urinary infection stones carcinoma of the prostate and carcinoma *in situ* of the bladder (1242, Bailey and Love, 23rd edn).

Investigation of choice
Pressure-flow urodynamic studies

Immediate management
Suprapubic catheterisation

Treatment of choice
Prostatectomy.

Your Notes:

130. A man having adenocarcinoma prostate which has already spread to pelvic side walls has to be given chemotherapy.

Diagnosis: Metastatic prostate carcinoma

Clinchers
- *Adenocarcinoma:* This is the most common variety of carcinoma prostate and is usually well-differentiated. Occasionally anaplastic variety is seen.
- *Spread to pelvic side walls:* Carcinoma prostate is more usually discovered at a stage when it has already spread beyond its capsule and may well have involved other organs, particularly the pelvic cellular tissues, bladder base and bone. The mainstay of this disease is androgen suppression or the use of specific androgen antagonists, which will produce symptomatic relief in disseminated prostatic cancer is about 75% of patients.

CONFUSA
This chemotherapy in this case is most probably stilbesterol, an oestrogen analogue, which is used as primary therapy is majority of cases. It may have feminising side effects such as gynaecomastia, nipple and scrotal pigmentation and testicular atrophy. More importantly, it may result in fluid retention and precipitate congestive cardiac failure, so that in elderly patients with cardiovascular disease bilateral orchidectomy should be performed.

Investigation of choice
Transrectal USG (can assess extracapsular spread)

Immediate management
Rule out heart disease

Treatment of choice
Stilbesterol.

Your Notes:

131. An elderly female has history of uncontrollable loose stools many times a day. On examination, packed solid faeces in rectum.

Diagnosis: Fecal impaction with overflow diarrhoea

Clinchers
- *Elderly female:* Fecal impaction usually occurs in the elderly with constipation.
- *Loose stools many times a day:* It is fecal incontinence and is a major problem in the elderly infirm or demented patient. It is often secondary to faecal loading and impaction (overflow incontinence).

CONFUSA
Fecal incontinence in younger patients, is most commonly due to neurological disorders or childbirth trauma. Fecal impaction is rare in them.

Investigation of choice
To find the cause for constipation so vary from patient to patient.

Immediate management
Rule out dementia

Treatment of choice
Manual removal of impacted faeces.

Your Notes:

132. A 30-year-old female has history of alternating constipation and diarrhoea, for 7 months. She told that she is passing hard pellet like stools.

Diagnosis: Irritable bowel syndrome (IBS)

Clinchers
- *30-year-old females:* Patients are usually 20-40 years old and females are more frequently affected.
  Note: Since this disorder is chronic, patients can present at any age often teens.
- *Alternating constipation and diarrhoea:* This is the most common symptom of the altered bowel habit in IBS. Other symptoms of IBS are:
  - Central or lower abdominal pain (relieved by defecation)
  - Abdominal bloating
  - Tenesmus
  - Mucus per rectum
- *Passing pellet like stools:* This can be due to abnormal colonic motility frequently present in IBS.
- *For 7 months:* Symptoms should be present for > 6 months for diagnosis.

CONFUSA
Half of all patients with this disorder who seek medical care have comorbid psychiatric disorders. IBS is usually a diagnosis of exclusion. There are markers of organic disease, which are usually present in this condition. These markers can represent some organic disease which will manifest itself over the time. The organic markers are:
- Age > 40 years
- History < 6 months
- Anorexia
- Weight loss
- Waking at night with pain/diarrhoea
- Mouth ulcers
- Rectal bleeding
- Abnormal investigations

Note: Presence of any of these question the diagnosis of IBS.

Investigation of choice
Follow the following flow chart.
Any marker of organic disease?
- Yes → Barium enema or Colonoscopy
- No ↓

Diarrhoea
- Yes → Stool culture, TSH, Faecal fats
- No ↓

Constipation?
- Yes → Plasma Ca^{2+}, TSH
- No ↓

Anemia or weight loss?
- Yes → Endomysial antibodies (for coeliac disease)
- No ↓

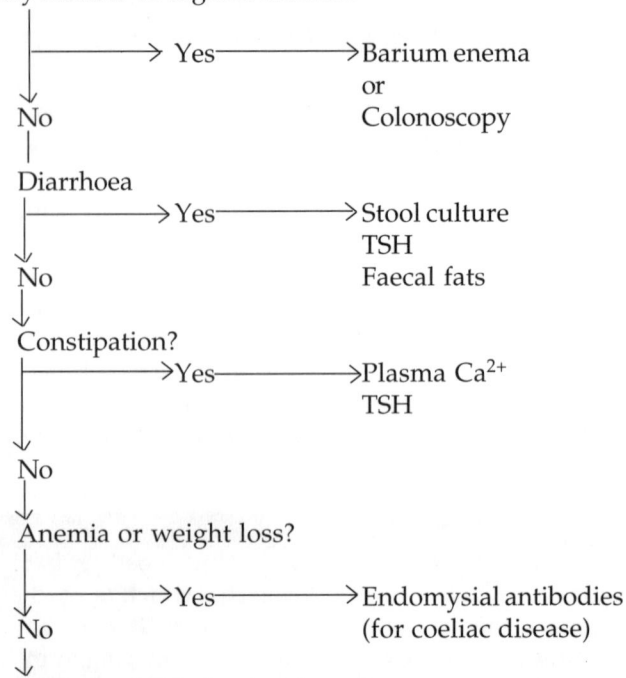

Rule out other diseases by:
- Upper GI endoscopy (GERD)
- Jejunal biopsy and aspirate (coeliac disease, giardiasis)
- Small bowel radiology (Crohn's)
- ERCP (chronic pancreatitis)
- Transit studies and anorectal physiological studies

Immediate management
Reassurance.

Treatment of choice
Treatment should be directed the predominant symptom, i.e.
- Food intolerance—exclusion diets
- Constipation—high fibre diet
- Diarrhoea—bulking agent + loperamide
- Colic and bloating—antispasmodics (mebeverine, alvarine citrate)
- Dyspepsia—Metoclopramide or antacids
- Psychiatric symptoms—Anxiolytics + cognitive therapy.

133. Female, 22-year-old, with bleeding and mucus per rectum, fever, loss of weight, has never been abroad.

Diagnosis: Inflammatory bowel disease (IBD)

Clinchers
- *22-year-old female:* The incidence of IBD peaks between 15 to 35 years, although it has been reported in every decade of life. Both the sexes are affected equally.
- *Bleeding and mucus per rectum:* Mucus per rectum is a symptom present both in IBD and IBS. Blood diarrhoea is more frequently seen in UC rather than CD.
- *Fever:* Fever is almost invariably present in IBD and differentiates it from IBS.
- *Loss of weight:* It is due to malabsorption in IBD.
- *Never been abroad:* This probably rules out infective causes of hemorrhagic diarrhoea i.e. *Shigella* and *E. coli*.

CONFUSA

IBD is a very frequent topic in PLAB exam and the questions are often difficult. Some students often have confusion in differentiating UC from CD. These are:

	Ulceratives colitis (UC)	Crohn's disease (CD)
Most common site	Colon	Ileocaecal
Rectum	Always involved	Often spared
Inflammation	Mucosa and submucosa	Transmural
Diarrhoea	Often bloody	Often not blood
Fistulas	Rare	Common
Perianal fissures	Absent	Present
Nephrolithiasis	Absent	Often present
Skin lesions	Absent	Present
Colon cancer risk	Markedly increased	Mildly increased

Investigation of choice
- *Screening:* Colonoscopy
- *Definitive:* Biopsy

Immediate management
Antipyretics for fever
+
Bulking agents for diarrhoea

Treatment of choice
- Sulfasalazine
- Refractory disease: Corticosteroids
- Surgery
  - UC—curative
  - CD—if perforation likely

134. An 80-year-old woman, fever 39 degrees centigrade, acute generalized abdominal pain, diarrhoea and vomiting, slightly dehydrated.

Diagnosis: Acute gastroenteritis (GE)

Clinchers
- *80-year-old woman:* Susceptibility to infection increases in old age and debilitation.
- *Fever 39° C:* It is a common accompaniment of many GE organisms.
- *Acute generalised abdominal pain:* Crampy and diffuse abdominal pain is there in acute GI.
- *Diarrhoea and vomiting:* It is the most common symptom of GI infection seen in almost every infection. Usually it is due to activation of specific GI receptors by toxins produced by organisms.
- *Slightly dehydrated:* It is due to fluid loss in diarrhoea.

CONFUSA

Vomiting without diarrhoea is present with:
- Clostridium botulinum

Diarrhoea without vomiting is present with:
- Clostridium perfringens
- Campylobacter (bloody)
- Cryptosporidium
- Yersinia enterocolitica
- Shigella (bloody)

* Source: 558, OHCM, 5th edn

Investigation of choice
Stool microscopy and culture.

Immediate management
Fluid resuscitation (oral in mild to moderate dehydration IV in severe dehydration)

Treatment of choice
- Antibiotics (as she is systemically unwell)
- Antidiarrhoeals (as symptoms of dehydration present)
- Antiemetics (contraindicated in dysentery, but here it is not specified whether the stools are bloody).

Your Notes:

135. A 55-year-old man, history of altered bowel habit from 2 months, anaemia, loss of weight.

Diagnosis: Colon carcinoma.

Clinchers
- *55-year-old man:* Colon carcinoma are the second most common cause of death from malignancy in UK. Tumors may occur at any age. Females are affected more than males (Note: The incidence of rectal cancer is roughly equal in two sexes). The peak in incidence occurs after 50 years.
- *Altered bowel habit for two months:* The most common symptom is a change in bowel habits, either constipation, diarrhoea or two alternating with each other.
- *Anaemia and loss of weight:* More common in caecal carcinoma (see   below).

CONFUSA
Tumors of the left side of the colon, where the contained stool is solid, are typically constricting growths, so obstructive symptoms predominate along with constipation. In contrast, tumors of the right side tend to be proliferative and here the stools are semi-liquid, therefore obstructive symptoms are relatively uncommon and the patient with a carcinoma of the caecum or ascending colon often presents with anaemia and loss of weight.

Investigation of choice
- *Screening:* Barium enema
- *Definitive:* Colonoscopy with biopsy.

Immediate management
Correct anaemia with haematinics or blood transfusion.

Treatment of choice
Surgical excision.

Your Notes:

---

136. A 4-year-old boy has fever since 2 days, presents with convulsions since 5 min, still convulsing in the ambulance, IV line has been established.

Diagnosis: Febrile convulsions

Clinchers
- *Boy:* Febrile convulsions occur in about 3% of children between the ages of 5 months and 5 years.
- *Fever:* They are thought to be caused by viraemia and often recurrent.
- *Convulsions × 5 min:* The child may present with prolonged fitting or there may have been a short period of clonic or tonic activity.
- *Still convulsing in the ambulance IV line has been established:* The first preference is to protect the convulsing child from harm If the child is still convulsing, give diazepam (or larazepam) emulsion 0.3 mg per kg slow IV. This can be repeated after a few minutes if fitting continues.

CONFUSA
Give 0.5 mg per ke diazepam per rectally if IV access is delayed. The usual progression of treatment (if fitting does not stop) should be

Diazepam—IV/per rectal
↓
Paraldehyde—per rectum (diluted 50:50 with arachis oil)
↓
Phenytoin—18 mg/kg IV over 15 minutes (with EEG monitoring
↓
IV thiopentone—for intractable fitting

Investigation of choice
Blood glucose (all cases)

Immediate management
IV lorazepam

Treatment of choice
- Criteria for hospital admission
  - Prolonged
  - Recurrent } Febrile convulsion
  - First
- Paracetamol or Ibuprofen after fitting has stopped.

Your Notes:

137. A 2-year-old boy with past and family history of febrile convulsions. He is ok now.

Diagnosis: Recurrent febrile convulsions

Clinchers
- *History of febrile convulsions:* A febrile convulsion is diagnosed if the following occur together:
  - A tonic/clonic, symmetrical generalised with no focal feature
  - Occurring as the temperature rises rapidly in a febrile illness
  - In a normally developing child between 5 months and 5 years of age
  - With no signs of CNS infection or previous history of epilepsy
  - When there are less than 3 seizures, each lasting < 5 min.
- *He is OK now:* This means that he require no active treatment now.
- *Family history positive:* The chances of recurrence of a febrile convulsion are about 50% if first degree relative is also affected.

CONFUSA
Apart from being taught the use of rectal diazepam, the patient should be explained to bring down any future fever promptly with oral paracetamol and tepid sponging. Since the child is only 2-year-old, he will undergo MMR and pertussis vaccination at 4 years age, both of which can cause fever. Explain them to be ready for immediate intervention then.

Immediate management
Rectal diazepam use explained to parents especially the mother, e.g. with one 5 mg tube (stesolid).

Treatment of choice
Control of convulsions have been explained in previous question.

Your Notes:

138. Young girl on Na valproate, parents come with complaints of increased seizure frequency and frequent absences from school. On examination, she is mildly obese.

Diagnosis: Side effects of valproate.

Clinchers
- *Young girl:* Valproate is often not the first line drug in children. Carbamazepine is a recommended effective first line drug for partial and generalized tonic-clonic seizures. It has the advantage of very few side effects.
- *Increased seizure frequency:* This signifies the refractiveness of valproate in this patient. If any drug fail to relieve seizures with monotherapy, addition of a second drug is necessary. If there is presence of side effects to first drug, then it should be discontinued after tapering the dose gradually.
- *Frequent absences from school:* Do not confuse this with absence seizures. This only signify increased frequency of the illness.
- *Mildly obese:* Sodium valproate causes weight gain as its adverse effect. So, this case requires a replacement of sodium valproate with another drug.

CONFUSA
If seizures continue despite gradual increases to the maximum tolerated dose and documented compliance, then it becomes necessary to switch over to another antiepileptic drug. This is usually done by maintaining the patient on the first drug while a second drug is added. The dose of the second drug should be adjusted to decrease seizures frequency without causing toxicity. Once this is achieved, the first drug can be gradually withdrawn (usually over weeks unless there is significant toxicity). The dose of the second drug is then further optimized based on seizures response and side effects.

Investigation of choice
Drug levels.

Immediate management
Evaluation by an expert.

Treatment of choice
Replace valproate with an appropriate drug.

Your Notes:

139. A 12-year-old girl, one episode of grandmal seizure of 3 min duration in her sleep.

Diagnosis: Probable epileptic seizure.

Clinchers
- *12-year-old girl:* Epilepsy commonly has its onset in adolescence. The incidence is slightly more in girls.
- *One episode:* Most probably this is her first episode. Thus it warrants admission for 24 hrs for investigations and observation. But the available text is unclear about admission criteria for seizures occurring in sleep.
- *Grand mal seizures:* These are tonic clonic seizures which cannot be referred to any part of cerebral hemispheres. Limbs stiffen (the tonic phase) and then jerk forcefully (clonic phase), with loss of consciousness. There is a definitive postictal phase (with drowsiness and confusion). They are usually of 1-5 minute duration.
- *In her sleep:* Generally seizures in sleep are virtually diagnostic of epilepsy.

CONFUSA
Epilepsy is always investigated by EEG (done by an expert). CT is done only if there are:
- Infantile spasms
- Unusual features
- CNS signs
- Partial or intractable epilepsy

MRI may be more sensitive, but is not so available and may require anaesthesia or sedation.

Investigation of choice
EEG (shows generalized burst of spikes and irregular 4-6 Hz spike-wave complexes)

Immediate management
Check blood glucose and protect child from immediate harm if there is a convulsion.

Treatment of choice
Carbamazepine if epilepsy is diagnosed (phenobarbitone if child < 1 year age)

Your Notes:

140. A 14-year-old girl has had been academically brilliant, lately has had difficulty with her school work. She has be caught day dreaming in class on a number of occasions.

Diagnosis: Petit mal epilepsy (absence seizures)

Clinchers
- *14-year-old:* It almost invariably begins in childhood.
- *Academically brilliant:* This rules out her being not interested in studies and voluntarily indulging in day dreaming.
- *Lately has had difficulty with her school work:* This suggests a problem of recent origin
- *Day dreaming:* In petit mal, the child ceases activity, stares and pales slightly. An attack lasts a few seconds. The eyelids twitch; a few muscle jerks may occur. After an attack, the child resumes normal activity. As these seizures generally do not produce much external effects, they can pass unrecognised or mistakenly taken as "day dreaming", a decline in school performance recognised by a teacher.

CONFUSA
Children with typical absence attacks may in adult life developed generalized seizures. Typical absence attacks are never due to acquired lesions such as tumors. They are a developmental abnormality of neuronal control. Petit mal describes only 3 Hz seizures, rather than clinically similarly absence attacks which are partial attacks.

Investigation of choice
EEG (3 Hz spike and wave EEG).

Immediate management
Rule out any focal signs or symptoms to differentiate from atypical absence seizures (partial seizures).

Treatment of choice
Ethosuximide

Side effects
- Ataxia
- Lethargy
- Headache
- Skin rash
- GI irritation
- Bone marrow suppression

Your Notes:

141. A 55-year-old lady with history of intermittent postmenopausal bleeding. Vaginal and speculum examinations are normal.

Diagnosis: Endometrial carcinoma

Clinchers
- *A 55-year-old:* Mean age of presentation is 56 years. It is rare under the age of 40.
- *Intermittent postmenopausal bleeding:* This symptom should always be assumed to be caused by carcinoma of endometrium until proven otherwise.
- *Vaginal and speculum examination are normal:* This has ruled out any local cause of bleeding (e.g. vaginal trauma) so this warrants examination of the endometrium now.

CONFUSA
Endometrial carcinoma is associated with hyperestrogenic states, i.e.
- Obesity
- Diabetes
- Late menopause
- Prolonged use of unopposed oestrogens
- Oestrogen secreting tumors

Investigation of choice
- *Screening:* Ultrasound (to assess dimensions of any tumor and to show endometrial thickness)
- *Definitive:* Uterine sampling or curettage

Immediate management
Perform staging to decide the line of treatment.

Treatment of choice
Usually surgical

Uterus	Tumor	Surgery
Small	Well differentiated	Total abdominal hysterectomy + bilateral salpingo-oophorectomy + internal iliac node frozen section biopsy
Enlarged	Confined to upper part of corpus	Extended hysterectomy + bilateral salpingo-oophorectomy + removal of a cuff of vagina + lymph node sampling
Cervix invaded		Wertheim's (Removal of upper half of the vagina and pelvic lymph node)

- *Radiotherapy*
  - If node is involved
  - If there is deep invasion of myometrium
- *Hormone therapy:* Progestogens inhibit the rate of growth and spread of endometrial carcinoma.

142. Young girl has put on weight, hirsutism, oligomenorrhoea.

Diagnosis: Polycystic ovary syndrome (PCOS).

Clinchers
- *Young girl:* 5-10% of the premenopausal women are affected by this common syndrome.
- *Put on weight:* PCOS is related to insulin resistance, so hyperinsulinemia is a feature. As a result the patient can become obese.
- *Hirsutism:* In PCOS, hormonal cycling is disrupted because of ovarian, hypothalamic-pituitary and adrenal dysfunction. As a result virilisation with hirsutism and acne usually occurs.
- *Oligomenorrhoea:* It is also a component of virilization. Often there is amenorrhoea (secondary) (Stein-Leventhal syndrome). The patient may present with infertility.

CONFUSA
Hirsutism is common (10% of women) and is usually benign. It implies hair growth in women in male pattern. Differential diagnosis of hirsutism depends on menses:
- Menstruation abnormal—cause is ↑ testosterone
- Menstruation normal—cause is other than of ↑ testosterone

Investigation of choice
- *Screening:* LH ↑, testosterone ↑
- *Definitive:* USG/laparoscopy (characteristic ovaries)

Immediate management
Advice weight loss

Treatment of choice
Symptomatic
- Infertility—clomiphene
- Bleeding—combined pill
- Hirsutism—cyproterone
- Insulin resistance—metformin

Your Notes:

143. Female on OCPs complains of postcoital bleeding.

Diagnosis: Cervical ectropion

Clinchers
- *OCP:* Ectocervix contain a transformation zone, where the stratified squamous epithelium of the vagina meets the columnar epithelium of the cervical canal. The anatomical site of this squamocolumnar junction fluctuates under hormonal influence, and the high turnover of this tissue is important in the pathogenesis of cervical carcinoma. The columnar epithelium is normally visible with the speculum during
  - Ovulatory phase of menstrual cycle
  - Pregnancy
  - OCP use
- *Postcoital bleeding:* It may give rise to postcoital bleeding, as fine blood vessels, within the columnar epithelium are easily traumatised.

CONFUSA
Cervical ectropion is sometimes termed as cervical erosion. Usually the main complaint of cervical ectropion is excessive nonpurulent discharge, as the surface area of the columnar epithelium containing mucus glands is increased. It may give rise to spotting during pregnancy in which case it is usually left untreated till after the pregnancy.

Investigation of choice
Per speculum exam (red ring around OS because the endocervical epithelium has extended its territory over the paler epithelium of the ectocervix).

Immediate management
Reassurance about cause and treatment.

Treatment of choice
Usually none required.
If symptoms are distressing
- Thermal cautery (sometimes confusingly called cold coagulation).

Your Notes:

144. An 18-year-old university student with history of 3 months of amenorrhoea and starvation.

Diagnosis: Anorexia nervosa

Clinchers
- *18-year-old:* Anorexia mainly affects females (sex ratio 10:1). The average age of onset is 15-16 years. The prevalence in the UK is about 1% in females aged 12-18.
- *University students:* It precipitates because of well-marked stressors, such as new school or colleges, first sexual encounters and examinations.
- *3 months of amenorrhoea:* Anorexia nervosa may lead to pituitary damage and thus to permanent amenorrhoea and sterility. The endocrinal disturbances include elevated cortisol and growth hormone levels.
- *Starvation:* There is deliberately weight loss, induced primarily by restriction of food intake. Weight is > 15% below normal and BMI is < 17.5.

CONFUSA
In anorexia nervosa, periods cease before weight loss becomes apparent (lecture notes, gynae-obs, pg 29, 1st edn). If the onset is before puberty, there is delay in secondary sexual development. In menstruating females, always rule out amenorrhoea due to OCP usage. In early stages the weight loss must be distinguished from other causes of weight loss.
The psychiatric differential diagnosis include:
- Depressive disorder
- Substance misuse
- Obsessive-compulsive disorder

The medical disorders in differential diagnosis as:
- Inflammatory bowel disease
- Malabsorption syndromes
- Hypopituitarism
- Cancer.

Investigation of choice
BMI

Immediate management
If extreme weakness, fainting, K^+ ↓ or glucose ↓, then prompt admission to hospital.

Treatment of choice
Cognitive-behavioural therapy.

Your Notes:

145. A woman on the contraceptive pill for several years has a slight whitish vaginal discharge. On inspection she is found to have a pinkish coloration of the outer cervix.

Diagnosis: Cervical ectropion

Clinchers

Note: See Q 143 of this theme also.
➤ *Contraceptive pill:* It increases the incidence of cervical ectropion as the hormonal inthence imparted by it causes to squamocolumnar junction to shift due to outgrowth of columnar epithelium.
➤ *Discharge:* Discharge in cervical ectropion is due to excessive mucus secretion as the surface area of the columnar epithelium containing mucus glands is increased. If the discharge becomes troublesome to the patient, discontinuing the contraceptive pill, or alternatively ablative treatment under local anaesthesia using a thermal probe can reduce it.
➤ *Pinkish coloration of outer cervix:* This is the typical appearance of the columnar epithelium on ectocervix. Other than ectropion, columnar epithelium is visible during pregnancy and ovulatory phase of menstrual cycle.

CONFUSA
The appearance of the cervix in ectropion is sometimes inappropriately termed as cervical erosion. It should be avoided as it conveys quite the wrong impression of what is really a normal phenomenon.

Investigation of choice
Per speculum examination (already done in this patient)

Immediate management
Reassurance (that it is a completely normal phenomenon)

Treatment of choice
Indicated only if the discharge is troublesome
- Thermal ablation under LA (heat the tissue to 100 °C, destroying epithelium to a depth of 3-4 mm)

Note: It is also known as cold agglutination.

Your Notes:

146. Patient with long-standing Parkinson's disease with intractable dysphagia.

Diagnosis: Intractable dysphagia

Clinchers
➤ *Long-standing Parkinson's disease:* The patient now must be having severe impairment of mental foulties so as to compound the already existing dysphagia in Parkinsons's disease.
➤ *Intractable dysphagia:* GI symptoms in parkinsons' disease are usually:
- Heart burn
- Dysphagia
- Constipation
- Weight loss

Since malnutrition and weight loss can severely affect the quality of life of a demented elderly patient, it need some definitive management, i.e. parenteral nutrition. Any patient requiring enteral nutrition for long periods should have a gastrostomy done and feeding is done with liquid diet through PEG tube.

CONFUSA
Examine for the state of hydration also, as dehydration and malnutrition go hand-in-hand. Overhydration can mask the appearance of malnutrition, so keep this fact in mind. Usually any patient requiring enteral nutrition in excess of one day should be feeded with a nasogastric tube and in excess of two weeks should be considered for PEG tube feeding.

Investigation of choice
Endoscopy to rule out any obstruction to oesophagus.

Treatment of choice
PEG tube feeding (gastrostomy).

Your Notes:

147. Patient after a stroke, 5 days later, fluids still being aspirated from stomach.

Diagnosis: Paralytic ileus.

Clinchers
- *Fluid still being aspirated from stomach:* This mean that there is no functioning bowel obstruction due to reduced bowel motility. It can be differentiated clinically from mechanical obstruction as there is no pain and bowel sounds are absent (hyperdynamic bowel sounds in mechanical obstruction). This adynamic bowel leads to no drainage of secretions of stomach and hence fluid can be aspirated from stomach. This sign along with no passage of any flatus are the clinical hallmarks of paralytic ileus. Postsurgical paralytic ileus can improve in 24-48 hours but in post-stroke patients (as is this case) it can extend for longer periods.

CONFUSA
The main confusion is among choosing between enteral and parenteral feedings. The criteria is quite clear cut, i.e. for enteral feeding to be successful, a dynamic and functioning GIT is required. That means if there is a paralytic ileus or bowel obstruction, parenteral feeding is the only choice.

Investigation of choice
Serum electrolytes (to rule out hyperkalemia, which also causes paralytic ileus)

Immediate management
NG aspiration of stomach contents.

Treatment of choice
Correction of electrolyte balance IV
   +
Parenteral feeding.

Your Notes:

148. Man after large bowel resection and ileostomy is septicaemic.

Diagnosis: Septicaemia

Clinchers
- *Large bowel resection and ileostomy:* GI surgeries especially resections produce a hyperkalemic state which produces adynamic bowel for a few days post-operatively. Also after ileostomies, a few days rest to bowel are given to allow the ileostomy to "ripe".
- *Septicemic:* In any septicemic condition, enteral feeding is usually not given as there decreased absorption of food from GIT. This is due to decreased tissue perfusion. This produces bloating and abdominal distension.

CONFUSA
Septicemia or localised abscess formations (most common—pelvic abscess) are common after GI surgeries because of high septic load of the intestinal contents.

Investigation of choice
Blood culture.

Immediate management
Nasogastric tube to drain contents of stomach.

Treatment of choice
Intravenous parenteral nutrition.
   +
Antibiotics (broad spectrum initially, thereafter depending upon culture reports).

Your Notes:

149. Man with jaundice and ascites suddenly deteriorates.

Diagnosis: Hepatic encephalopathy.

Clinchers
- *Jaundice and ascites:* This signifies hepatic disease. Most probably it is cirrhosis of liver of which the most common cause is chronic alcoholism.
- *Suddenly deteriorates:* Sudden deterioration of the condition in the setting of chronic liver failure strongly suggests encephalopathy is failure of liver to detoxify ammonium ions into readily excretable urea, a low protein diet given prophylactically, can present it.

CONFUSA
The pathogenesis of the development of ascites in liver disease is controversial, but is probably secondary to renal sodium and water retention. Portal hypertension is also contributive as it exerts a local hydrostatic pressure and leads to increased hepatic and splanchnic production of lymph and transudation of fluid into peritoneal cavity.

Investigation of choice
Serum albumin, bilirubin urea.

Immediate management
Refer patient to specialised unit.

Treatment of choice
There is no specific treatment but only support therapy,

Note: Dexamethasone is of no value. Low protein, low salt diet should be given in this condition irrespective of the presence of encephalopathy.

Your Notes:

150. Girl with diarrhoea and jejunal villous atrophy.

Diagnosis: Coeliac disease

Clinchers
- *Girl:* It is marginally more common in females. It can present at any age. In infancy it appears after weaning on to gluten-containing foods. The peak incidence in adults is in third and fourth decades but it is shifting towards younger ages over the years.
- *Diarrhoea:* Common GI symptoms are diarrhoea and steatorrhoea, abdominal discomfort or pain and weight loss.
- *Jejunal villous atrophy:* The mucosal appearance of a jejunal biopsy specimen in diagnostic. The mucosa of the proximal small bowel is predominantly affected, the mucosal damage decreasing in severity towards the ileum as the gluten is digested into smaller non-toxic fragments.

CONFUSA
Other causes of flat mucosa (subtotal villous atrophy)
- Zollinger-Ellison syndrome
- Hypogammaglobulinaemia

Note: The lesion in coeliac disease is subtotal villous atrophy. True atrophy of the mucosa is not present because the crypt hyperplasia compensates for villous atrophy and the total mucosal thickness is normal.

Investigation of choice
- *Screening:* Anti-reticulin antibodies
- *Definitive:* Jejunal biopsy

Immediate management
Compensate for malabsorption and weight loss with gluten free diets.

Treatment of choice
Lifelong gluten-free diet.

Your Notes:

151. An elderly busy man with indigestion, acute pain lateral side of hip.

Diagnosis: Probable osteoarthritis (OA).

Clinchers
- *Elderly:* The peak incidence of OA is in 6th decade. The disease is frequently bilateral, usually with more advanced pathology or more severe symptoms on one side. It is symptomatic three times more in women.
- *Busy man:* This require immediate pain relief so that the disease does not affect his day to activities.
- *Indigestion:* This is a contraindication for NSAID use which are often used for pain relief in OA.
- *Acute pain lateral side of hip:* Pain is the predominant symptom in OA and although the disease is bilateral in manifest earlier on one side. The most common joints to involves in OA are the weight bearing joints, i.e. hip and knee joints. Pain is felt over greater trochanter (as in this case) or groin.

CONFUSA
OA management also involves use of walking aids. It is held in:
- Contralateral hand—for hip arthritis
- Ipsilateral hand—for knee arthritis

for nocturnal pain in OA, low dose tricyclics can be used.

Investigation of choice
Radiology (loss of joint space; subchondral sclerosis and cysts marginal osteophytes).

Immediate management
Local steroid injection (although it may complicate things if used for long-time).

Treatment of choice
Exercises and physiotherapy
Arthrodesis/osteotomy/arthroplasty in severe disease.

Your Notes:

152. Patient with symmetrical polyarthritis, pain does not decrease with simple analgesia.

Diagnosis: Rheumatoid arthritis.

Clinchers
- *Symmetrical:* Since RA is a systemic autoimmune disease, it ought to be symmetrical.
- *Polyarthritis:* Small bones of the hand bilaterally are involved initially in RA bringing a picture of polyarthritis.
- *Pain does not decrease with simple analgesia:* This mean that an additional drug is required to bring pain relief. NSAIDs are the first line drug in RA and control pain and stiffness (but do not reducing the underlying inflammatory relapse or the acute flare reactants in the serum).

CONFUSA
"*Simple analgesic*" in UK paracetamol (or a combination of dextropropoxyphene and paracetamol). Drugs used in RA does not qualify as simple analgesia. While starting with NSAIDs in RA, always start with a familiar drug. Methotrexate is drug of choice is USA and not much used in UK.

Investigation of choice
ESR and Hb.

Immediate management
Refer to physiotherapy unit for occupational therapy and regular exercise (counselling).

Treatment of choice
Ibuprofen 400-800 mg/8h after food.

Your Notes:

153. Patient with hot swollen metatarsal joint, pain does not decrease with paracetamol.

Diagnosis: Acute gout

Clinchers
- *Hot swollen metatarsal joint:* Involvement of this joint is almost pathognomic of gout and is known publically as *podagra*. In acute stage there is severe pain, redness and swelling in the affected joint. Attack is due to deposition of sodium monourate crystals in joints.
- *Does not decrease with paracetamol:* Usually the pain of gout is severe and does not respond to simple analgesia. NSAIDs are often required. But note that aspirin is contraindicated as it increases serum urate.

CONFUSA

Here is the UK protocol of treatment of an episode of acute gout:

NSAID (Ibuprofen, naproxen)
↓
If contraindicated (peptic ulcers, etc)
↓
Colchicine 1 mg PO, thereafter 0.5 mg/2-3 h PO
↓
If both of above drugs contraindicated (e.g. renal failure)
↓
Steroids

Investigation of choice
Synovial fluid microscopy (negatively birefingent crystals and neutrophils with ingested crystals).

Immediate management
Pain relief

Treatment of choice
NSAIDs.

Your Notes:

154. Pregnant woman with numbness, tingling on lateral side of hand.

Diagnosis: Carpal tunnel syndrome (CTS)

Clinchers
- *Pregnancy:* CTS is associated with
  - Pregnancy
  - Rheumatoid arthritis
  - DM
  - Hypothyroidism
  - Dialysis
  - Trauma
- *Numbness, tingling on lateral side of hand:* There is aching pain in the hand and arm (especially at night), and paraesthesiae in the thumb, index and middle fingers (lateral side of hand in anatomical position).

CONFUSA

The paresthesiae and pain in CTS are relieved by dangling the hand over the edge of the bed and shaking it. There may be sensory loss and weakness of abductor pollicis brevis with associated wasting of thenar eminence. Light touch, two point discrimination and sweating may be impaired.

Investigation of choice
Neurophysiology (to assess axonal degeneration and find level of brim)

Immediate management
Phalen test or tinel test can be used on screening tests but are unreliable.

Treatment of choice
Splinting ± Yoga (Namaste posture)
If the symptoms do not improve after pregnancy, the following may be used
- Local hydrocortisone injection
- Surgical decompression

Your Notes:

155. A 35-year-old woman treated one year ago for a breast cancer with 12/20 nodes positive, presents with a two day history of increasing confusion. She is drowsy and disoriented. Her husband reports that she has been complaining of severe thirst for the past week.

Diagnosis: Hypercalcaemia.

Clinchers
- *35-year-old woman treated one year ago for a breast cancer with 12/20 nodes positive:* This status suggest a high risk of recurrence as nodal status is the best indicator of metastatic disease.
- *Two day history of increasing confusion ...... severe thirst:* Signs and symptoms of hypercalcaemia of malignancy are:
  - Lethargy
  - Anorexia
  - Nausea
  - Polydipsia
  - Polyuria
  - Constipation
  - Dehydration
  - Confusion
  - Weakness.

CONFUSA
The signs and symptoms of hypercalcemia of malignancy are most obvious with serum calcium > 3 mmol/L. Diuretics should always be avoided in it. It is caused by:
- Lytic bone metastases
- Production of osteoclast activating factor by tumor
- PTH like hormones by tumor.

Investigation of choice
Serum calcium.

Immediate management
Bisphosphonate IV (if resistant: calcitonin).

Treatment of choice
Control of underlying malignancy.

Your Notes:

156. Patient with intractable hiccups.

Diagnosis: Intractable hiccups.

Clinchers
- *Intractable hiccups:* Hiccups are due to involuntary diaphragmatic contraction with closure of the glottis and are extremely common. Occasionally, patients present with persistent hiccups. This can be result of:
  - Diaphragmatic irritation (e.g. subphrenic abscess)
  - Metabolic cause (e.g. uraemia)

In palliative care hiccups are seen more commonly after chemotherapy as a side effects (mechanism metabolic).

CONFUSA
Hiccups are also a feature of vertebrobasilar circulation emboli. But it will be accompanied by more prominent focal defects. For it remember that vomiting, hiccup and excessive yawning indicate a lower brainstem lesion in a stuporose patient.

Investigation of choice
Serum electrolytes, urea and uric acid.

Immediate management
Adequate hydration if chemotherapy is the cause.

Treatment of choice
- Chlorpromazine 50 mg TDS
  +
  Diazepam 5 mg TDS
- Haloperidol if it due to metabolic causes (as in this case).

Your Notes:

157. Patient cannot cough up bronchial secretions. Noise is distressing to attendants.

Diagnosis: Bronchial rattles

Clinchers
- *Bronchial secretions:* In palliative exaggerated bronchial secretions are there in case of bronchial malignancies. It is due to increase in surface area and number of glands in bronchial epithelium. Such patients are usually debilitated and cannot cough up the secretions. Such profuse secretions require regular endotracheal suction to keep the passages clear and provide symptomatic relief to the patient. Often it produces noisy bronchial rattles which can be quite distressing to the patient and the attendant. To prevent these problems and to give symptomatic relief to the patient, anticholinergics can be given to dry up the respiratory secretions.

CONFUSA
Partial bronchial obstruction can also produce noisy breathing. But that needs palliative surgery to treat the condition, although prednisolone can provide symptomatic relief.

Investigation of choice
Chest X-ray

Immediate management
Endotracheal suction

Treatment of choice
Hyoscine hydrobromide 0.4-0.8 mg/8h Sc
or
0.3 mg sublingual.

Your Notes:

158. Patient after radiotherapy for bowel adenocarcinoma comes with bright red rectal bleeding.

Diagnosis: Radiation proctitis

Clinchers
- *Radiotherapy for bowel adenocarcinoma:* It means that pelvic irradiation was given in this patient. Radiation proctitis, which may present as a localized area of colitis, is usually found in the setting of radiation prcotitis.
- *Bright red rectal bleeding:* Whenever rectal bleeding is the presenting complaint, a colonic source should be considered. Radiation damage to rectum (proctitis) produces diarrhoea, with or without blood and tenesmus.

CONFUSA
The onset of radiation proctitis may be months to years after irradiation. Characteristic features on sigmoidoscopy include:
- Mucosal atrophy
- Telangiectasia
- Friability
- Small ulceration

GI desquamation after radiation can be differential diagnosis but its main presenting feature is a profuse non-bloody diarrhoea.

Investigation of choice
Sigmoidoscopy (proctoscopy is seldom sufficient in proctitis due to any cause).

Immediate management
Blood transfusion if anaemic and massive blood loss.

Treatment of choice
- Symptomatic
- Local steroids sometimes help (per rectal prednisolone)

Your Notes:

159. Patient with superior vena cava obstruction after radiotherapy.

Diagnosis: Superior vena cava (SVC) obstruction

Clinchers
- *SVC obstruction after radiotherapy:* It is commonly due to:
  - Lung carcinoma
  - Lymphoma

  Since for lymphoma and small cell lung carcinoma chemotherapy is generally is used, the condition must be a radiosensitive lung carcinoma, i.e. non-small cell lung cancer.

Signs and symptoms of SVC obstruction are:
- Dysphnoea
- Orthopnoea
- Facial and upper limb swelling
- Cough
- Plethora
- Cyanosis
- Headache
- Venous enlargement.

CONFUSA
Bronchoscopy should be avoided in all cases of SVC obstruction as it can be hazardous and can lead to vena caval perforation.

Investigation of choice
Venography (SVC stenting)

Immediate management
Dexamethasone 4 mg/6h PO

Treatment of choice
SVC stenting + debulking of tumor later on

Your Notes:

160. Female with fungating breast carcinoma with a bad odour.

Diagnosis: Fungating breast carcinoma

Clinchers
- *Fungating breast carcinoma:* This must be an inoperable tumor and may require palliative surgery and radiotherapy.
- *Bad odour:* Metronidazole 400 mg/8h PO mitigates unpleasant odours from tumors. Charcol dressings such as actisorb also absorb the bad odour. The etiology of bad odour in a fungating carcinoma invariably is infection by anaerobic organisms. The odour can be very distressing to the patient, attendants and health care workers.

CONFUSA
Occasionally toilet mastectomy or radiotherapy is required to control a fungating tumor, but often incision through microscopically permeated tissues makes the outcome worse than original.

Investigation of choice
None required

Immediate management
Charcoal dressing

Treatment of choice
Metronidazole (400 mg/8h PO or gel)

Your Notes:

March—2002

161. A middle-aged man with hepatosplenomegaly, fatigue, immature cells seen in blood film.

Diagnosis: Chronic myeloid leukemia (CML)

Clinchers

- *Middle-aged man:* CML occurs most often in middle-age. There is a slight male predominance.
- *Hepatosplenomegaly:* In CML there is a marked splenomegaly (produces abdominal discomfort due to enlargement). Hepatomegaly is variable.
- *Fatigue:* Unlike most other leukemias, CML present with chronic insidious and nonspecific symptoms, e.g.
  - Weight loss
  - Tiredness
  - Gout
  - Fever
  - Sweats
  - Bleeding
  - Abdominal pain
- *Immature cells:* Blood film shows raised WCC with, characteristically the whole spectrum of myeloid precursors, including a few blast cells visible on blood film.
- *Anemia:* Hb levels are either low or normal in CML.

CONFUSA

Before causing death, CML transforms into an acute leukemia which is rapidly fatal (within 6 months). But unlike de novo acute leukemia, with acute phase of CML is characterised by the development of acute leukaemia which may be myeloid (60%), lymphoid (30%) or erythroid (10%) in origin. Moreover in CML this phase is refractory to treatment.

Investigation of choice
- *Screening:* Peripheral blood smear
- *Definitive:* Bone marrow biopsy and demonstration of Ph chromosome

Immediate management
Register for allogenic transplantation if patient is less than < 55 years.

Treatment of choice
Hydroxyurea (in chronic phase).

Your Notes:

162. Man returns from Ghana presents with fever with rigors

Diagnosis: Malaria

Clinchers

- *Ghana:* Most of the African countries are endemic for malaria. Appropriate malarial prophylaxis should be given for travel to endemic countries.
- *Fever with rigors:* Typical presentation of malaria is with fever, rigors, headaches, dizziness, flu like symptoms, diarrhoea and thrombocytopenia. The rule of thumb is to suspect any patient presenting with unexplained fever and rigors with a travel history should be suspected to have malaria until proven otherwise.

CONFUSA

P.ovale has been reported predominantly from east and west Africa P.vivax is the major species in temperate zones, whereas in the topics all forms of malaria are seen. But with present day ease and speed of travel, sporadic cases of malaria are being increasingly recognised. Mosquitoes may stowaway in luggage causing malaria in non-tropical areas.

Investigation of choice
Thick and thin blood films:
- Thick film—for demonstration of parasite
- Thin film—for identification of parasite
- Two to three blood smears taken each day for three to four days and found to be negative and necessary before a patient is declared malaria free.

Immediate management
Analgesics and antipyretics are given as necessary. IV fluids may be required to combat dehydration and shock.

Treatment of choice

Species	Treatment	Resistant to
P. falciparum	Quinine + tetracycline	Chloroquine
P. vivax/ovale	Chloroquine + Primaquine	-

Note:
- If species unknown   treat as P. falciparum
  If mixed species
- if doubt over resistance—treat as resistant

163. A 60-year-old man presents with fatigue and backache with localised tenderness. He also have decreased visual acuity.

Diagnosis: Myeloma

Clinchers
- *60-year-old:* Myeloma usually occurs in older age group. The peak age is 70 years.
- *Man:* Sex ratio is equal for myeloma.
- *Fatigue:* It occurs because of anaemia, renal failure or dehydration via proximal tubule dysfunction from light chain precipitation.
- *Backache with localised tenderness:* Bone pain or tenderness is the most common presentation and is often postural, e.g. back, ribs, long bones and shoulder.
- *Decreased visual acuity:* Visual acuity is decreased in myeloma (most probably due to hyperviscosity complications). On fundoscopy hemorrhages or exudates may be seen.

CONFUSA
Bone pain or tenderness in myeloma is never found in extremities. If alkaline phosphate is raised, suspect a healing pathological fracture somewhere (most common: rib). Bone scintigrams which demonstrate lesions in many other tumors are usually normal in myeloma.

Investigation of choice
Serum/gel electrophoresis.

Immediate management
Analgesia and transfusion as needed.

Treatment of choice
Solitary lesions—radiotherapy
Multiple myeloma—chemotherapy

Your Notes:

---

164. Old lady with Hb—3g/dl, MCV—120 fl, family history presents with fatigue, lethargy.

Diagnosis: Megaloblastic anemia.

Clinchers
- *Old lady:* Incidence of pernicious anaemia (the most common cause of megaloblastic anemia: which is MCV > 110 fl) increases in old age. Female to male ratio is 1.6:1.
- *Hb 3g/dL:* Hb is usually between 3-11 g/DL in pernicious anemia.
- *MCV 120 fL:* MCV has to be greater than 110 fL to qualify as a megaloblastic type.
- *Family history:* Pernicious anemia has a higher incidence in blood group A. It is secondary to atrophic gastritis and lack of gastric intrinsic factor, both of which are probably of autoimmune origin and may have a familial preponderance.
- *Fatigue, lethargy:* Most common symptom of pernicious anemia is tiredness and weakness (seen in 90%). The second most common feature is dyspnoea (70%), sore red tongue (25%), diarrhoea and lemon tinge to skin. There may be prematurely grey hair and neuropsychiatric symptoms.

CONFUSA
A typical feature of pernicious anemia is presence of a lemon yellow tinge to skin. This colour is produced whenever there is jaundice (mild) with a coexisting pallor (anemia) in a fair skinned individual. One other condition producing this colour is mild hemolytic anemia. B_{12} deficiency anemia can be clinically differentiated from folate deficiency anemia by the absence of neurological signs in the latter.

Investigation of choice
Schilling test
Antibodies to intrinsic factor (most specific test)

Immediate management
Immediate blood transfusion as Hb is 3

Treatment of choice
Hydroxocobalamin (B_{12}) therapy

Your Notes:

March—2002

165. An elderly female with past history of rectal bleeding, normal on endoscopy and enema studies done previously presents with profuse fresh rectal bleeding.

Diagnosis: Chronic intestinal ischaemia.

Clinchers

- *Elderly female:* It frequently occurs in elderlies because of increased incidence of atherosclerotic vaso-occlusive diseases in them.
- *Past history of rectal bleeding:* It suggest that there must be some definitive predisposing factor which is giving rise to recurrent emboli and hence repeated infractions. A heart lesion (atrial fibrillation) or liver disease can be the culprits here. Other cause can be superior mesenteric artery disease.
- *Normal on endoscopy and enema studies:* Because there is no intrinsic GI pathology, there studies will always be normal.
- *Profuse fresh rectal bleeding:* It is due to ischaemic necrosis of the infarcted bowel area.

CONFUSA
Mesenteric infarction can be differentiated from other GI pains by ↑ Hb, WCC and a moderately raised plasma amylase. There will also be a persistent metabolic acidosis. In chronic disease (as in this question) there is typical postprandial pain which is relieved by passing stools.

Investigation of choice
Mesenteric angiogram (Barium enema if mesenteric infaction is suspected).

Immediate management
Rule out—vasculitis/trauma/radiotherapy/strangulation.

Treatment of choice
Surgery.

Your Notes:

166. An 85-year-old with 14 children, severe heart failure, complains of dysuria, feeling of pressure in lower abdomen.

Diagnosis: Genital prolapse

Clinchers

- *85-year-old:* Prolapse is more evident in older age (i.e. late after menopause) when there is general weakening and shrinking of the supports of the pelvic organs.
- *With 14 children:* Each labour increases the risk of prolapse. It is due to overstretching of the uterine supports during labour.
- *Severe heart failure:* This patient is unfit for operation on medical grounds. So pessary treatment is indicated here.
- *Dysuria:* Urinary symptoms in genital prolapse are:
  - *Frequency of* micturition is common and is often only at day time. Nocturnal frequency may be present if there is added cystitis
  - *Urgency* of micturition due to weakness of the bladder sphincter mechanism and urge incontinence may occur in some cases
  - *Difficulty in emptying:* The bladder completely
  - *Retention of urine* following urethral overstretch
  - *Stress incontinence.*
- *Feeling of pressure in lower abdomen:* A dragging sensation or bearing down in the back or lower abdomen is a common complaint in prolapse. Other associated complaints can be:
  - A feeling of fullness of vagina
  - A lump coming down

CONFUSA
Symptoms similar to those of prolapse may be caused by:
- Varicose veins of the vulva
- Haemorrhoids
- Rectal prolapse
- Cystitis
- Vaginitis with congestion of vulva
- Pressure form a large abdominal tumor

There are a few cases where a ring pessary fails to control prolapse and operation cannot be performed. In these cases use: *Cup and stem pessary.*

Investigation of choice
- Colposcopy
- Urine microscopy and culture if UTI is also suspected

Immediate management
Reassurance that the condition is treatable

Treatment of choice: Plastic ring pessary.

167. Female with well-controlled diabetes mellitus type 2 with recurrent urinary tract infection (UTI).

Diagnosis: Chlamydial UTI

Clinchers
- *Well-controlled diabetes:* Infections in persons with diabetes may not occur more frequently than in non-diabetics but they tend to be more severe, possibly because of impaired leucocyte function, a frequent accompaniment of poor control. But since this case has a well-controlled diabetes, this is also ruled out. Most probably this is a case of recurrent UTI with no identifiable source.
- *Recurrent UTI:* Females have a higher incidence of UTI because of a short urethra which is prone to entry of bacteria during intercourse poor perineal hygiene and the occasional inefficient voiding ability (due to diabetic neuropathy).

CONFUSA
In women with recurrent acute urinary symptoms, pyuria and urine that is sterile (even when obtained by suprapubic aspiration), sexually transmitted urethritis—producing agents such as *Chlamydia trachomatis*, *Neisseria gonorrhoeae*, and herpes simplex virus are etiologically important.

Investigation of choice
- *Screening:* MSU—nitrate stick test
- *Definitive:* MSU—culture (pure growth of more than 10^5 organisms per ml urine).

Immediate management
Rule out diabetic neuropathy (i.e. bladder involvement) and pyelonephritis).

Treatment of choice
Recurrent UTI for which an identifiable source has not been found may be managed by long-term low dose antimicrobial therapy, such as trimethoprim. Ciprofloxacin or norfloxacin can be alternatives.

Your Notes:

---

168. A young female with long-standing irregular bowel habit and persistent UTI.

Diagnosis: Probable Crohn's disease (CD)

Clinchers
- *Young female:* CD has peak incidence at between 20 and 40 years. It is uncommon before the age of 10 years and both sexes are equally affected.
- *Long-standing irregular bowel habit:* The major symptom of inflammatory bowel disease (including CD) is irregular bowel habit. Mainly it presents as diarrhoea, abdominal pain and weight loss.
- *Persistent UTI:* Fistula formation is common in CD and it may atypically present with symptoms of fistula rather than those of bowel. Although uncommon a persistent UTI in the setting of CD, should be suspected to be due to enterovesical fistula.

CONFUSA
Pneumaturia (air in the urine) present as bubbling while micturition and is a definitive symptom of enterovesicle fistula. Other causes of enterovescile fistula can be malignancy and regional enteritis (chronic). Irritable bowel disease can also cause UTI (due to impaired local hygiene) but that will be recurrent rather than persistent.

Investigation of choice
Small bowel barium enema

Immediate management
High dose urinary antibacterials

Treatment of choice
Surgical closure of fistula

Your Notes:

169. An 80-year-old sexually active woman with dyspareunia and recurrent dysuria.

Diagnosis: Atrophic vaginitis

Clinchers
- *80-year-old:* This condition is always seen postmenopausally because of lack of oestrogens.
- *Sexually active women:* Because of vaginal wall dryness and thinning, there can be discomfort during intercourse. If the woman would not have been sexually active, atrophic vaginitis, if mild, would have been asymptomatic.
- *Dyspareunia:* There is *superficial* dyspareunia in this condition.
- *Recurrent dysuria:* Low grade infection can coexist with atrophic vaginitis.

CONFUSA
Hormone replacement therapy postmenopausally produces withdrawal bleeds. Topical estorgens are enough to thicken the epithelium and reduce the pH, but insufficient to produce excessive endometrial stimulation or other causes of bleeding.

Investigation of choice
Urine culture and sensitivity

Immediate management
Advice topical lubrication during coitus.

Treatment of choice
- If there is secondary infection, antibiotics to which the organism is sensitive may be given
- Topical oestrogen creams or pessaries (e.g. dienoestrol or premarin (once or twice a week)

Your Notes:

170. A middle-aged woman with a vaginal discharge is found to have several ulcers at the vaginal introitus.

Diagnosis: Herpes labialis

Clinchers
- *Middle-aged woman:* Herpes labialis is most common in sexually active females, so its incidence is characteristically minimal in children and elderly.
- *Vaginal discharge:* Pain, itching, dysuria, vaginal and urethral discharge, and tender inguinal lymphadenopathy are the predominant local symptoms.
- *Several ulcers of the vaginal introitus:* Widely spaced bilateral lesions of the external genitalia are characteristic. In it painful vesicles develop initially which then coalesce into multiple ulcers.

CONFUSA
First episodes of genital herpes in patients who have had prior HSV-1 infection are associated with less frequent systemic symptoms and faster healing than primary genital herpes. In primary herpes, if the case is seen very early it may only affect a small part of the vulva appearing to be a recurrent episode. It is sensible therefore to routinely prescribe a course of antiviral medication for five days for all patients presenting with first attack, even if the clinical suspicion is of a secondary episode.

Investigation of choice
Culture/electron microscopy.

Immediate management
Rule out any past history of genital herpes.

Treatment of choice
Aciclovir 200 mg, 5 times a day for five days
+ Analgesics
+ bathing in salt water
+ lignocaine gel.

Your Notes:

171. Female with bilateral varicose veins, lipodermato-sclerosis. She is using compression stockings. Despite that increase in itching and eczema. BMI is 27.

Diagnosis: Bilaterally symptomatic varicose veins

Clinchers
- *Females:* Females are most frequently affected than man. Inheritance is also a major factor. Women in whom neither parent has varicose veins have a 10 percent risk of developing varices, but when both parents are affected there is an 80 percent chance.
- *Bilateral varicose veins:* Bilaterality of the condition rules out any local cause or obstruction producing them in one limb.
- *Using compression stockings:* Graded compression stockings are indicated for minor varicosities and is the first line of management. They may also be indicated in:
  - Elderly
  - Pregnant
  - Unfit people for surgery.

  The stocking is elasticated and specially fitted to ensure that it delivers gradual compression along its length such that at the ankle the elastic compression of the leg is much higher than that at the thigh.
- *Increased itching and eczema:* A proportion of patients develops skin complications. These range from mild eczema to severe ulceration. Since the condition is occurring in this female, despite using graded compression stockings, it implies failure of first line of management and that the disease is progressive. Surgery is definitely indicated now as the patient is symptomatic and this eczema may lead to severe venous ulceration.
- *BMI is 27:* She is mildly overweight. Varicose veins usually benefit by losing weight in the initial stages (more difficult to improve now in this patient). Although, still help the patient in losing weight as it may be beneficial in preventing recurrence after treatment. Also a normal weight reduces risk of other disease.

CONFUSA
Sclerotherapy will not be used in this patient because it is mainly indicated for:
- Cosmetic reasons (acid not symptomatic)
- Small and moderate sized varices below the knee
- It may complicate the already existing eczema.

Investigation of choice
Venography or Duplex scanning

Immediate management
Loose weight

Treatment of choice
- For cosmetic reasons—sclerotherapy
- For symptomatic condition—surgery (as is this case)

Note: Varicose vein surgery is one of the most commonly performed elective surgical procedures in UK.

Your Notes:

172. 75-year-old, underwent 2 operations for varicose veins, presents with painful legs, has history of heart failure. On examination bilateral gross varicose veins, lipodermatosclerosis, no ulcers.

Diagnosis: Complicated varicose veins.

Clinchers
- *75-year-old:* Incidence of varicose vein increases with age, as accumulation of environmental factors also contribute to its pathogenesis.
- *Underwent 2 operations for varicose veins:* This means the condition is recurrent and another operation will be useless.
- *History of heart failure:* A relative contraindication for surgery now.
- *Lipodermatosclerosis:* It is a late and serious complication in which palpable indication develops in the skin and subcutaneous tissues. This particularly affects the gaiter area of the leg, just above the malleoli, and may be precursor for leg ulceration. Contraction of the skin and subcutaneous tissues is seen and the ankle becomes narrower (*champagne bottle leg*).
- *No ulcers:* This rules out a relative contraindication for sclerotherapy. Hence it can be safely given.

CONFUSA
The basis of sclerotherapy is that a solution which destroys the endothelial lining of the veins is injected. In the UK the most widely employed drug is sodium tetradecyl (STD), which chemically is a soap. To be effective the sclerosant has to be given into an empty vein that is compressed immediately after the injection has been given to avoid the development of thrombosis with vein. Sclerotherapy is treatment of choice for recurrent varicose veins because:
- The vein sclerose to form a fibrous cord incapable of recanalisation and recurrence
- Remove the risk and damage produce by repeated operations
- Easily manageable as an OPD treatment.

Investigation of choice
Venography/Duplex scanning

Immediate management
Gradual compression stockings (not if ulcers are present)

Treatment of choice
Injection sclerotherapy.

173. Female with BMI 33, comes with complaints of varicose veins and eczema.

Diagnosis: Varicose veins due to obesity.

Clinchers
- *Female:* Varicose veins are twice as common in females as in males.
- *BMI 33:* She is grossly overweight. She should loose weight and aim for a BMI of 20-25. Obesity is a definitive risk factor. Other risk factors are:
  - Family history
  - Prolonged standing
  - Female sex
- *Bilateral:* Thus rules out any local pathology in one leg leading to this condition.
- *Eczema:* This is the first stage of development of complication. She may not require invasive treatment later on if she act now to lose weight.

CONFUSA
Pregnancy per se is not a risk factor. It only accentuates an existing condition and may bring to notice the insignificant varicosities. It is partly as a result of enlarged uterus or the iliac veins and partly due to relaxation of smooth muscle under the influence of hormones such as progesterone.

Investigation of choice
Doppler USG/venography

Immediate management
Counselling to loose weight

Treatment of choice
Aim for BMI of 20-25 by loosing weight.

Your Notes:

174. Man with varicose veins has to fly for 20 hours. His father has a history of pulmonary embolism after flying.

Diagnosis: High-risk case for pulmonary embolism.

Clinchers
- *Varicose veins:* Thrombosis is a common complication for varicose veins and is referred to as superficial thrombophlebitis. Usually this remain in the superficial veins and only cause considerable discomfort. Sometimes thrombosis extends into the deep venous system to cause deep vein thrombosis (DVT) although this in infrequent. DVT is the most common risk factor for pulmonary embolism (PE).
- *Fly for 20 hours:* Prolonged sitting as in a long flight increases the risk for DVT considerably in a predisposed.
- *Father has a history of PE after flying:* This increases the risk of family history is also positive.

CONFUSA
Since in this case three definite risk factors for PE are present, this person need to take precautions. He should be prescribed graded compression stocking for the period of immobility and should be given a proper advice on how to keep himself mobile during flight.

Investigation of choice
Patients with a family history of thromboembolism should be investigated for thrombophilia.

Immediate management
Counselling

Treatment of choice
Graded compression stockings.

Note: Prophylactic anticoagulation is only indicated if the patient himself had any past history of PE or DVT.

Your Notes:

---

175. A patient presents with a shallow ulcer, with no in rolled edges, situated over the medical malleolus. It has been reducing in size with compression bandaging. There is some evidence of lipodermatosclerosis and varicose veins in the distribution of the greater saphenous veins.

Diagnosis: Venous ulcer

Clinchers
- *Shallow ulcer:* Venous ulcers are always shallow and superficial.
- *No in rolled edges:* Rules out basal cell carcinoma which has rolled out edges.
- *Situation over the medical malleolus:* Venous ulcers are typically found in gaiter area of the leg, especially around the medial malleolus.
- *Reducing in size with compression bandaging:* It is due to improving deep venous competence due to compression bandaging. Note that compression bandaging is absolutely contraindication in arterial ulcers as it will worsen the condition. So preferably avoid them in all ulcers.
- *Lipodermatosclerosis:* It is a late complication of varicose veins and signify that the disease is long-standing.
- *Varicose veins in the distribution of greater saphenous vein:* This explains the anatomical location of ulcer over the medial malleolus.

CONFUSA
- *Venous ulcers*—painless, shallow, over medial malleolus (i.e. gaiter area of leg)
- *Arterial ulcers*—painless, deep and punched out, over dorsum of foot and toes.

Investigation of choice
Venography or Duplex scan

Immediate management
Calculate BMI

Treatment of choice
Sclerotherapy
(surgery is reversed for more symptomatic conditions).

Your Notes:

176. Man returned from trip to Asia, complains of anorexia, malaise, dark urine, pale stools.

Diagnosis: Hepatitis B (most probably)

Clinchers
- *Trip to Asia:* Hepatitis A is the most common type of viral hepatitis worldwide, often in epidemics. The disease is commonly seen in autumn and affects children and young adults. Spread of infection is mainly by the faecal-oral route and arises from the ingestion of contaminated food or water (e.g. shellfish). Overcrowding and poor sanitation facilitate spread. It is common in developing countries in Asia.
- *Anorexia malaise:* The viraemia causes the patient to feel unwell with nonspecific symptoms that includes nausea, anorexia and a distaste for cigarettes. Jaundice develops after one or two weeks.
  Note: Many recover at this stage and remain anicetric.
- *Dark urine, pale stools:* As the jaundice deepens, the urine becomes dark and stools pale owing to intrahepatic cholelithiasis.

CONFUSA
Clinically the differential diagnosis is from all other causes of jaundice—but in particular from other types of viral and drug induced hepatitis. Common cause of jaundice in travellers are:
- Viral hepatitis
- Cholangitis
- Liver abscess
- Leptospirosis
- Typhoid
- Malaria
- Dengue fever
- Yellow fever
- Haemoglobinopathies

Investigation of choice
Viral serology and LFT
- Serum transaminases rise 22-40 days after exposure
- IgM rises from day 25 and signifies recent infection
- IgG remains detectable for life.

Immediate management
Symptomatic and advise to avoid alcohol
Notify health authorities as it is a notifiable disease in UK

Treatment of choice
Supportive
If fulminant hepatitis—interferon α

177. An 80-year-old man has never been out of UK, one month history of epigastric pain, dark urine, pale stools, jaundice.

Diagnosis: Common bile duct obstruction (CBD obstruction).

Clinchers
- *80-year-old man:* The age point more towards malignancy than a stone as the cause of obstruction of CBD.
- *Never been out of UK:* Rules out infective causes like cholangitis or hepatitis.
- *One month history:* It signify that the symptomatology is chronic and rules out infective causes and acute cholecystitis.
- *Epigastric pain:* Gallbladder pathologies produce continuous picture of any obstructive jaundice. Dark urine is due to bilirubinuria and pale stools due to decreased bile pigments.

CONFUSA
A young person is more likely to have hepatitis, so questions should be asked about drug and alcohol se, and sexual behaviour. An elderly person with gross weight loss is more likely to have a carcinoma. All patients may complain of malaise. Abdominal pain occurs in patients with biliary obstruction by gallstones and sometimes with an enlarged liver there is pain resulting from distension of the capsule.

Investigation of choice
ERCP

Immediate management
Heme test of stools (if positive, suspect malignancy)

Treatment of choice
Depends on diagnosis
- Stones—cholecystectomy
- Malignancy—surgery/palliation

Your Notes:

178. Female with fever, rigors, right upper quadrant pain, jaundice, USG is normal.

Diagnosis: Acute cholecystitis.

Clinchers
- *Female:* Female sex is a risk factor for cholesterol stones in gallbladder, which is the usual cause for acute cholecystitis. The disease can occur at any age.
- *Fever, rigors:* The patient is usually ill with a fever and shallow respirations.
- *Right upper quadrant (RUQ) pain:* The main symptoms are severe pain in the epigastrium and right hypochondrium. The pain is continuous, increasing in intensity over 24 hours. It can radiate to back and shoulder. It may be accompanied by nausea and vomiting. Right hypochondrium tenderness is present, being worse on inspiration (Murphy's sign). There is guarding and rebound tenderness.
- *Jaundice:* Mild jaundice occurs in 20% of cases owing to accompanying common duct stones or to surrounding oedema occluding the CBD.
- *USG is normal:* Although can accurately diagnose stones as small as 2 mm, it may be false negative in 2-4 percent of cases.

CONFUSA
A less severe case of acute pancreatitis simulates acute cholecystitis. The fever in acute cholecystitis is more marked than pancreatitis and is in range of 38-39° C with marked toxaemia and leucocytosis. Rigors are almost nerve seen in acute pancreatitis.

Investigation of choice
Oral cholecystography (OCG)
OCG is a useful procedure for diagnosis of gallstones but has been diagnosis replaced by USG. However, OCG is still useful for
- Selection of patients for nonsurgical therapy of gallstone disease such as
  - Lithotripsy
  - Bile duct dissolution therapy
- When USG is inconclusive

Immediate management
Nil by mouth + analgesia

Treatment of choice
Cefuroxime 1.5 g/8 h IV
In suitable candidates do cholecystectomy (laparoscopic if no question of GB perforation).

179. Female 50-year-old, 5 years history of mild pruritus history of pale stools, dark urine, jaundice.

Diagnosis: Primary biliary cirrhosis (PBC).

Clinchers
- *50-year-old female:* Ninety percent of those affected are women in the age range 40-50 years. It used to be rare but now being diagnosed more frequently in its milder forms.
- *5 years history of mild pruritus:* Pruritus is often the earliest symptom, preceding jaundice by a few years.
- *Pale stools, dark urine, jaundice:* This is a characteristic picture of obstructive jaundice. It signifies a late stage of PBC—the patient is jaundiced with severe pruritus. Pigmented xanthelasma on eyelids or other deposits of cholesterol in the creases of the hands may be seen. Hepatosplenomegaly may be present.

CONFUSA
PBC is usually associated with:
- Autoimmune disorders
  - Sjögren's syndrome
  - Scleroderma
  - Rheumatoid arthritis
- Keratoconjunctivitis sicca (dry eyes and mouth) is seen in 70% of cases
- Renal tubular acidosis
- Membranous glomerulonephritis

Mitochondrial antibodies (measured routinely by ELISA—in titres more than 1:160) are present in over 95% of patients. M2 antibody is specific. Other nonspecific antibodies (e.g. ANA and SMA) may also be present.

Investigation of choice
- *Screening:* ELSIA for mitochondrial antibodies
- *Definitive:* Liver biopsy

Immediate management
USG (in a jaundiced patient, extrahepatic biliary obstruction should be excluded)

Treatment of choice
Symptomatic:
- Pruritus: colestyramine
- Diarrhoea: codeine phosphate
- Malabsorption: prophylactic fat soluble vitamin supplements
  - In case serum bilirubin > 100 µmol/L—consider liver transplantation.

180. Man with history of hemochromatosis and alcohol addiction presents with jaundice, ascites, variceal bleed. USG is unequivocal, high ferritin level.

Diagnosis: Hereditary haemochromatosis (HHC)

Clinchers
- *Mass:* Middle-aged males are more frequently and severely affected than women.
- *Haemochromatosis:* HHC is one of the most common inherited (autosomal recessive) single gene disorders in northern Europeans.
- *Alcohol addiction:* The course of the disease depends on a number of factors including sex, dietary iron intake, presence of associated hepatoxins (especially alcohol) and genotype.
- *USG unequivocal:* USG will not demonstrate anything significant. A liver biopsy is definitive (with Perl's stain).
- *High ferritin level:* Serum ferritin is elevated, usually >500µg/L or 240 nmol/L.

CONFUSA
Haemochromatosis tend to present about 10 years later in females than males on the menstrual blood loss is protective. So while in males, its peak incidence is in middle-ages, in case of females it is usually postmenopausal. Iron overload may be present in alcoholics, but alcohol excess per se does not cause HHC. There is a history of excess alcohol intake in 25% of patients.

Investigation of choice
- *Screening:*
  - Homozygotes
    - Serum iron (↑↑)
    - Serum ferritin (↑↑)
  - Heterozygotes
    - Serum ferritin (↑)
    - Transferrin saturation (↑)
- *Definitive*
  - Liver biopsy/MRI

Immediate management
Manage cirrhotic symptoms

Treatment of choice
Venesection routinely
If venesection not tolerated, chelation therapy.

181. Man after trip to Asia presents with red, swollen scrotum.

Diagnosis: Epididymo-orchitis

Clinchers
- *Trip to Asia:* He might have caught gonococcal infection from sex workers in Thailand. Or it could be TB also but that needs a primary infection somewhere else.
  Chlamydia can also cause epididymo orchitis in < 35 years old.
- *Red, swollen scrotum:* The patient will have a very painful swelling of the epididymis, often with a secondary hydrocele and constitutional effects (pyrexia, headaches and leucocytosis). There may be a history of dysuri suggesting a UTI, or urethral discharge suggesting a sexually transmitted organism.

CONFUSA
Examination of urine may reveal the presence of organisms and pus cells, but the urine need not be abnormal. Rectal examination of the prostate may reveal coexistent prostatitis. Always look for urethral discharge in a patient of epididymo-orchitis. A 'first-catch' is more likely to show abnormalities than MSU.

Investigation of choice
Urethral swab for culture

Immediate management
Rule out torsion of testis which usually present like epididymo-orchitis
- It the patient is in his teens, torsion is more likely; if he is in his twenties and sexually active, epidymitis is more likely.
- In torsion the testes like high in scrotum and pain is a bit relieved by lifting testes (worsens in epididymo-orchitis).

Treatment of choice
Erythromycin for chlamydia
For others—ciprofloxacin.

Your Notes:

182. Man with painful red scrotum and vomiting.

Diagnosis: Torsion of testis.

Clinchers
- *Painful red scrotum:* The differential diagnoses are:
  - Mumps orchitis
  - Epididymo-orchitis
  - Torsion of testes
  - Torsion of testicular appendage
- *Vomiting:* Of all the above conditions, only torsion produces a pain severe enough to produce vomiting. There may be associated abdominal pain also which is because the nerve supply of the testis is mainly from T_{10} sympathetic pathway.

CONFUSA
Torsion of the testis can also present as a pain in lower abdomen (can mimic appendicitis if on right side) torsion of appendicular appendage can present in similar way but on examination the testis does not lie high in scrotum and a dark blue pea like swelling may be visible through the scrotal skin. Torsion may also mimic a strangulated inguinal hernia.

Investigation of choice
The diagnosis is entirely clinical. The only investigation is to see whether the testis is still viable or not and that is possible only on surgical exploration (usually viability maintained till 6 hours).

Immediate management
Inform surgeons.

Treatment of choice
Urgent surgical exploration.

Your Notes:

183. Man with painless testicular swelling since 2 months.

Diagnosis: Suspected testicular tumor.

Clinchers
- *Painless testicular swelling:* Tumors of the testes usually present as a painless, swollen testicle or lump on a testicle which is hard and may be associated with an overlying secondary hydrocele, which sometimes contains blood stained fluid.
- *Since two months:* Tumors usually become noticeably in a considerable time and one to two months after appearance are taken by the patient to realise that it is abnormal. Age of the man is not specified in this question otherwise a clinical differentiation between suspected seminoma (30-40 years) and teratoma (20-30 years) might have been possible.

CONFUSA
Tumors of testes may present with a misleading history of recent trauma, and rarely it may present having undergone torsion. Occasionally gynaecomastia may be a presenting feature, due to production of paraneoplastic hormones.

Investigation of choice
Scrotal USG may reveal a solid tumor in a hydrocele but a negative finding can not exclude malignancy. Also
- Seminomas—β hCG
- Teratomas—AFP

Immediate management
Staging is essential. Conduct all necessary investigations. (CXR, CT and excision biopsy).

Treatment of choice
Orchidectomy.

Your Notes:

March—2002

184. Man with a swelling of scrotum since 3 years.

Diagnosis: Sebaceous cyst (most probably)

Clinchers
- *Swelling of scrotum:* Since the question is not about testicular swelling but only a scrotal swelling, we are left with a handful of diagnosis, i.e.
  - *Filarial elephantiasis of the scrotum:* It is due to obstruction of pelvic lymphatics by *Wuchereria bancrofti*. But it is rarely seen in UK and is associated with penile swelling also. So it can be safely excluded as a diagnosis.
  - *Sebaceous cysts:* These are common in scrotal area. Although they are often multiple, a solitary scrotal sebaceous cyst is not an infrequent finding.

CONFUSA
A sebaceous cyst can remain as it is (i.e. with no increase in size) for many years. In scrotal area, they are often small (unlike-skull) and thus do not produce any problem to the patient (except cosmetic). They are painful only when they are infected.

Investigation of choice
The diagnosis of a sebaceous cyst is entirely clinical.

Immediate management
None

Treatment of choice
Complete excision along with cyst wall if:
- Patient ask for it
- Cosmetic reasons
- Infected
- Producing discomfort.

Your Notes:

185. Man with no history of unsafe sex presents with dysuria and urinary frequency.

Diagnosis: Urinary tract infection (UTI)

Clinchers
- *History of unsafe sex:* It is the main risk factor for acquisition of UTI in sexually active population. Exposure to commercial sex workers increases the risk much more.
- *Dysuria:* It is a feature of cystitis. Other features of cystitis are:
  - Frequency
  - Urgency
  - Strangury
  - Haematuria
  - Suprapubic pain
- *Urinary frequency:* Also a feature of cystitis in UTI.

CONFUSA
The most common organism causing UTI is *E. coli*. (>70% in community but $\leq$ 41% in hospital). Among sexually transmitted diseases (like this one) *Chlamydia* is the main culprit (in < 35 years).

Investigation of choice
MSU—send it for lab culture if urine dipsticks show leucocytes, nitrite, proteinuria or haematuria.

Immediate management
Take a detailed history.
If this is not the first UTI of his life, try to differentiate between:
- Recurrent UTI: further infection with new organisms
- Relapse of UTI: further infection with same organisms

Treatment of choice
Trimethoprim 200 mg/12 h PO × 3 days is the DOC for cystitis.
Alternative: cephalexin.

Your Notes:

186. Condition that can cause necrosis, formation of fluid-filled spaces that can get infected.

Diagnosis: Acute pancreatitis.

Clinchers
- *Necrosis formation of fluid filled space that can get infected:* Acute pancreatitis is an unpredictable disease which if not treated early can become severe and fatal. Due to self-perpetuating pancreatic inflammation (and of other retroperitoneal tissues). Litres of extracellular fluid are trapped in the gut, peritoneum and retroperitoneum. There may be a rapid progress from a phase of mild oedema to one of necrotising pancreatitis. In fulminating cases the pancreas is replaced by black fluid. Death may be from shock, renal failure, sepsis, or respiratory failure, with contributory factors being protease-induced activation of complement, kinin, and the fibrinolytic and coagulation cascades.

CONFUSA
Acute pancreatitis may present as a hypovolemic shock which may confuse a fresh SHO as there is no evident source of bleed or blood loss. Also the serum amylase levels should be more than 1000 IU/mL as many other disease processes may produce mild rise in it.

Investigation of choice
Serum amylase (> 1000 IU/ml)

Immediate management
Plasma expanders (Haemaccel) and 0.9% saline until vital signs are satisfactory and urine flow at > 30 mL/h.

Treatment of choice
Laparotomy ± debridement on suspect abscess formation or pancreas necrosis.

Your Notes:

---

187. Condition associated with gatroesophageal reflux, epithelial metaplasia, increased risk of carcinoma.

Diagnosis: Barret's oesophagus.

Clinchers
- *Gastroendophageal reflux:* The predisposing condition to Barret's is chronic reflux oesophagitis.
- *Epithelial metaplasia:* Squamous mucosa of the oesophagus shows metaplastic change and the squamocolumnar junction (ora serrata) migrates upwards in response to chronic reflux oesophagitis. The length affected may be a few can only or all of the oesophagitis.
- *Increased risk of carcinoma:* It carries a 40 fold increase in risk of adenocarcinoma.

CONFUSA
The most common carcinoma in the middle third of oesophagus is squamous cell carcinoma, whereas in the lower third it is adenocarcinoma.

Investigation of choice
Endoscopy

Immediate management
Exclude malignant change by biopsy.

Treatment of choice
- *If premalignant changes are found:* Oesophageal resection (especially in younger, fit patients)
- *If no premalignant changes:* Regular endoscopy
  +
  Intensive antireflux measures
  ±
  Epithelial laser ablation/photodynamic therapy.

Your Notes:

March—2002

188. Condition associated with epigastric pain radiating to the back, pale loose stools, associated with alcohol consumption.

Diagnosis: Chronic pancreatitis.

Clinchers

➤ *Epigastric pain radiating to the back:* In chronic pancreatitis the epigastric pain 'bores' through to the back. It is relieved by:
  - Sitting forward
  - Hot water bottles on epigastrium/back: look for *erythema ab ignes* dusky greyness here.

➤ *Pale loose stools:* These signify steatorrhoea a common finding in this condition. It is due to pancreatic insufficiency and also results in malabsorption (hence bloating) and weight loss.

➤ *Alcohol consumption:* Chronic alcohol intake is the most common cause of chronic pancreatitis. Although rarely it can be produced by:
  - Cystic fibrosis
  - Haemochromatosis
  - Pancreatic duct obstruction
      - Stones
      - Pancreatic cancer
  - Hyperparathyroidism
  - Familial.

CONFUSA
Serum amylase estimations performed during attacks of pain may be elevated, but in long-standing disease are often normal, there being insufficient pancreatic tissue remaining to cause a large rise. The differential diagnosis of chronic pancreatitis from a pancreatic carcinoma is usually possible only at laparotomy.

Investigation of choice
USG (dilated biliary tree; stones)
Note: If USG is normal consider CT or ERCP

Immediate management
Blood glucose (as chronic pancreatitis can produce diabetes)

Treatment of choice
Stop alcohol
  +
Analgesia
  +
Low fat diet with pancreatic enzyme (pancreatin) by mouth
Pancreatico-jejunostomy/total pancreatectomy for refractive cases.

189. Condition associated with persistent inflammation, can cause lymphoma.

Diagnosis: *Helicobacter pylori* infection.

Clinchers

➤ *Persistent inflammation:* Initially, H. pylori infection produces acute gastritis which rapidly becomes chronic active gastritis and in some peptic ulcer disease may develop. Some strains or H. pylori (Cag A positive strains) may be particular associated with gastroduodenal disease *H. pylori* causes tissue damage by releasing toxins—Vac A (vacuolating toxin) and Cag A (cytotoxin associated protein).

➤ *Can cause lymphoma:* Over 90% of patients with gastric B cell lymphomas (mucosal associated lymphoid tissue—MALT lymphoma) have *H. pylori*. Low grade tumors have been shown to regress with *H. pylori* eradication.

CONFUSA
The exact mode of transmission is unlcear, but intrafamilial clustering suggests person to person spread, either oral-oral or faeco-oral. Childhood acquisition of *H. pylori* is prevalent in developing countries and its presence is also associated with lower socioeconomic status worldwide. Between one-third and two-third of the western populations have this infection and prevalence is higher in older population—presumably acquired in their childhood.

Investigation of choice
- *Screening:* Urea breath test ^{13}C or ^{14}C (using urea as substrate)
- *Definitive:* Serological IgG antibody tests

Treatment of choice
Triple therapy (for one week)
Omeprazole + metronidazole + clarithromycin
or
Omeprazole + metronidazole + amoxycillin.

Your Notes:

190. Condition associated with megaloblastic anemia, increased risk of carcinoma.

Diagnosis: Pernicious anemia

Clinchers
- *Megaloblastic anemia:* Megaloblastic anemia is caused by:
  - Vit B_{12} or folate deficiency
  - Hydroxyurea (hydroxycarbamide)

  In B_{12} deficiency, synthesis of thymidine, and hence DNA, is impaired and consequently red cell production is reduced.
- *Increased risk of carcinoma:* Since pernicious anemia is due to malabsorption of B_{12} resulting from atrophic gastritis and lack of gastric intrinsic factor secretion, risk of carcinoma stomach increases manifold. So one should have a low threshold for endoscopy while investigating it. Since it is an autoimmune disease, risk of other autoimmune diseases also increases. Some of such classical associations are:
  - Thyroid disease
  - Vitiligo
  - Addison's disease

CONFUSA
Note that pernicious anemia is manifestation of a disease which affects all cells of the body. Note that megaloblasts are macrocytes with MCV > 110 fL, so many conditions can lead to macrocytic anemia (MCV > 96 fL), only a couple of them lead to megaloblastic anemia (enumerated above). Also beware of diagnosing pernicious anemia in those below 40 years (malabsorption more common).

Investigation of choice
- *Screening:* Peripheral blood film
- *Definitive:* Antibodies to intrinsic factor

Immediate management
Rule out thyroid disease (present in 25% cases of pernicious anemia).

Treatment of choice
- *Initial:* Hydroxocobalamin (B_{12}) 1 mg IM alternate days for weeks (or, if CNS signs, until improvement occurs)
- *Maintenance:* Hydroxocobalamin 1 mg IM every 2 month for life

191. Female, 41-year-old, presents with hard, irregular fixed swelling, stridor, dysphagia since 3 months.

Diagnosis: Anaplastic carcinoma thyroid

Clinchers
- *Female:* ♀ : ♂ ≈ 3:1
- *41-year-old:* Its risk and incidence increases with age and mainly occurs in elderly women.
- *Hard, irregular fixed swelling:* It is a typical presentation from anaplastic carcinoma. It needs to be differentiated from sarcoma or lymphoma. Multinodular goitre can also present like this.
  Note: Anaplastic carcinoma tissues do not concentrate iodine.
- *Stridor:* Due to tracheal compression by the rapid internal growth of the tumor. It may also invade the trachea.
- *Dysphagia:* Due to oesophageal compression due to mass effect of the tumor.
- *Since 3 months:* Anaplastic carcinomas are very fast growing and highly malignant.

CONFUSA
Usually the more malignant tumors of thyroid occur in younger age and tumors occurring in elderly patients are usually benign. But anaplastic carcinoma is an exception to this state of affairs as it occurs more in the elderly and is highly malignant (both locally and hematogeneously). Always make it a point to rule out thyroid lymphoma and sarcoma because their presentation is very similar.

Investigation of choice
Biopsy.

Immediate management
Tracheostomy for stridor (if it worsens).

Treatment of choice
- Radical thyroidectomy
- Inoperable tumors
  palliative radiotherapy.

Your Notes:

March—2002

192. Old lady with smooth neck swelling, bradycardia, spare coarse hair, macrocytic anemia.

Diagnosis: Hashimoto's thyroiditis.

Clinchers
- *Old lady:* It usually occurs in women aged 60-70 years.
- *Smooth neck swelling:* The gland is usually uniformly enlarged and firm, although it may occasionally be a symmetrical and irregular.
- *Bradycardia:* It is due to hypothyroidism which may be a feature of Hashimoto's thyroiditis (although the patient is mostly euthyroid).
- *Sparse coarse hair:* The patients of hypothyroidism have a slow, deep voice and are usually overweight and apathetic, with a dry, coarse skin and thin hair, especially in the lateral third of the eyebrows.
- *Macrocytic anemia:* Hypothyroid patients often have normochromic macrocytic anemia.

CONFUSA
It is important to diagnose the condition correctly by demonstrating the presence of thyroid antibodies and if necessary, by biopsy, because thyroidectomy will precipitate severe hypothyroidism in these cases. Occasionally lymphoma occurs in such glands. Note that in
- Graves' disease—TSH autoantibody ↑
- Hashimoto's thyroiditis—thyroglobulin autoantibody increased

Investigation of choice
Autoantibody titres (thyroglobulin)

Immediate management
Exclude lymphoma in thyroid and other autoimmune diseases.

Treatment of choice
T_4 replacement therapy upto 0.3 mg/day will shrink the gland and the symptoms of myxoedema should disappear.

Your Notes:

193. Female on treatment for supraventricular tachycardia complains of seeing dots and glare on driving at night, exophthalmos, no goitre.

Diagnosis: Drug induced thyrotoxicosis.

Clinchers
- *Female:* Thyroid disorders are overall more prevalent in females, however drug induced thyrotoxicosis have an equal incidence in both sexes:
- *On treatment for SVT:* Given her existing clinical profile, she must be on treatment with amiodarone. Amiodarone is used in a wide range of ventricular and supraventricular arrhythmias. However, because of its toxic potential, its use is limited to resistant VT and recurrent VF. It is also used to maintain sinus rhythm in AF when other drugs here failed. Rapid termination of ventricular and supraventricular arrhythmias can be obtained by IV injection. WPW tachyarrhythmia is obtained can be obtained by suppression of both normal and aberrant pathways. Its long duration of action make it suitable for long-term prophylactic use; but close monitoring is required.
- *Complains of seeing dots and glare on driving at night:* This is due to corneal oedema occurring due to inflammatory reaction in thyrotoxicosis. Otherwise also it can be due to corneal microdeposits occurring due to long-term use of amiodarone.
- *Exophthalmos, no goitre:* Absence of goitre excludes a primary thyroid abnormality. Exophthalmos is due to retro-orbital inflammatory and oedema characteristically seen in thyrotoxicosis.

CONFUSA
Had she not been taking drugs for SVT, this clinical profile would have qualified for a diagnosis of Graves' disease. Amiodarone is an iodine containing highly lipophilic long acting antiarrhythmic drug. It interferes with thyroid function in many ways including inhibition of peripheral conversion of T_4 to T_3.

Investigation of choice
Serum T_4.

Immediate management
Review SVT treatment by a cardiologist.

Treatment of choice
Discontinue amiodarone

194. Female, swelling in the neck, tremor irritability, diarrhoea, bruit.

Diagnosis: Graves' disease

Clinchers
- *Female:* Graves' disease is more prevalent in females, especially in women aged 30-50 years (♀: ♂ ≈ 9:1)
- *Swelling in neck:* The thyroid gland is usually smoothly enlarged but not invariably so.
- *Tremor:* Fine tremor of the outstretched hands is present and reflects the increased sympathetic activity.
- *Irritability:* It is due to the emotional lability commonly seen in hyperthyroidism. Frank psychosis may also develop.
- *Diarrhoea:* It is due to increased sympathetic activity.
- *Bruit:* The thyroid may have a bruit because of its increased vascularity in this condition.

CONFUSA
Additional signs in Graves' disease which differentiate it from other hyperthyroid conditions are:
- Bulging eyes (exophthalmos)
- Thyroid bruit
- Ophthalmoplegia
- Vitiligo
- Pretibial myxedema
- Thyroid acropachy

Investigation of choice
TSH receptor autoantibodies.

Immediate management
Rule out IDDM and pernicious anemia as these are usually associated with Graves' disease.

Treatment of choice
Graves' disease may be treated with antithyroid drugs or radioiodine treatment; subtotal thyroidectomy is rarely indicated.
DOC—carbimazole.

Your Notes:

195. A 35-year-old woman who was diagnosed as having coeliac disease at the age of 12 years has had good control of her abdominal symptoms for a number of years. She presents with a recent history of weight loss, tiredness, diarrhoea and abdominal pain.

Diagnosis: Small bowel lymphoma (probable).

Clinchers
- *35-year-old:* Incidence of lymphomas peak after 30 years
- *Coeliac disease:* The risk of small bowel lymphoma is increased in patients with a prior history of:
  - Malabsorption conditions (e.g. celiac sprue)
  - Regional enteritis
  - Depressed immune function
    - Congenital immunodeficiencies
    - Prior organ transplantation
    - Autoimmune disorders
    - AIDS
- *Good control of abdominal symptoms for a number of years:* Coeliac disease symptoms are very amenable to diet control and since the symptoms are in control in this patient for many years, there is no reason that they should relapse. Considering her age and high risk, lymphoma should be ruled out.
- *Weight loss, tiredness, diarrhoea and abdominal pain:* Characteristic of any malabsorption syndrome (in this case induced by lymphoma).

CONFUSA
Primary intestinal lymphoma accounts for 20% of malignancies of small bowel. Essentially all these neoplasms are non-Hodgkin's lymphoma. Its incidence is: Ileum > jejunum > duodenum (mirrors the relative amount of normal lymphoid cells in these anatomic areas).

Investigation of choice
- *Screening:* Contrast radiographs (infiltration and thickening of mucosal folds, mucosal nodules, ulcerations)
- *Definitive:* Surgical exploration and resection for tissue diagnosis.

Immediate management
Rule out ethnic relation (Jews and Arabs) which produce a nonresectable immunoproliferative small intestinal disease and any non-compliance on gluten free diet.

Treatment of choice
Surgical exploration +
Postresection radio/chemotherapy.

196. Female with breast carcinoma 3 years back, was treated with mastectomy and lymph node clearance on the left side, presents with a swollen limb and decreased hand movements.

Diagnosis: Acquired lymphoedema of arm.

Clinchers

- *Breast carcinoma:* The late oedema of the arm is a troublesome complication of breast cancer treatment. It is seen more commonly when radical axillary lymph node dissection and radiotherapy are combined.
- *3 years back:* It usually present late but can occur anytime from months to years after treatment.
- *Mastectomy and lymph node clearance on left side:* It involves massive removal of lymphatics which hampers the lymphatic drainage of arm. Radical axillary dissection is now rarely combined with radiotherapy (radiotherapy produced postradiation fibrosis which when compounded by impaired lymphatic drainage due to block dissection, increases the risk of lymphoedema by several times) because of this complication, but still it does occur with either modality of treatment alone.
- *Swollen arm:* Due to impaired lymphatic drainage.
- *Decreased hand movements:* It is due to compression of the nerves supplying the hand in compartments of arm and forearm.

CONFUSA

There is usually no precipitating cause but recurrent tumor must be excluded as neoplastic infiltration on the axilla can cause arm swelling due to both lymphatic and venous blockage. The differentiating features is that the neoplastic infiltrations are often painful due to nerve involvement. The diagnosis of lymphoedema also depends on exclusion of other causes of oedema, e.g. venous oedema. Lymphoedema cannot be differentiating from venous oedema by "pitting sign" in acute stage (as both will pit on pressure). However, when lymphoedema becomes chronic the subcutaneous tissue become indurated from fibrous tissue replacement, the pitting will not then occur.

Investigation of choice

Lymphangiography using radio-opaque contrast or radioactive isotope will confirm lymphatic obstruction, and contrast lymphangiography may demonstrate megalymphatics.

Immediate management

Rule out recurrence of carcinoma.

Treatment of choice

Treatment of late oedema is difficult but limb-elevation, elastic arm stockings and pneumatic compression devices can be useful.

Your Notes:

197. Presents with thirst, confusion, constipation.

Diagnosis: Hypercalcemia of malignancy.

Clinchers
> *Thirst, confusion, constipation:* signs and symptoms of hypercalcemia of malignancy are:
> - Lethargy
> - Anorexia
> - Nausea
> - Polydipsia
> - Polyuria
> - Constipation
> - Dehydration
> - Confusion
> - Weakness

These signs and symptoms are most obvious with serum calcium > 3 mmol/L.

Hypercalcemia of malignancy is the most common paraneoplastic endocrine syndrome and is responsible for about 40% of all hypercalcemia.

CONFUSA
Hypercalcemia of malignancy can occur by one of the two mechanisms:
1. Humoral hypercalcemia—caused by circulating hormones (e.g. PTH)
2. Local osteolytic hypercalcemia—caused by local paracrine factors secreted by cancers within bone. This type occurs in relation with breast carcinoma which produces lytic bone metastases. Other cancers involved are kidney, ovary and skin.

Investigation of choice
Serum calcium.

Immediate management
Rehydrate with 3-4 litres of 0.9% saline IV (over 24 hours).
Note: Avoid diuretics

Treatment of choice
Bisphosphonate pamidronate (60-90 mg IV) decreases osteoclastic bone resorption.

Alteration of mental status (as in this case) is indicated of severe hypercalcemia and require treatment with calcitonin in addition to all of the above measures.

Your Notes:

198. Presents with weakness of both legs, difficulty walking, urine retention.

Diagnosis: Vertebral compression fracture due to metastases.

Clinchers
> *Breast carcinoma:* Bone is a common site for the disposition of secondary tumors usually of epithelial origin. Breast metastases are common in
> - Ribs
> - Thoracic vertebrae
> - Clavicles
>
> *Weakness of both legs:* Vertebral fractures involving the cord may entrap cord to produce paraplegia below the level of the fracture. Usually legs are involved in fracture of thoracic vertebrae. Upper limbs are also involved if there is cervical vertebral fracture.
>
> *Difficulty walking:* Due to paraplegia.
>
> *Urinary retention:* Bladder tone is lost immediately after cord injury. Distension leads to ureteric reflux and renal damage. Later on the bladder may become automatic or neurogenic bladder. Bowel dysfunction will also be present.

CONFUSA
Causes of spinal cord compression can be either extension of tumor from vertebral body (osteoblastic metastases) or crush fracture (osteoclastic metastases). Breast carcinoma commonly produces osteoclastic metastases though it can produce osteoblastic metastases too. Prostatic carcinoma produces osteoblastic metastases.

Investigation of choice
- *Screening:* Urgent plain X-ray spine
- *Definitive:* MRI/myelogram

Immediate management
Get neurosurgery and clinical oncology opinions.

Treatment of choice
Dexamethasone 8-16 mg IV then 4 mg/6h PO
Surgical decompression is the definitive treatment.

Your Notes:

199. Presents with headache, confusion. On examination, papilledema present.

Diagnosis: Raised intracranial pressure (ICP) due to cerebral metastases.

Clinchers
- *Headache:* It is the most common symptom of raised intracranial pressure. It is often worse in the morning and is accompanied by nausea and vomiting. Fits or focal neurological signs may appear as the ICP rises.
- *Confusion:* It is due to cerebral edema secondary to brain metastases.
- *Papilledema:* It is due to edema of retinal nerve layer and a common finding on fundoscopy (in both the eyes) in increased ICP.

CONFUSA
Breast carcinoma commonly metastasizes to brain, bone and liver. Brain metastases are usually solitary and produce reactive cerebral edema.

Investigation of choice
CT scan

Immediate management
Ventilatory support.

Treatment of choice
Dexamethasone 4 mg/6h PO
Radiotherapy/surgery for isolated metastases.

Your Notes:

200. Presents with features of fracture femur.

Diagnosis: Metastatic tumor producing pathological fracture.

Clinchers
- *Fracture femur:* Breast carcinoma (and most other epithelial tumors) commonly metastasizes to bone. Usually it is the local bones which are involved but arterial spread may result in deposition anywhere in the skeleton, particularly the flat bones, vertebrae and proximal ends of femur and humerus. Usually the breast carcinoma produces osteolytic (clastic) metastases which increases the risk of fractures especially in weight bearing bones like femur and vertebrae.

CONFUSA
Presence of bony metastases usually means a poor prognosis for life. So the priority in treating any pathological fracture is not restoration of bone congruity but the improvement of life's quality.

Investigation of choice
- *Screening:* X-ray femur (radiolucency)
- *Definitive:* Whole body bone scan

Immediate management
Splinting and take opinion of an orthopaedician and a clinical oncologist.

Treatment of choice
Pathological fractures are normally best treated by internal fixation to enable the patient to mobilize early. Still the best treatment is to treat the primary. Breast carcinoma may respond to hormone therapy, e.g. oophorectomy, androgen or steroid treatment. Tamoxifen is a common antiestrogen drug used for this purpose.

Your Notes:

November—2001

RxPG Analysis

Total themes:	**40**
Repeat themes:	**4**
Repeat themes with different header:	**7**

November 2001

KgPC Analysis	
Total themes,	10
Repeat themes.	1
Repeat theme with different header.	7

November—2001

THEME 1: DIAGNOSIS OF PERSONALITY DISORDERS

OPTIONS
a. Histrionic personality disorder
b. Borderline personality disorder
c. Schizotypal personality disorder
d. Schizoid personality disorder
e. Panic attack disorder
f. Paranoid personality disorder
g. Obsessive-compulsive personality disorder
h. Avoidant personality disorder
i. Antisocial personality disorder
j. Dependent personality disorder
k. Manic-depressive illness

INSTRUCTIONS

*For each patient described below choose the **single most likely diagnosis** from the list of options above. Each option may be used once, more than once or not at all.*

QUESTIONS

1. A 20-year-old man keeps cleaning his hands every time he shakes his partners hands. He was a high achiever in high school.

2. A 56-year-old farmer believes his 34-year-old neighbour is killing his farm animals despite the local veterinary's advice that the death is due to an outbreak of anthrax. He spends hours watching his neighbour through pair of binocular lens, hoping to catch in the act.

3. A 16-year-old girl is described as 'queer' by her mates. She is unfriendly and has no close friends despite numerous attempts by boys in her college. She lacks empathy and is largely introspective.

4. A 16-year-old girl in high school always comes late to class wearing strong perfume in a vain attempt to attract attention. She laughs loudly at jokes, many of her mates do not find particularly hilarious.

5. A 32-year-old man always gives in to his wife over any decision even when he knows this is not right. He insists on having his wife prepare his every meal, wash him and put him to sleep. He cries whenever his wife is away.

THEME 2: DIAGNOSIS OF DIABETIC COMPLICATIONS

OPTIONS
a. Hyperglycemia
b. Hypoglycemia
c. Urinary tract infection
d. Somatic neuropathy
e. Autonomic neuropathy
f. Intermittent claudication
g. Atherosclerosis
h. Possible infection
i. Lactic acidosis
j. Ketoacidosis
k. Amyotrophy

INSTRUCTIONS

*For each of the patients listed below, choose the **most likely complication** from the list of options above. Each option may be used once, more than once, or not at all.*

QUESTIONS

6. A 48-year-old female, insulin dependent diabetic, who has been on treatment for 20-year presents with a history of three episodes of severe hypoglycemia. She has not changed her insulin requirement, diet or exercise pattern.

7. A 48-year-old female, insulin dependent diabetic, who has been on treatment for 20-years, presents with urinary frequency but no dysuria or urgency. Her blood glucose is 17.5 mmol/L.

8. A 30-year-old female, insulin dependent diabetic, presents with failure to pass urine.

9. A 68-year-old diabetic on treatment for the last 5-year presents with calf pain exacerbated by movement.

10. A 70-year-old diabetic on treatment with metformin presents with severe epigastric pain, drowsiness and confusion.

First Aid for the PLAB

THEME 3: DIAGNOSIS OF PNEUMONIA ORGANISMS

OPTIONS
a. Aspiration
b. Bronchiectasis
c. Fungal
d. *Haemophilus influenzae*
e. *Klebsiella*
f. Lung cancer
g. *Mycoplasma pneumoniae*
h. *Pneumocystitis carinii*
i. *Staphylococcus aureus*
j. *Streptococcus pneumoniae*
k. Tuberculosis

INSTRUCTIONS
For each patient described below, choose the **single most likely** underlying cause from the above list of options. Each option may be used once, more than once, or not at all.

QUESTIONS

11. A 35-year-old woman presents with a four-month history of cough, productive o sputum, and recent haemoptysis. She has lost 5 kg in weight. The chest X-ray shows right upper lobe consolidation.

12. A previously well 18-year-old girl has had influenzae for the last two weeks. She is deteriorating and has a swinging fever. She is coughing up copious purulent sputum. Chest X-ray shows cavitating lesions.

13. A 65-year-old man, currently undergoing chemotherapy for chronic leukemia, has felt unwell with fever and an unproductive cough for two weeks despite treatment with broad spectrum intravenous antibiotics. The chest X-ray shows an enlarging right sided, mid-zone consolidation.

14. A 27-year-old male prostitute has felt generally unwell for two months with some weight loss. Over the last three weeks he has noticed a dry cough with increasing breathlessness. Two courses of antibiotics from his GP has produced no improvement. The chest X-ray shows bilateral interstitial infiltrates.

15. On return to university, a 20-year-old student presented with the onset of fever, malaise and a dry cough. The student health service gave him amoxycillin. After a week he felt no better and his chest X-ray showed patchy bilateral consolidation.

THEME 4: DIAGNOSIS OF SUDDEN VISUAL LOSS

OPTIONS
a. Acute glaucoma
b. Cataract
c. Central retinal artery occlusion
d. Cerebral embolism
e. Cerebral haemorrhage
f. Chronic (simple) glaucoma
g. Hypertensive encephalopathy
h. Polymyalgia rheumatica
i. Retinal detachment
j. Temporal arteritis
k. Uveitis

INSTRUCTIONS
For each patient described below, choose the **single most likely diagnosis** from the above list of options. Each option may be used once, more than once, or not at all.

QUESTIONS

16. A 78-year-old man has had a painful scalp and headache for three weeks, and is generally unwell, complains of acute onset of blindness in his right eye.

17. A 50-year-old woman complains of sudden loss of vision in one eye. She describes the incident, like a curtain coming down.

18. An 84-year-old woman notices sudden increased visual impairment. She is found to have homonymous hemianopia.

19. A 68-year-old smoker suddenly notices markedly reduced vision in one eye. He cannot read any letter on visual acuity chart but can count fingers. The fundus is pale.

20. A 30-year-old man has recurrent episodes of an acutely painful red eye with reduced vision.

November—2001

THEME 5: DIFFERENTIAL DIAGNOSIS OF DEMENTIA

OPTIONS
a. Alcoholic dementia
b. Alzheimer's dementia
c. Creutzfeldt-Jakob's disease
d. Head trauma
e. Human immunodeficiency virus (HIV)
f. Huntington's chorea
g. Parkinsonism
h. Pick's disease
i. Repeated trauma
j. Vascular dementia
k. Substance induced dementia

INSTRUCTIONS
*For each patient described below, choose the **single most likely diagnosis** from the above lists of options. Each option may be used once, more than once or not at all.*

QUESTIONS

21. A 56-year-old man with no previous history is brought to the accident and emergency department by his wife who says that he has become progressively more forgetful, tends to lose his temper and is emotionally labile. There is no history of infectious diseases or trauma.

22. A 74-year-old man presents with weakness in his arm and leg (from which he recovered within a few days) and short-term memory loss. He has an extensor plantar response. He had a similar episode two years ago and became unable to identify objects and to make proper judgements.

23. A 38-year-old hemophiliac who received several blood transfusions a few years ago presents with irritability and increasing memory deficit. He is unable to speak properly. He is on antitubercular treatment.

24. A 34-year-old woman presents with memory loss, poor concentration and inability to recognize household objects. On examination she has a right handed involuntary writhing movement. There is a strong family history of similar complaints.

25. A 62-year-old patient with chronic schizophrenia presents with mask-like face and involuntary pill rolling movement in both hands. He complains of chronic cough and forgetfulness.

THEME 6: PRESCRIBING AND RENAL FAILURE

OPTIONS
a. Ciclosporin
b. Bendrofluazide
c. Spirinolactone
d. Cyclophosphamide
e. Captopril
f. Gentamycin
g. Calcium
h. Magnesium
i. Metoprolol
j. Furosemide
k. Paracetamol

INSTRUCTIONS
For each patient described below, choose the single most appropriate drug to prescribe from the above list of options. Each option may be used once, more than once, or not at all.

QUESTIONS

26. A 60-year-old woman hypertensive was started on antihypertensive 2 weeks ago. Now has a creatinine level of 500 micromol/L

27. A child with recurrent nephrotic syndrome is brought for treatment. 3 weeks after start of treatment, he now has massive haematuria.

28. A patient in severe renal failure has potassium level of 2. 5 mmol/L.

29. Patient with complaint of ataxia and tinnitus and mild hearing loss. He has moderate renal failure.

30. A fit 50-year-old man is prescribed oral Acetazolamide by an Ophthalmologist for suspected glaucoma. He presents with lethargy and shortness of breath on exertion. Sodium 140 mmol/L, Potassium 3.2 mmol/L, Bicarbonate 18 mmol/L, Chloride 115 mmol/L, Urea 6.7 mmol/L, Creatinine 114 mmol/L.

| THEME 7: IMMEDIATE MANAGEMENT IN TRAUMA | THEME 8: TREATMENT OF ASTHMA IN CHILDHOOD |

OPTIONS (Theme 7)
a. Plain abdominal X-ray
b. Asses airway and stabilize spine
c. CT scan of abdomen
d. Transfer to operating theatre
e. Burr hole(s) should be drilled
f. Chest drain after needle thoracocentesis
g. Normal saline infusion
h. Immediate blood transfusion
i. Splint limb
j. Bolus of 50% dextrose followed by a saline infusion
k. Computed tomography (CT) brain scan

OPTIONS (Theme 8)
a. As required oral bronchodilator
b. Adrenaline
c. Desensitisation
d. Inhaled long acting bronchodilator
e. Inhaled sodium cromoglycate
f. Inhaled steroid
g. Intermittent inhaled bronchodilation
h. Intravenous (IV) aminophylline
i. Milk free diet
j. Oral steroids
k. Nebulised bronchodilators

INSTRUCTIONS (Theme 7)
*For each patient described below choose the **single most likely immediate action** from the above options. Each option may be used once, more than once, or not at all.*

INSTRUCTIONS (Theme 8)
*For each condition described below, choose the **single most appropriate treatment** from the above list of options. Each option may be used once, more than once, or not at all.*

QUESTIONS (Theme 7)

31. A 43-year-old man is brought to the accident and emergency department delirious, following and injury at a rugby match. His Glasgow Coma Scale (GCS) at the scene of injury is 13. On examination, his right pupil is fixed and dilated and GCS is now 7. Initial resuscitation has been done. The neurosurgeon is 30 minutes away.

32. A 22-year-old motorist arrives in the accident and emergency department after an accident. His airway is patent. He is noted to have a splinted right leg.

33. A 30-year-old man is involved in a fight. He has a bruise on the cheek. He complains of an acute abdominal pain and is vomiting. He had a herniorraphy two weeks ago. He is conscious and fundoscopy has not been done.

34. A 29-year-old motorist, in the accident and emergency department resuscitation room, appears to be stable after an accident. While standing up, he becomes progressively dyspnoeic. There is reduced air entry on the left side of his chest.

35. An 18-year-old girl is being resuscitated after an accident. Her airway is secure. She complains of neck pain. Her pulse rate is 100 beats/min and blood pressure is 110/70 mmHg. Glasgow Coma Scale is 13. She has a deformed left thigh.

QUESTIONS (Theme 8)

36. A nine-year-old boy has a mild cough and wheeze after playing football in the cold weather.

37. A six-year-old girl with asthma uses her bronchodilator twice a day to relieve her mild wheeze. Her parents refuse to give her any treatment containing corticosteroids.

38. A nine-year-old girl with chronic asthma presents to the. A and E department with rapidly worsening wheeze not relieved with inhaled bronchodilators.

39. A four-year-old boy with eczema and recurrent wheeze whenever he gets a viral infection has now developed night cough, there has been no improvement in spite of using inhaled bronchodilator twice each night.

40. A 14-year-old boy, with well-controlled asthma, using inhaled steroids and a bronchodilator comes to the A and E department with breathlessness and swollen lips after eating a peanut, butter-sandwich.

November—2001

THEME 9: DIAGNOSIS OF COMPLICATIONS OF CHOLECYSTECTOMY

OPTIONS
a. Acute pancreatitis
b. Acute renal failure
c. Biliary peritonitis
d. Inferior vena cava thrombosis
e. Myocardial infarction
f. Pulmonary embolism
g. Small bowel obstruction
h. Stone in common bile duct
i. Subphrenic abscess

INSTRUCTIONS
For each test result below, choose the single most likely complication of cholecystectomy from the above list of options. Each option may be used once, more than once or not at all.

QUESTIONS
41. Chest X-ray shows raised right diaphram with small pleural effusion above.

42. Ultrasound scan shows intra-abdominal free fluid with paralytic ileus.

43. Liver function tests show raised alkaline phosphates, raised bilirubin, normal albumin and normal hepatocellular enzymes.

44. Ultrasound scan shows dilated common bile duct with no free intra-abdominal fluid or bowel distension.

45. Chest X-ray shows signs of left ventricular dilatation and an electrocardiograph (ECG) shows Q waves with ST elevation.

THEME 10: POSTOPERATIVE COMPLICATIONS

OPTIONS
a. DVT
b. Setticaemyocardial infarctiona
c. Impending wound dehiscence
d. Wound infection
e. Urinary tract infection
f. Myocardial infarction
g. Acute tubular necrosis
h. Transfusion reaction
i. Cardiac failure
j. Pelvic abscess
k. Pulmonary collapse

INSTRUCTIONS
For each patient described below, choose the single most likely postoperative complication from the above list of options. Each option may be used once, more than once, or not at all.

QUESTIONS
46. A 50-year-old woman underwent an anterior resection for carcinoma of the rectum one week ago. Has low grade fever and with complaint of pain in the calf + tenderness in the calf.

47. A young woman underwent emergency appendicectomy days ago for perforated appendix. She appeared to be making a good recovery but has developed intermittent pyrexia (up to 39 deg. C). On examination—no obvious cause found, but he is tender anteriorly on rectal examination

48. An elderly man underwent an emergency repair of an abdominal aortic aneurysm. Had been severely hypotensive before and during surgery. After surgery, his blood pressure was satisfactory, but urine output only 5 ml/hr in the first 2 hours.

49. An elderly woman underwent emergency laparotomy for peritonitis. Fourth post-operatively day she is noted to have sero-sanuinous discharge from the wound, but there is no erythema or tenderness around the wound.

50. A 60-year-old with features of septicaemia (warm peripheries, low BP etc.)

THEME 11: THE DIAGNOSIS OF ABDOMINAL PAIN

OPTIONS
a. Familial polyposis
b. Food poisoning
c. Anorexia-bulaemia
d. Irritable bowel syndrome
e. Crohn's disease
f. Ulcerative colitis
g. Diverticular disease
h. Gallstone ileus
i. Rectal carcinoma
j. Colonic cancer
k. Pelvic abscess

INSTRUCTIONS
From the list of options given above choose the **diagnosis that fully and accurately** reflects the details of the presentations given below. You may use each option once, more than once, or not at all.

QUESTIONS

51. For the past two weeks a middle-aged railway engineer has complained of acute constipation. His stools are dark, but not apparently blood stained. Abdominal palpation detects a mass with moderate tenderness.

52. A 43-year-old man says he cannot finish his stool and that what he does pass is streaked with blood. He says he has always been regular. He wants to know if a laxative will help.

53. A 49-year-old lawyer complains of blood and diarrhoea. She is also suffering from abdominal pain, fever, and general ill-health. On palpation you find tenderness in the lower abdomen.

54. A young woman presents with recurrent abdominal pain, episodic diarrhoea, malaise, and fever. Over the past few years she has felt her health to be declining. At presentation she complains of severe abdominal pain and constipation.

55. A young woman complains of cramp like abdominal pain, and difficulties with bowel movements. Acute abdominal pain is frequently relieved by embarrassing flatulence. Barium studies and sigmoidoscopy have proved inconclusive.

THEME 12: DIAGNOSIS OF HIP PAIN

OPTIONS
a. Fracture neck of femur
b. Perthes disease
c. Slipped femoral epiphysis
d. Osteoarthritis
e. Septic arthritis
f. Congenital dislocation of the hip
g. Transient synovitis
h. Osteogenesis imperfecta
i. Osteomyelitis

INSTRUCTIONS
For each of the patients described below, choose the **single most likely diagnosis** from the list of options above. Each option may be used once, more than once or not at all.

QUESTIONS

56. A 7-year-old boy presents with a history of acute onset of pain in the knee. On examination, the left lower limb is flexed, abducted, internally rotated.

57. A 67-year-old woman complains of right hip pain. On examination the right hip is adducted, externally rotated and flexed.

58. A 10-year-old girl is febrile. On examination it is difficult to abduct the thighs.

59. A child presents with right hip pain. On examination the hip is flexed, abducted and externally rotated.

60. A five-year-old girl complains of progressively increasing severe pain in her left hip and upper leg for 6 days. She is able to walk but limps visibly. Blood tests are as follows: WCC 19/fl, ESR 72 mm/hr and CRP 94 mg/l. X rays and ultrasound scans of the hip are normal.

THEME 13: THE MANAGEMENT OF RED EYE

OPTIONS
a. No treatment
b. Check blood pressure and do coagulation studies
c. Immediate antibiotic therapy
d. Enucleation
e. 0.5% prednisolone drops 4 hourly
f. 0.5% prednisolone drops 2 hourly and cyclopentolate drops
g. 3% pilocarpine drops and acetazolamide
h. 500 mg acetazolamide
i. Acyclovir drops
j. Total iridectomy 15 % flourescein drops

INSTRUCTIONS
For each patient described below, choose the single **most appropriate mode of management** from the above list of options. Each option may be used once more than once or not at all.

QUESTIONS

61. A 69-year-old patient presented to his GP with sudden onset of redness in the right eye. There was no pain and vision was unaffected.

62. A 60-year-old patient complains of severe pain in his left eye with severe deterioration of vision. He had noticed haloes around street lights at night for a few days before the onset of the pain.

63. A mother brings her 2-year-old child with a squint. On examination a leucokoric right pupil is seen with an absent red reflex.

64. A 12-year-old Libyan boy gave a two weeks history of discomfort, redness and mucopurulent discharge affecting both eyes. His two siblings have a similar problem.

65. A 23-year-old man has a history of recurrent attacks of blurring of vision associated with redness, pain and photophobia. Both eyes have been affected in the past. His brother is currently being investigated for bowel disease and a severe backache.

THEME 14: THE DIAGNOSIS OF WEAKNESS AND ILL HEALTH

OPTIONS
a. Teratoma
b. Seminoma
c. Chronic infection
d. Multiple myeloma
e. Burkitt's lymphoma
f. Non-Hodgkin's lymphoma
g. Hodgkin's disease
h. Thrombocytopenia
i. Chronic myeloid leukaemia
j. Waldenstrom's macroglobinaemia
k. Acute lymphoblastic leukaemia

INSTRUCTIONS
From the list of options given above choose the **diagnosis that most fully and accurately** corresponds to the clinical details of the individual presentations given below. You may use each option once, more than once, or not at all.

QUESTIONS

66. A child is brought to you with weakness, malaise, and bone pain. On physical examination you find painfully enlarged lymph nodes and hard and enlarged testicles. He has a history of sore throats and chest infections.

67. A 51-year-old lecturer presents with lethargy, abdominal pain, fever, and weight loss. On physical examination you find a large spleen. A blood examination shows normocytic normochromic anaemia with a very high white cell count.

68. An elderly man presents with backache, pallor, and shortness of breath. He has suddenly had some difficulties with his vision. Blood examination demonstrates a high ESR, and normochromic normocytic anaemia. There is rouleux formation.

69. A young woman complains of weakness, fatigue, and anorexia. Her cervical lymph nodes are enlarged, painless, and rubbery. Her skin itches and she sometimes has night sweats. On physical examination you find her spleen and liver to be enlarged.

70. A 44-year-old man presents with ill-health. He complains of wasting, fever and sweats. He does not have a skin rash, but he does have skin nodules. On physical examination you find disparate groups of lymph nodes to be enlarged.

THEME 15: PHARMACOLOGY AND TOXICOLOGY

OPTIONS
a. Tricylic antidepressants
b. Opiate
c. Naloxone
d. Warfarin
e. Specific antidote
f. Heparin
g. Cyanide
h. Ethanol
i. Vitamin A
j. Paracetamol
k. 100% O_2

INSTRUCTIONS
Choose the most appropriate answer. You may use each option once, more than once, or not at all.

QUESTIONS
71. A homeless patient presents to A and E with drowsiness. On examination, abrasions and puncture marks were found on his arm. He has pin point pupil. What would you give?
72. This drug competes with vitamin K.
73. A man was found in his car with a hose directed from the exhaust. What would you give?
74. A patient who has overdosed on an unknown medication presents with palpitations. What is the most likely cause?
75. This interferes with metabolism at the mitochondrial level.

THEME 16: DIAGNOSIS OF MALABSOPTION AND DIARRHOEA IN CHILDREN

OPTIONS
a. Lactose intolerance
b. Chronic disease
c. Acrodermatitis enteropathica
d. Chronic nonspecific diarrhoea
e. Coeliac disease
f. Ulcerative colitis
g. *Giardia lamblia* infection
h. *Enterobius vermicularis* infection
i. *Ascaris lumbricoides*
j. Hirschsprungs's disease
k. Irritable bowel syndrome

INSTRUCTIONS
*For each patient described below, choose the **single most likely diagnosis** from the options listed above. Each option may be used once, more than once, or not at all.*

QUESTIONS
76. A 4-year-old Irish girl looks wasted and appears short for her age. The mother reports the daughter has been vomiting on several occasions in the past, with associated diarrhoea. The SHO thinks he has an enteropathy and on serology IgA gliadin and Endomysial antibodies are found.
77. A mother brings her 5-year-old son who has been passing bloody stool associated with severe abdominal pain. On examination he is found to have mildly swollen tender wrists and red nodular tender lesions were found on his forearms.
78. An 8-year-old girl has got repeated episodes of diarrhoea. On each occasion the stool contains segments of undigested vegetables. The paediatrician recommends restricting fluids to meal times. The girls condition improves and she is thriving.
79. A mother and her daughter have just returned from a tropical holiday and is concerned that her daughter has an STD, since she complains of constant perianal and vulval irritation. There is no associated vaginal discharge. She has worms coming out of her bottom at night.
80. A 15-year-old girl complains of episodic diarrhoea which typically starts in the morning with a constant urge to go to the toilet on waking, and after breakfast. She says there is associated abdominal pain in the right iliac fossa relieved by defaecation or flatus. She has had the symptoms for 3 months.

THEME 17: MANAGEMENT OF PAIN IN LABOUR

OPTIONS
a. Spinal anaesthesia
b. Epidural anaesthesia
c. Pudendal nerve block
d. General anaesthesia
e. Pethidine injection
f. Nitrous oxide
g. Local anaesthesia
h. Naloxane
i. Transcutaneous electrical nerve stimulation (TNES)
j. Aspirin
k. Omeprazole

INSTRUCTIONS
For each of the patients described below, **choose the most appropriate option**, from the list of options above. Each option may be used once, more than once or not at all.

QUESTIONS
81. A 20-year-old primigravida at 40 weeks, is 6 cm dilated and she requests pain relief. She dislikes injections.

82. A 39-year gravida 3 para 2 + 0, presents at 39 weeks. Her cervix is 8 cm dilated but she complains of severe pain. Her baby is in occipito-posterior position.

83. A 28-year-old woman wants to be able to move around during labour, pain free.

84. A gravida 4 para 2 + 1, has been in labour for 4 hours. She is 3 cm dilated and has already received 2 injections of pethidine. She stills complains of pain.

85. A 31-year-old woman has a retained placenta, following a spontaneous vaginal delivery.

THEME 18: THE DIAGNOSIS OF FACIAL PAIN

OPTIONS
a. Migraine
b. Abscess
c. Coryza
d. Serous otitis media
e. Glaucoma
f. Iritis
g. Trigeminal neuralgia
h. Sinusitis
i. Systemic lupus erythematosus
j. Temporal arteritis
k. Herpes zoster

INSTRUCTIONS
Examine the following five cases of facial pain and decide which of the above mentioned diagnoses is most likely given the somewhat limited information you have before you. You may use each diagnosis once, more than once, or not at all.

QUESTIONS
86. A 53-year-old nurse complains of facial pain. A week earlier she had a red rash and blisters around her right eye. This area of her face has now become acutely painful.

87. A 31-year-old man complains of facial pain between the eyes and on one side of the face. His nose and the affected eye are congested. He says the pain is severe.

88. A 20-year-old man says his face hurts, especially around the eyes and cheeks. When he bends forwards it worsens and makes him cry.

89. A 57-year-old teacher says she has facial pain, especially in the temples at night. On the right side of her face it throbs. For the past three weeks she has felt unwell and had to miss classes. Also, combing her hair has become painful.

90. A 43-year-old mechanic complains of left sided facial pain. The pain is stabbing and runs up and down his face, especially at meal times. He has been to the dentist, but the dentist has found his teeth to be in good order.

THEME 19: THE DIAGNOSIS OF DIFFICULTIES WITH MICTURITION

OPTIONS
a. Pregnancy
b. Infection
c. Gylcosuria
d. Congenital abnormalities
e. Bladder tumour
f. Childbirth
g. Urethral syndrome
h. Urge incontinence
i. Stress incontinence
j. True incontinence
k. Vesicovaginal fistula

INSTRUCTIONS
For each of the patient cases given below choose an *appropriate and accurate diagnosis* from the list of options given above. You may use each options once, more than once, or not at all.

QUESTIONS

91. An overweight woman complains of having to go to the toilet more than usual. She says she does drink a lot of tea but that she is always thirsty and tired. She needs the energy.

92. A young mother with chronic bronchitis says that every time she coughs, she pees, and she would like you to do something about it. She is on a course of antibiotics at the moment.

93. A middle-aged woman complains of having to urinate frequently. She says that unless she rushes to the toilet she wets herself and she finds wetting herself most embarrassing.

94. A 36-year-old sales executive says she wets herself without warning all the time. Before the birth of her third child she had no complaints but now she says she has no control whatsoever.

95. A 27-year-old travel guide wants something done about the pain she feels on micturition, especially when it is cold. Repeated urine cultures have all been negative. Sometimes, she says, going to the toilet is very painful for her.

THEME 20: INVESTIGATION OF BREAST DISEASE

OPTIONS
a. Open biopsy
b. Fine needle aspiration cytology
c. Ultrasound
d. Reassurance
e. Mammography
f. Wide excision
g. Computed tomography (CT)
h. Magnetic resonance imaging (MRI)
i. Lymphnagiography

INSTRUCTIONS
For each of the patients described below, **choose the single most useful option** from the list above. Each option may be used once, more than once, or not at all.

QUESTIONS

96. A 35-year-old woman comes to the clinic for screening of her breasts.

97. A 45-year-old woman presents with a mass in the right upper quadrant of her right breast. A round smooth mass is found in the axilla.

98. A 36-year-old woman comes with a hard mass in her breast. The skin is tethered. Ultrasound and mammography were inconclusive. The patient wants to be satisfied that this is not malignant.

99. A 36-year-old woman presents with itching of her left nipple. On examination, no ulceration is seen, but a scaly lesion around the nipple is observed.

100. A 23-year-old woman says she feels lumps in her breasts during the time of her periods. She also feels anxious and irritable.

THEME 21: THE MANAGEMENT OF PATIENTS IN A COMA

OPTIONS
a. Alcohol level
b. Angiography
c. Arterial blood gases
d. Blood cultures
e. Blood sugar
f. Computed tomography (CT)
g. Naloxone
h. Paracetamol screen
i. Plasma osmolality
j. Toxicology
k. Urea and electrolytes

INSTRUCTIONS
For each patient described below, **choose the single most appropriate intervention** from the options above. Each option may be used once, more than once, or not at all.

QUESTIONS
101. A 25-year-old found deeply unconscious is brought to the accident and emergency Department. He has an abrasion over his left temple and puncture marks on his left forearm.

102. A 37-year-old alcoholic is found wandering in a park. His partner says he has had a number of falls recently and in the accident and emergency the patient is confused. The blood sugar level is normal.

103. A young diabetic is admitted in a comatose state. his plasma glucose level is 17mmols and he is dehydrated.

104. A middle-aged woman remains unconcious 12 hours following a cholecystectomy. On examination both pupils are seen to be pinpoint.

105. A young diabetic is admitted in a comatose state. His plasma glucose level is 2 mmols.

THEME 22: TRANSMISSION OF DISEASE

OPTIONS
a. Brucellosis
b. *Staphylococcus aureus*
c. *Escherichia coli*
d. *Klebsiella pneumoniae*
e. Hepatitis C
f. *Pseudomonas aeruginosa*
g. *Neisseria meningitidis*
h. Typhoid
i. Scabies
j. Hepatitis A
k. Tuberculosis

INSTRUCTIONS
For each of the conditions below, **choose the most likely answer** from the list of options above. Each option may be used once, more than once or not at all.

QUESTIONS
106. A 45-year-old sheep farmer complains of headache, anorexia, muscle and joint pain. He has as 'undulating' fever.

107. It is a skin to skin contact disease.

108. A 32-year-old woman presents with dysuria, swinging fever and loin pain.

109. It spread by faecal-oral route.

110. A 67-year-old man has lost 10 kg in weight, over the last 6 months. In addition he has a 5 months history of a productive cough.

THEME 23: ECG INTERPRETATION

OPTIONS
a. Hypothermia
b. Pyrexia
c. Right atrial hypertrophy
d. Left atrial hypertrophy
e. Right ventricular hypertrophy
f. Left ventricular hypertrophy
g. Conduction defect
h. Myocardial infarction
i. Ischaemic heart disease
j. Pulmonary hypertension
k. Myocarditis

INSTRUCTIONS
*Choose an option from the above list of **diagnoses that most fully and accurately** corresponds to the ECG changes described below. You may use each option once, more than once, or not at all.*

QUESTIONS
111. A teenage boy with dyspnoea and chest pain is brought into accident and emergency. He has a history of rheumatic fever. An ECG demonstrates left atrial hypertrophy and left ventricular hypertrophy. It also demonstrates Q waves and raised ST segment.
112. An elderly woman is found unconscious at home. An ECG demonstrates sinus bradycardia. J waves, ST depression, and flattened T waves.
113. A patient's ECG shows a biphasic P wave.
114. A patient's ECG shows T wave inversion and ST depression.
115. A 25-year-old woman complains of tiredness and malaise. Her T waves are widespread and deep.

THEME 24: DIZZINESS FITS AND CONFUSION

OPTIONS
a. Nephrotic syndrome
b. Tuberculosis
c. Intestinal hurry'
d. Recurrence of carcinoma
e. Glucose-6-phosphatase deficiency
F Pernicious anaemia
g. Nephroblastoma
h. Wilms' tumour
i. Secondaries
j. Benign postural hypotension
k. Alkalosis

INSTRUCTIONS
*Choose an option from the list of diagnoses given above that **accurately and fully captures** the details of the presentations given below. You may use each option once, more than once, or not at all.*

QUESTIONS
116. A 45-year-old man is diagnosed as having a kidney condition and treated. He soon develops postural hypotension with ankle oedema. His serum sodium is high, his potassuim normal, his urea normal, and he has heavy proteinuria.
117. A 20-year-old teacher is restless and confused. She is pale and sweaty and tachyapnoeic. Her arterial oxygen is high and her carbon dioxide is low.
118. A baby has anumber of fits, each occurring in the morning on four consecutive days. On physical examination you find the liver to be enlarged. His fasting blood sugar is low and his uric acid is high.
119. A 30-year-old salesman complains of night sweats and dizziness. His ESR is high and his blood sugar is low. He has a normocytic anaemia and sterile pyuria.
120. A 50-year-old man is brought in by his wife who says he is always fatting. He has a fresh abdominal scar. His haemoglobin is low. His mean corpuscular volume is low. His mean corpuscular haemoglobin concentration is low. And his glucose tolerance test shows lag storage.

November—2001

THEME 25: NON-ACCIDENTAL INJURY

OPTIONS
a. Elderly abuse
b. Child physical abuse
c. Child sexual abuse
d. Emotional abuse
e. Henoch schonlein purpura
f. Immune thrombocytopenic purpura
g. Child neglect
h. Coeliac disease
i. Osteogenesis imperfecta
j. Osteoporosis
k. Sickle cell anaemia
l. Accidental injury

INSTRUCTIONS
For each patient described below, choose the **single most likely diagnosis** from the above list of options. Each option may be used once, more than once, or not at all.

QUESTIONS

121. A mother 16-years, brings her baby for immunisation. The nurse notices the baby has multiple bruises along both arms and legs and is crying excessively. The house officer notices multiple fractures and that the baby has blue sclerae.

122. A 70-year-old man is receiving treatment for Alzheimer's disease. A 23-year-old grand daughter looks him after. He has recently developed faecal incontinence. The SHO notices bruises on both wrists and back.

123. An anxious mother brings her 6-year-old daughter who is bleeding per vaginum. Six months prior to this presentation the girl had a confirmed streptococcal sore-throat infection. She is otherwise normal.

124. A 4-day-old girl is brought to casualty by the maternal grandparent who is worried about two dark bluish patches on the child's buttocks. Child's mother is white and the father is black.

125. An 8-year-old girl is noted to have fresh bloody staining of her pants. She also suffers from enuresis. She has recently started horse-riding lessons.

THEME 26: DIFFERENTIAL DIAGNOSIS OF ANGINA

OPTIONS
a. Unstable angina
b. Stable angina
c. Syndrome X
d. Myocardial infarction
e. Pericarditis
f. Peptic ulcer disease
g. Arrythmia
h. Spontaneous pneumothorax
i. Acute cholecystitis
j. Chronic pancreatitis
k. Tuberculosis

INSTRUCTIONS
For each of the patients below, choose the **single most appropriate diagnosis** from the list of options above. Each option may be used once, more than once or not at all.

QUESTIONS

126. An obese 34-year-old man complains of epigastric pain, which seems to exacerbated by eating his favourite meal, fish and chips. He get temporary relief when hungry.

127. An obese 45-year-old man complains of recurring chest pain which radiates to his neck lasting 20 minutes. It coincides with his weekly executive board meetings.

128. An obese 29-year-old woman complains of with a cough of two weeks complains of right upper quadrant pain. She is mildly febrile. There was no abdominal tenderness on examination.

129. Condition associated with epigastric pain radiating to the back, pale loose stools, associated with alcohol consumption.

130. Female with fever, rigors, right upper quadrant pain, jaundice, ultrasound is normal.

THEME 27: THE IMMEDIATE MANAGEMENT OF MENINGITIS

OPTIONS
a. Lumbar puncture
b. CT skull
c. X-ray
d. Immunisation
e. Immediated hydration
f. Rifampicin prophylaxis
g. MRI spine
h. Contact tracing
i. Isoniazid prophylaxis
j. Transfer to ITU
k. Reassure
l. Serum urate

INSTRUCTIONS
For each patient described below, **choose the single most urgent first step** from the above list of options. Each option may be used once, more than once or not at all.

QUESTIONS
131. An HIV patient develops a severe headache and confusion. She is discovered to have bilateral papilloedema.
132. An 8-year-old boy with acute leukemia is admitted in a comatose state. He is found to have lymphoblast depletion prevention.
133. A 14-year-old boy presents with drowsiness and generalised headache. He is recovering from a bilateral parotitis. His CT scan is normal.
134. An intravenous drug abuser presents with suspected meningitis. The organism is confirmed in the CSF by India ink preparation.
135. An anxious mother called you to say that her son's best friend in school has caught meningitis.

THEME 28: PRESCRIPTION AND DISEASE

OPTIONS
a. Vancomycin
b. Benzyl penicillin
c. Erythromycin
d. Actinomycin
e. Metronidazole
f. Amoxycillin
g. Glyceryl trinitrate (GTN)
h. Co-trimoxazole
i. Zidovudine (AZT)
j. Ondansetron
k. Trimethoprim

INSTRUCTIONS
For each of the disease conditions mentioned below, **choose the drug of choice** from the above list of possible options. Each option may be used once, more than once or not at all.

QUESTIONS
136. Uncomplicated urinary tract infection (UTI).
137. Pseudomembranous colitis (Patient allergic to vancomycin).
138. Sinusitis in patient allergic to penicillin.
139. Acute otitis media.
140. Acute streptococcal sore throat (patient allergic to penicillin).

THEME 29: CLINICAL MANAGEMENT OF HYPERTENSION IN PREGNANCY

OPTIONS
a. Low dose aspirin
b. A period of observation for blood pressure
c. 24 hour urinary protein
d. Foetal ultrasound
e. Retinoscopy
f. Induction of labour
g. Renal function tests
h. Intravenous antihypertensive
i. Recheck blood pressure in seven days
j. Immediate caesarean section
k. Oral antihypertensive

INSTRUCTIONS
For each patient described below, choose the **single most appropriate action** from the above list of options. Each option may be used once, more than once or not at all.

QUESTIONS
141. A patient in her third pregnancy presents to her GP at 12-weeks gestation. She was mildly hypertensive in both of her previous pregnancies. Her BP is 150/100 mmHg. Two weeks later at the hospital antenatal clinic her BP is 150/95 mmHg

142. A 22-year-old Nigerian woman has an uneventful first pregnancy to 30 weeks. She is then admitted as an emergency with epigastric pain. During the first 2 hours her BP rises from 150/105 to 170/120 mmHg. On dipstick she is found to have 3+ proteinuria. The foetal cardiotocogram (CTG) is normal.

143. At an antenatal clinic visit at 38-weeks gestation, a 36-year-old multiparous woman has a BP of 140/90 mmHg. She has no proteinuria, and is otherwise well.

144. At 32 weeks, a 22-year-old primigravida is found to have a BP of 145/100 mmHg. She has no proteinuria, but she is found to have oedema to her knees.

145. At 34 weeks, a 86 kg woman complains of persistent headaches and 'flashing lights'. There is no hyperreflexia and her BP is 150/100 mmHg. Urinalysis is negative but she has finger oedema.

THEME 30: DIAGNOSIS OF CONSTIPATION

OPTIONS
a. Carcinoma of the colon
b. Parkinsonism
c. Anorexia nervosa
d. Myxoedema
e. Bulimia
f. Diverticulosis
g. Chronic pseudo-obstruction
h. Systemic sclerosis
i. Hypercalcemia
j. Diabetic neuropathy
k. Irritable bowel syndrome

INSTRUCTIONS
For each patient described below, choose the **single most likely diagnosis** from the above list of option. Each option may be used once, more than once, or not at all.

QUESTIONS
146. A 42-year-old woman complains of excessive thirst, polyuria, polydipsia and constipation. She admits to losing weight. Her fasting blood glucose is 5.4 mmol/L.

147. A 23-year-old man being treated for myeloma is brought to the A and E department, confused. This followed a hour history of severe abdominal pain, vomiting. Prior to this, the patient had complained of polyuria, polydipsia and constipation.

148. A 16-year-old frail girl complains of constipation. Her body mass index (BMI) is found to be 17. She is extremely afraid of eating and admits to sticking a finger down her throat to induce vomiting after meals. She is unusually sensitive to cold.

149. A 60-year-old man with a history of weight loss, presents with bleeding per rectum. He also reports a history of diarrhoea which seems to alternate with constipation. His haemoglobin is 10g/dl.

150. A 65-year-old woman presents with constipation, and reports difficulty in starting or stopping to walk. She has dysarthria and dribbling.

First Aid for the PLAB

THEME 31: HUMAN IMMUNODEFICIENCY VIRUS

OPTIONS
a. Prophylactic AZT
b. Needle exchange
c. Refer to social worker
d. Refer to your consultant
e. Methadone
f. Counselling
g. Condoms
h. Combination therapy
i. Pentamidine
j. Pyridoxine and sulphadiazine
k. Cotrimoxazole

INSTRUCTIONS
For each of the patients described **choose the single most appropriate intervention** from the list of options above. Each option may be used once, more than once or not at all.

QUESTIONS
151. A 23-year-old woman has been using heroin (IV) for 4 years. She is not willing to stop using the heroin.
152. A third-year medical student was drawing blood from a known HIV positive patient gets a needle stick injury.
153. A healthy 20-year-old pregnant woman whose partner is a haemophiliac.
154. A 28-year-old haemophiliac with a history of 20 previous blood transfusions presents with a dry cough and fever. His chest X-ray shows widespread mottling.
155. A 20-year-old sexually active woman who is going to Thailand for a holiday.

THEME 32: DIAGNOSIS OF RENAL DISEASE

OPTIONS
a. Acute hypothyroidism
b. Type iv renal tubular acidosis
c. Acute adrenal insufficiency
d. Central nervous lesion with panhypopituitarism
e. Cytomegalovirus disease
f. Type I renal tubular acidosis
g. Syndrome of inappropriate ADH secretion (SIADH) with nephrotic syndrome
h. None of the answers
i. Membranous nephropathy
j. Type II Renal tubular acidosis

INSTRUCTIONS
For each patient described low, **choose the single most appropriate diagnosis** from the above list of options. Each option may be used once, more than once or not used at all.

QUESTIONS
156. A 30-year-old man with AIDS presented in shock. Serum biochemistry reveals: Potassium 6.7 mmol/L, bicarbonate 20 mmol/L, chloride 84 mmol/L, creatinine 160µmol/L.
157. A 41-year-old Londoner developed a temperature of 41°C, 5 weeks after cadaveric renal transplantation. WBC is $2.1 \times 1,000,000,000/L$, Hb is 8.8 g/dl, creatinine 177µmol/L. Aspartate aminotransferase (AST) 82 U/L. Alanine aminotransferase (ALT) 132 U/L.
158. A 36-year-old woman with leukemia has been treated with Amphotericin B for a fungal pneumonia. She presents with muscle weakness. Sodium 137 mmol/L, potassium 2.7 mmol/L, bicarbonate 19 mmol/L, chloride 110 mmol/L, creatinine 84µmol/L, urine pH 6.8 mmol/L.
159. An 83-year-old woman with small cell lung cancer presents with ankle oedema and is found to have 8 g/day, urine proteinuria. He is started on frusemide. 10 days later his blood pressure is 115/75 mmHg lying and 85/65 mmHg standing. Serum biochemistry was; sodium 121 mmol/L, bicarbonate 24 mmol/L, potassium 3.6 mmol/L, creatinine 113 µmol/L, chloride 95 mmol/L, urea 11.5 mmol/L, glucose 5.7 mmol/L, albumin 27g, osmolality 263 mOs m/L, urine osmolality 417 mOs m/L.
160. A fit 50-year-old man is prescribed oral acetazolamide by an opthalmologist for suspected glaucoma. He presents with lethargy and shortness of breath on exertion. Sodium 140 mmol/L, potassium 3.2 mmol/L, bicarbonate 18 mmol/L, chloride 115 mmol/L, urea 6.7 mmol/L, creatinine 114 mmol/L

THEME 33: RISK FACTORS FOR DEEP VEIN THROMBOSIS (DVT)

OPTIONS
a. Dehydration
b. Hormone replacement therapy (HRT)
c. Immobility
d. Inherited clotting abnormality
e. Malignancy
f. Multiple myeloma
g. Polycythaemia rubra vera
h. Pregnancy
i. Varicose veins

INSTRUCTIONS
For each patient described below who presents with a DVT, choose the **single most likely underlying risk factors** from the above lists of options. Each option may be used once, more than once or not at all.

QUESTIONS
161. A 60-year-old man presents with malaise and back pain which has been present for three months. He is found to have significant proteinuria.

162. A 30-year-old woman presents with a three month history of amenorrhoea.

163. A 60-year-old man with a plethoric appearance presents with pleuritic chest pain. He has palpable splenomegaly.

164. A 70-year-old man presents with back pain and jaundice.

165. A 25-year-old woman with a family history of deep vein thrombosis was prescribed a combined oral contraceptive pill six months ago and has not missed any tablets.

THEME 34: DIAGNOSIS OF A RASH

OPTIONS
a. Pulmonary tuberculosis
b. Sarcoidosis
c. Reiter's syndrome
d. Urticaria
e. Lyme disease
f. Dystonia myotonica
g. Herpes simplex
h. Behcet's syndrome
i. Myasthenia
j. Dermatomyositis
k. Smallpox

INSTRUCTIONS
For each of the patients with a rash described below, choose the **single most likely diagnosis** from the above list of options.

QUESTIONS
166. A 29-year-old man with known arthritis presented with a painful red eye and a brownish rash on his feet. He has recently been treated for dysentery.

167. A 30-year-old woman presented to the family GP complaining of difficulty in lifting her arms up. She also reported having difficulty getting up and down stairs. A scaly, erythematous rash was noticed on the dorsum of the hand, and knuckles. She had earlier complained dysphagia.

168. A mother brought her 10-year-old son to the GP, with a history of joint pains and recurrent oral ulcers. On examination the boy had hypopyon and mild conjuctivitis.

169. A 40-year-old sheep farmer from Kent presented to her GP complaining of muscle and joint pain with an associated chronic headache, which has been present for 3 weeks. On examination, she had an erythematous annular rash with a central clear area, on her abdomen.

170. A 30-year-old woman presented with tender, red nodules on both lower limbs and forearms. She had painful joints and was febrile. She had a month history of a productive cough and investigations revealed raised, angiotensin converting enzyme levels.

THEME 35: ASSOCIATION OF SKIN LESIONS AND SPECIFIC DISEASE

OPTIONS
a. Hyperthyroidism
b. Diabetes mellitus
c. Liver disease
d. Coeliac disease
e. Hypogonadism
f. *Borrelia burgdorferi* infection
g. Carcinoma of tail of pancreas
h. Measles
i. Deep vein thrombosis
j. Psoriasis
k. Leptospirosis

INSTRUCTIONS

*For each of the patients described below, choose the **most likely association** from the options given above. Each option may be used once, more than once, or not at all.*

QUESTIONS

171. A fit 55-year-old gentleman, complains of recurrent episodes of 'seeing visible veins on his body', which are tender. He has started to lose weight and attributes this to his diarrhoea. The consultant dermatologist thinks he has thrombophlebitis migrans.

172. A 49-year-old woman complains of itchy blisters, which are occurring in groups on her knees and elbows. The itch is becoming unbearable and she is contemplating suicide. She responds to 180 mg of dapsone within 48 hours of treatment.

173. A Welsh farmer with malaise and arthralgia is increasingly anxious about a skin lesion which started as a papule (Diameter approx 1 mm) which has progressed to a red ring (Diameter approx 50 mm) with central fading.

174. A 42-year-old woman who reports a loss in weight, presents with a shiny erythematous lesion on her skin. Its centre appear yellowish and edges are beginning to ulcerate with undermining. (Fasting blood glucose is 5.3 mmol/L).

175. A 32-year-old woman complains of palpitations and is found to have red oedematous swellings above both lateral malleoli, which she says are beginning to affect her feet. She is found to have digital clubbing and periorbital puffiness.

THEME 36: NATURAL HISTORY CERVICAL CANCER

OPTIONS
a. 3-6 months
b. 12 months
c. 24-36 months
d. 3-10 years
e. 20 years
f. 30 years
g. 45 years
h. 50 years
i. 55 years
j. 65 years
K. 80 years

INSTRUCTIONS

*For each scenario below, choose the **single most likely time or time interval** from the above list of options. Each option may be used once, more than once, or not at all.*

QUESTIONS

176. The time span over which a percentage of women with cervical intraepithelial neoplasia (CIN) untreated will develop cancer.

177. The age at which the peak incidence of cervical carcinoma occurs.

178. The interval for cervical smears to be taken in a woman treated one year previously for cervical intraepithelial neoplasia.

179. The age at which screening stops for women with a normal smear history.

180. The timescale within which the 50% of patients with recurrent disease will present, following treatment for stage 1B cervical cancer.

November—2001

THEME 37: DIAGNOSIS OF COMMON GENETICAL DISORDERS

OPTIONS
a. Klinefelter's syndrome
b. Patau syndrome
c. Down's syndrome
d. Turner's syndrome
e. Cri-du-chat syndrome
f. Fragile X-syndrome
g. Sickle cell disease
h. Sickle cell trait
i. Beta thalassaemia
j. Williams syndrome
k. Prader-Willi syndrome
l. Di George syndrome
m. Acute myeloid leukemia
n. Edward's syndrome

INSTRUCTIONS
For each patient described below choose the **single most appropriate diagnosis** from the list of options above. Each option may be used once, more than once, or not at all.

QUESTIONS

181. A 15-year-old boy has very poor grades at school despite being very attentive and hard working. His mother reckons its because he is teased at school because his breasts look like a girl's. On further examination he is found to have small firm testes. He is mildly asthmatic.

182. A 5-year-old South African boy is brought to the accident and emergency department deeply jaundiced. He is found to have mildly swollen, tender feet and hands. His mucosae are pale.

183. A 6-year-old Asian boy gets regular blood transfusion for his haematological abnormality. His mucosae are pale and skull is grossly bossed. Haematological investigations were done and showed; MCHC 25g/dl, Hb 8g/dl, MCV 74fl.

184. A 10-year-old boy is brought to the accident and emergency department with a swollen right arm. His temperature is 38.5°C and is unable to move his arm due to severe pain. Blood culture confirms *Salmonella typhi* osteomyelitis. This is his second presentation this month and earlier presented with an acute onset hepatosplenomegaly associated with severe pallour. The SHO does a Sodium Metabisulphite test on the patient's blood which turns out to be positive.

185. A 39-year-old male is getting progessively forgetful and is later found to have Alzheimer's disease. He has small ears and an IQ score of 67.

THEME 38: MANAGEMENT OF ACUTE CHEST PAIN

OPTIONS
a. Glyceryl trinitrate (0.5 mg) sublingually
b. IV 50 ml of 50% dextrose
c. High flow O_2 and ramipril 2.5 mg/12 hr PO
d. High flow O_2, 10 mg IV morphine + anticoagulation
e. Crossmatch blood and inform surgeons
f. Insert a 16 G cannula in second intercostal space
g. IV heparin 5000-10,000 iu over 5 min
h. Underwater seal drainage
i. 10 mg IV diamorphine
j. Nifedine
k. Ramipril

INSTRUCTIONS
For each patient described below, choose the **single most appropriate immediate measure** to take from the above list of options. Each option may be used once, more than once or not at all.

QUESTIONS

186. A tall young man developed sharp pain on one side of his chest two days ago. Since then he has been short of breath on exertion.

187. After a heavy bout of drinking a 56-year-old man vomits several times and develops chest pain. When you examine him, he has a crackling feeling under the skin around his neck.

188. A 23-year-old woman on the oral contraceptive pill suddenly gets tightness in her chest and becomes very breathless.

189. A 30-year-old man with Marfan's syndrome has sudden central chest pain going through to the back.

190. A 57-year-old man develops crushing pain in the chest associated with nausea and profuse sweating. The pain is still present when he arrives in hospital an hour later.

THEME 39: INVESTIGATIONS OF PATIENT WITH HAEMOPTYSIS

OPTIONS
a. Computed tomography
b. Fibreoptic bronchoscopy
c. Fine needle aspiration
d. Mediastinoscopy
e. Mediastinotomy
f. Magnetic resonance imaging (MRI)
g. Pulmonary angiogram
h. Selective arteriogram
i. Sputum culture
j. Sputum cytology
k. Ventilation perfusion scan

INSTRUCTIONS
For each suspected diagnosis below, choose the **single most definitive investigation** from the above list of options. Each option may be used once, more than once, or not at all.

QUESTIONS
191. Tuberculosis.
192. Carcinoma of the right main bronchus.
193. Pulmonary embolism
194. Bronchiectasis.
195. Bronchial carcinoid.

THEME 40: ANTIBIOTIC PROPHYLAXIS OF SURGICAL PATIENTS

OPTIONS
a. Angiography
b. Bronchoscopy
c. Colle's fracture
d. Dental treatment of a cardiac patient
e. Dislocated shoulder
f. Emergency appendicectomy
g. Heart valve replacement
h. Sigmoid colectomy
i. Splenectomy
j. Thyroidectomy

INSTRUCTIONS
For each prophylactic regimen given below, choose the **single most likely indication** from the above list of options. Each option may be used once, more than once or not at all.

QUESTIONS
196. 3 gm sachet of amoxicillin one hour before the procedure.
197. Three days of intravenous broad spectrum antibiotics beginning with induction of anaesthesia.
198. Clear fluids by mouth and two sachets of sodium picosulphate on the day before the operation plus broad spectrum intravenous antibiotics at induction.
199. Long-term oral penicillin and immunisation against pneumococcal infection.
200. One dose of metronidazole at induction of anaesthesia.

November—2001

General Medical Council PLAB Test Part 1

First Aid for the PLAB

DO NOT WRITE IN THIS SPACE

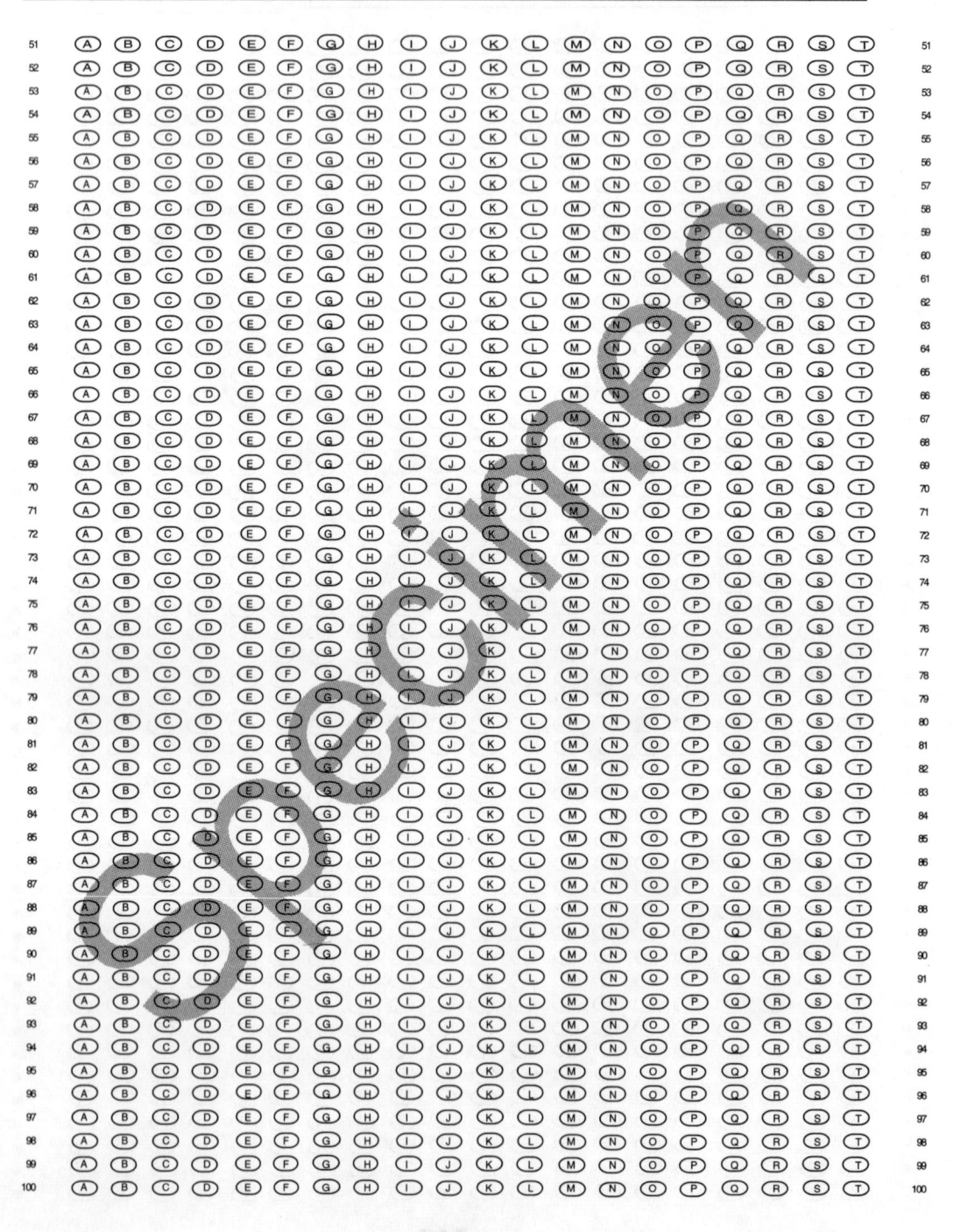

November—2001

DO NOT WRITE IN THIS SPACE

First Aid for the PLAB

DO NOT WRITE IN THIS SPACE

November—2001

Answers

1	g	Obsessive compulsive personality disorders
2	f	Paranoid personality disorders
3	d	Schizoid personality disorder
4	a	Histrionic personality disorder
5	j	Dependent personality disorder
6	h	Possible infection
7	a	Hyperglycaemia
8	e	Autonomic neuropathy
9	f	Intermittent Claudication
10	i	Lactic acidosis
11	k	Tuberculosis
12	i	Staphylococcus Aureus
13	c	Fungal Pneumonia
14	h	Pneumocystitis carinii pneumonia
15	g	Mycoplasma pneumoniae
16	j	Temporal arteritis
17	i	Retinal detachment
18	e	Cerebral haemorrhage
19	c	Central retinal artery occulsion
20	k	Uveitis
21	b	Alzheimer;s dementia
22	j	Vascular dementia
23	e	HIV
24	f	Huntington's chorea
25	g	Parkinsonim (drug induced)
26	e	Captopril
27	d	Cyclo phosphamide
28	j	Frusemide
29	f	Gentamicin
30	i	Acetazolamide
31	e	Burr hole(s) should be drilled
32	g	Normal saline infusion
33	d	Transfer to operating theatre
34	f	Chest drain after needle thoracocentesis
35	i	Splint limb
36	k	Nebulization
37	e	Inhaled sodium chromoglycate
38	k	Nebulized Bronchodiltor
39	e	Inhaled sodium chromoglycate
40	a	As required oral bronchodilator
41	i	Subphrenic abscess
42	c	Biliary peritonitis
43	h	Stone in common bile duct
44	h	Stone in common bile duct
45	e	Myocardial Infarction
46	a	DVT
47	j	Pelvic abscess
48	g	Acute tubular necrosis
49	c	Impending wound dehiscence
50	b	Septicaemia
51	j	Colonic cancer (left side)
52	i	Rectal carcinoma
53	f	Severe ulcerative colitis
54	e	Crohn's Disease
55	d	Irritable bowel syndrome (IBS)
56	b	Perthes disease
57	a	Fracture neck of femur
58	e	Septic arthritis
59	c	Slipped femoral epiphyses
60	i	Osteomyelitis

61	a	No treatment
62	g	3% pilocarpine and accetazolamide
63	d	Enucleation
64	c	Immediate antibiotic therapy
65	f	05% prednisolone drops 2 hourly and cyclopentolate drops
66	k	Acute lymphoblastic leukaemia
67	i	Chronic myeloid leukaemia
68	d	Multiple myeloma
69	g	Hodgkin's disease
70	f	Non Hodgkin's lymphoma
71	c	Naloxone
72	d	Warfarin
73	k	100% O2
74	a	Tricyclic antidepressents
75	g	Cyanide
76	e	Coeliac disease
77	f	Ulcerative colitis
78	d	Chronic non specific diarrhea
79	h	Entrobius vermicularis
80	k	IBS
81	f	Nitrous oxide
82	b	Epidural anaesthesia
83	c	Pudendal nerve block
84	b	Epidural anaesthesia
85	d	General anaesthesia
86	k	Herpes zoster
87	g	Trigeminal neuralgia
88	h	Sinusitis
89	j	Temporal arteritis
90	g	Trigeminal neualgia
91	c	Glycosuria
92	i	Stress incontinence
93	h	Urge incontinence
94	j	True incontinence
95	g	Uretheral syndrome
96	e	Mammography
97	b	Fine needle aspiration cytology
98	b	Fine needle aspiration cytology
99	d	Reassurance
100	d	Reassurance
101	g	Naloxone
102	f	CT scan
103	i	Plasma osmolality
104	g	Nalaxone
105	e	Blood sugar
106	a	Brucellosis
107	i	Scabies
108	c	Escherichia coli
109	j	Hepatitis A
110	k	Tuberculosis
111	h	Myocardial infarction
112	a	Hypothermia
113	d	LAH
114	i	IHD
115	k	Myocarditis
116	a	Nephrotic syndrome
117	k	Alkalosis
118	e	G6PD deficiency
119	b	Tuberculosis
120	c	Intertinal hurry
121	i	Osteogenesis imperfecta
122	a	Elderly abuse
123	c	Child sexual abuse

November—2001

124	b	Child physical abuse		156	c	Acute adrenal insufficiency
125	l	Accidental injury		157	e	CMV disease
126	f	Peptic ulcer disease		158	f	Type I RTA
127	b	Stable angina		159	h	None of the answers
128	k	Tuberculosis		160	j	Type II RTA
129	j	Chronic pancreatitis		161	f	Multiple Myeloma
130	i	Acute cholecystitis		162	h	Pregnancy
131	b	CT skull		163	g	Polycyathemic rubravera
132	g	Immediate hydration		164	e	Malignancy
133	a	Lumbar puncture		165	d	Inherited clotting abnormality
134	j	Transfer to ITU		166	c	Reiter's syndrome
135	k	Reassure		167	j	Dermatomyositis
136	k	Trimethoprim		168	h	Behcet's syndrome
137	e	Metronidazole		169	e	Lymes disease
138	c	Erythromycin		170	b	Sarcoidosis
139	f	Amoxycillin		171	g	Carcinoma of tail of pancreas
140	c	Erythromycin		172	d	Cocliac disease
141	c	24 hours urinary protein		173	f	Borrelia burghdorferi
142	h	IV antihypertensive		174	b	Diabetes mellitus
143	b	A period of observation of BP		175	a	Hyperthyroidism
144	d	Foetal USG		176	d	3-10 years
145	c	24 hours urinary protein		177	f	30 years
146	i	Hypercalcaemia		178	b	12 months
147	i	Hypercalcaemia		179	j	65 years
148	c	Anorexia nervosa		180	b	12 months
149	a	Carcinoma colon		181	a	Klinefelters's syndrome
150	b	Parkinsonism		182	g	Sickle cell disease
151	b	Needle exchange		183	i	Beta thalassemia
152	a	Prophylactic AZT		184	g	Sickle cell disease
153	f	Counselling		185	c	Down's syndrome
154	k	Cotrimoxazole		186	h	Underwater seal drainage
155	g	Condoms		187	e	Cross match blood and inform surgeons

188	c	High flow O2 + 10 mg IV morphine + anticoagulation	194	a	CT
189	e	Cross match blood and inform surgeons	195	a	CT
			196	d	Dental treatment of a cardiac patient
190	c	High flow O2 + 10 mg IV morphine + anticoagulation	197	g	Heart value replacement
191	i	Sputum culture	198	h	Sigmoid colectomy
192	b	Fibreoptic bronchoscopy	199	i	Spelectomy
193	g	Pulmonary angiogram	200	f	Emergency appendicectomy

November—2001

EXPLANATIONS

1. A 20-year-old man keeps cleaning his hands every time he shakes his partners' hands. He was a high achiever in high school.

Diagnosis: Obsessive compulsive personality disorder (OCD).

Clinchers
- *20-year-old:* The onset of OSD is usually in early 20's. It is slightly more common in unmarried people.
- *Man:* OCD is equally common in men and women.
- *Keeps cleaning his hands every time he shakes his partners' hands:* Washers are the most common type. Here the obsession is of contamination with dirt, germs, body excretions and the like. The compulsion is washing of hands or the whole hand, repeatedly many times a day. It usually spreads on to washing of clothes, washing of bathroom, door knobs and personal articles, gradually. The person tries to avoid contamination but is unable to, so washing becomes a ritual.
- *High achiever in school:* This disorder is more common in persons from upper social strata and with high intelligence.

CONFUSA
The differential diagnosis is from depressive disorder (in which obsessional symptoms are common), psychotic disorder (since obsessions can be hard to distinguish from delusions) and anankastic personality disorder.

Investigation of choice
Clinical diagnosis.

Immediate management
Specialist evaluation.

Treatment of choice
Behavioural therapy
 +
Drug treatment
(TCA/SSRI/clomipramine).

Your Notes:

2. A 56-year-old farmer believes his 34-year-old neighbour is killing his farm animals despite the local veterinary's advice that the death is due to an outbreak of anthrax. He spends hours watching his neighbour through pair of binocular lens, hoping to catch in the act.

Diagnosis: Paranoid personality disorder.

Clinchers
- *56-year-old farmer:* It occurs at early age in adult life with a stable course over the years.
- *Believes his 34-year-old neighbour is killing his farm animals despite the local veterinary's advice that the death is due to an outbreak of anthrax:* In it, the person may have excessive sensitiveness to setbacks and rebuffs. There is tendency to bear grudges persistently, e.g. refusal to forgive insults and injuries or slights. There may be recurrent suspicious, with out justification and contrary to evidence (as in this case).
- *Spends hours watching his neighbour* There is preoccupation with unsubstantiated conspirational explanation of events and the patient may go to any length to prove them.

CONFUSA
Paranoid personality disorder is more common in men. It is more common in minority groups and immigrants. Psychodynamically the underlying defense mechanism is projection. For the diagnosis of this disorder, clear evidence is usually required of the presence of at least three of the traits or behaviours given in clinical description by ICD-10 (CDDG). This disorder is found premorbidly in some patients of paranoid schizophrenia.

Investigation of choice
Clinical diagnosis.

Immediate management
Exclude delusional (paranoid) disorder.

Treatment of choice
Individual and supportive psychotherapy.

Your Notes:

3. A 16-year-old girl is described as 'queer' by her mates. She is unfriendly and has no close friends despite numerous attempts by boys in her college. She lacks empathy and is largely introspective.

Diagnosis: Schizoid personality disorder.

Clinchers
- *16-year-old girl:* Like all personality disorder, schizoid personality disorder has an onset in early childhood with stable course over the years. It is more common in men.
- *Described as 'queer' by her mates:* There is almost invariable preference for solitary activities in this disorder. The patient lacks close friends or confiding relationships (or having only one) and of desire of such relationships. There is also marked insensitivity to prevailing social norms and conventions.
- *Unfriendly and has no close friends:* See above.
- *Despite numerous attempts by boys in her college:* There is little interest on the part of the patient in having sexual experiences with another person (taking into account her age).
- *Lacks empathy:* There is emotional coldness, detached or flattened affectivity and limited capacity to express either warm, tender feelings or anger towards others.
- *Largely introspective:* There is excessive preoccupation with fantasy and introspection.

CONFUSA
The features of this disorder may overlap with paranoid and schizotypal personality disorders, but can be differentiated clinically as psychotic features are absent. Psychodynamically it is supposed to result from 'cold and aloof' parenting in a child with introverted temperament. However, this hypothesis is far from proven in the research conducted so far.

Investigation of choice
Clinical diagnosis.

Immediate management
Specialist evaluation.

Treatment of choice
Individual psychotherapy.
+
Psychoanalysis
+
Gradual involvement in group psychotherapy

4. A 16-year-old girl in high school always comes late to class wearing strong perfume in a vain attempt to attract attention. She laughs loudly at jokes, many of her mates do not find particularly hilarious.

Diagnosis: Histrionic personality disorder

Clinchers
- *16-year-old:* Like all personality disorders, it has an onset in early childhood with stable course over the years.
- *Girls:* More common in females.
- *Always comes late + strong perfume + laughs loudly:* These are exhibitionistic traits which signify an attention seeking attitude, a characteristic feature. There is also continual seeking for excitement and appreciation by others. Dramatic emotionally, i.e. self dramatization, theatricality and exaggerated expression of emotions is usually present. There is an attempt to look charming, beautiful and seductive. Suicidal gestures may be made.

CONFUSA
Associated features may include egocentricity, self-indulgence, continuous longing for appreciation, feelings that are easily hurt and persistent manipulative behaviour to achieve own needs. Interpersonal relationships of such persons are often stormy and ungratifying. Psychodynamically, there are intense dependency needs. The defence mechanisms used most are acting out and dissociation.

Investigation of choice
Clinical diagnosis.

Immediate management
Specialist evaluation.

Treatment of choice
Psychoanalysis
+
Psychoanalytic psychotherapy.

Your Notes:

5. A 32-year-old man always gives in to his wife over any decision even when he knows this is not right. He insists on having his wife prepare his every meal, wash him and put him to sleep. He cries whenever his wife is away.

Diagnosis: Dependent personality disorder

Clinchers
- *32-year-old man:* Like all personality disorders, it has an onset in early childhood with sable course over the years.
- *Always gives in to his wife over any decision even when he knows this is not right:* In this disorder the patient encourage or allow others to make most of one's important life decisions. There is limited capacity on the patient's part to make everyday decisions without an excessive amount of advice and reassurance from others.
- *Insists on having his wife prepare his every meal, wash him and put him to sleep:* These suggest dependence on her wife as the patient usually think himself as incompetent.
- *Cries whenever his wife is away:* There is feeling of being uncomfortable or helplessness when alone or abandoned by person with who he has a close relationship. It is because of exaggerated fears of inability to care for onself.

CONFUSA
Dependent personality disorders may overlap with avoidant and passive aggressive personality disorders. Some patients exhibit masochistic character. They repetitively establish close interpersonal relationships which result in punishment.

Investigation of choice
Clinical diagnosis

Immediate management
Specialist evaluation

Treatment of choice
Individual psychotherapy
 +
Group psychotherapy
 +
Behaviour therapy in the form of assertiveness training is useful

6. A 48-year-old female, insulin dependent diabetic, who has been on treatment for 20-year presents with a history of three episodes of severe hypoglycemia. She has not changed her insulin requirement, diet or exercise pattern.

Diagnosis: Possible infection

Clinchers
- *48-year-old female with IDDM:* As IDDM usually have an onset at a younger age, she must be having a long history of diabetes.
- *Three episodes of severe hypoglycaemia:* Non-compliance to therapy or diet and exercise changes can induce such attacks. But since these have been specifically ruled out in this question, a possible systemic infection seems to be most probable.

CONFUSA
Infections in persons with diabetes may not occur more frequently than in nondiabetics, but they tend to be more severe, possibly because of imparied leukocyte function. In addition to common infections of the skin, urinary tract, lungs and blood stream infections like malignant external otitis, Rhinocerebral mucormycosis, emphysematous cholecystitis and emphysematous pyelonephritis, appear to have a specific relationship with diabetes.

Investigation of choice
Blood culture

Immediate management
Detailed history

Treatment of choice
Treat the infection if present, with broad spectrum antibiotics

Your Notes:

7. A 48-year-old female, insulin dependent diabetic, who has been on treatment for 20 years, presents with urinary frequency but no dysuria or urgency. Her blood glucose is 17.5 mmol/L.

Diagnosis: Hyperglycaemia

Clinchers
- *48 year old female + IDDM:* IDDM patients prone to insulin resistance after a few years and require a greater dose of insulin else they get hyperglycemic
- *Urinary frequency but no dysuria or urgency:* Urinary frequency alone is feature of diabetes mellitus as polyuria would be reported as incresed urinary frequency.
- *17.5 mmol/L blood glucose:* Significant hyperglycaemia.

CONFUSA
Among the given list of options, the confusion can be with—Urinary tract infection, but absence of dysuria and urgency go less in its favour.

Investigation of choice
- Blood sugar fasting.
- Urine culture and sensitivity to rule out concomitant infection since blood glucose has already been done.

Immediate management
Increase dose of insulin.

Treatment of choice
Better diabetic control.

Your Notes:

8. A 30-year-old female, insulin-dependent diabetic, presents with failure to pass urine.

Diagnosis: Autonomic neuropathy

Clinchers
- *IDDM patient:* Such patients are more prone to autonomic neuropathy.
- *Failure to pass urine:* Retention of urine is suggestive of autonomic involvement of the bladder. That occurs with a long-standing history of diabetes. Since the patient is now 30-year-old and IDDM usually have a juvenile onset, one must be having a long history to substantiate our diagnosis.

CONFUSA
Diabetic neuropathy may affect every part of the nervous system, with the possibei exception of brain. While rarely a direct cause of death, neuropathy is a major cause of morbidity. Most common picture is that of a peripheral polyneuropathy.

Investigation of choice
Pelvic USG.

Immediate management
Urinary catheterisation.

Treatment of choice
Chronic catheter drainage.

Your Notes:

9. A 68-year-old diabetic on treatment for the last 5-year presents with calf pain exacerbated by movement.

Diagnosis: Intermittent claudication

Clinchers
- *Calf pain exacerbated by movement:* This is a typical history of intermittent claudication. The pain is initially relieved by rest.
- *68-year-old diabetic:* this female has a high chances of having atherosclerosis secondary to diabetes or as a primary disease. This produces the vascular disease with diminished blood supply which cause intermittent claudication and foot ulcers.

CONFUSA
Hypertriglyceridaemia is common in diabetes and is due both to overproduction of VLDL in the liver and to a disposal defect in the periphery.

Investigation of choice
Doppler USG lower limb (or Duplex USG)

Immediate management
Instruction about proper foot care in an attempt to prevent ulcers.

Treatment of choice
Maintain diabetic control properly to keep hypertriglyceridaemia under control
  +
Symptomatic management.

Your Notes:

---

10. A 70-year-old diabetic on treatment with metformin presents with severe epigastric pain, drowsiness and confusion.

Diagnosis: Lactic acidosis

Clinchers
- *Metformin:* Lactic acidosis is a common side effect of metformin.
- *Severe epigastric pain + drowsiness + confusion:* The usual side effects of metformin are abdominal discomfort, anorexia, nausea, metallic taste, mild diarrhoea and tiredness. Lactic acidosis is the most serious complication of metformin intake.

CONFUSA
Ketoacidosis can be a confusing option, but ketoacidosis is very uncommon in NIDDM patients Alcohol intake in a patient or metformin therapy precipitate severe lactic acidosis.

Investigation of choice
Arterial blood gases.

Immediate management
IV Fluids.

Treatment of choice
$NaHCO_3$.

Your Notes:

11. A 35-year-old woman presents with a four-month history of cough, productive of sputum, and recent haemoptysis. She has lost 5 kg in weight. The chest X-ray shows right upper lobe consolidation.

Diagnosis: Tuberculosis

Clinchers
- *35-year-old woman:* Reactivation of primary TB occurs in usually mid-adult life (usually acquired in childhood).
- *Four-month history of cough:* Any prolonged history of cough should make one suspicious of TB.
- *Productive of sputum:* Cough in TB is almost always productive and the sputum may be mucoid, purulent or blood-stained.
- *Recent haemoptysis:* It is an regular finding in pulmonary TB.
- *Lost 5 kg weight:* It is due to associated loss of appetite.
- *Right upper lobe consolidation:* The CXR typically shows patchy or nodular shadows in the upper zones, loss of volume and fibrosis with or without cavitation.

CONFUSA
An abnormal CXR is often found with no symptoms in pulmonary TB but pulmonary TB is extremely unlikely in the absence of any radiographic abnormality. The X-ray appearances alone may strongly suggest TB, but every effort must be made to obtain microbiological evidence. A single X-ray does not given an indication of the activity of the disease. Very similar CXR appearances occur in:
- Histoplasmosis
- Cryptococcosis
- Coccidioidomycosis
- Aspergillosis

Investigation of choice
Sputum microscopy and culture

Immediate management
Exclude HIV after consent
+
Contact tracing

Treatment of choice
Anti TB drug regimen

Your Notes:

---

12. A previously well 18-year-old has had influenzae for the last two weeks. She is deteriorating and has a swinging fever. She is coughing up copious purulent sputum. Chest X-ray shows cavitating lesions.

Diagnosis: *Staphylococcus aureus*

Clinchers
- *Previously well:* Exclude any pre-existing bacterial infection.
- *18-year-old:* S. aureus affects all age groups.
- *Has had influenzae for the last two weeks:* S. aureus normally causes a pneumonia only after a preceding influenzae viral illness.
- *Deteriorating:* The infection starts in the bronchi, leading to patchy areas of consolidation in one or more lobes, which break down to form abscesses, and thus the condition deteriorates during the course of infection.
- *Has a swinging fever:* It is due to abscess formation.
- *Coupious purulent sputum:* Characteristic of it.
- *Cavitating lesions:* It causes a bilateral cavitating bronchopneumonia.

CONFUSA
Staphylococcal pneumonia may complicate influenza infection or occur in the young, elderly, IV drug users or patients with underlying disease (e.g. leukaemia, lymphoma, cystic fibrosis). It can lead to development of septicaemia with metastatic abscesses in other organs. In IV drug abusers symptoms of septicaemia predominates over the respiratory symptoms.

Investigation of choice
Sputum culture

Immediate management
O_2 to maintain $PaO_2 > 8$ kPa

Treatment of choice
Flucloxacillin

Your Notes:

13. A 65-year-old man, currently undergoing chemotherapy for chronic leukemia, has felt unwell with fever and an unproductive cough for two weeks despite treatment with broad spectrum intravenous antibiotics. The chest X-ray shows an enlarging right sided, mid-zone consolidation.

Diagnosis: Fungal pneumonia

Clinchers
- *65-year-old man + chemotherapy + chronic leukaemia:* All these factors suggest immunocompromised state which predispose to fungal infections.
- *Felt unwell with fever:* Malaise and pyrexia are usually present.
- *Unproductive cough:* This suggest a non-bacterial cause of the pneumonia.
- *For two weeks despite treatment with broad spectrum antibiotics:* This almost confirms the suspicious of non-bacterial pneumonia.
- *CXR shows an enlarging right sided, mid-zone consolidation:* This is the lung abscess due to fungal infection.

CONFUSA
Candida and Cryptococcus cause pneumonia in the immunosuppressed. Aspergillus gives rise to a widespread invasion of lung tissue in immunocompromised patients. *Pneumocystis carinii* occurs along with AIDS. Other fungal pneumonias can be due to *Actinomyces israelii* and *Nocardia asteroides*.

Investigation of choice
- *Screening:* CXR
- *Definitive:* Bronchoalveolar lavage (as the cough is unproductive)

Immediate management
FBC (to evaluate status of leukaemia)

Treatment of choice
Antifungals

Your Notes:

14. A 27-year-old male prostitute has felt generally unwell for two months with some weight loss. Over the last three weeks he has noticed a dry cough with increasing breathlessness. Two courses of antibiotics from his GP has produced no improvement. The chest X-ray shows bilateral interstitial infiltrates.

Diagnosis: Pneumocystitis carinii pneumonia (PCP)

Clinchers
- *27-year-old male prostitute:* Strongly suspect AIDS in this patient.
- *Generally unwell for two months:* Malaise and constitutional upset is common with *P. carinii* pneumonia.
- *Weight loss:* This can be both due to AIDS and *P. carinii* infection.
- *Last three weeks:* It usually presents with a prolonged course.
- *Dry cough with increasing breathlessness:* It presents with a dry cough, exertional dyspnoea, fever and bilateral crepitations.
- *Two courses of antibiotics.... no improvement:* Rules out a bacterial course.
- *CXR shows bilateral interstitial infiltrates:* The typical radiographic appearance of PCP is of a diffuse bilateral alveolar and interstitial shadowing beginning in the perihilar regions and spreading out in a butterfly pattern.

CONFUSA
Other CXR appearance of PCP include a localized infiltrate, nodule, cavity or a pneumothorax. In patients receiving aerosolized pentamidine for prophylaxis, infiltrates may be localized to the upper zones. In early infection the CXR is normal but high-resolution CT scans of the chest can demonstrate a characteristic ground-glass appearance even then. Definitive diagnosis rests on demonstrating the organisms in the lungs via bronchoalveolar lavage. As the organism cannot be cultured in vitro it must be directly observed either with silver staining or immunofluorescent techniques.

Investigation of choice
- *Screening:* CXR
- *Definitive:* Bronchoalveolar lavage

Immediate management
CD4 lymphocyte count (as PCP is usually not seen until CD4 < 200)

Treatment of choice
IV co-trimoxazole for 21 days (side effect: typical allergic rash).

15. On return to university, a 20-year-old student presented with the onset of fever, malaise and a dry cough. The student health service gave him amoxycillin. After a week he felt no better and his chest X-ray showed patchy bilateral consolidation.

Diagnosis: *Mycoplasma pneumoniae.*

Clinchers

- *20-year-old:* It often occurs in patients in their teens and twenties.
- *On return to university:* It is frequent amongst those living in boarding institutions.
- *Onset of fever, malaise and dry cough:* Generalised features such as headaches and malaise often precede the chest symptoms by 1-5 days. Cough may not be obvious initially and physical signs in the chest may be scanty.
- *Amoxicillin:* It responds to erythromycin or tetracycline but not to amoxicillin. Since after a week, he is not feeling any improvement, our suspicion of mycoplasma is becoming almost certain.
- *Patchy bilateral consolidation:* This is characteristic and confirms our suspicion.

CONFUSA
On CXR, usually only one of the lower lobes is involved but sometimes there may be dramatic shadowing in both lower lobes. There is frequently no correlation between the X-ray appearances and the clinical state of the patient. Complication of *Mycoplasma pneumoniae* can be skin rash (erythema multiforme), Steven-Johnson syndrome, meningoencephalitis Guillain-Barré syndrome.

Investigation of choice
Mycoplasma serology

Immediate management
Rule out extrapulmonary complications

Treatment of choice
Erythromycin 500 mg QID for 7-10 days
(Alternative : Tetracycline)

Your Notes:

16. A 78-year-old man has had a painful scalp and headache for three weeks, and is generally unwell, complains of acute onset of blindness in his right eye.

Diagnosis: Temporal arteritis

Clinchers

- *Painful scalp and headache:* Interruption of blood flow to visual cortex causes sudden greying of vision, and other symptoms that mimic migraine.
    Transient monoocular blindness usually occurs from a retinal embolus or severe ipsilateral carotid stenosis.
- *Acute onset blindness in right eye:* Anterior ischaemic optic neuropathy (AION) is an infarction of the optic nerve head due to inadequate perfusion via the posterior ciliary arteries. Patient has sudden loss, often upon awakening, and painless swelling of the optic disc. Arteric AION is caused by *temporal arteritis*.

CONFUSA
Malignant hypertension can cause visual loss from exudates, haemorrhages, cotton wool spots (focal nerve fibre layer infarct) and optic disc edema.

Investigation of choice
Visual field mapping
Ophthalmoscopy
ESR

Immediate management
Immediate glucocorticoid therapy

Treatment of choice
Glucocorticoid therapy for atleast 2 years.

Your Notes:

17. A 50-year-old woman complains of sudden loss of vision in one eye. She describes the incident, like a curtain coming down.

Diagnosis: Retinal detachment

Clinchers

- *50-year-old woman:* Retinal detachment is most common between 40 and 60 years, though it may occur at any age. F:M (3:2) ratio.
- *Sudden painless loss of vision:* Causes of sudden painless loss of vision are:
  - Retinal detachment
  - Central retinal artery/vein occlusion
  - Vitreous haemorrhage
  - Central serous retinopathy
  - Optic neuritis
  - Methyl alcohol amblyopia
- *Curtain coming down (in one eye):* Appearance of dark cloud, or veil like curtain in front of eye suddenly is the sign of retinal detachment (large and central).

CONFUSA

Retinal detachment should be differentiated from the other causes of sudden painless loss of vision (given above). In early cases of retinal detachment patient notices a localised relative loss in the field of vision (of detached retina) which progresses as detachment proceeds towards the macular area.

Investigation of choice

- *Ophthalmoscopy:* Detached retina gives grey reflex instead of normal pink reflex
- *Visual field charting*
- *USG* confirms the diagnosis.

Treatment of choice

- Sealing of retinal breaks
- Bring the sclerochoroid and detached retina near to each other

High risk factors for retinal detachment: Myopia, aphakia, retinal detachment in fellow eye, history of retinal detachment in family.

Your Notes:

18. An 84-year-old woman notices sudden increased visual impairment. She is found to have homonymous hemianopia.

Diagnosis: Cerebral haemorrhage

Clinchers

- *84-year-old woman:* Incidence of rupture of cerebral vessel aneurysms increases with age. These aneurysms are common in females.
- *Sudden increased visual impairment:* Since the defect is of sudden onset, it rules out tumors or other chronic disease processes as a causation. There is no given history of trauma cerebral embolism can be ruled out as it usually do not produce permanent changes.
- *Homonymous hemianopia:* Most commonly it results from lesions in optic tract (tumours pressing it), geniculate body and optic radiations (cerebral haemorrhage). Since we have ruled out tumors to be cause, cerebral haemorrhage is a safe answer.

CONFUSA

Hemianopia denotes loss of half of the field of vision. The most common clinical form is homonymous hemianopia, in which the right of left half of the binocular field of vision is lost, owing to loss of the temporal half of one field and the nasal half of the other, a condition due to a lesion situated in any part of the visual paths from the chiasma to the occipital lobe. Right hemianopia is more quickly discovered than left owing to the fact that reading is impossible; left hemianopia is often discovered when the patient does not see food on the left side of the plate.

Investigation of choice
MRI/CT

Immediate management
Admit and specialist evaluation

Treatment of choice
Symptomatic + as per radiological findings.

Your Notes:

19. A 68-year-old smoker suddenly notices markedly reduced vision in one eye. He cannot read any letter on visual acuity chart but can count fingers. The fundus is pale.

Diagnosis: Central retinal artery occlusion (CRAO)

Clinchers
- *68-year-old smoker:* These are the risk factors for CRAO. More commonly seen in patients suffering from hypertension and other cardiovascular diseases. It is usually unilateral, but rarely be bilateral (1-2% cases).
- *Notices reduced vision in one eye:* CRAO is usually unilateral. Sudden painless loss of vision is suggestive of central retinal artery occlusion.
- *Fundus is pale:* Retina becomes milky white due to oedema. Retinal arteries are markedly narrowed. Fundus is pale.

CONFUSA
Sudden painless loss of vision occur in central retinal artery occlusion, vitreous haemorrhage, retinal detachment, central retinal vein occlusion, central serous retinopathy, optic neuritis and methyl alcohol amblyopia.

Investigation of choice
Investigate for the cause.

Immediate management
- Immediate lowering of IOP (IV mannitol)
- Vasodilators and inhalation of a mixture of 5% CO_2 and 95% O_2 (may help in relieving angiospasm)
- Anticoagulants
- Intravenous steroids

Treatment of choice
Treatment is unsatisfactory as retinal tissue cannot survive ischaemia for more than a few hours. Emergency treatment (as above) should be followed.

Your Notes:

---

20. A 30-year-old man has recurrent episodes of an acutely painful red eye with reduced vision.

Diagnosis: Uveitis

Clinchers
- *Acutely painful red eye reduced vision:* These symptoms are suggestive of anterior uveitis (iridocyclitis).
- *Pain:* It is a dominating symptom of anterior uveitis, typically worsen at right.
- *Redness:* It is due to circumcorneal congestion, which is a result of active hyperaemia of anterior ciliary, vessels.
- *Reduces vision:* Defective vision in patient with iridocyclitis may vary from slight blur in early phase to marked deterioration in late phase.
- Look for corneal edema and keratic precipitates (KP) at back of cornea.

CONFUSA
Acute congestive glaucoma and acute conjunctivitis should be kept in mind here, and should be differentiated from iridocyclitis. Other conditions that may cause sudden painful visual loss are chemical or mechanical injuries to the eyeball.

Investigation of choice
Includes battery of tests due to its varied etiology.

Immediate management
1 per cent atropine sulphate eye ointment or drops 2-3 times day. In case of atropine allergy other cycloplegics should be used

Treatment of choice
Local treatment with mydriatic-cycloplegic drugs and corticosteroids (reduce inflammation).

Systemic therapy with corticosteroids (especially in non-granulomatous iridocyclitis). NSAIDs where steroids contraindicated. Adrenocorticotrophic hormone where steroids fail to act.

Finally treat the cause.

Your Notes:

21.
A 56-year-old man with no previous history is brought to the Accident and Emergency Department by his wife who says that he has become progressively more forgetful, tends to lose his temper and is emotionally labile. There is no history of infectious diseases or trauma.

Diagnosis: Alzheimer's dementia (AD)

Clinchers

- *56-year-old":* The onset can be in middle adult life or even earlier (of presenile onset) but the incidence is higher in later life.
- *No previous history:* It is insidious in onset and usually have no precipitating or prodromal symptoms.
- *Brought by wife:* The patients are not insightful enough to present themselves.
- *Progressively more forgetful:* There is impaired ability to learn new information or to recall previously learned information.
- *Tends to lose his temper and is emotionally labile:* Behavioural changes are common and include wandering, agitation and aggression. Paranoia with persecutory delusions occurs in upto 50% of patients.
- *No history of infectious diseases or trauma:* Though AD can develop long after head trauma, majority have no risk factors.

CONFUSA
Apraxia (as impaired ability to carry out motor activities despite intact motor function) and agnosia (the failure to recognize or identify objects despite intact sensory functions) are characteristic of AD.

Investigation of choice
Histology (rarely used)

Immediate management
Rule out other dementia (with neuroimaging, B_{12}, TSH).

Treatment of choice
MRC menu (see page 536, OHCM, 5th edn).

Your Notes:

22.
A 74-year-old man presents with weakness in his arm and leg (from which he recovered within a few days) and short term memory loss. He has an extensor plantar response. He had a similar episode two years ago and became unable to identify objects and to make proper judgements.

Diagnosis: Vascular dementia (multi-infarct dementia)

Clinchers

- *74-year-old:* Prevalence and severity of vascular dementia increases with age as the incidence of cerebrovascular accidents (which predispose to it). increases.
- *Man:* Male have more prevalence of vascular diseases.
- *Weakness in his arm and leg (from which he recovered within a few days):* This represents a stroke which is the predisposing factor for vascular dementia.
- *Short-term memory loss:* This signifies dementia which is most probably of new onset.
- *Extensor plantar:* It signify a pyramidal lesion as the normal flexor plantar has become extensor.
- *Similar episode two years ago..... judgements:* There is usually a history of TIAs with brief impairment of consciousness, fleeting paresis or visual loss. The dementia may follow a succession of acute CVAs or less commonly a single major stroke.

CONFUSA
Vascular dementia is the second most common cause of dementia is distinguished from Alzheimer's disease by its history of onset, clinical features and subsequent course. Vessel occlusion is the most common cause of vascular dementia, and this may produce a variety of cognitive deficits depending on the site of the ischaemic damage. It is typically associated with signs of cortical dysfunction.

Investigation of choice
Clinical ± MRI + Psychometric testing (e.g. Wechsler scale)

Immediate management
Counselling of family

Treatment of choice
None

Your Notes:

23. A 38-year-old haemophiliac who received several blood transfusions a few years ago presents with irritability and increasing memory deficit. He is unable to speak properly. He is on antitubercular treatment.

Diagnosis: HIV (AIDS-dementia complex)

Clinchers
- *38-year-old haemophiliac:* Prevalence of AIDS and HIV is more in older haemophiliacs who have been treated with transfusions before mid 80's (i.e. before the advent of HIV testing).
- *Irritability and increasing deficit + unable to speak properly:* This is a diffuse, progressive usually fatal HIV-related dementia, sometimes associated with a cerebellar syndrome. It is thought to be due cerebral HIV infection.
- *He is on anti TB treatment:* TB is frequently associated with AIDS that represents symptomatic state of HIV infection.

CONFUSA
AIDS dementia complex (ADC) has varying degrees of severity, ranging from mild memory impairment and poor concentration through to severe cognitive deficit, personality change and psychomotor slowing. Changes in effect are common and depressive or psychotic features may be present. The spinal cord may show vacuolar myelopathy. In severe cases brain CT scan shows atrophic changes. MRI changes consists of lesions in white matter (T_2 section). EEG may show non-specific changes consistent with encephalopathy. CSF neopterin concentration may be raised.

Investigation of choice
CT scan/MRI

Immediate management
Rule out distal sensory polyneuropathy which is frequently associated with ADC.

Treatment of choice
Zidovudine has a beneficial effect on HIV neurological disease, with startling improvement in cognitive function in many patients with ADC.

Your Notes:

---

24. A 34-year-old woman presents with memory loss, poor concentration and inability to recognize household objects. On examination she has a right handed involuntary writhing movement. There is a strong family history of similar complaints.

Diagnosis: Huntington's chorea (HC)

Clinchers
- *34-year-old:* The onset is usually in middle age. Death usually occurs between 10 and 20 years after the onset.
- *Woman:* Both sexes have equal incidence as it is an autosomal dominant trait.
- *Presents with memory loss, poor concentration and inability to recognize household objects:* This is dementia.
- *Right handed involuntary writhing movements:* This is chorea. Relentlessly progressive chorea and dementia in middle life are the hallmarks of this inherited disease.
- *Strong family history of similar complaints:* Inheritance of HC is an autosomal dominant trait with full penetrance, the children of an affected parent have a 50% chance of inheriting the disease.

CONFUSA
The family history of the disease in previous generations is often concealed, either by design or default. There is steady progression, of both the dementia and chorea. No treatment arrests the disease, although Phenothaizines (e.g. sulpiride) may reduce the chorea, by causing drug induced Parkinsonism. Tetrabenazine helps to control the movements. Mutation analysis, which is accurate and specific, is available for presymptomatic testing of family members.

Investigation of choice
Neuroimaging (if possible with the chorea, will show atropy of caudate nucleus).

Immediate management
Patient and family counselling.

Treatment of choice
Phenothiazines +/or tetrabenazine.

Your Notes:

25. A 62-year-old patient with chronic schizophrenia presents with mask-like face and involuntary pill rolling movement in both hands. He complains of chronic cough and forgetfulness.

Diagnosis: Parkinsonism (drug induced)

Clinchers

- *62-year-old:* The disease is common and worldwide, with prevalence increasing sharply with age to about 1 in 200 in those above 70 years.
- *Chronic schizophrenia:* This suggests a chronic use of antipsychotics which can induce parkinsonism as a long term side effects.
- *Mask like face:* This is the impassive facial expression which is typical of parkinsonism.
- *Involuntary pill rolling movement in both hands:* This athetosis and characteristically seen in parkinsonism (between thumb and forefingers).
- *Chronic cough:* This is due to anticholinergic side effects of antipsychotics (laryngeal dryness causes cough).
- *Forgetfulness:* Dementia usually accompanies it (but not present as such in parkinsonism).

CONFUSA
In Parkinson's disease a stoop is characteristic and the gait is shuffling and festinant and with poor arm swinging. The posture is sometimes called 'simian' to describe the ape-like forward flexion, immobility of the arms and lack of facial expression.

Investigation of choice
There is no laboratory test for the disease. The diagnosis is made by recognising the clinical pattern.

Immediate management
Rule out other brain diseases

Treatment of choice
Levodopa

Your Notes:

26. A 60-year-old woman hypertensive was started on antihypertensive 2 weeks ago. Now has a creatinine level of 500 micromol/L.

Diagnosis: Acute renal failure

Clinchers

- *On antihypertensive 2 week ago:* Angiotensin converting enzyme activity inhibition (ACE inhibitors) and renal prostaglaind biosynthesis (cyclooxygenase inhibitor) inhibitors are the major culprits, leading to renal hypoperfusion, leading to prerenal azotemia.
  Captopril is an ACE inhibitor that lowers the BP.
  Captopril induces hypotension as a result of decrease in total peripheral resistance. Both systolic and diastolic BP falls.
- *Creatinine level of 500 Hmol/L:* Normal value of creatinine in plasma ranges between 70-≤ 150 mmol/L. Recent increase in the plasma urea and creatinine concentration are the biochemical indictors of acute renal failure.

CONFUSA
On captopril, renal blood flow is not compromised even when BP falls substantially, but for in patients with bilateral renal artery stenosis due to dilatation of efferent arterioles and fall in glomerular filtration pressure, therefore contraindicated in such patients.

Investigation of choice
- Blood tests: U&E, FBC, creatinine, blood culture.
- Urine: Microscopy & biochemical tests.
- ECG (hyperkalemia).

Immediate management
- Change in antihypertensive therapy.
- Adjust doses of renally excreted drugs.

Manage complications, (hyperkalemia, pulmonary edema, bleeding). Seek specialist help sooner rather than later.

Drug producing this condition
Captopril.

Your Notes:

27. A child with recurrent nephrotic syndrome is brought for treatment. Three weeks after start of treatment, he now has massive haematuria.

Diagnosis: Haemorrhagic cystitis

Clinchers
- *Child with recurrent nephrotic syndrome:* Minimal change disease accounts for 80% of nephrotic syndrome in children. MCD is highly steroid responsive, but relapses occur in 50% of cases following withdrawal of glucocorticoids. In such patients upto fail to achieve lasting remission, alkylating agents are usual. *Cyclophosphamide* (2 to 3 mg/kg per day) or chlorambucil (0.1 to 0.2 mg/kg per day) is started after steroid induced remission and continued for 8 to 12 weeks.
- *Now develops massive haematuria:* Microscopic haematuria may be present in MCD (in 20-30 percent cases). But massive haematuria here is a sign of cystitis, which may occur with the use of cyclophosphamide.

CONFUSA
The benefits of cyclophosphamide must be balanced against risk of infertility, cystitis, alopecia, infection and secondary malignancies.

Investigation of choice
Cystoscopy

Immediate management
Stop cyclophospamide

Treatment of choice
Long term renal and patient survival is excellent in MCD. Titrate the risk of cyclophosphide, otherwise MCD is highly steroid.

Drug producing this condition
Cyclophosphamide

Your Notes:

28. A patient in severe renal failure has potassium level of 2.5 mmol/L.

Diagnosis: Hypokalemia (Answer: Frusemide)

Clinchers
- *Severe renal failure:* May be due to glomerulonephritis, pyelonephritis, interstitial nephritis, DM, hypertension, cystic diseases, etc. In CRF there is usually, irreversible and long-standing loss of renal function. In CRF treatment is aimed at treating reversible causes (relieve obstruction, stop nephrotoxic drugs, treat hypercalcemia). High does of loop diuretics (frusemide) are used to treat edema.
- *Potassium level of 2.5:* Normal range of potassium is 3.5-5 mmol/L. Hypokalaemia is the most significant problem with high ceiling diuretics (frusemide) and thiazides. Usual manifestations of hypokalemia are weakness, fatigue, muscle cramps and cardiac arrhythmias.

CONFUSA
Hypokalemia is less common with standard doses of high ceiling diuretics (frusemide), than with thiazides, possibly because of shorter duration of action of the former which permits intermittent operation of compensatory reflection mechanism.

Investigation of choice
- Blood: FBC, ESR, U and E, Creatinine, Serum calcium
- Urine: Microscopy, creatinine clearance
- Renal ultrasound

Immediate management
Change frusemide with potassium sparing Diuretics

Treatment of choice
For hypokalaemia: Attempt to maintain serum K^+ at or above 3.5 mEq/L, by:
- High dietary K^+ intake
- Supplements of KCl (24-72 mEq/day) or
- Concurrent use of K^+ sparing diuretics

Your Notes:

29. Patient with complaint of ataxia and tinnitus with mild hearing loss. He has moderate renal failure.

Diagnosis: Ototoxicity (Answer: Gentamycin).

Clinchers
Aminoglycoside antibiotics (gentamycin) have a narrow therapeutic index. Most important side effects being nephrotoxocity and ototoxicity. Rarely respiratory depression may be observed.

Nephrotoxicity is manifested clinically by a gradual rise in serum creatinine levels after a few days of therapy.

Ototoxicity from aminoglycosides therapy presents as either auditory or vestibular damage.

CONFUSA
Fear to toxicity should not prevent the use of aminoglycosides for a legitimate indication, since toxicity is usually mild and reversible.

Investigation of choice
- Serum concentration of gentamycin
- Blood urea or Serum creatinine

Immediate management
Stop gentamycin. When serum concentration are monitored and duration of therapy kept minimum, then adverse effect are unlikely.

Treatment of choice
Substitute gentamicin with a safe drug.

Your Notes:

---

30. A fit 50-year-old man is prescribed oral Acetazolamide by an Ophthalmologist for suspected glaucoma. He presents with lethargy and shortness of breath on exertion. Sodium 140 mmol/L, Potassium 3.2 mmol/L, Bicarbonate 18 mmol/L, Chloride 115 mmol/L, Urea 6.7 mmol/L, Creatinine 114 mmol/L.

Diagnosis: Type II renal tubular acidosis (Proximal RTA)

Clinchers
- *Fit 50 year old man:* Excludes any pre-existing pathology to be the cause of this condition.
- *Oral acetazolamide:* Acetazolamide causes increased renal bicarbonate losses. Hence it is the most probable cause in this case.
- *Lethargy and shortness of breath on exertion:* These are due to hypokalemia and acidosis respectively.
- *Sodium 140 mmol/L:* Normal.
- *Potassium 3.5 mmol/L:* Low, as hypokalaemia is a feature.
- *Bicarbonate 18 mmol/L:* Low as acetazolamide ↑ renal losses.
- *Urea 6.7 mmol/L:* Normal, but still on higher side (range 2.5-6.7 mmol/L).
- *Creatinine 114 mmol/L:* Normal.

CONFUSA
Renal tubular acidosis generally may be secondary to immunological drug-induced or structural damage to the tubular cells, an inherited abnormality, or an isolated (primary) abnormality. As with most disorders which are not well understood, the nomenclature is confusing.

Investigation of choice
Urinary pH and serum electrolytes

Immediate management
Discontinue acetazolamide if still taking

Treatment of choice
Sodium bicarbonate (massive doses may be required to overcome the renal 'leak').

Your Notes:

31. A 43-year-old man is brought to the Accident and Emergency Department delirious, following and injury at a rugby match. His Glasgow Coma Scale (GCS) at the scene of injury is 13. On examination, his right pupil is fixed and dilated and GCS is now 7. Initial resuscitation has been done. The neurosurgeon is 30 minutes away.

Diagnosis: Extra-dural hemorrhage (EDH).

Clinchers
- *Following injury:* EDH is common after direct head injuries, although subdural hematoma may also occur.
- *A lucid interval, where GCS is initially 13 and later 7:* This is a hallmark of a significant EDH.
- *Right pupil fixed and dilated:* Since ipsilateral pupillary dilatation occurs but it is a late sign.
- *Initial resuscitation has been done:* It means that now secondary management is required which in this case is management of EDH.
- *Neurosurgeon is 30 minutes away:* Since he will take time to come and evaluate this patient, immediate drilling of burr-holes should be the urgent step.

> **CONFUSA**
> CT brain scan can be definitive in forming a diagnosis but no time should be lost in conducting the investigation since GCS is rapidly decreasing.

Investigation of choice
CT—Head.

Immediate management
Drilling of burr holes.

Treatment of choice
Drilling of burr holes followed by neurosurgical ligation of bleeding vessels.

Your Notes:

32. A 22-year-old motorist arrives in the Accident and Emergency Department after an accident. His airway is patent. He is noted to have a splinted right leg.

Diagnosis: Normal saline infusion.

Clinchers
- *22-year-old motorist:* Young motorists constitute a high risk group for RTA.
- *Airway patent:* This suggest that managment of primary survey is over.
- *Splinted right leg:* This suggests that there may be a femoral fracture and also the fact that secondary survey is also over. Femoral fractures are associated with profuse blood loss and no time should be wasted in restoring the blood volume.

> **CONFUSA**
> Restoration of blood volume is best done by blood transfusion but arranging blood and cross-matching have taken time. So the first priority in such patients should be to start with a plasma expander immediately (i.e. haemaccel) and transfuse blood later on. But since it is not given as an option, infusion of normal saline is the safest answer here.

Investigation of choice
X-ray (right thigh).

Immediate management
Haemaccel/Normal saline
+
Admit.

Treatment of choice
Surgical/conservative management of fracture femur.

Your Notes:

November—2001

33. A 30-year-old man is involved in a fight. He has a bruise on the cheek. He complains of an acute abdominal pain and is vomiting. He had a herniorraphy two weeks ago. He is conscious and fundoscopy has not been done.

Diagnosis: Wound dehiscence

Clinchers
- *30-year-old is involved in a fight:* This necessiates the exclusion of occult head or abdominal injuries to rule out serious trauma.
- *Bruise on cheek:* Most probably this signifies no fatal head injury.
- *Acute abdominal pain:* It could be due to blunt abdominal trauma or wound dehiscence.
- *Herniorraphy two weeks ago:* This suggests that the wound of the operation, though sealed by now, is weak and prove to dehiscence.
- *Conscious:* Rules out head injury for the moment but continuous observation is required.

CONFUSA
Fundoscopy has not been done in this patient. It is usually done to rule out raised ICT which is represented by papilloedema. But since our suspicioun of head injury or haematoma formation is minimal and abdominal injury is high, this investigation can be postponed or even excluded in the order of priorities.

Investigation of choice
USG.

Immediate management
Take the patient to OT.

Treatment of choice
Surgical repair.

Your Notes:

---

34. A 29-year-old motorist, in the Accident and Emergency Department resuscitation room, appears to be stable after an accident. While standing up, he becomes progressively dyspnoeic. There is reduced air entry on the left side of his chest.

Diagnosis: Tension pneumothorax

Clinchers
- *29-year-old motorist:* The incidence of RTA is maximum in young motorcylists. The accident must have caused chest trauma and hence a rib fracture which could've been easily missed in presence of other serious and more evident injuries.
- *Progressively dyspnoeic:* Progressive dyspnoea suggests a tension pneumothorax. It is a medical emergency and can lead to a fatal outcome if not treated urgently.
- *While standing up:* The process of mobilisation might have pushed the sharp end of a fractured rib against the pleura and thereby puncturing it to produce this condition.
- *Reduced air entry on left side of chest:* This confirms our diagnostic suspicion, or at least provide as enough clinical ground to proceed a head with management of tension pneumothorax

CONFUSA
Traumatic pneumothoraxes can result from both penetrating and nonpenetrating chest trauma. Tension pneumothorax usually occurs during mechanical ventilation or resuscitative efforts. Tension pneumothorax must be treated as a medical emergency. If the tension in the pleural space is not relieved, the patient is likely to die from inadequate cardiac output or marked hypoxaemia. A large bore needle should be inserted into the plerual space through the second anterior intercostal space. If large amounts of gas escape from the needle after insertion, the diagnosis is confirmed. The needle should be left in place until a thoracostomy tube can be inserted.

Investigation of choice
CXR (but after needle thoracocentesis).

Immediate management
Immediate needle thoracocentesis.

Treatment of choice
Chest drain (must in all cases of traumatic pneumothorax).

35. An 18-year-old girl is being resuscitated after an accident. Her airway is secure. She complains of neck pain. Her pulse rate is 100 beats/min and blood pressure is 110/70 mmHg. Glasgow Coma Scale is 13. She has a deformed left thigh.

Diagnosis: Polytrauma

Clinchers
- *18-year-old girl:* Young patients can be resuscitated successfully most of the time after RTA. All she needs is urgent and coordinated medical care.
- *Airway secure:* This means that primary survey is over and we now need to focus on secondary survey.
- *Neck pain:* This could be due to spinal, vertebral or soft tissue injuries of neck which are very common after RTA e.g Whiplash injuries. Since primary survey has been over the neck must have been stabilised. This complaint thus does not require any urgent intervention
- *Pulse 100 bpm:* This is tachycardia and an indication to rule out hypovolemia or continuing blood loss.
- *BP 110/70:* This is normal but can be deceptive as BP does not fall till about 25% of circulating blood volume is lost.
- *GCS 13:* This may indicate a concussion injury or a severe head injury. Definitive care will require urgent evaluation of neurological condition and head injuries by a neurosurgeon after stabilising ABC (Airway, breathing and circulation).
- *Deformed left thigh:* This could be the source of continuing blood loss so its splintage now has a priority over almost everything (as it constitutes management of C in ABC)

CONFUSA
Gross swelling of thigh after RTA should always arouse suspicion of a rupture of the femoral artery. Otherwise shock is rare with an isolated fracture, but blood replacement may be necessary. Sciatic nerve injury occasionally occurs.

Investigation of choice
X-ray cervical spine and femur.

Immediate management
Splint the limb +
Neurosurgical referral +
Haemaccel.

Treatment of choice
Fixation of fracture + treatment of other injuries.

36. A nine-year-old boy has a mild cough and wheeze after playing football in the cold weather.

Diagnosis: Exercise induced asthma

Clinchers
- *Nine year old boy:* Exercise induced asthma is most commonly present in childhood.
- *Mild cough and wheeze:* These are the diagnostic symptoms of asthma.
- *After playing football in cold weather:* Cold weather and exercise are both precipitants of asthma. Exercise is one of the most common precipitants of acute episodes of asthma. Exercise probably provokes bronchospasm to some extent in every asthmatic patients, and in some it is the only trigger that produces symptoms. There is a significant interaction between the ventilation produced by exercise, the temperature, and the water content of the inspired air and the magnitude of the postexertional obstruction.

CONFUSA
Cromoglycate is used prophylaxis is mild and exercised asthma (always inhaled), especially in children. Note that it may precipitate asthma. Exercise induction differs from other naturally occurring provocations of asthma, such as antigens or viral infections, in that it does not evoke any long-term sequelae nor does it change airway reactivity.

Investigation of choice
PEFR

Immediate management
Nebulisation.

Treatment of choice
Prophylactic inhaled sodium cromoglycate.

Your Notes:

37. A six-year-old girl with asthma uses her bronchodilator twice a day to relieve her mild wheeze. Her parents refuse to give her any treatment containing corticosteroids

Diagnosis: Asthma

Clinchers
- *Six-year-old girl:* Sodium cromoglycate is preferred treatment for mild cases of asthma in children.
- *Uses her bronchodilator twice a day to relieve her mild wheeze:* If occasional short acting bronchodilators are required for symptom relief for more than once daily or night time symptoms, go to step 2 of British thoracic society guidelines (BTS guidelines).
- *Refuse to give her any treatment containing corticosteroids:* Since step 2 and step 3 of BTS guidelines are based on steroids, we will proceed to step 4 which recommends sodium cromoglycate for children.

CONFUSA
Usually all the questions pertaining to treatment of asthma in PLAB exam are based upon BTS guidelines. Refer to them on page 172, OHCM, 5th edn or www.bnf.org.

Investigation of choice
PEFR monitoring

Immediate management
Evaluate for antigens precipitants

Treatment of choice
Inhaled sodium cromoglycate
(addition of it to the existing bronchodilator treatment)

Your Notes:

38. A nine-year-old girl with chronic asthma presents to the. A and E department with rapidly worsening wheeze not relieved with inhaled bronchodilators.

Diagnosis: Acute episode of severe asthma

Clinchers
- *Nine-year-old girl:* In childhood there is a 2:1 male/female preponderance, but the sex ratio equalizes by age 30.
- *Chronic asthma:* This increases the risk of status asthmatics.
- *Rapidly worsening wheeze:* This suggest urgent intervention as the condition is worsening.
- *Not relieved with inhaled bronchodilators:* Acute attacks need to be treated with steroids if bronchodilators are not effective.

CONFUSA
Glucocorticoids are not bronchodilators, and their major use in asthma is in reducing airway inflammation. Systemic or oral steroids are most beneficial in acute illness when severe airway obstruction is not resolving or is worsening despite intense optimal bronchodilator theory, and in chronic disease when there has been failure of a previously optimal regimen with frequent recurrences of symptoms of increasing severity.

Investigation of choice
None required

Immediate management
Nebulised bronchodilators

Treatment of choice
Oral steroids.

Your Notes:

39.
A four-year-old boy with eczema and recurrent wheeze whenever he gets a viral infection has now developed night cough, there as been no improvement in spite of using inhaled bronchodilator twice each night.

Diagnosis: Asthma

Clinchers
- *Four-year-old boy:* In young children, the most important infections agents are respiratory syncytial virus and parainfluenza virus.
- *Eczema and recurrent wheeze:* Well-controlled studies have demonstrated that respiratory viruses and not bacteria or allergy are the major etiologic factors. Although asthma is most commonly associated with atropy (e.g. eczema).
- *Viral infection:* Respiratory viral infections, are the most common of the stimuli that evoke acute exacerbations of asthma.
- *Night cough despite bronchodilators twice each night:* This suggest that the bronchodilators should be changed to long acting ones or additional drugs are required.

CONFUSA
Cromolyn and nedocromil, like the inhaled steroids, improve lung function and reduce symptoms and lower airway reactivity in asthmatics. They are most effective in atopic patients who have either seasonal disease or perennial airway stimulation.

Investigation of choice
PEFR before sleep.

Immediate management
Rule out any heart disease.

Treatment of choice
Inhaled sodium cromoglycate (Additional).

Your Notes:

40.
A 14-year-old boy, with well controlled asthma, using inhaled steroids and a bronchodilator comes to the A and E. Department with breathlessness and swollen lips after eating a peanut, butter-sandwich.

Diagnosis: Anaphylaxis

Clinchers
- *Well controlled asthma, using inhaled steroids and a bronchodilator:* This is step 2 treatment in BTS guidelines. Since it is well controlled a severe acute attack of asthma is unlikely is this patient.
- *Breathlessness and swollen lips after eating a peanut butter-sandwich:* This is an anaphylactic reaction to peanut which is common among caucasians. It requires management on its guidelines. But since he is an asthmatic, oral bronchodilator can be added on as required basis.

CONFUSA
It is a type I IgE mediated hypersensitivity reaction to peanut. Release of histamine and other agents.

Causes: Capillary leak, wheeze, cyanosis, oedema of larynx, lids, tongue and lips, urticaria. These more common in atopic individuals. Other foods which are commonly involved are eggs, fish and strawberries.

Investigation of choice
ECG monitoring

Immediate management
Admit + IM adrenaline (Not IV unless the patient is severely ill or has no pulse).

Treatment of choice
As required oral brochodilator.

Your Notes:

41. Chest X-ray shows raised right diaphragm with small pleural effusion above.

Diagnosis: Subphrenic abscess

Clinchers
- *Chest X-ray shows....:* In subphrenic abscess the chest X-ray may show the following:
  - Elevation of the diaphragm on the affected side.
  - Pleural effusion and/or collapse of the lung base.
  - Gas and fluid level below the diaphragm.

CONFUSA
A localized collection of pus may occur in the subphrenic region following general peritonitis. Usually the underlying cause is a peritonitis involving the upper abdomen—leakage following biliary or gastric surgery or a perforated peptic ulcer. Rarely, infection occurs from haematogenous spread or from direct spread from a primary chest lesion, e.g. emphysema.

Investigation of choice
- *Screening:* CXR (already done in this case)
- *Definitive:* CT scan

Immediate management
Find the cause (evident in this case)

Treatment of choice
Broad spectrum antibiotics
↓
If fails
↓
Ultrasound/CT guided percutaneous drainage

Your Notes:

42. Ultrasound scan shows intra-abdominal free fluid with paralytic ileus.

Diagnosis: Biliary peritonitis

Clinchers
- *Intra-abdominal free fluid:* In advanced peritonitis the abdomen becomes distended and tympanitic, signs of free fluid are present, the patient becomes increasingly, toxic with a rapid, feeble pulse, vomiting is faeculent and the skin is moist, cold and cyanosed (the Hippocratic Facies).
- *Paralytic ileus:* Because of it the abdomen is silent in peritonitis or the transmitted sounds of the heart beat and respiration may be detected.

CONFUSA
Bile peritonitis is only a rare accompaniment of acute cholecystitis, because unlike the appendix, which when inflamed rapidly undergoes gangrene, the inflamed gallbladder is usually thickened and walled off by adhesions. In addition, again unlike the appendix, which only receives an end-artery supply from the ileo-colic artery, the gallbladder has an additional blood supply from the liver bed, therefore, frank gangrene of the inflamed gallbladder is unusual.

Investigation of choice
Erect CXR.

Immediate management
IV morphine.

Treatment of choice
Laparotomy (required to deal with the underlying cause, but the mortality is approximately 50%).

Your Notes:

43. Liver function tests show raised alkaline phosphatase, raised bilirubin, normal albumin and normal hepatocellular enzymes.

Diagnosis: Stone in common bile duct (choledocholithiasis)

Clinchers
- *Liver function tests:* They are performed whenever jaundice, part or present, is a feature.
- *Raised alkaline phosphatase:* Persistently raised alkaline phosphatase is always suspicious of choledocholithiasis.
- *Raised bilirubin:* Stone in CBD is associated with jaundice in 75% cases.
- *Normal albumin and hepatocellular enzymes:* This rules out lives injury and hence suggest a CBD pathology.

CONFUSA
Differential diagnosis of stone in the CBD is as follows:
- With jaundice (75%)
  - Carcinoma pancreas or other malignant obstruction of CBD
  - Acute hepatitis
  - Other causes of jaundice
- Without jaundice (25%)
  - Renal colic
  - Intestinal obstruction or angina pectoris

Investigation of choice
USG

Immediate management
IV vitamin K (as depressed absorption of this fat soluble vitamin lower the serum prothrombin with consequent bleeding tendency).

Treatment of choice
Conservative management with subsequent exploration of CBD or emergency endoscopic sphincterectomy if severe.

Your Notes:

44. Ultrasound scan shows dilated common bile duct with no free intra-abdominal fluid or bowel distension.

Diagnosis: Stone in common bile duct

Clinchers
- *Dilated CBD:* USG demonstrate dilatation of the duct system suggesting distal duct obstruction and hence is an invaluable investigation in this case.
- *No free intra-abdominal fluid or bowel distention:* This rules out any biliary leakage or peritonitis. Still barium meal or upper GI endoscopy are advisable in cases of chronic cholecystitis to exclude an associated peptic ulcer or hiatus hernia.

CONFUSA
Unfortunately, USG, like CT scan, is unreliable in detecting stones in the bile ducts, especially at the lower ends.

Investigation of choice
USG

Immediate management
IV vitamin K (see previous Q)

Treatment of choice
See previous Q.

Your Notes:

45. Chest X-ray shows signs of left ventricular dilatation and an electrocardiograph (ECG) shows Q waves with ST elevation.

Diagnosis: Myocardial infarction

Clinchers
- *Left ventricular dilatation:* Cardiomegaly may be identified on CXR is cases of MI.
- *Q waves:* Acute Q waves signify transmural infarction. T wave inversion and the development of Q waves follow over hours to days.
- *ST elevation:* Hyperacute T waves, ST elevation or new LBBB occur with hours of acute Q waves.

CONFUSA
This complication most often occurs in older patients because of preexisting pathology. Cholecystectomy may be adviced when the patient is young and other wise well, as symptomless stones may eventually produce the numerous problems. If the patient is elderly and unfit, symptomless stones are left untreated.

Investigation of choice
ECG

Immediate management
High flow O_2 + IV morphine

Treatment of choice
Thromblysis.

Your Notes:

46. A 50-year-old woman underwent an anterior resection for carcinoma of the rectum one week ago. Has low grade fever and with complaint of pain in the calf + tenderness in the calf.

Diagnosis: Deep vein thrombosis

Clinchers
- *50-year-old:* Incidence of this complication is particularly more in:
  - Elderly
  - Obese
  - Those with malignant disease
  - Who have varicose veins
  - History of previous DVT
  - Those undergoing
    - Abdominal surgery
    - Pelvic surgery
    - Hip surgery (most common)
  - Women on
    - OCP
    - HRT
  - Presence of predisposing factors
    - Reduced levels of endogenous anticoagulants
      - protein C
      - protein S
      - antithrombin III
    - Possession of the Leiden mutation of coagulation factor V
- *Anterior resection for carcinoma of rectum:* Pelvic surgeries have the highest incidence of DVT post-operatively
- *One week ago:* DVT typically occurs in the second post-operative week (see confusa also)
- *Low grade fever:* DVT is often associated with a mild pyrexia. The skin temperature of the affected calf is invariably raised (due to dilatation of the superficial veins of the leg and inflammatory reaction).
- *Complaint of pain in calf:* It is the major presenting feature and is usually associated with swelling and redness.
- *Tenderness in calf:* This confirm that pain is due to DVT only.

CONFUSA
DVT usually occurs during the second postoperative week. Earlier thrombosis particularly occurs when the patient has already been in hospital for some time preoperatively. Radioiodine studies have confirmed that the thrombotic process usually commence at, or soon after, the operation. The classical *Homan's sign*

(↑ resistance to forced foot dorsiflexion, which may be painful) is positive in less than 20% cases and cannot be relied upon. On the contrary, it may dislodge thrombus giving rise to thromboembolism.

Investigation of choice
Doppler USG/venogram.

Immediate management
Enoxapain 1 mg/kg BD or 1.5 mg/kg/OD.

Treatment of choice
Heparin for 3 months.

Your Notes:

47. A young woman underwent emergency appendicectomy 6 days ago for perforated appendix. She appeared to be making a good recovery but has developed intermittent pyrexia (up to 39°C). On examination—no obvious cause found, but she is tender anteriorly on rectal examination.

Diagnosis: Anterior pelvic abscess

Clinchers
- *Appendicectomy:* A pelvic abscess may follow any general peritonitis, but it is particularly common after acute appendicitis (75%), or after gynaecological infections.
- *Perforated appendix:* This increases the chances of development of the abscess manifold as there is direct exposure of the septic load.
- *Good recovery:* Rules out any systemic involvement.
- *Intermittent pyrexia (upto 39°C):* This is the characteristic swinging pyrexia and points towards an abscess somewhere in body.
- *Tender anteriorly on rectal examination:* This suggests that the abscess in situated anteriorly between the uterus and posterior fornix of vagina.

CONFUSA
In the male the abscess lies between the bladder and the rectum, in the female between the uterus and posterior fornix of the vaginal anteriorly, and the rectum posteriorly (pouch of Douglas). An early pelvic cellulitis may respond rapidly to a short cause of chemotherapy, but there is the risk that the prolonged antibiotic treatment of an unresolved infection may produce a chronic inflammatory mass. It is safer therefore, where there is an established pelvic abscess, to withhold chemotherapy and await pointing into the vagina (as in this case) or rectum through which surgical drainage can be carried out.

Investigation of choice
USG/CT scan.

Immediate management
Chemotherapy (see confusa also).

Treatment of choice
Drainage of abscess.

Your Notes:

48. An elderly man underwent an emergency repair of an abdominal aortic aneurysm. He had been severely hypotensive before and during surgery. After surgery, his blood pressure was satisfactory, but urine output only 5 ml/hr in the first 2 hours.

Diagnosis: Acute tubular necrosis (Ischaemic).

Clinchers

- *Emergency repair of an abdominal aortic aneurysm:* This means that the repair was undertaken after an aneurysmal rupture or acute aortic expansion. Either of these produce a severe hypotension. Moreover, during the surgery the renal arterial ostia are often compressed when the aorta is clamped and are thus rendered ischaemic for the duration of cross clamping. The left renal vein may be ligated and divided as part of the operative procedure. Hypotension pre-or post-operatively may exacerbate the renal injury.
- *Severely hypotensive before and during surgery:* Circulatory compromise produces renal hypoperfusion and thence ischaemic necrosis of the tubules.
- *After surgery, his BP was satisfactory:* This rules out any continuing ischaemia and a need for urgent intervention. Also it suggests a definitive injury to the kidney.
- *Urine output only 5 ml/hr in first 2 hours:* Urine output should be >30 mL/hr postoperatively. A value significantly lower than this suggests renal dysfunction (due to hypoperfusion or ATN).

CONFUSA

Low urine output (if there is no ATN) postoperatively is almost always due to inadequate infusion of fluid. One should check JVP, and review for sings of cardiac failure. Treat by increasing IVI rate unless patient is in heart or renal failure, or profusely bleeding (in that case, blood should be transfused). If in doubt a fluid challenge may be indicated: ½-1 L over 30-60 minutes, with monitoring of urine output. Then the IVI rate may be increased to 1 litre/h for 2-3 h. Only if output does not increase should a diuretic be considered; a CVP line may be needed if estimation of fluid balance is difficult. A normal value is 0-5 cm of water relative to the sternal angle.
Note: If not catheterised exclude retention.

Investigation of choice
Urinary sodium concentration (It differentiates whether the oliguria is prerenal and amenable to fluid therapy or a result of acute tubular necrosis—urinary Na >40 mmol/L.

Immediate management
Perform an aseptic catheterisation
+
early specialist (nephrologist and interminist) referral

Treatment of choice
Supportive until spontaneous recovery of renal function occurs.

Your Notes:

49. An elderly woman underwent emergency laparotomy for peritonitis. Fourth postoperative day she is noted to have serosanguinous discharge from the wound, but there is no erythema or tenderness around the wound.

Diagnosis: Impending burst abdomen.

Clinchers
- *Elderly women:* Incidence of wound dehiscence is more in elderly patients because of poor wound healing and weak abdominal muscles.
- *Peritonitis:* It implies a high septic load in the peritoneal cavity. It can have a significance in etiology of burst abdomen indirectly by inducing wound infection (not likely in this case).
- *Fourth postoperative day:* The abdomen usually dehiscence on about the 10th day. But the warning signs may be visible much before.
- *Serosanguinous discharge from the wound:* This is the blood-tinged serous effusion (which is always present during the first week or two within the abdominal cavity after operation). It usually seeps through the breathing-down wound and serves as a warning of impending burst abdomen.
- *No erythema or tenderness around the wound:* this rules out wound infection and leaves us with only the above diagnosis.

CONFUSA
Sometimes, the deep layer of the abdominal incision gives way but the skin sutures hold; such cases result in a massive incisional hernia.

Investigation of choice
Clinical diagnosis, no investigation required.

Immediate management
Place a sterile dressing over the wound + call seniors.

Treatment of choice
Reassessment of wound in OT.

Your Notes:

---

50. A 60-year-old with features of septicaemia (warm peripheries, low BP etc.) after an abdominal surgery.

Diagnosis: Postoperative septicaemia

Clinchers
- *60-year-old:* Septicaemia is a common postoperative complication among elderly and children because of incomplete immune system
- *Features of septicaemia after an abdominal surgery:* Gram negative septicaemia is particularly seen after colonic, biliary and urological surgery. The principal effect of endotoxins is to cause vasodilatation of the peripheral circulation together with increased capillary permeability. The effects are partly direct, and partly indirect due to activation of normal tissue inflammatory responses such as the complement system and mediators such as tumor necrosis factor.

CONFUSA
Septicaemia is often overlooked as:
- The temperature may not be raised
- The WBC count may be normal or low
- Blood cultures may be negative

The hallmark is impaired tissue perfusion

Investigation of choice
Blood culture (take sample before starting antibiotics).

Immediate management
Colloid/crystalloid IVI + refer to ITU for monitoring ± ionotropes.

Treatment of choice
Cefuroxime 1.5 g/8h IV.
+
Metronidazole 500 mg/6h IV.

Your Notes:

51. For the past two weeks a middle aged railway engineer has complained of acute constipation. His stools are dark, but not apparently blood stained. Abdominal palpation detects a mass with moderate tenderness.

Diagnosis: Colonic cancer (left side)

Clinchers

- *Middle aged railway engineer:* Colon cancer may occur at any age, but it more common after 40.
- *Acute constipation for past two weeks:* In it, typically an adult with presiously regular bowel habit suddenly develops irregularity. There may be increasing difficulty in getting the bowels to move, requiring laxatives. The episodes of constipation may be followed by attacks of diarrhoea.
- *Stools are dark, but not apparently blood stained:* This is malaena, signifying blood loss high in the colon. Otherwise bleed may be bright, malaena or occult.
- *Mass with moderate tenderness:* This confirms our suspicious as there is usually a mass palpable either per abdomen or per rectum.

CONFUSA
Tumors of the left side of the colon, where the contained stool is solid, are typically constricting growths, so obstructive features predominate. In contrast, tumors of the right side tend to be proliferative and here the stools are semi-liquid therefore obstructive symptoms are relatively uncommon and the patient with a carcinoma of the caecum or ascending colon often presents with anaemia and loss of weight. In carcinoma of left side of colon, the lump that is felt on abdominal, rectal or bimanual palpation is sometimes not the tumor itself, but impacted faeces above it. When the tumor is situated in a pendulous pelvic colon, a hard movable swelling may be felt in the rectovesical pouch on rectal examination.

Investigation of choice
Colonoscopy

Immediate management
Laxatives for constipation

Treatment of choice
Surgery

52. A 43-year-old man says he cannot finish his stool and that what he does pass is streaked with blood. He says he has always been regular. He wants to know if a laxative will help.

Diagnosis: Rectal carcinoma

Clinchers

- *43-year-old man:* The sexes are equally affected and it occurs in any age group from the twenties onwards, but is particularly common in age range 50-70 years.
- *He cannot finish his stool:* The patients bowels open but there is a sensation that there are more faeces to be passed. This sense of incomplete defecation is typical of rectal carcinoma.
- *What he does pass is streaked with blood:* The patient may endeavour to empty the rectum several times a day (spurious diarrhoea), often with the passage of flatus and a little blood stained mucus (blood slime).
- *He says he has always been regular:* This signify that the alteration in bowel habits is of recent onset and excludes any pre-existing pathology.
- *Wants to know if a laxative will help:* The patient may find it necessary to start taking an aperient, or to supplement the usual dose and as a result the tendency towards diarrhoea ensues.

CONFUSA
Sence of incomplete defecation results in tenesmus which is a painful straining to empty the bowels without resultant evacuation. This "sense" is a very important early symptom and is almost invariably present in tumours of the lower half of the rectum. Pain is a late symptom. Weight loss is suggestive of hepatic metastases. In approximately 90% of cases the neoplasm can be felt digitally.

Investigation of choice
- *Screening:* Proctosigmoidoscopy
- *Definitive:* Biopsy

Immediate management
Laxatives

Treatment of choice
Surgery —upper 1/3—Anterior resection
　　　　　—middle 1/3—± Anterior resection
　　　　　—lower 1/3—Abdominoperineal resection

53. A 49-year-old lawyer complains of blood and diarrhoea. She is also suffering from abdominal pain, fever, and general ill health. On palpation you find tenderness in the lower abdomen.

Diagnosis: Severe ulcerative colitis (UC)

Clinchers
- *49-year-old lawyer (she):* The sex ratio is equal. It is uncommon before the age of 10 and most patients are between the ages of 20 and 40 at diagnosis.
- *Blood and diarrhoea:* The first symptom is watery or bloody diarrhoea. There may be a rectal discharge of mucus which is either blood-stained or purulent.
- *Abdominal pain, fever, general ill health:* Pain as an early symptom is unusual and suggest severe disease. Other indicators of severe diseases are:
  - more than four motions a day, together with
  - one or more signs of systemic illness, i.e
    - fever over 37.5°C
    - tachycardia > 90/m
    - hypoalbuminemia < 30 g/l
    - weight loss > 3 kg
- *Tenderness in lower abdomen:* May or may not be present in UC.

CONFUSA
Diarrhoea usually implies that there is active disease proximal to the rectum. In 95 percent of cases the disease starts in the rectum and spreads proximally. Bad prognosis is indicated by:
- a severe initial attack
- disease involving whole colon
- increasing age, especially after 60 years

If the disease remains confined to the left colon, the out look is better.

Investigation of choice
- *Screening:* Barium enema
  (findings: • loss of haustrations, • granularity, • pseudopolyps)
- *Definitive:* Colonoscopy and biopsy

Immediate management
Examine for extraintestinal manifestations i.e. arthritis/skin lesions/eye problems/liver and bile duct diseases).
  +
Admit (this case is a medical emergency since this is a severe attack, 1040, Bailey, 23 edn).

Treatment of choice
IV hydrocortisone 100-200 mg QID + rectal infusion of prednisolone + sulfasalazine maintenance/surgery

54. A young woman presents with recurrent abdominal pain, episodic diarrhoea, malaise, and fever. Over the past few years she has felt her health to be declining. At presentation she complains of severe abdominal pain and constipation.

Diagnosis: Crohn's disease (CD)

Clinchers
- *Young woman:* It is slightly more common in females than in males but is more commonly diagnosed in young patients between the ages of 25 and 40. There does seem to be a second peak of incidence around the age of 17.
- *Recurrent abdominal pain, episodic diarrhoea, malaise, and fever:* There is often a history of mild diarrhoea extending over many months occurring in bouts accompanied by intestinal colic. Patients may complain of pain, particularly in the right iliac fossa and there may be a tender mass palpable. Intermittent fevers, secondary anaemia and weight loss are common.
- *Over the past few years she has felt her health to be declining:* It is due to generalised systemic nonspecific effects like loss of appetite, weight loss, anaemia, etc.
- *Severe abdominal pain and constipation:* This could be due to intestinal obstruction after formation of adhesions. Constipation is otherwise rare in this disease.

CONFUSA
Constipation in CD is rare and can be due to:
• After months of repeated attacks with acute inflammation of the affected area of intestine begins to narrow, with fibrosis causing abdominal pain on eating, giving rise to 'food fear' which leads to no formation of stools.
• Delay and dilatation of small intestine causing partial obstruction
• Intestinal adhesions or strictures.

Investigation of choice
Small bowel enema
  ±
Technetium labelled leucocyte scan

Immediate management
Pain relief

Treatment of choice
Mesalazine (for acute attack like this)

55. A young woman complains of cramp-like abdominal pain, and difficulties with bowel movements. Acute abdominal pain is frequently relieved by embarrassing flatulence. Barium studies and sigmoidoscopy have proved inconclusive.

Diagnosis: Irritable bowel syndrome (IBS).

Clinchers

- *Young woman:* Symptoms of IBS typically begin young adulthood (esp. females) and the prevalence of IBS is similar in elderly and young adults.
- *Cramp like abdominal pain and difficulties with bowel movements:* Abdominal pain and altered bowel habits are non-specific symptoms found in patients with a wide variety of illnesses including IBS.
- *Acute abdominal pain is frequently relieved by embarrassing flatulence:* "Manning criteria" for IBS include abdominal pain or discomfort that is relieved by defecation or associated with a change in stool frequency or consistency, abdominal distension, the sensation of incomplete evacuation, and the passage of mucus.
- *Barium studies and sigmoidoscopy have proved inconclusive:* A diagnosis of IBS is based on a careful history to identify characteristic symptoms (e.g. Manning criteria), physical examination, selected laboratory tests, and if necessary, further testing to exclude other disorders.

> **CONFUSA**
> Patients presenting with abdominal pain in the absence of abdominal pain may be considered to have IBS if no alternative explanation for the symptoms is found. However, patients with otherwise unexplained chronic constipation in the absence of abdominal pain are generally considered to have a distinct disorder.

Investigation of choice
All required to exclude other diseases (but not always).

Immediate management
Reassurance + counselling.

Treatment of choice
Symptomatic.

Your Notes:

---

56. A 7-year-old boy presents with a history of acute onset of pain in the knee. On examination, the left lower limb is flexed, abducted, internally rotated.

Diagnosis: Perthes disease.

Clinchers

- *7-year-old:* The condition usually presents at age 7-8, although it may occur at any age from 3 years (or occasionally younger) upto 11 to 12.
- *Boy:* Boys are affected more commonly than girls. 15% of cases are bilateral.
- *History of acute of pain in the knee:* Pain and limb are the usual presenting features. Pain is often slight and may have been present over several weeks.
- *Left lower limb is flexed, abducted and internally rotated:* The clinical signs are usually minor, perhaps slight restriction of movements of the hip, especially internal rotation associated with some spasm.

> **CONFUSA**
> The prognosis of perthes' disease which is sometimes known as Legg-Calve-Perthes disease, is better in younger child and when only part of the head is involved. Girls fare worse than boys for any given age. Many of the difficulties centre around treating a condition which quickly becomes symptom-free and is then only manifest as a senses of changes on X-rays.

Investigation of choice
Radiology.

Immediate management
Bed rest + refer to specialist.

Treatment of choice
Traction (in bed or an abduction frame).

Your Notes:

57. A 67-year-old woman complains of right hip pain. On examination the right hip is adducted, externally rotated and flexed.

Diagnosis: Fracture neck of femur.

Clinchers
- *67-year-old:* In elderly people, the fracture occurs with a seemingly trivial fall. Osteoporosis is considered an important contributory factor at this age.
- *Woman:* Incidence of osteoporosis is more in post menopausal females.
- *Right hip pain:* The elderly patient with fracture neck of femur is usually brought to the casualty department with complaints of pain in the groin and inability to move his limb or bear weight on the limb following a 'trivial' injury like slipping on the floor, missing a step, etc.
- *Right hip is adducted, externally rotated are flexed:* The affected leg may be shortened and externally rotated but this classical appearance is dependent on the grade of the fracture.

CONFUSA
A more valuable sign in fracture neck of femur is pain on gentle passive rotation of the extended leg. If the fracture has impacted, other movements may be good with minimal pain including even straight leg raising. Tenderness is most marked posteriorly.

Investigation of choice
AP and lateral views of hips.

Immediate management
Admit + box splint + analgesia.

Treatment of choice
Internal fixation/hemiarthroplasty.

Your Notes:

58. A 10-year-old girl is febrile. On examination it is difficult to abduct the thighs.

Diagnosis: Septic arthritis.

Clinchers
- *10-year-girl:* In children the most common cause of septic arthritis is osteomyelitis. Minor trauma, soft tissue infection or a non-specific joint inflammation can also lead to it.
- *Difficult to abduct the thighs:* The most common joints to become infected are the interphalangeal joints and the knee. The joint is held in flexion and all movements are restricted by intense pain.
- *Febrile:* This denotes the systemic reaction to sepsis.

CONFUSA
If there is doubt then the patient should be assumed to have a septic arthritis until provided otherwise. Diagnostic joint aspiration is not recommended in the ED. Admission must be arranged under the care of either the orthopaedic or the rheumatology departments, as seems most appropriate from the likely underlying pathology.

Investigation of choice
Radiograph + joint aspiration under specialist care.

Immediate management
Admit.

Treatment of choice
Antibiotics.

Your Notes:

November—2001

59. A child presents with right hip pain. On examination the hip is flexed, abducted and externally rotated.

Diagnosis: Slipped femoral epiphyses

Clinchers
- *Child:* It occurs more commonly in very fat and sexually underdeveloped or tall, thin sexually normal children. It occurs at puberty, between 12-14 years.
- *Right hip pain:* Pain in the groin, often radiating to the thigh and the knee is the common presenting complaint.
- *Hip is flexed, abducted and externally rotated:* On examination, the leg is found to be externally rotated and 1-2 cm short. A limitation of the hip movements is characteristic—there is limited abduction and internal rotation. When the hip is flexed, the knee goes towards the ipsilateral axilla. Muscle bulk may be reduced. Trendelenburg's sign may be positive.

CONFUSA
Often in the initial stages, the symptoms are considered due to a 'sprain', and disregarded. They soon disappear only to recur. Limp occurs early and is more constant. It is more common in boys and in patients with endocrine abnormalities.

Investigation of choice
Radiology.

Immediate management
Prophylactic pinning of the unaffected side.

Treatment of choice
Closed reduction + pinning.

Your Notes:

60. A five-year-old girl complains of progressively increasing severe pain in her left hip and upper leg for 6 days. She is able to walk but limps visibly. Blood tests are as follows: WCC 19/fl, ESR 72 mm/hr and CRP 94 mg/l. X rays and ultrasound scans of the hip are normal.

Diagnosis: Osteomyelitis (acute).

Clinchers
- *Five year old girl:* Acute osteomyelitis occur mainly in children. Poor lining conditions predipose to it, and there may be an obvious primary focus of infection such as a boil, sore throat etc.
- *Progressively increasing severe pain in her left hip and upper leg for 6 days:* Pain is usually localized to the metaphyseal region of the bone.
- *Able to walk but limps visibly:* There is an unwillingness to move because of pain. There may be a visible limp if area of hip and femur and involved.
- *WCC 19/fl, ESR 72 mm/hr and CRP 94 mg/l:* All the inflammatory markers rise as it is as infective condition.
- *X-rays and ultrasound scans of the hip are normal:* X-ray changes are not apparent for few days but then shows haziness and loss of density of affected bone—subperiosteal reaction—sequesterum and involucrum.

CONFUSA
Osteomyelitis can be difficult to differentiate clinically from septic arthritis. But a typical difference between the two is in walking. In osteomyelitis the child may still be able to walk which is not the case with septic arthritis. Also the pain in osteomyelitis is more chronic in onset and less severe than septic arthritis.

Investigation of choice
MRI.

Immediate management
Send blood culture (positive in 60%).

Treatment of choice
Flucloxacillin 250-500 mg/6hr IVI or IM till sequesterum culture reports are known.

Open surgery to drain abscess and remove sequestera.

61. A 69-year-old patient presented to his GP with sudden onset of redness in the right eye. There was no pain and vision was unaffected.

Diagnosis: Subconjunctival haemorrhage

Most appropriate management: No treatment.

Clinchers
Red eye may be due to variety of conditions, but here since there is no pain and the vision is unaffected, no active intervention is required. Though in this case we must check the blood pressure of the patient. No need to go for coagulation studies, as one of the options in this questions suggests.

Subconjunctival haemorrhage may be due to rupture of conjunctival capillaries, due to raised pressure, e.g. in whooping cough, strangulation, epileptic fits, etc. May also be seen in vascular diseases such as arteriosclerosis, hypertension and diabetes mellitus.

CONFUSA
Checking the blood pressure and observation are the main line of treatment in this patient. If any underlying cause is established or suspected, it should be investigated and managed.

Investigation of choice
Not required.

Immediate management
No treatment.

Treatment of choice
Treat the cause when discovered. Assurance to the patient is must. No other active intervention required. Cold compresses can be given in the beginning if bleeding.

Your Notes:

---

62. A 60-year-old patient complains of severe pain in his left eye with severe deterioration of vision. He had noticed haloes around street lights at night for a few days before the onset of the pain.

Diagnosis: Angle closure glaucoma (ACG)

Most appropriate management: 3% pilocarpine drops and acetazolamide.

Clinchers
- *69-year-old patient:* Angle closure glucoma is comparatively most common in 5th to 6th decades of life.
- *Severe pain and deterioration of vision:* Causes of painful (sudden) loss of vision are:
  - Acute congestive glaucoma
  - Acute iridocyclitis
  - Chemical injury to eyeball
  - Mechanical injury to eyeball
- *Coloured haloes:* These are seen around the light due to corneal edema.

CONFUSA
Though the management in this case is essentially surgical, medical therapy of 3% pilocarpine drops and acetazolamide is instituted as an emergency.

Investigation of choice
Gonioscopy

Immediate management
3% pilocarpine and acetazolamide

Treatment of choice
Peripheral iridectomy or filtration surgery. In the interval between confirmation of the diagnosis and surgery use give 3% pilocarpine drops and acetazolamide.

Your Notes:

63. A mother brings her 2-year-old child with a squint. On examination a leucokoric right pupil is seen with an absent red reflex.

Diagnosis: Retinoblastoma

Most appropriate management: Enucleation

Clinchers
- *2-year-old child:* Retinoblastoma is the most common intraocular tumor of childhood. Though congenital, it is not recognised at birth, and is usually seen between 1-2 years of age, with no sex predisposition.
- *Squint:* Usually convergent may develop in retinoblastoma.
- *Leucokoric right pupil:* Conditions other than retinoblastoma that present as leucocoria are: congenital cataract, inflammatory deposits in vitreous following a plastic cyclitis or choroiditis, coloboma of the choroid, retrolental fibroplasia, toxocara endophthalmitis and exudative retinopathy of coats.

CONFUSA
Retinoblastoma should be differentiated from other conditions that present as leukocoria.

Investigation of choice
Fundus examination and ophthalmoscopy
Plain X-ray orbit shows calcification
USG and CT are very useful

Treatment of choice
Enucleation (excision of the eyeball)
Absolute indications of enucleation are:
- retinoblastoma, and
- malignant melanoma

Indications of evisceration (removal of the contents of the eyeball leaving behind the sclera) are
- panophthalmitis
- expulsive choroidal haemorrhage, and
- bleeding anterior staphyloma.

Your Notes:

64. A 12-year-old Libyan boy gave a two-week history of discomfort, redness and mucopurulent discharge affecting both eyes. His two siblings have a similar problem.

Diagnosis: Acute mucopurulent conjunctivitis

Most appropriate management: Immediate antibiotic therapy

Clinchers
- *12-year-old Libyan boy:* Infective conjunctivitis is still common in developing countries.
- *Discomfort, redness, mucopurulent discharge:* There are the symptoms of acute mucopurulent conjunctivitis. Discomfort and foreign body sensation due to engorgement of vessels.
- *Time siblings have similar problem:* Mucopurulent conjunctivitis may be caused by *Staphylococcus aureus* Koch-Weeks bacillus, Pneumococcus or streptococcus. It is infective in nature.

CONFUSA
Conjunctival congestion is more marked in palpebral conjunctiva, fornices and peripheral part of bulbar conjunctiva. Circumcorneal congestion is seen in iridocyclitis.

Investigation of choice
Conjunctival cytology and bacterial examination of secretions and scrapings.

Immediate management
Topical broad spectrum antibiotics to control the infection.

Treatment of choice
Topical antibiotics
- Irrigation of conjunctival sac with sterile warm saline once or twice a day
- Dark goggles
- No bandage
- No steroids (infection may flare up).

Your Notes:

65. A 23-year-old woman has a history of recurrent attacks of blurring of vision associated with redness, pain and photophobia. Both eyes have been affected in the past. She is currently being investigated for bowel disease and a severe backache.

Diagnosis: Multiple sclerosis

Most appropriate management: 0.5% prednisolone drops 2 hrly and cyclopentolate drops

Clinchers
- *23-year-old man:* Multiple sclerosis has female preponderance. Mean age of onset is 30 years.
- *Recurrent attacks of blurring of vision:* Early picture of multiple sclerosis is usually one of relapses followed by remissions become incomplete. In multiple sclerosis, plaques of demyelination are seen at the sites through at the CNS.
- *Bowel disease of severe backache:* Bowel (constipation), fatigue, motor weakness, optic neuritis, incontinence, numbness, tingling in limbs, cerebellar symptoms may be seen in multiple sclerosis.

CONFUSA
Isolated neurological deficits are never diagnostic, but may become so, if a careful history reveals previous episodes.

Investigation of choice
MRI is sensitive

Immediate management
Treat the complication

Treatment of choice
No cure but following may help
- Methylprednisolone (shortens relapses), use sparingly. It does no alter overall prognosis.
- β-interferon: ↓ relapse rate by 1/3.

Your Notes:

66. A child is brought to you with weakness, malaise, and bone pain. On physical examination you find painfully enlarged lymph nodes and hard and enlarged testicles. He has a history of sore throats and chest infections.

Diagnosis: Acute lymphoblastic leukaemia (ALL).

Clinchers
- *Child:* ALL is predominantly a disease of children.
- *Weakness, malaise and bone pain:* Apart from non-specific symptoms like weakness and malaise, there are also specific symptoms like bone pain, arthritis, splenomegaly, lymphadenopathy, thymic enlargement, CNS involvement, e.g. cranial nerve palsies.
- *Painfully enlarged lymph nodes and hard and enlarged testicles:* Patients with ALL can present with infiltration of spleen, lymph nodes, liver, skin or CNS. Involvement of testis as a foci or as an extramedullary site of relapse is not uncommon.
- *History of throats and chest infections:* This increased risk of infection occurs with absolute neutrophil counts less than 500/μL and is the leading cause of death. Infections commonly involve mucosal sites such as the pharynx and perianal area as well as the lungs and skin—particularly IV line sites.

CONFUSA
Patients with ALL present with signs and symptoms of marrow failure. These include pallor and fatigue, bleeding and neutropaenia respectively. With platelet transfusions, haemorrhage is no longer a major cause of death, although alloimmunization can limit optimal platelet support of patients particularly when patients have been heavily transfused.

Investigation of choice
Peripheral blood films and bone marrow biopsy.

Immediate management
Enrol him in national trials.

Treatment of choice
Chemotherapy (page 654, OHCM, 5th edn).

Your Notes:

67. A 51-year-old lecturer presents with lethargy, abdominal pain, fever, and weight loss. On physical examination you find a large spleen. A blood examination shows normocytic normochromic anaemia with a very high white cell count.

Diagnosis: Chronic myeloid leukaemia (CML).

Clinchers

- *51-year-old lecturer:* It occurs most often in middle age with a slight male predominance.
- *Lethargy, abdominal pain, fever, weight loss:* Characteristically CML presents with constitutional symptoms.
- *Large spleen:* In most patients the abnormal finding on physical examination at diagoisis is minimal to moderate splenomegaly; mild hepatomegaly is found occasionally.
- *Normocytic normochromic anaemia:* Platelet counts are almost always elevated at diagnosis and mild degree of normochromic nomocytic anaemia is present.
- *Very high white cell count:* Elevated white blood cell counts with various degrees of immaturity of the granulocytic series are observed at diagnosis.

CONFUSA

The clinical onset of the CML is generally insidious. Accordingly, some patients are diagnosed while asymptomatic, during health screening tests; other patients present with fatigue, malaise, and weight loss or have symptoms resulting from splenic enlargement, such as early satiety and LUQ pain or mass. Less common infections, thrombosis, or bleeding. Occasionally, pateints present with leukostatic manifestations due to severe leukocytosis or thrombosis such as vaso-occlusive disease, CVA, MI, venous thrombosis, priapsim, visual disturbances and pulmonary insufficiency.

Investigation of choice
Blood film.

Immediate management
Cytogenic study to find Philadelphia chromosome whose absence mean poor prognosis.

Treatment of choice
Hydroxyurea.
 +
Allogenic transplantation of bone marrow (Always considered if patient is < 55 yrs).

68. An elderly man presents with backache, pallor, and shortness of breath. He has suddenly had some difficulties with his vision. Blood examination demonstrates a high ESR, and normochromic normocytic anaemia. There is rouleaux formation.

Diagnosis: Multiple myeloma.

Clinchers

- *Elderly:* Myeloma increases in incidence with age. The median age at diagnosis is 68 years. It is rare under age 40.
- *Man:* Males are slightly more commonly affected than females and Blacks have nearly twice the incidence of Whites.
- *Backache:* Bone pain is the most common symptom in myeloma. The pain usually involves the back and ribs.
- *Pallor + shortness of breath:* Due to anaemia and pneumonia respectively.
- *Difficulties with his vision:* Hyperviscosity may lead to headache, fatigue, visual disturbances and retinopathy.
- *High ESR:* Characteristic of multiple myeloma.
- *Normochromic, normocytic anaemia:* It ocucrs in about 80% of myeloma patients and is related both to the replacement of normal marrow by expanding tumor cells and to the inhibition of haematopoiesis by factors made by tumor.
- *Rouleaux formation:* Due to hyperviscosity state seen.

CONFUSA

Unlike the pain of metastatic carcinoma, which often is worse at night, the pain of myeloma is precipitated by movement. Persistent localized fracture. The bone lesions are lytic in nature and are rarely associated with osteoblastic new bone formation; therefore, radioisotope bone scanning is less useful in diagnosis than plain radiography.

Investigation of choice
- *Screening:* ESR
- *Definitive:* Bone marrow biopsy.

Immediate management
Analgesia + transfusion.

Treatment of choice
Chemotherapy
(Melphalan—alone or as ABCM regimen).

69. A young woman complains of weakness, fatigue, and anorexia. Her cervical lymph nodes are enlarged, painless, and rubbery. Her skin itches and she sometimes has night sweats. On physical examination you find her spleen and liver to be enlarged.

Diagnosis: Hodgkin's disease (HD)

Clinchers
- *Young woman:* In Hodgkin's disease the age-specific incidence curve is characteristically bimodal, with an initial peak in young adults (15 to 35 years) and a second peak after age 50. There is increased male prevalence which is most prominent in young adults.
- *Weakness, fatigue and anorexia:* 25 to 30 per cent of patients have some constitutional symptoms at presentation. The most common is low grade fever, which can be associated with recurrent night sweats. Another important presenting symptom is unexplained weight loss of greater than 10 percent over 6 months or less. Fatigue, malaise and weakness are other frequent symptoms.
- *Cervical lymph nodes are enlarged, painless and rubbery:* HD commonly presents with a newly-detected mass or group of lymph nodes that are firm, freely movable and usually nontender. Approximately half of the patients presents with adenopathy in the neck or supraclavicular area, and over 70% of patients present with superficial lymph node enlargement. Because these are frequently non-painful, detection by the patient may be delayed until the lymph nodes are quite large
- *Skin itches:* Pruritus occurs in approximately to 10 per cent of patients of initial diagnosis; it is usually generalized may be associated with a skin rash, and rarely may be the only disease manifestation.
- *Night sweats:* Most common constitutional symptom at presentation is a low grade fever, which can be associated with recurrent night sweats, for same patients night sweats may be the sole complaint. These symptoms ar more commonly seen in older patients and in those with more advanced stage disease.
- *Spleen and liver enlarged:* In HD, primary abdominal disease with hepatomegaly, splenomegaly and massive adenopathy is uncommon, and other neoplastic diseases, especially non-Hodgkin's lymphoma must be excluded under these circumstances.

CONFUSA
Nodes involved by HD tend to be contiguous and or axila in contrast to non-Hodgkin's lymphomas, which have a tendency to be noncontinuous and centrifungal and involve epitrochelar, Waldeyer's and abdominal nodes.

Investigation of choice
Lymph node biopsy.

Immediate management
Immediate symptomatic management.

Treatment of choice
Radiotherapy for stages I_A and II_A
Chemotherapy for II_A to IV_B (ABVD regimen)

Your Notes:

70. A 44-year-old man presents with ill health. He complains of wasting, fever and sweats. He does not have a skin rash, but he does have skin nodules. On physical examination you find disparate groups of lymph nodes to be enlarged.

Diagnosis: Non-Hodgkin's lymphoma (NHL)

Clinchers

- *44-year-old man:* Can occur at any age and with variable expressions in sexes as it constitutes a heterogenous group of lymphomas.
- *Presents with ill health + wasting, fever and sweats:* Unlike patients with Hodgkin's disease who present with weight loss, fever or night sweats, fewer than 20 percent of patients with NHL present with mediastinal adenopathy.
- *Does not have a skin rash, but the does have skin nodules:* Absence of skin rash excludes HD. Skin nodules represent cutaneous lesions found in aggressive NHLs.
- *Disparate groups of lymph nodes to be enlarged:* Unlike HD, which have centripetal (axial) and contiguous lymphadenopathy. NHL is characterised by centripetal (non-axial) and non-contiguous (disparate) lymphadenopathy.

CONFUSA
In teenages and young adults, infections mononucleosis and HD should be placed high in the differential diagnosis. Regarding any lymphadenopathy, it is generally agreed that a firm lymph node larger than 1 cm that is not associated with a documentable infection and that persists longer than 4 weeks should be considered for biopsy.

Investigation of choice
Histology (lymph node biopsy).

Immediate management
Staging of the disease.

Treatment of choice
Since this tumor is appearing to be of a high grade—CHOP regimen chemotherapy.

Your Notes:

71. A homeless patient presents to A and E with drowsiness. On examination, abrasions and puncture marks were found on his arm. He has pin-point pupil.

Diagnosis: Opioid poisoning

Antidote: Naloxone

Clinchers

- *Homeless patient:* Risk factor for drug addiction.
- *Drowsiness:* Stupor, coma, fall in BP, shallow and occasional breathing are all signs of acute opioid poisoning.
- *Abrasions and puncture marks:* Further support the diagnosis of drug injection.
- *Pin-point pupil:* This confirms the diagnosis of opioid poisoning.

CONFUSA
Drowsiness, coma can be caused by benzodiazepines, alcohol, opiates, tricyclic or barbiturates.
Constricted pupils are seen opiates or insecticides (organophosphates). On the other hand dilated pupils are seen in amphetamines, cocaine, quinine or tricyclic.

Investigation of choice
Take blood. Always check for paracetamol and salicylate levels. Diagnosis is mainly from history.

Immediate management
Naloxone e.g. 0.8-2 mg IV repeat every 2 minutes, until breathing adequate.

Treatment of choice
Advocate supportive measures
Start the antidote
Referral to psychiatrist.

Your Notes:

72. This drug competes with vitamin K.

Most appropriate answer: Warfarin

Clinchers
Warfarin is the most commonly used coumarin. It is used twice daily (oral) as long-term anticoagulation. It has a narrow therapeutic range, which varies with the condition being treated. It is measured as a ratio compared with standard prothrombin time (international normalized ratio, INR).

Warfarin produces a state analogous to vitamin K deficiency, by inhibiting the reductase enzyme responsible for regenerating the active form of vitamin K. In UK warfarin tablets are 1 mg (brown), 3 mg (blue), 5 mg (pink).

Contraindications for warfarin
- Peptic ulcer
- Bleeding disorders
- Severe hypertension
- Liver failure
- Endocarditis
- Cerebral aneurysms

Main indications for anticoagulation
- DVT; pulmonary emboli
- Stroke prevention: AF, or prosthetic heart valves (treat indefinitely)
- Prevention of thromboembolism postoperatively in high risk patient.

Your Notes:

73. A man was found in his car with a hose directed from the exhaust. What would you give?

Diagnosis: Carbon monoxide poisoning

I would give: 100% O_2

Clinchers
In CO poisoning despite hypoxaemia skin is pink (or pale), not blue as carboxyhemoglobin (COHb) displaces O_2 from Hb binding sites. These is tachycardia, tachypnoea. If COHb >50%, fits, coma and cardiac arrest.

Investigation of choice
Confirm diagnosis with heparinized blood sample (CO Hb > 10%) quickly (as levels become normal quickly)

Immediate management
Remove the source
Give 100% O_2

Treatment of choice
In severe cases, anticipate cerebral oedema. Give mannitol IV
- Monitor ECG
- Hyperbaric O_2
- Discuss with poisons service.

Your Notes:

74. A patient who has overdosed on an unknown medication presents with palpitations. What is the most likely cause?

Diagnosis: Tricyclic antidepressants overdose.

Clinchers
Acute poisoning due to overdose of tricyclic antidepressant is not infrequent and it may endanger life. It is usually self-attempted by the depressed patients.

Manifestations include ECG changes, ventricular arrhythmia, tachycardia.

Excitement, delirium and other anticholinergic symptom as seen in atropine poisoning along with respiratory depression with low BP may be present/

CONFUSA
Atropine poisoning should be kept in mind, as it also presents with anticholinergic symptoms.

Investigation of choice
Blood tests
ECG

Immediate management
Physostigmine (0.5-2 mg IV), reversed central and peripheral anticholinergic effects.

Treatment of choice
Treatment is primary supportive
- Correct acidosis by bicarbonate infusion
- Physostigmine
- Propranolol/lidocaine (for arrhythmias)
- Diazepam IV (for convulsions and delirium).

Your Notes:

75. This interferes with metabolism at the mitochondrial level.

Diagnosis: Cyanide poisoning

Clinchers
Cyanide blocks electron transport, resulting in decreased oxidative metabolism and oxidative utilization, decreased ATP production and lactic acidosis.

Lethal dose
- Sodium cyanide 200-300 mg
- Hydrocyanic acid 500 mg

Early effects: Headache, vertigo, excitement, anxiety, burning of mouth and throat, dyspnoea, tachycardia, hypertension.

Later effects: Coma, seizures, opisthotonus, trismus, paralysis, respiratory, arrhythmia, hypotension and death.

Immediate management
100% O_2 and GI decontamination.

Treatment of choice
Amyl nitrite inhaled for 30 sec each min.
Sodium nitrite 3% solution IV, 2.5-50 ml/min then 50 ml of 25% sodium thiosulphate is given IV over 1-2 min, producing sodium thiocyanide, excreted in urine.

If symptom persist, repeat half the dose of sodium nitrite and sodium thiosulfate.

Your Notes:

76. A 4-year-old Irish girl looks wasted and appears short for her age. The mother reports the daughter has been vomiting on several occasions in the past, with associated diarrhoea. The SHO thinks he has an enteropathy and on serology IgA gliadin and Endomysial antibodies are found.

Diagnosis: Coeliac disease

Clinchers
- *Frequent episodes of diarrhoea with vomiting:* These are precipitated by diets containing gluten such as wheat, barley, rye.
- *Wasting:* It is failure to thrive due to malabsorption
- *α-Gliadin and anti-endomysial (IgA) antibodies:* These are almost 95% specific to coeliac disease.

CONFUSA
Other causes of malabsorption and failure to thrive such as lactose intolerance and chronic non-specific diarrhoea, which are excluded by positive anti-endomysial antibodies.

Investigation of choice
- α-gliadin and anti-endomysial (IgA) antibodies are used for screening.
- Jejunal biopsy (villous atrophy seen) is definitive

Immediate management
Correction of fluid and electrolyte imbalance due to malabsorption.

Treatment of choice
Life-long gluen free diet, such as rice, maize, soya, potato, etc.

Your Notes:

---

77. A mother brings her 5-year-old son who has been passing bloody stool associated with severe abdominal pain. On examination he is found to have mildly swollen tender wrists and red nodular tender lesions were found on his forearms.

Diagnosis: Ulcerative colitis

Clinchers
- *Bloody stools associated with abdominal pain:* This points towards a colonic pathology, most probably an inflammatory bowel disease.
- *Mildy swollen tender wrists:* since ulcerative colitis is associated with large joint arthritis.
- *Red nodular tender lesions on forearm:* These are suggestive of erythema nodosum a dermatological association of ulcerative colitis

CONFUSA
Giardia lamblia infection is a common cause of dysentery and must be excluded. Differentiation of ulcerative colitis from colonic Crohn's disease may be particularly difficult, even when the resected colon is examined by an expert pathologist.

Investigation of choice
- Procto-sigmoidoscopy: Inflammed friable mucosa.
- Barium enema: Loss of haustra, granular mucosa seen.

Immediate management
Counselling of mother about taking proper care of the son

Treatment of choice
Initially this is medical in the uncomplicated case (Sulfasalazine and steriods), but surgery is required when medical treatment fails or when complications supervene.

Your Notes:

78. An 8-year-old girl has got repeated episodes of diarrhoea. On each occasion the stool contains segments of undigested vegetables. The paediatrician recommends restricting fluids to meal times. The girls condition improves and she is thriving.

Diagnosis: Chronic non-specific diarrhoea

Clinchers
- *Repeated episodes of diarrhoea:* It is without any associated complaints.
- *Stool containing undigested vegetables:* Suggests gastric hurrying as the cause of diarrhoea, probably due to excess fluid intake in between meals
- *Improvement on restricting fluids to meal times:* Implies better regulation of diet.

CONFUSA
Lactose intolerance can be a confusing option which is excluded by resolution of symptomatology on restricting fluids to meal times.

Investigation of choice
Stool microscopic examination and culture to rule out any infective pathology.

Immediate management
Refer to a dietician

Treatment of choice
Fluids and electrolyte management.

Your Notes:

---

79. A mother and her daughter have just returned from a tropical holiday and is concerned that her daughter has an STD, since she complains of constant perianal and vulval irritation. There is no associated vaginal discharge. She has worms coming out of her bottom at night.

Diagnosis: Enterobius vermicularis infection

Clinchers
- *Returning from a tropical holiday:* Suggests imroper sanitary conditions while at holiday, conducive to feco-oral transmission of pinworms.
- *Peiranal and vulval irritation:* Occurs due to worms coming out of bowel to lay eggs.
- *Worms coming out of bottom at night:* To lays eggs.

CONFUSA
Acrodermatitis enteropathica is due to zinc deficiency, where a perianal rash may occur, although worms would not be seen

Investigation of choice
Apply sticky take to the perineum and identify eggs microscopically.

Immediate management
Anti-pruritis.

Treatment of choice
T. Mebendazole 100 mg PO stat repeated at 2 weeks if $\geq$ 2 years of age.
- Treatment of whole family
- Sanitary hygiene.

Your Notes:

80. A 15-year-girl complains of episodic diarrhoea which typically starts in the morning with a constant urge to go to the toilet on waking, and after breakfast. She says there is associated abdominal pain in the right iliac fossa relieved by defaecation or flatus. She has had the symptoms for 3 months.

Diagnosis: Irritable Bowel Syndrome (IBS)

Clinchers
- Some characteristics of IBS are:
  - Episodic diarrhoea on walking.
- Urge of pass stool in morning, after breakfast.
  - Abdominal pain releived by defaecation or flatus. Since all these are present in this patient, we can safely label it as IBS, but it is better to avoid labelling as Irritable Bowel Syndrome if symptoms are present for less than 6 months.

CONFUSA
Diarrhoea of chronic disesae
- The young age goes against colorectal carcinoma which may present similarly with diarrhoea alternating with constipation and tenesmus
- Absence of per-rectal bleed goes against ulcerative colitis

Investigation of choice
Stool microscopic examination sigmoidoscopy, colonoscopy and Barium studies to exclude organic pathology.

Immediate management
Exclusion of organic pathology

Treatment of choice
- High fibre diet
- Psychotherapy.

Your Notes:

81. A 20-year-old primigravida at 40 weeks, is 6 cm is dilated and she requests pain relief. She dislikes injections.

Management of pain: Nitrous oxide

Clinchers
Relaxation is the best nondrug analgesia that is safe for mother and fetus, but this is not always sufficient. Epidural anaesthesia can be set up once labour is established (cervix > 3 cm).

Nitrous oxide (inhaled) can be used throughout the labour. Nitrous oxide 50% in oxygen is self administered using demand value. It is contraindicated in pneumothorax.

CONFUSA
This female dislikes injections, therefore injectable forms of anaesthesia can be ruled out. Nitrous oxide (an inhalational agent) should be the best option here.

Contraindication of nitrous oxide: Pneumothorax.

Treatment of choice
In this question, the best option seem to be nitrous oxide. (Entonox)

Your Notes:

82. A 39-year gravida 3 para 2 + 0, presents at 39-weeks. Her cervix is 8 cm dilated but she complains of severe pain. Her baby is in occipitoposterior position.

Diagnosis: Occipitoposterior presentation

Preferred analgesia: Epidural anaesthesia

Clinchers

➤ *Gravida 3 para 2+0:* Currently pregnant, with two live births and no miscarriages.
➤ 73% occipitoposterior delivery will be spontaneous vaginal delivery, 22% will require forceps and 5% a caesarean section.

In occipitoposterior deliveries, labour tends to be prolonged, because of the degree of rotation needed, so adequate hydration and analgesia (consider epidural) are important.

During labour (occipitoposterior presentation):
- 65% rotate 130° to become occipitoanterior
- 20% rotate to transverse and then arrest (deep transverse arrest)
- 15% rotate so that occiput lies posterior, here birth is be flexion of head

CONFUSA
Pudendal block is used for instrumental delivery, but analgesia is insufficient for rotational forceps.
Epidurals may be helpful in:
- Occipitoposterior position
- Breech/multiple pregnancies
- Preterm delivery
- Pre-eclampsia
- Forceps delivery, and
- Incoordinate uterine contractions

Problems with epidural anaesthesia
- Postural hypotension
- Urinary retention (catheterize irregularly)
- Paralysis
- After delivery
  - urinary retention
  - headache.

Your Notes:

83. A 28-year-old woman wants to be able to move around during labour, pain free.

Preferred analgesia: Pudendal nerve block

Clinchers
Block pudendal nerve with xylocaine 0.5 or 1% as its two or three branches circumnavigate the ischial spine. It numbs the area on right only. Here women can more around freely, without pain.

Pudendal block is used with perineal infiltration, for instumental delivery, but analgesia is insufficient for rotational forceps. It is basically used for outlet manipulation in second stage of labour.

CONFUSA
Nitrous oxide due to its effect on consciousness (impaired) and sedative affect can be ruled out in this question.

Your Notes:

84. A Gravida 4 para 2 + 1, has been in labour for 4 hours. She is 3 cm dilated and has already received 2 injections of pethidine. She stills complains of pain.

Preferred analgesia: Epidural anaesthesia

Clinchers
Pethidine 50-150 mg IM can be tried in labour pain, but not when birth is expected in < 2-3 hours as neonatal respiratory depression may occur (reversible with naloxone).

Since cervix is 3 cm dilated epidural anaesthesia can be considered. In anaesthetizes the fibers carried by T_{11}-S_5. Constant monitoring is required once epidural is set up. She has been in labour for four hours, so epidural will be of great help. For other indications of epidural refer to Q 82, Nov. 2001 paper.

CONFUSA
Narcotic injections (pethidine) are tried in the first stage, with onset of analgesia within 20 minutes and lasts 3 hours. They are contraindicated in mothers on MAOIs (page 340, OHCS).

Problems with epidural
Refer question no 82, (PLAB November 2001).

Your Notes:

85. A 31-year-old woman has a retained placenta, following a spontaneous vaginal delivery.

Diagnosis: Retained placenta

Preferred anaesthesia: General anaesthesia

Clinchers
Placenta not delivered in 30 minutes after delivery will probably not be expelled. Physiological third stage takes 30 minutes.

Danger with retained placenta is haemorrhage, therefore active intervention is required.

For manual removal, call on anaesthetist. Manual removal can be done under epidural if *in situ*, halothane assists by relaxing the uterus.

CONFUSA
Retained placenta is an emergency. Delay may precipitate postpartum haemorrhage.

Immediate management
Set up IVI and cross match blood (24)

Treatment of choice
Remove placenta manually. This can be done under epidural anaesthesia, if *in situ*, halothane assists by relaxing the uterus. Rarely placenta does not separate manually (placenta accreta) and hysterectomy may be necessary.

Your Notes:

86. A 53-year-old nurse complains of facial pain. A week earlier she had a red rash and blisters around her right eye. This area of her face has now become acutely painful.

Diagnosis: Herpes zoster

Clinchers

- *53-year-old:* The episodes of herpes zoster become increasingly common with advancing age.
- *Nurse:* This increases the chances of acquiring chickenpox which is the primary cause of herpes zoster.
- *Facial pain:* Pain heralds an acute episode. At least 50% of patients > 50 years old with zoster reports pain months after resolution of instances lesions.
- *Red rash and blisters around her right eye:* Erythematous maculopapules which rapidly evolve into vesicles in the distribution of a dermatome is characteristic of zoster.
- *Acutely painful:* This is acute neuritis which is seen with an acute episode of zoster

CONFUSA
The Tzanck preparation has a sensitivity of only ~60% and does not distinguished varicella, herpes zoster virus from herpes simplex virus infection. Serologic tests include fluorescent antibody to membrane antigen (FAMA) and ELISA. Confirmation is possible with viral isolation in tissue culture VZV takes longer to isolate than HSV.

Investigation of choice
- *Screening:* FAMA/ELISA
- *Definitive:* Virus isolation in tissue culture

Note: Investigations are not usually required as the diagnosis is clinically easy.

Immediate management
Analgesia (oral)

Treatment of choice
Aciclovir for skin lesions
Low dose amitriptiline if pain relief not possible with simple analgesics.

Your Notes:

---

87. A 31-year-old man complains of facial pain between the eyes and on one side of the face. His nose and the affected eye are congested. He says the pain is severe.

Diagnosis: Trigeminal neuralgia

Clinchers (Note: See Q 90 of this theme also)

- *31 years old man:* It is chiefly a condition of those over 50 years old. Male to female ratio is >1.
- *Facial pain between the eyes and on one side of face:* The pain is unilateral affecting the mandibular and maxillary divisions most often and the ophthalmic division only rarely.
- *His nose and the affected eyes are congested:* It is due to vasodilatation seen along with pain.
- *Pain is severe:* There are severe paroxysms of knife like or electric-shock-like pain, lasting seconds. The face may screw up with pain (hence tic douloureux).

CONFUSA
The pain of trigeminal neuralgia characteristically does not occur at right (Reference: Kumar and Clark, 1021, 5th edn). There is controversy on this point as OHCM mentions it on the contrary (page 333, OHCM, 5th edn). The recurrence are inevitable although spontaneous remissions last for months or years. Secondary trigeminal neuralgia occurs due to multiple sclerosis (especially in young). Vascular malformation, or a cerebello-pontine angle tumors.

Investigation of choice
Clinical diagnosis

Immediate management
High dose analgesia for pain relief

Treatment of choice
Carbamazepine
If drugs fail, surgery.

Your Notes:

88. A 20-year-old man says his face hurts, especially around the eyes and cheeks. When he bends forwards it worsens and makes him cry.

Diagnosis: Sinusitis (maxillary)

Clinchers
- *20-year-old:* Sinusitis is common at all ages in adults (as the sinuses are well developed and accumulate the predisposing pathologies by the adult age).
- *Man:* Males are slightly more affected.
- *Face hurts, especially around the eyes and cheeks:* Typically it is situated over the upper jaw, but may be referred to the gums or teeth. For this reason patient may primarily consult a dentist. Pain is aggravated by stooping, coughing or chewing. Occasionally pain is referred to the ipsilateral supraorbital region and thus may simulate frontal sinus infection.
- *Makes him cry:* That signifies that the pain is severe as is the case with it.

CONFUSA
Sinusitis is an infection of the paranasal sinuses that often complicate, upper respiratory tract infections (e.g. coryza and allergic rhinitis). Acute infections are usually caused by *Streptococcus pneumoniae* and *Haemophilus influenzae*. Symptoms include frontal headache and facial pain and tenderness, usually with nasal discharge but are often difficult to differentiate from symptoms of the common cold.

Investigation of choice
X-rays (Water's view)

Immediate management
Steam inhalation

Treatment of choice
Antimicrobial drugs + nasal decongestants.

Your Notes:

---

89. A 57-year-old teacher says she has facial pain, especially in the temples at night. On the right side of her face it throbs. For the past three weeks she has felt unwell and had to miss classes. Also, combing her hair has become painful.

Diagnosis: Temporal arteritis (TA)

Clinchers
- *57-year-old:* It is common in elderly, it is rare under 55 years.
- *Facial pain, especially in the temples at night:* Pain in invariable and is felt over the inflamed superficial temporal or occipital arteries. Touching the skin over the inflamed vessel (e.g. combing the hair) causes pain.
- *On right side of her face it throbs:* Arterial pulsation is felt initially but is soon last and the artery becomes hard, tortuous and thickened.
- *For three weeks:* It signifies a chronic condition that it is.
- *Combing her hair has become painful:* See above.

CONFUSA
Generalised muscle pains, proximal limb girdle pain and tenderness, without joint effusion, i.e. polymyalgia rheumatica occur in under half the patients. Rare complications of TA can be brainstem ischaemia, cortical blindness, ischaemic neuropathy of peripheral or cranial nerves, and involvement of the aorta, coronary, renal and mesenteric arteries are sometimes seen.

Investigation of choice
- *Screening:* ESR (60-100 mm/h)
- *Definitive:* Biopsy of temporal artery

Immediate management
Oral steroids (immediately)

Treatment of choice
Steroid maintenance therapy (for at least 2 years).

Your Notes:

90. A 43-year-old mechanic complains of left sided facial pain. The pain is stabbing and runs up and down his face, especially at meal times. He has been to the dentist, but the dentist has found his teeth to be in good order.

Diagnosis: Trigeminal neuralgia (TN)

Clinchers (Note: See Q 87 of this theme also)
- *43 years old:* It appears in middle or old age.
- *Left sided facial pain:* It is almost always unilateral.
- *Stabbing pain:* Severe paroxysm of knife-life or electric shock like pain, lasting seconds occur in the distribution of the fifth nerve.
- *Especially at meal times:* Each paroxysm is stereotyped, brought on by stimulation of a specific and often tiny trigger zone in the face. Washing, shaving, a cold wind or eating are examples of the trivial stimuli and provoke the intense pain.
- *He has been to dentist....:* This excludes dental causes. Very often the patient presents to dentists as they mistook the pain to be dental in origin.

> **CONFUSA**
> Onset in young adulthood raises the possibility of multiple sclerosis. Carbamazepine is effective in 75% of cases of TN or nonresponders, phenytoin or baclofen can be tried. When medications fail, surgical gangliolysis or suboccipital craniectomy for decompression of trigeminal nerve are options. Microvascular decompression is recommended (where available) if a tortuous or redundant blood vessels is found in the posterior fossa near the trigeminal nerve.

Investigation of choice
Clinical diagnosis

Immediate management
High dose analgesia for pain relief

Treatment of choice
Carbamazepine (see confusa also).

Your Notes:

---

91. An overweight woman complains of having to go to the toilet more than usual. She says she does drink a lot of tea but that she is always thirsty and tired. She needs the energy.

Diagnosis: Glycosuria

Clinchers
- *Overweight:* Glycosuria can occur in diabetes mellitus or otherwise. NIDDM usually presents in overweight adults.
- *Woman:* DM is slightly more common in females because of its possible autoimmune aetiology
- *Having to go to toilet more than usual:* This is a polyuria and occurs due to hyperglycaemia.
- *She does drink a lot of tea but that she is always thirsty:* This is polydipsia, again due to hyperglycaemia.
- *Tired + needs the energy:* Generalised weakness, feeling unwell and fatigue are the common complaints initially. Weight loss also occurs due to fluid depletion and the accelerated breakdown of fat and muscle secondary to insulin deficiency.

> **CONFUSA**
> Correlation between urine tests and simultaneous blood glucose is poor for three reasons:
> - Changes in urine glucose lag behind changes in blood glucose.
> - The mean renal threshold is around 10 mmol/L but the range is wide (7-13 mmol/L). The threshold also rises with age.
> - Urine tests can give no guidance concerning blood glucose levels below the renal threshold.

Investigation of choice
Blood glucose (see confusa)

Immediate management
Dipstick test for glucose in urine

Treatment of choice
As per the findings, but weight loss and diet control is most important.

Your Notes:

92. A young mother with chronic bronchitis says that every time she coughs, she pees, and she would like you to do something about it. She is on a course of antibiotics at the moment.

Diagnosis: Genuine stress incontinence (GSI)

Clinchers
- *Chronic bronchitis:* This gives a repeatitive stress factor to the patient i.e. cough.
- *Everytime she coughs, she pees:* On clinical examination. GSI may be demonstrated when the patient coughs. It occurs when the bladder pressure exceeds the maximum uretheral pressure in the absence of any detrusor contraction.
- *On a course of antibiotics:* This suggest that her bronchitis is severe. Also it suggest that she is undergoing treatment for the basic cause and now we need to treat the incontinence.

CONFUSA
The aetiology of GSI after child birth is due to damage to the nerve supply of the pelvic floor and uretheral sphincter (caused by child birth). It leads to progressive changes in these structures resulting in altered function. In addition, mechanical trauma to the pelvic floor musculature and endopelvic fascia and ligaments occurs as a consequence of vaginal delivery. Prolonged second stage, large bodies and instrumental deliveries cause the most damage.

Investigation of choice
Urodynamic studies

Immediate management
Clinical examination by an expert

Treatment of choice
Pelvic floor exercises/physiotherapy
±
Surgery

Your Notes:

93. A middle aged woman complains of having to urinate frequently. She says that unless she rushes to the toilet she wets herself and she finds wetting herself most embarrassing.

Diagnosis: Urge incontinence (UI)

Clinchers
- *Middle aged woman:* The most common cause of urge incontinence is such females is bladder unstability following child births.
- *Having to urinate frequently:* This is "frequency", a common finding in UI. It is due to detrusor instability.
- *Unless she rushes to toilet she wet herself:* This is "urgency" which is characteristic of urge incontinence. It is due to contraction of bladder while the patient is attempting to inhibit micturition.
- *Embarrassing:* Since the condition is symptomatic and embarrasing, it require urgent treatment.

CONFUSA
Urge incontinence can be present alone or association with GSI in which case it is called mixed incontinence. The cause of the unsuppressible or unhibited bladder contractions is usually idiopathic, but bacterial cystitis, bladder tumour, bladder outlet obstruction and neurogenic bladder must be excluded.

Investigation of choice
Urodynamic studies

Immediate management
Exclude UTI and glycosuria

Treatment of choice
Bladder training (gradually increasing the time interval between voiding).

Your Notes:

94. A 36-year-old sales executive says she wets herself without warning all the time. Before the birth of her third child she had no complaints but now she says she has no control whatsoever.

Diagnosis: True incontinence

Clinchers
- *36-year-old:* True incontinence presenting in this age is due to acquired causes i.e. obstetric injuries.
- *Wets herself without warning all the time:* In true incontinence of urine, due to a vesicovaginal or ureterovaginal fistula, the urine is discharged involuntarily and continuously so that the patient is constantly wet.
- *No complaints before birth of her third child:* This suggests obstetric trauma to be the cause, i.e. prolonged labour, forceps application etc.

CONFUSA
The bladder is always empty without residual urine in the case of a vesicovaginal fistula and only contains half the expected normal in the case of a ureterovaginal fistula.

Investigation of choice
Micturition cysto-uretherography

Immediate management
Detailed obstetric history

Treatment of choice
Surgery.

Your Notes:

95. A 27-year-old travel guide wants something done about the pain she feels on micturition, especially when it is cold. Repeated urine cultures have all been negative. Sometimes, she says, going to the toilet is very painful for her.

Diagnosis: Urethral syndrome (US)

Clinchers
- *27-year-old:* US is mostly seen in the sexually active females and is often associated with intercourse.
- *Pain she feels on micturition, especially when it is cold:* This is dysuria, a common manifestation of cystitis.
- *Repeated urine cultures have all been negative:* Characteristically MSU are all negative in cystitis causing US. It may be due to subinfective numbers of organisms being massaged into the urethra during the intercourse.
- *Going to the toilet is very painful:* This suggest a symptomatic cystitis and hence an indication for active treatment.

CONFUSA
Mildly symptomatic US can be managed by using proper lubrication during the intercourse. Micturating before and after intercourse, different coital positions (her on top) can help.

Investigation of choice
None

Immediate management
Exclude glycosuria

Treatment of choice
Trimethoprim.

Your Notes:

96. A 35-year-old woman comes to the clinic for screening of her breasts.

Diagnosis: Normal

Clinchers
- *35-year-old:* The UK national health service offers 3 yearly single view of mammography to those between 55 and 64 years old. (Other age groups above 30 years may be screened if they want, but are not sent for).
- *Screening:* Mammography uses negligible radiation and cancer pick-up rate is 5 per 1000 'healthy' woman screened. It is a good screening examination. The patient should also be taught monthly self-examination and advised to report if she finds and discrete lump

CONFUSA
Mammogram is a soft tissue X-ray of the breast, which may reveal small carcinomas that typically show as an area of speckled calcification. It is also be helpful in reassuring the patient that a lesion is benign. Mammograms may reveal malignancies that are impalpable, but may mislead in some malignant lesions and inter a benign nature and vice-versa. Biopsy is the safest policy in any doubtful case.

Investigation of choice
Mammography

Immediate management
Teach local self examination

Treatment of choice
Depends on the investigation result.

Your Notes:

---

97. A 45-year-old woman presents with a mass in the right upper quadrant of her right breast. A round smooth mass is found in the axilla.

Diagnosis: Breast mass (suspected malignancy)

Clinchers
- *45-year-old:* There is an increased incidence of breast cancer with age. Any age may be affected, but it is rare below the age of 30 years.
- *Mass in the right upper quadrant of her right breast:* This is the most common site of a breast malignancy.
- *Woman:* Females are 100 times more likely to have a breast carcinoma than men.
- *Round smooth mass in axilla:* The main lymphatic drainage of breast is through axillary nodes, so this could be a metastatic node. Lymph node metastases usually present as smooth, firm, painless, swelling.

CONFUSA
There is a high degree of clinical error (around 25%) in estimating whether a tumor is stage I or II—axillary lymph nodes may be involved, although they cannot be felt. Conversely axillary nodes that are palpable may prove free from tumor. However it does not make much of a difference in management as both stages I and II lesions are usually submitted to curative surgery (III and IV—palliative surgery)

Investigation of choice
FNAC

Immediate management
Examine contralateral axilla

Treatment of choice
Curative surgery if FNAC shows malignant cells.

Your Notes:

Breast LUMP

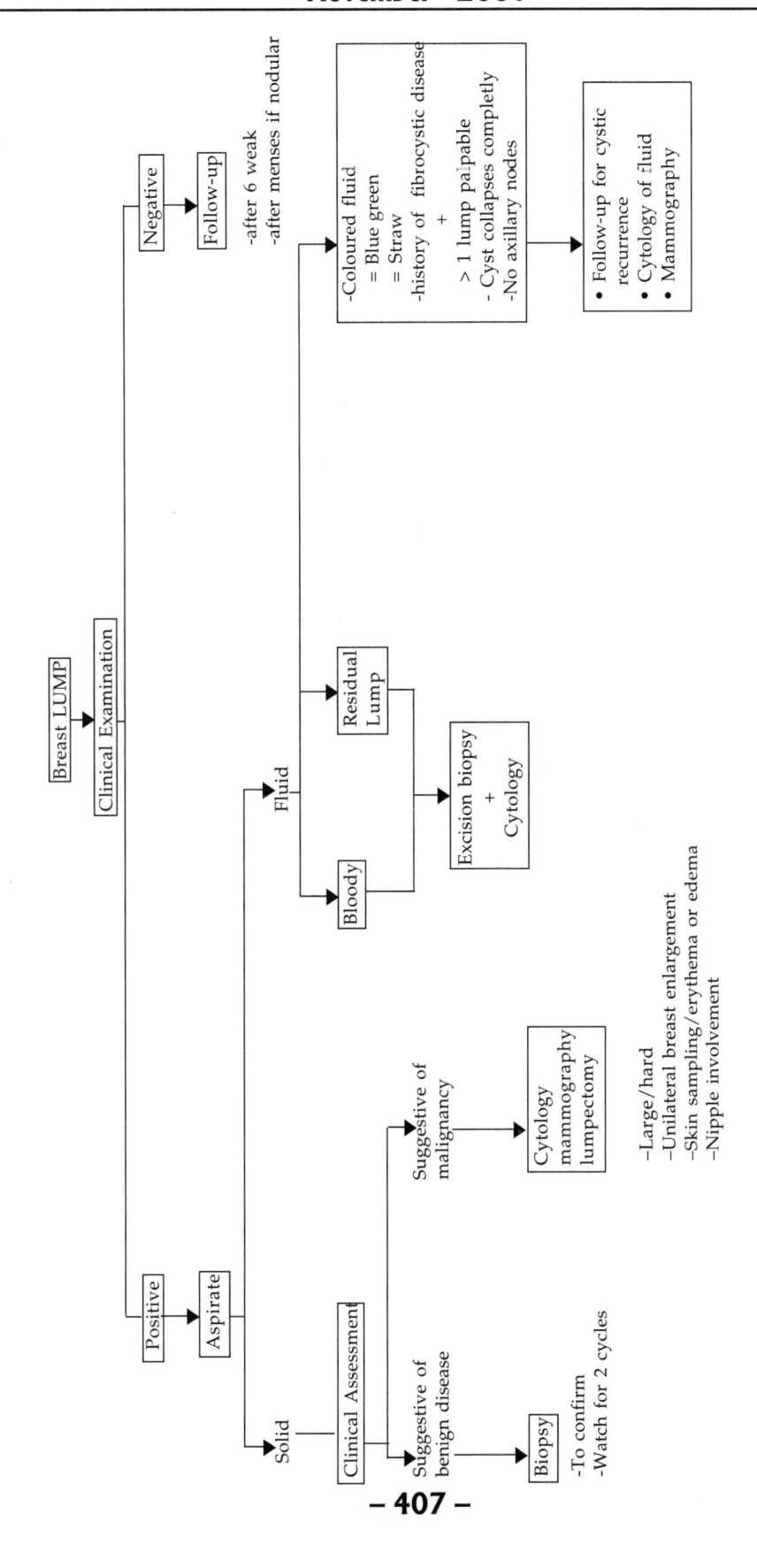

Clinical Examination

Positive → Aspirate

Solid → Clinical Assessment

- **Suggestive of benign disease** → Biopsy
  - To confirm
  - Watch for 2 cycles

- **Suggestive of malignancy** → Cytology, mammography, lumpectomy
  - Large/hard
  - Unilateral breast enlargement
  - Skin sampling/erythema or edema
  - Nipple involvement

Fluid

- **Bloody** → Excision biopsy + Cytology
- **Residual Lump** → Excision biopsy + Cytology

- Coloured fluid
  - = Blue green
  - = Straw
- history of fibrocystic disease
  +
- > 1 lump palpable
- Cyst collapses completly
- No axillary nodes

  →
  - Follow-up for cystic recurrence
  - Cytology of fluid
  - Mammography

Negative → Follow-up
- after 6 weak
- after menses if nodular

98. A 36-year-old woman comes with a hard mass in her breast. The skin is tethered. Ultrasound and mammography were inconclusive. The patient wants to be satisfied that this is not malignant.

Diagnosis: Breast mass (probable malignancy)

Clinchers
- *36-year-old:* There is an increased incidence of breast cancer with age. Any age may be affected, but it is rare below the age of 30 years.
- *Hard mass:* Usually malignant tumors are hard in feeling on palpation.
- *Skin is tethered:* Involvement of skin and subcutaneous tissues leads to skin dimpling, retraction of the nipple and eventually ulceration.
- *USG and mammography where inconclusive:* These are preliminary noninvasive screening tests. If these are inconclusive and the condition is suggestive of malignancy, cytological diagnosis (through FNAC) is the only option left.
- *Patient wants to be satisfied:* This also necessiates FNAC as the patient is demanding the proof.

CONFUSA
Skin fixation is a strong supporting evidence of carcinoma, although it may be seen rarely over an area of fibroadenosis and may accompany fat necrosis or follow chronic abscess.

Investigation of choice
FNAC

Immediate management
Respect the patient's wishes and proceed for FNAC

Treatment of choice
Surgery according to cytological diagnosis and staging.

Your Notes:

99. A 36-year-old woman presents with itching of her left nipple. On examination, no ulceration is seen, but a scaly lesion around the nipple is observed.

Diagnosis: Eczema/fungal infection

Clinchers
- *36-year-old:* It can occur in any age group after puberty as it is a primarily allergic disorder.
- *Itching of her left nipple:* It is invariably associated with any eczematous disease.
- *No ulceration:* It is usually absent. Its presence in eczema may signify the excerations due to scratching.
- *Scaly lesion around the nipple:* This confirms our diagnostic suspicion somewhat. But a fungal infection can also present in the same way.

CONFUSA
Eczema of nipple is rare and is usually bilateral. It is usually associated with eczema elsewhere on body whereas in case of fungal infection, the lesion might be solitary. Paget's disease always needs to be ruled out before dignosing eczema (Paget's disease also have an additional feature of discharge from surface). Psoriasis can also be a diagnosis but it is never so localized.

Investigation of choice
KOH examination of smear

Immediate management
Reassurance

Treatment of choice
As per the diagnosis.

Your Notes:

100. A 23-year-old woman says she feels lumps in her breasts during the time of her periods. She also feels anxious and irritable.

Diagnosis: Fibrocystic breast disease (FCBD)

Clinchers

- *23-year-old:* FCBD are more common in the young females.
- *Feels lumps in her breasts:* This is a complaints that require a complete evaluation to rule out any disease (see confusa).
- *During the time of her periods:* This is characteristic of FCBD and is due to cyclical developmental changes in young women.
- *Anxious and irritate:* This could be secondary to FCBD or primarily due to the accompanying pre-menstrual syndrome (PMS).

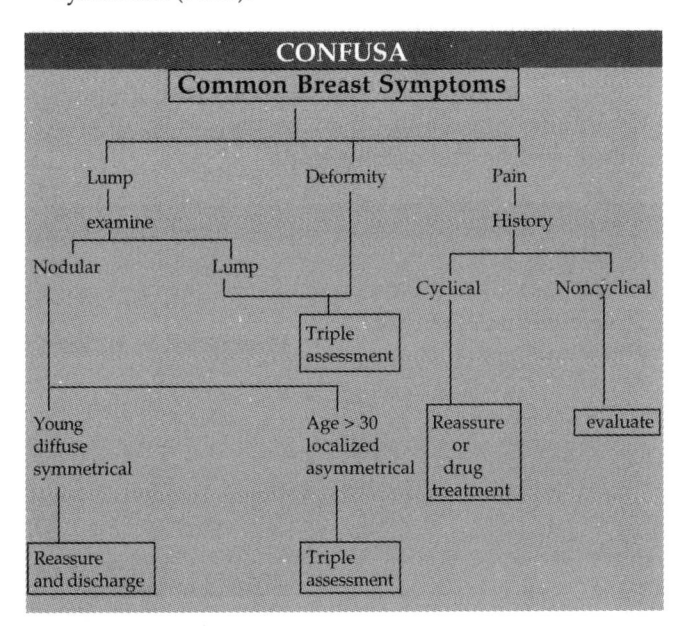

CONFUSA
Common Breast Symptoms

```
                Lump      Deformity      Pain
                  |                        |
               examine                  History
                  |                    /      \
         Nodular    Lump          Cyclical    Noncyclical
            |         |              |            |
            |      Triple         Reassure     evaluate
            |    assessment         or
         /      \                  drug
     Young    Age > 30          treatment
     diffuse  localized
    symmetrical asymmetrical
        |          |
    Reassure     Triple
    and discharge assessment
```

Investigation of choice
Clinical examination

Immediate management
Reassurance

Treatment of choice
None required. Dischage her after proper evaluation

101. A 25-year-old found deeply unconscious is brought to the Accident and Emergency Department. He has an abrasion over his left temple and puncture marks on his left forearm.

Diagnosis: Suspected head injury after IV drug abuse

Clinchers

- *25-year-old:* Incidence of drug abuse is highest in teens and twenties.
- *Deeply unconscious:* This can be either due to head injury or due to opiate overdose.
- *Abrasion over his left temple:* This raises the suspicion of a head injury. Since the patient is unconscious and thus cannot be evaluated clinically properly, it necessiates an urgent CT scan to rule out brain injury.
- *Puncture marks on left forearm:* These are highly likely to be needle marks from IV drug abuse. The suspicion is increased by the fact that the marks are on left arm (as majority of population is right handed and thus use it to self inject on the other arm).

CONFUSA
A drug addict can sustain physical injuries from falls, burns or other trauma because of altered state of consciousness. Also there is an increased possibility of them being assaulted because of a high crime rate in their community.

Investigation of choice
CT scan skull

Immediate management
IV naloxone (to rule out opiate intoxication)

Treatment of choice
As per the diagnosis.

Your Notes:

102. A 37-year-old alcoholic is found wandering in a park. His partner says he has had a number of falls recently and in the Accident and Emergency the patient is confused. The blood sugar level is normal.

Diagnosis: Head injury (probable).

Clinchers

- *Alcoholic:* Subdural hematomas are commonly seen in alcoholics. There may be no apparent injury. The first sign may be a failure to wake up after an episode of heavy drinking.
- *History of number of falls recently:* Frequent falls weakne the bridging veins which traverse the subdural space. They can bleed to give rise to subdural hematomas. This mechanism is responsible for their frequent incidence in alcoholics. Subdural hematomas are also common among elderly and HIV patients. But in them the pathogenesis is cerebral atropy → shrinkage of brain → stretching of bridging veins → rupture → hematoma.
- *Confused:* A CT scan is indicated in all cases of clouding on consciousness or low GCS in an alcoholic, as the clinical assessment is difficult in an intoxicated patient.

CONFUSA
A normal blood sugar rules out hypoglycemia which is a more common cause of confusion in an alcoholic. On the other hand this patient could be plainly showing only the features of intoxication, but CT scan is still essential from medicolegal point of view in UK.

Investigation of choice
CT scan (subdural hematoma—inner concave border).

Immediate management
Admit in hospital (at least overnight).

Treatment of choice
Depends on CT findings.

Your notes:

---

103. A young diabetic is admitted in a comatose state. His plasma glucose level is 17 mmols and he is dehydrated.

Diagnosis: Diabetic ketoacidosis (DKA).

Clinchers

- *Young diabetic:* DKA coma only cocurs with type I diabetes, so it is more common in young diabetics (as type I diabetes usually presents in childhood).
- *Comatose state:* Apart from coma other symptoms are polyuria, polydipsia, lethargy, anorexia, hyperventilation, ketotic breath (smells like peach), dehydration, vomiting, abdominal pain, etc.
- *Plasma glucose level is 17 mmols:* Normal range of blood glucose is 3.5-5.5 mmol/l. Usually in DKA it is > 20 mmol/L. But 17 mmol/l is also a very high value.
- *Dehydrated:* Gross hyperglycemia causes an osmotic diuresis, decreased tissue perfusion and circulatory collapse. It produces dehydration. Dehydration is more life-threatening than any hyperglycemia—so its correction takes precedence.

CONFUSA
Some students get confused between DKA and HONK coma (hyperglycemic hyperosmolar nonketotic coma).

DKA	HONK
1. Occurs only in IDDM	1. Occurs only in NIDDM
2. History of 2-3 days	2. Longer history (eg 1 wk)
3. Glucose usually > 20 mmol/l	3. Glucose >35 mmol/l
4. Acidosis present (pH <7.3)	4. Acidosis absent
5. Ketotic breath present	5. No ketotic breath
6. Younger patients	6. Patient often old
7. Insulin given immediately in treatment	7. Insulin is given late, cautiously and in lower dosage

Investigation of choice
Plasma osmolality (2[Na$^+$] + [urea] + [glucose])

Immediate management
IV access and start fluid (0.9% NS) immediately.

Treatment of choice
Fluid replacement (0.9%NS) + 10U soluble insulin IV (if plasma glucose > 20 mmol/L).
↓
Insulin sliding scale.

Your Notes:

104. A middle-aged woman remains unconcious 12 hours following a cholecystectomy. On examination both pupils are seen to be pinpoint.

Diagnosis: Opiate overdosage.

Clinchers
- *Middle-aged woman:* Maximum incidence of gallstones is in middle-aged women. In the UK they are found in approximately 10% of women in their forties increasing to 30% after the age of 60 years. They are about half as common in men (aphorism: fair, fat, fertile, females of forty).
- *Remains unconcious 12 hours following a cholecystectomy:* Opiate overdosage (prescribed postoperatively for analgesia) can produce coma, respiratory depression and acidosis.
- *Both pupils are seen to be pinpoint:* Pinpoint pupils are seen in opiate overdose and hence our suspicion is confirmed.

CONFUSA
The other common etiology of pinpoint pupils is pontine hemorrhage. But that is very unlikely in postoperative middle-aged patient. Moreover no indication of any hypertensive disease is given in this question (Hypertension is associated with pontine hemorrhage).

Investigation of choice
Respiratory rate.

Immediate management
Respiratory support (oxygen/IPPV)

Treatment of choice
Immediate reversal by naloxone.

Your notes:

105. A young diabetic is admitted in a comatose state. His plasma glucose level is 2 mmols/L

Diagnosis: Hypoglycemia

Clinchers
- *Young diabetic:* The most common cause of hypoglycemia is insulin or sulfonylurea treatment in a known diabetic. It can also be due to insufficient food or change in routine of insulin (i.e. site of injection, type of insulin, new syringe size). It is more so in younger patients because there is usually no set lifestyle.
- *Comatose state:* Initially, a hypoglycemic patient is restless and agitated but, if untreated, rapidly becomes unresponsive. There is pallor profuse sweating and a bounding pulse. Aggression can be such that the patient arrives in police custody and may be thought to be intoxicated. False neurological signs are sometimes seen.
- *His plasma glucose level is 2 mmols:* Hypoglycemia by definition is < 2.5 mmol/L.

CONFUSA
The other two conditions which can produce comatose state in a diabetic are:
- Nonketotic (HONK) coma
- Diabetic ketoacidosis (DKA)

Investigation of choice
- Venous blood glucose
- In case of unexplained hypoglycemia
  - Liver function tests
  - Insulin assay
  - C peptide assay
  - Toxicology (paracetamol) screen

Immediate management
Start treatment after taking blood sample.

Treatment of choice
- 50 ml of 50% dextrose solution (adults)
- 2-5 ml/kg of 10% dextrose solution (child)
- If venous access is delayed:
  - Glucagon 1-2 mg IM (20 µg/kg for children)
- 50% dextrose harms veins, so follow by 0.9% saline flush.
- If there is no prompt recovery after treatment, give dexamethasone 4 mg/4h IV to combat cerebral edema after prolonged hypoglycemia.
- Once conscious, give sugary drinks.

106. A 45-year-old sheep farmer complains of headache, anorexia, muscle and joint pain. He has as 'undulating' fever.

Diagnosis: Brucellosis

Clinchers
- *45-year-old sheep farmer:* Brucellosis is a zoonosis and often occurs in workers in close contacts with animals or carcasses. Otherwise spread is largely by ingestion of raw milk from infected cattle or goats.
- *Headache, anorexia, muscle and joint pain:* The onset is insidious, with malaise, headache, weakness, generalized myalgia and night sweats.
- *Undulating fever:* The fever pattern is classically undulant, although continuous and intermittent patterns are frequent.

> **CONFUSA**
> Brucellosis has a worldwide distribution. It has been virtually eliminated from cattle in the UK. The organism does not withstand pasteurization. The organisms usually gain entry into the human body via the mouth, though less frequently they may enter via the respiratory tract, genital tract or abraded skin. The bacilli travel in the lymphatics and infect lymph nodes. This is followed by haematogenous spread with ultimate localization of the bacilli in the reticuloendothelial system.

Investigation of choice
Blood culture/bone marrow culture

Immediate management
Take travel history

Treatment of choice
Doxycycline 100 mg/12 h PO
+
Streptomycin 1 g/day IM for 2-3 weeks.

Your Notes:

---

107. It is a skin-to-skin contact disease.

Diagnosis: Scabies

Clinchers
Scabies is spread by prolonged close contact such as within households or institutions, and by sexual contact. It presents clinically with itchy red papules (or ocassionally vesicles and pustules) which can occur anywhere in the skin but rarely on the face, except in neonates.

> **CONFUSA**
> Crusted scabies (Norwegian scabies) is a clinical variant that occurs in immunosuppressed individuals where huge number of mites are carried in the skin. The patient is extremely infections after relatively minimal contact. Clinically this presents as hyperkeratotic crusted lesions especially on the hands and feet. Itch is often absent or minimal. Lesions may progress such that the patient has a widespread erythema with irregular crusted plaques. It can therefore mimic eczema or psoriasis.

Investigation of choice
Microscopy (demonstration of a mite is definitive)

Immediate management
Trace all contacts

Treatment of choice
Topical scabicide
(malathion or 5% permerthrin to the whole body and washed off after 24 hours).

Your Notes:

108. A 32-year-old woman presents with dysuria, swinging fever and loin pain.

Diagnosis: Escherichia coli (urinary tract infection)

Clinchers

- *32-year-old:* UTI are common in sexually active females.
- *Dysuria:* The most typical symptoms of UTI are:
  - Frequency of micturition by day and night
  - Painful voiding (dysuria)
  - Suprapubic pain and tenderness
  - Haematuria
  - Smelly urine
- *Swinging fever and loin pain:* Swinging fever typically represents a foci of pus in the body. Loin pain and tenderness, with fever and systemic upset, suggest extension of the infection to the pelvis and kidney, known as pyelitis and pyelonephritis.

CONFUSA

Organisms causing UTI in domicilliary practice:

• E. coli and other coliforms	68%+
• Proteus mirabilis	12%
• Klebsiella aerogenes	4%
• Enterococcus faecalis	6%
• Staphylococcus saprophyticus or epidermidis	10%

Investigation of choice
- *Screening:* MSU
- *Definitive:* IVU (as pyelonephritis is suspected)

Immediate management
Rule out complicated disease

Treatment of choice
Trimethoprim.

Your Notes:

109. It spread by faecal-oral route.

Diagnosis: Hepatitis A virus (HAV)

Clinchers
Spread of infection is mainly by the faeco-oral route and arises from the ingestion of contaminated food or water (e.g. shellfish). Overcrowding and poor sanitation facilitate spread. There is no carrier state. In the UK it is a notifiable disease.

CONFUSA
No HAV carries state has been identified after acute type A hepatitis; perpetuation of the virus in nature depends presumably on nonepidemic, inapparent subclinical infection. Hepatitis A tends to be more symptomatic in adults. Travel to endemic areas is a common source of infection for adults from nonendemic areas. More recently recognized epidemiologic foci of HAV infection include child care centres, neonatal ICU, promiscuous homosexual men and IV drug abusers. Although HAV is rarely blood borne, several outbreaks have been recognized in recipients of clotting factor concentrates.

Investigation of choice
Serum transaminases, IgM

Immediate management
Notify relevant authorities

Treatment of choice
Supportive
Rarely interferon α for fulminant hepatitis.

Your Notes:

110. A 67-year-old man has lost 10 kg in weight, over the last 6 months. In addition he has a 5 month history of a productive cough.

Diagnosis: Tuberculosis (TB)

Clinchers

- *67-year-old man:* Reactivation of TB is seen in old age debility or immunosuppressed states.
- *Lost 10 kg weight over last 6 months:* It is due to the chronic disease producing a generalised ill health and loss of appetite.
- *5 month history of productive cough:* In the majority of cases, cough eventually develops—perhaps initially non-productive and subsequently accompanied by the production of purulent sputum. Blood streaking of the sputum is frequently documented.

CONFUSA
Physical findings are of limited use in pulmonary tuberculosis. Many patients have no abnormalities detectable by chest examination, while others have detectable rales in the involved areas during inspiration, especially after coughing. Occassionally, ronchi due to partial bronchial obstruction and classical amphrotic breath sounds in areas with large cavities may be heard. The most common haematological findings are mild anaemia and leukocytosis. Hyponatraemia due to SIADH has also been found.

Investigation of choice
Sputum microscopy and culture

Immediate management
CXR

Treatment of choice
Anti TB drug regimen for 6 months.

Your Notes:

---

111. A teenage boy with dyspnoea and chest pain is brought into Accident and Emergency. He has a history of rheumatic fever. An ECG demonstrates left atrial hypertrophy and left ventricular hypertrophy. It also demonstrates Q waves and raised ST-segment.

Diagnosis: Myocardial infarction (MI)

Clinchers

- *Teenage boys:* Although the incidence of MI is increasing in younger age, an acute MI in teenage is rare. In this case suspicion should be raised for familial hypercholesterolemia or cocaine use which can produce MI at such a young age.
- *Dyspnoea and chest pain:* The cardinal feature of AMI.
- *History of rheumatic fever:* Aortic insufficiency due to residual heart damage after rheumatic fever can cause MI as a major coronary blood supply from aorta is compromised.
- *ECG: LAH + LVH + Q waves + raised ST segment:* LAH and LVH confirms our suspicion of aortic stenosis (and hence aortic insufficiency) to be the cause of MI. Q waves signify a transmural infarct. Total occlusion of the infarct artery produces ST-segment elevation, and most such individuals ultimately evolve a Q-wave MI.

ECG progression in MI

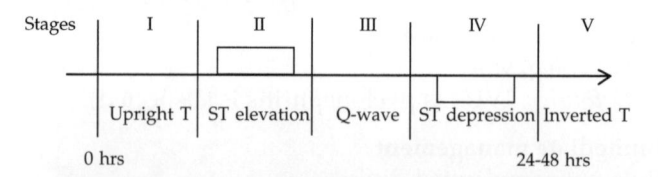

Stages	I	II	III	IV	V
	Upright T	ST elevation	Q-wave	ST depression	Inverted T
0 hrs					24-48 hrs

CONFUSA
ECG pathologic correlation are far from perfect and, therefore a more rational nomenclature for designating electrocardiographic infarction is now commonly in use, with the terms Q-wave and non-Q-wave infarction replacing the terms transmural and non-transmural infarction, respectively. A small population may sustain only a non-Q wave MI. When the obstructing thrombus is subtotally occlusive obstruction is transient or a rich collateral network is present, no ST-segment elevation is seen.

Investigation of choice
12 lead ECG

Immediate management
High flow O_2 + IV morphine

Treatment of choice
Anticoagulation

112. An elderly woman is found unconscious at home. An ECG demonstrates sinus bradycardia. J waves, ST-depression, and flattened T waves.

Diagnosis: Hypothermia (Urban or subacute hypothermia)

Clinchers

- *Elderly woman:* Old age and no one to look after are important predisposing factors for hypothermia. The victim is usually exposed to moderate cold for days, often with several predisposing factors.
- *Unconscious at home:* The most common cause in UK of an elderly to be found unconscious at home with no obvious injuries is hypothermia. Upto 3% of medical patients admitted to UK hospitals during winter months have core temperature below 35°C.
- *ECG: sinus bradycardia + ST depression + flattened T waves:* There all suggest prolonged repolarization, a characteristic features of hypothermia.
- *J waves:* It is characteristic notching of the S-wave (usually seen in V4). It is also called osborn wave and is present in 80% of patients with severe hypothermia.

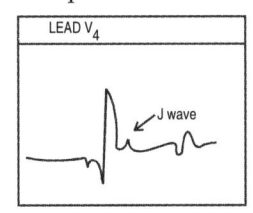

Figure

CONFUSA
- Do not assume that if vital signs seem to be absent, the patient must be dead:rewarm and re-examine.
- Do not rewarm too fast, causing peripheral vasodilatation, shock and death. Thermal blankets may cause too rapid warming in old patients.
- Treat the patient gently the most common precipitant of VF hypothermia is mechanical irritation of the body.

Investigation of choice
Core tempeature (< 35°C) +
Urgent U & E, plasma glucose and amylase, TFT +
ECG (definitive if J waves present)

Immediate management
Slowly rewarm after removal of cold stimuli (½°C increase per hour)

Treatment of choice
Warming + treatment of complications (if any)

113. A patient's ECG shows a biphasic P-wave.

Diagnosis: Left atrial hypertrophy (LAH)

Clinchers

Left atrial overload typically produces a biphasic P-wave in V_1 with a broad negative component or a broad ($\geq$ 120 ms), often notched P-wave in one or more leads.

Lead	Normal	LAH
II	RA → ⌒ ← LA	RA → ⌒⌒ ← LA
V_1	RA ⌒ LA	RA ⌒ / LA

Figure

CONFUSA
Biphasic P-wave in lead V_1 is with a prominent negative component representing delayed depolarization of the LA.

Investigation of choice
- *Screening:* ECG
- *Definitive:* Echocardiography

Immediate management
Specialist referral

Treatment of choice
As per the cause of LAH.

Your Notes:

114. A patient's ECG shows T-wave inversion and ST depression.

Diagnosis: Ischaemic heart disease

Clinchers
- *T-wave inversion:* It may signify previous MI. T-wave inversions due to chronic ischaemia correlate with prolongation of repolarisation and are often associated with QT lengthening.
- *ST depression:* It is found in myocardial ischaemia, as a digoxin side effect or in the ventricular "strain pattern" which is found with right or left ventricular hypertrophy. The ST segments are also inverted in bundle branch blocks.

(*Note:* MI cannot be diagnosed from ECG in left bundle branch block).

CONFUSA
Negative T waves can be sign of a sub-endocardial myocardial infarction. They are found in the resolution phase of myocardial infarction and in ischaemic heart disease without evidence of myocardial death.
Note:
- Horizontal depression of ST segment—ischaemia
- Down sloping depression of ST segment—digoxin

Investigation of choice
ECG

Immediate management
Specialist evaluation

Treatment of choice
As per the cause.

Your Notes:

---

115. A 25-year-old woman complains of tiredness and malaise. Her T waves are widespread and deep.

Diagnosis: Myocarditis

Clinchers
- *25-year-old-woman:* Although most common cause of myocarditis is infection in females autoimmune disease results in significant number of cases.
- *Tiredness and malaise:* Symptoms of myocarditis are usually fatigue, dyspnoea, chest pain and palpitations.
- *T waves widespread and deep:* This signify T waves inversion which characteristically occurs in myocardial along with other T-wave abnormalities.

CONFUSA
In myocarditis, ECG demonstrates ST and T-wave abnormalities and arrhythmias. Head blocks may be seen with diphtheric myocarditis, while Chaga's disease produces both heart block and ventricular tachyarrhythmias.

Investigation of choice
Serology + ECG

Immediate management
Bedrest and eradication of any acute infection

Treatment of choice
Treatment of underlying cause
+
Supportive treatment.

Your Notes:

116. A 45-year-old man is diagnosed as having a kidney condition and treated. He soon develops postural hypotension with ankle oedema. His serum sodium is high, his potassium normal, his urea normal, and he has heavy proteinuria.

Diagnosis: Nephrotic syndrome (NS)

Clinchers

- *45-year-old man:* Although proliferative glomerulonephritis is more common than membranous disease, the later is the most common form of glomerulonephritis to cause nephrotic syndrome in UK. Diabetic glomerular disease can also cause it in a middle aged person.
- *Having a kidney condition and treated:* It must be a glomerular nephritis which was treated.
- *Postural hypotension:* It can occur due to autonomic dysfunction and hypovolemia.
- *Ankle oedema:* It is characteristically seen and is due to hypoalbuminaemia.
- *Serum Na^+ high, potassium normal, urea normal:* Activation of renin-angiotensin-aldosterone system produces hyperaldostereonism which promotes sodium and water reabsorption in the distal nephron.
- *Heavy proteinuria:* It occurs partly because structural damage to the glomerular basement membrane leads to an increase in size and number of pores, allowing passage of more and larger molecules. Reduction of fixed negative charge occurs in glomerular disease and is an important factor in genesis of heavy proteinuria.

CONFUSA
Neither elevation of JVP nor pulmonary oedema are features of nephrotic syndrome, through they either or both may be present if renal and/or cardiac failure are present in the nephrotic patient.

Investigation of choice
- *Screening:* 24-hour urinary protein (>3-4 g/day)
- *Definitive:* Transcutaneous renal biopsy

Immediate management
Diuresis (but is contraindicated here because of postural hypotension).

Treatment of choice
Dietary sodium restriction + albumin infusion

117. A 20-year-old teacher is restless and confused. She is pale and sweaty and tachypnoeic. Her arterial oxygen is high and her carbon dioxide is low.

Diagnosis: Alkalosis (Hyperventilation)

Clinchers

- *20-year-old teacher:* Hyperventilation syndrome due to panic attacks is very common in young females.
- *Pale:* Due to sympathetic activation that decreases blood flow to skin and peripheries.
- *Confused:* The alkalemia associated with hypocapnia due to hyperventilation may produce neurologic symptoms (however in panic attacks usually the consciousness is preserved).
- *Tachypnoeic:* This confirms hyperventilation to be the cause of her symptoms.
- *Arterial oxygen is high and CO_2 low:* Due to hyperventilation itself.

CONFUSA
Alveolar hyperventilation decreases $PaCO_2$ and increases the $HCO_3^-/PaCO_2$ ratio, thus increasing pH. Nonbicarbonate cellular buffers respond by consuming HCO_3^-. Hypocapnia develops when a sufficiently strong ventilatory stimulus causes CO_2 output in the lungs to exceed its metabolic production by tissues. Plasma pH and (HCO_3^-) appear to vary proportionately with $PaCO_2$ over a range from 40 to 15 mmHg. Alkalosis thus produces also causes hypocalcaemia.

Investigation of choice
ABG

Immediate management
Reassurance + rebreathing from paper bag

Treatment of choice
Correct alkalosis (+ hypocalcaemia if present).

Your Notes:

118. A baby has a number of fits, each occurring in the morning on four consecutive days. On physical examination you find the liver to be enlarged. His fasting blood sugar is low and his uric acid is high.

Diagnosis: G6PD deficiency

Clinchers
- *Baby:* G6PD deficiency presents at a young age. Among the congenital shunt defects, it is the most common.
- *Number of fits each occurring in the morning on four consecutive days:* These suggest severe hemolytic crises. Since they are occurring at same time every day, the cause should be searched for which could be a breakfast of fava beans or simply circardias stress.
- *Liver to be enlarged:* It is a common finding in G6PD deficiency.
- *Fasting blood sugar low:* It could also be the stress as in newborns (age is not given in this questions), hypoglycemia can precipitate attacks.
- *Uric acid high:* Due to haemolysis.

CONFUSA
Although we are also not 100% convinced by this answer, among the given list of options it is the closest guess. May be some points in either the question or the options is missing. But if the question repeats in this form only, then you can safely mark it as an answer.

Investigation of choice
Characteristic cells in peripheral smear during an attack (Screening: Dye reduction tests)

Immediate management
Consider blood transfusion

Treatment of choice
As per the cause + symptomatic.

Your Notes:

119. A 30-year-old salesman complains of night sweats and dizziness. His ESR is high and blood sugar is low. He has a normocytic anaemia and sterile pyuria.

Diagnosis: Tuberculosis (Genitourinary)

Clinchers
- *30-year-old:* Reactivation of tuberculosis occurs usually in adult life.
- *Sales man:* Since the job profile includes outdoor work and intensive community contact, there is high risk of acquiring communicable diseases.
- *Night sweats and dizziness:* Early in the cause of disease, symptoms and signs are often nonspecific and insidious, consisting mainly of fever and night sweats, weight loss, anorexia, general malaise and weakness.
- *ESR high:* It is an acute phase reactant and is invariably raised (as with almost all chronic diseases).
- *Blood sugar low:* Partly due to loss of appetite and partly due to bacteremia.
- *Normocytic anaemia:* This is the typical anaemia of chronic disease and hence points towards an existing chronic symptomatology.
- *Sterile pyuria:* The documentation of culture-negative pyuria in acidic urine should invariably raise a suspicion of tuberculosis.

CONFUSA
Genitourinary TB accounts for about 15% of all extrapulmonary cases and may involve any portion of GU tract. The kidneys are mainly involved, but it is also a cause of painless, craggy swellings in the epididymis and salpingitis, tubal abscesses and infertility in females. Unlike other systems, in GU infection the local symptoms predominate. Urinary frequency, dysuria, haematuria and flank pain are common presentation although it may be asymptomatic till late in disease.

Investigation of choice
Culture of three morning urine specimens

Immediate management
Find out primary foci of infection (as in almost all cases GU tuberculosis is due to haematogenous spread from elsewhere)

Treatment of choice
Anti TB drug regimen (2+4 months)

120.
A 50-year-old man is brought in by his wife who says he is always farting. He has a fresh abdominal scar. His haemoglobin is low. His mean corpuscular volume is low. His mean corpuscular haemoglobulin concentration is low. And his glucose tolerance test shows lag storage.

Diagnosis: Intestinal hurry

Clinchers

- *50-year-old man:* Occurrence of hypermotility of intestines in this age is not common without an obvious cause.
- *Always farting:* Due to malabsorption.
- *Fresh abdominal scar:* Since intestinal hurry is usually seen after postgastrectomy (dumping), postvagotomy and gastrojejunostomy, it could be due to any of these operations.
- *Hb, MCV, MCHC are all low:* Due to malabsorption (due to HCl deficiency) and intrinsic factor deficiency causing pernicious anaemia.
- *GTT shows lag storage:* This is characteristic of postgastrectomy dumping syndromes and thus confirms our diagnosis.

CONFUSA
The dumping syndrome comprises attacks of fainting, vertigo and sweating after foot, rather like a hypoglycaemic attack. This is probably an osmotic effect due to gastric contents of high osmolarity passing rapidly into the jejunum, absorbing fluid into the gut lumen and producing a temporary reduction in circulating blood volume.

Investigation of choice
GTT

Immediate management
Bulk forming diets

Treatment of choice
Treatment of anaemia + symptomatic

121.
A 16-year-old mother brings her baby for immunization. The nurse notices the baby has multiple bruises along both arms and legs. The baby is crying excessively. The house officer notices multiple fractures and that the baby has blue sclerae.

Diagnosis: Osteogenesis imperfecta.

Clinchers

- *16-year-old mother:* Not of much significance except the fact that battered baby condition is more prevalent among teenage mothers.
- *Multiple bruises along both arms and legs:* Because of connective tissue involvement, the skin scars extensively.
- *Crying excessively:* Because of pain induced by fractures and generalised illness.
- *Multiple fractures:* It is the hallmark of severe osteogenesis imperfecta. But these are also found in battered baby syndrome (non-accidental injury).
- *Blue sclerae:* It is the differentiating feature from non-accidental injury as blue sclerae are almost pathognomic of osteogenesis imperfecta with this clinical profile.

CONFUSA
Non-accidental injury is the main differential diagnosis in this case. Other thing to be noted is that osteogenesis imperfecta is known by many different names and they can appear in the options as such, i.e. fragilitas ossium, brittle bone syndrome, Adair-Dighton syndrome.

Investigation of choice
Screening: X-ray (decrease in bone density)
Definitive: Absorptiometry (X-ray/photon)

Immediate management
Symptomatic treatment (i.e. fractures—traction followed by light cast).

Treatment of choice
Judicious exercise programme to prevent loss of bone mass secondary to physical inactivity.

Your notes:

122. A 70-year-old man is receiving treatment for Alzheimer's disease. He is looked after by a 23-year-old granddaughters. He has recently developed fecal incontinence. The SHO notices bruises on both wrists and back.

Diagnosis: Elderly abuse.

Clinchers
- *70-year-old:* Proves that he is an elderly person!
- *Alzheimer's disease:* Such patients are usually very difficult to look after and one usually requires the services of a trained nurse to care for such demented persons.
- *Fecal incontinence:* Must have compounded the problems of the young granddaughters who was looking after him.
- *Bruises on both wrists and back:* Bruises on both wrists strongly suggest towards use of handcuffs on him, (which his granddaughter might have used to prevent him from wandering aimlessly and getting lost—a frequent occurrence in dementia). The bruises on the back could result either from direct assaults or from the violent attempts of the patient to get free from the handcuffs (thereby bruising his back against wall/bed/chair).

CONFUSA
This is a straight forward question with only a mild confusion between some terminologies in the options. It can qualify as a physical abuse alos, but elderly abuse is more specific and his children rather than the granddaughter are more responsible for his condition.

Investigation of choice
Detailed history.

Immediate management
Admission in hospital and inform social services.

Treatment of choice
Rehabilitation.

Your notes:

123. An anxious mother brings her 6-year-old daughter who is bleeding per vaginum. Six months prior to this presentation the girl had a confirmed streptococcal sore-throat infection. She is otherwise normal.

Diagnosis: Sexual abuse.

Clinchers
- *6-year-old:* Usually such a young child cannot give a proper history of sexual abuse.
- *Bleeding per vaginum:* A common finding in children's sexual abuse. Other common finding is presence of veneral disease before puberty.
- *Confirmed streptococcal sore throat six months back:* This is important as it can be a precipitating factor of Henoch-Schölein purpura. However, it usually does not occur after so long as six months as it is IgA mediated. It usually presents within 2-6 weeks.
- *Otherwise normal:* Rules out any systemic disease.

CONFUSA
The main differential diagnosis in this case is HSP. However the main finding in HSP is a purpura on extensor surfaces which is excluded in this question (as the child is otherwise normal). So it is safe to answer as a childhood sexual abuse. (Also do not forget the theme is non-accidental injury).

Investigation of choice
Forensic specimens (pubic hair, vaginal swabs) by an expert.

Immediate management
Inform social services.

Treatment of choice
Follow local guidelines of the region.

Your notes:

124. A 4-day-old girl is brought to casualty by the maternal grandparent who is worried about two dark bluish patches on the child's buttocks. Child's mother is white and the father is black.

Diagnosis: Battered baby.

Clinchers
- *Brought to casualty by the maternal grandparent.* Always suspect abuse if accompanying adult is not a parent.
- *Two dark bluish patches on the child's buttocks.* Injury to buttocks is one of the most common finding in battered baby syndrome.
- *Child's mother is white and the father is black.* Inter-racial marriages are often a risk factor for battered baby syndrome.

CONFUSA
The main differential diagnosis in this case is 'birth marks' or congenital naevus. But they are usually present either at birth or after seven days (Strawberry angioma). Here the socio-cultural history is also raising suspicious of battered baby syndrome.

Investigation of choice
Detailed history from accompanying adult + complete physical examination.

Immediate management
Inform social services.

Treatment of choice
Follow local guidelines of region/hospital.

Your notes:

---

125. An 8-year-old girl is noted to have fresh bloody staining of her pants. She also suffers from eneuresis. she has recently started horse-riding lessons

Diagnosis: Accidental injury.

Clinchers
- *Fresh bloody staining of her pant:* Most probably from trauma as the history given in question does not potray any illness.
- *She also suffers from eneuresis:* Bedwetting occurs on most nights in 15% of 5-year-olds, and is still a problem in upto 3% of 15-year-olds (usually from delayed maturation of bladder control). So it is probably normal.
- *She has recently started horse-riding lessons:* It can be reason for trauma, most probably rupture of hymen, which is common in horse riding training for adolescent girls.

CONFUSA
GMC has tried to mislead us by putting the history of eneuresis in this question. But eneuresis has nothing to do with bleeding anywhere. So the question is still straight enough.

Investigation of choice
For bleeding: Local examination.

For eneuresis: Test for UTI, GU abnormality and DM.

Immediate management
Reassurance.

Treatment of choice
Desmopressin nasal spray.

Your notes:

126. An obese 34-year-old man complains of epigastric pain, which seems to exacerbated by eating his favourite meal, fish and chips. He get temporary relief when hungry.

Diagnosis: Peptic ulcer (PU) disease

Clinchers
- *Obese:* There is no *per se* relationship between obesity and PU disease. Although PU patients may gain weight due to high intake of milk to relieve symptoms.
- *34-year-old man:* In UK, ulcer rates are declining rapidly for young man and increasing rapidly for older individuals especially females DU are more common than GU in young man.
- *Epigastric pain:* The pain is typically epigastric occurs in attacks that last for days or weeks and interspersed with periods of relief. Pain that radiates into the back suggest a posterior penetrating ulcer.
- *Exacerbated by eating his favourite meal, fish and chips:* The pain is usually related to hunger, eating specific foods, or the time of the day. Often associated with heaviness, bloating or fullness after meals.
- *Get temporary relief when hungry:* The pain of duodenal ulceration is worse when hungry so this excludes it to be the cause.

CONFUSA
The relationship of the pain to food is variably and on the whole is not helpful in the diagnosis. It is a myth to say that one can differentiate between a gastric and duodenal ulcer merely on the time relationship of the pain. Peptic ulcer may come on immediately after a meal but more typically commences about 2 hours after food.

Investigation of choice
Upper GI endoscopy

Immediate management
Counselling (stop smoking + food advise)

Treatment of choice
Triple therapy (for *H. pylori*)
+
Acid suppression (proton-pump inhibitor).

Your Notes:

---

127. An obese 45-year-old man complains of recurring chest pain which radiates to his neck lasting 20 minutes. It coincides with his weekly executive board meetings.

Diagnosis: Stable angina

Clinchers
- *Obese:* Obesity, particularly central obesity, is associated with coronary artery disease, but it is not certain which obesity itself is independently linked to the condition.
- *45-year-old:* Coronary artery disease rates increase with age.
- *Man:* Males constitutes approximately 70% of cases
- *Recurring chest pain:* Indicates angina most in this clinical profile.
- *Radiates to neck:* Angina can radiate to the left shoulder and to both arms and especially to the ulnar surfaces of the forearm and hand. It can also arise in or radiate to the back, neck, jaw, teeth or epigastrium.
- *Lasting 20 minutes:* The pain fades quickly i.e. with 1-5 minutes and never last more than 20 minutes.
- *Consider with....:* This is the precipitant (i.e. stress) and hence it is stable angina.

CONFUSA
Stable angina is one which is precipitated by exertion (e.g. exercise, hurrying or sexual activity) or emotion (e.g. stress, anger, fright or frustration) and are relieved by rest. When it occurs at rest it is called unstable angina. Occasionally the pain of stable angina disappears with continued exertion. Cardiac syndrome X refers to these patients with a good history of angina, a positive exercise test and angiographically normal coronary arteries.

Investigation of choice
Exercise ECG (confirms the diagnosis)

Immediate management
GTN sublingual for termination of an acute attack.

Treatment of choice
Aspirin (75 mg daily).

Your Notes:

128. An obese 29-year-old woman complains of with a cough of two weeks complains of right upper quadrant pain. She is mildly febrile. There was no abdominal tenderness on examination.

Diagnosis: Tuberculosis (TB)

Clinchers
- *Obese:* These is no as such relationship.
- *29-year-old woman:* It can occur in any age group although and elderly (> 70 years) are more susceptible.
- *Cough of two weeks:* Prolonged cough without any major systemic manifestations is a strong indicator of TB.
- *RUQ pain:* Although classically TB involves upper lobes, in immunocompromised states it may involve any portion of lung (basilar lobe of right lung in this case).
- *Mildly febrile:* It manifest usually as a vague illness with mid evening rise of temperature.
- *No abdominal tenderness:* This rules out cholecystitis as a differential diagnosis.

CONFUSA
TB can cause disease when there is only minimal immunosuppression and thus often appears early in the course of infection. HIV related TB frequently represents reactivation of latent TB, but there is also clear evidence of newly acquired infection and nosocomial spread in HIV-infected populations. The response of tuberculosis testing is blunted in HIV-positive individuals and is unreliable. Sputum microscopy may be negative even in pulmonary infection and culture techniques are the best diagnostic tools.

Investigation of choice
Sputum microscopy and culture

Immediate management
HIV screening in suspected on history

Treatment of choice
Anti TB therapy.

Your Notes:

129. Condition associated with epigastric pain radiating to the back, pale loose stools, associated with alcohol consumption.

Diagnosis: Chronic pancreatitis.

Clinchers
- *Epigastric pain radiating to the back:* In chronic pancreatitis the epigastric pain 'bores' through to the back. It is relieved by:
  - Sitting forward
  - Hot water bottles on epigastrium/back: look for *erythema ab ignes* dusky greyness here.
- *Pale loose stools:* These signify steatorrhoea a common finding in this condition. It is due to pancreatic insufficiency and also results in malabsorption (hence bloating) and weight loss.
- *Alcohol consumption:* Chronic alcohol intake is the most common cause of chronic pancreatitis. Although rarely it can be produced by:
  - Cystic fibrosis
  - Haemochromatosis
  - Pancreatic duct obstruction
    - Stones
    - Pancreatic cancer
  - Hyperparathyroidism
  - Familial.

CONFUSA
Serum amylase estimations performed during attacks of pain may be elevated, but in long-standing disease are often normal, there being insufficient pancreatic tissue remaining to cause a large rise. The differential diagnosis of chronic pancreatitis from a pancreatic carcinoma is usually possible only at laparotomy.

Investigation of choice
USG (dilated biliary tree; stones)
Note: If USG is normal consider CT or ERCP

Immediate management
Blood glucose (as chronic pancreatitis can produce diabetes)

Treatment of choice
Stop alcohol
+
Analgesia
+
Low fat diet with pancreatic enzyme (pancreatin) by mouth
Pancreatico-jejunostomy/total pancreatectomy for refractive cases.

First Aid for the PLAB

130. Female with fever, rigors, right upper quadrant pain, jaundice, USG is normal.

Diagnosis: Acute cholecystitis.

Clinchers
- *Female:* Female sex is a risk factor for cholesterol stones in gallbladder, which is the usual cause for acute cholecystitis. The disease can occur at any age.
- *Fever, rigors:* The patient is usually ill with a fever and shallow respirations.
- *Right upper quadrant (RUQ) pain:* The main symptoms are severe pain in the epigastrium and right hypochondrium. The pain is continuous, increasing in intensity over 24 hours. It can radiate to back and shoulder. It may be accompanied by nausea and vomiting. Right hypochondrium tenderness is present, being worse on inspiration (Murphy's sign). There is guarding and rebound tenderness.
- *Jaundice:* Mild jaundice occurs in 20% of cases owing to accompanying common duct stones or to surrounding oedema occluding the CBD.
- *USG is normal:* Although can accurately diagnose stones as small as 2 mm, it may be false negative in 2-4 percent of cases.

CONFUSA
A less severe case of acute pancreatitis simulates acute cholecystitis. The fever in acute cholecystitis is more marked than pancreatitis and is in range of 38-39° C with marked toxaemia and leucocytosis. Rigors are almost nerve seen in acute pancreatitis.

Investigation of choice
Oral cholecystography (OCG)
OCG is a useful procedure for diagnosis of gallstones but has been diagnosis replaced by USG. However, OCG is still useful for
- Selection of patients for nonsurgical therapy of gallstone disease such as
  - Lithotripsy
  - Bile duct dissolution therapy
- When USG is inconclusive

Immediate management
Nil by mouth + analgesia

Treatment of choice
Cefuroxime 1.5 g/8 h IV
In suitable candidates do cholecystectomy (laparoscopic if no question of GB perforation).

131. An HIV patient develops a severe headache and confusion. She is discovered to have bilateral papillodema.

Diagnosis: Cerebral toxoplasmosis.

Clinchers
- *HIV patient:* The most common CNS infections in a HIV poistive patient are cerebral toxoplasmosis and cryptococcal meningitis.
- *Severe headache:* The clinical presentation of cerebral toxoplasmosis is of focal neurological features, convulsions, fever, headache and possible confusion.
- *Bilateral papilloedema:* It may be positive due to increased intracranial tensions as toxoplasmosis behave like a space occupying lesion.

CONFUSA
In addition to classic presentation as a CNS mass lesion, T. gondii has been reported to cause a variety of other clinical problems in HIV infected patients, including a CNS presentation more characteristic of herpes simplex with a negative CT scan, chorioretinitis, pneumonia, peritonitis with ascites, gastrointestinal tract involvement, cystitis and orchitis.

Investigation of choice
- *Screening:* CT scan—multiple ring enhancing lesions.
  Note:
  - A single lesion on CT may be found to be one of several on MRI
  - A solitary lesion on MRI mitigates against toxoplasmosis
- *Definitive:*
  Brain biopsy.

Immediate management
Medical management of raised ICT.

Treatment of choice
Pyrimethamine + Sulfadiazine
(side effects: Renal stones)

Your Notes:

132. An 8-year-old with acute leukemia is admitted in a comatose state. He is found to have lymphoblast depletion prevention of infectious diseases.

Diagnosis: Tumor lysis syndrome.

Clinchers
- *8-year-old leukaemias are the most common type of childhood:* Malignancies are over 95% of cases are of acute variety. In the acute series ALL accounts for 70-80% cases. The peak age of onset of ALL is 3-7 years.
- *Acute leukaemia:* As his diagnosis is known he must be on some treatment. Usually chemotherapy is given for ALL.
- *Lymphoblast depletion:* Since lymphoblasts rapidly proliferate in ALL, their depletion should raise a suspicion of any treatment with chemotherapeutic drugs. Tumor lysis syndrome is due to rapid cell death on starting chemotherapy for rapidly proliferating tumors like ALL. It results in rise in serum urate, potassium and phosphate, precipitating renal failure, which can lead to comatose condition if not treated urgently.

CONFUSA
Coma can also occurs in ALL as leukemic blast cells can infiltrate brain to produce leukemic meningitis.

Investigation of choice
Serum urate level (increased).

Immediate management
Immediate hydration.

Treatment of choice
Haemodialysis.

Your Notes:

---

133. A 14-year-old boy presents with drowsiness and generalised headache. He is recovering from a bilateral parotitits. His CT scan is normal.

Diagnosis: Viral meningitis (aseptic meningitis)

Clinchers
- *14-year-old boy:* Mumps is generally a childhood disease caused by RNA paramyoxovirus. Incidence of meningitis in males is three times more after mumps.
- *Drowsiness and generalised headache:* There are cardinal symptoms of increased ICP. Other symptoms can be:
  - Irritability
  - Vomiting
  - Fits
  - Bradycardia
  - BP increase
  - Impaired consciouness (confusion)
  - Coma
  - Irregular respiration
  - papilloedema (late sign)
- *Recovering from bilateral parotitis:* Meningitis secondary to mumps usually occur in convalescent phase. Mumps is characterised by painful swelling of the parotids, unilaterally at first, becoming bilateral in 70%.
- *CT scan is normal:* Rules out any space occupying lesion in the brain or ventricular dilatation, both of which are contraindication to lumbar puncture.

CONFUSA
In aseptic meningitis, CSF has cells but is Gram stain negative and no bacteria can be cultured on standard media. Mumps infection confers life-long immunity, so a documented history of previous infection excludes this diagnosis.

Investigation of choice
- *Screening:* Lumbar puncture, will show a picture of aseptic meningitis
- *Definitive:* Isolation of virus from CSF.

Immediate management
Symptomatic (hospital admission usually not required).

Treatment of choice
Bed-rest in a quiet and dark room.

Your Notes:

134. An intravenous drug abuser presents with suspected meningitis. The organism is confirmed in the CSF by India ink preparation.

Diagnosis: Cryptococcal meningitis.

Clinchers
- *IV drug abuser:* He must be having an undiagnosed HIV infection resulting in immunodeficient state. Cryptococcal meningitis does not occur in immunocompetent people.
- *Suspected meningitis:* CNS infections in HIV positive people are usually by toxoplasmosis, CMV and *Cryptococcus*. Toxoplasmosis causes a SOL and CMV causes encephalitis. *Cryptococcus* is associated with meningitis usually.
- *Organism confirmed in CSF in India Ink preparation:* This is characteristic of *Cryptococcus neoformans* (a fungi) whose thick capsule resist staining and can only be demonstrated as translucencies against black background in India ink preparations.

CONFUSA
Cryptococcal meningitis have an insidious onset and is often without neck stiffness. The etiology of neck stiffness is inflammation and it is often absent in immunodeficients and neonates. Conditions (other than meningitis) which can produce neck stiffness are *Shigella* gastroenteritis and subarachnoid hemorrhage.

Investigation of choice
India ink staining of CSF.
or
Detection of cryptococcal antigen in blood/CSF.

Immediate management
Transfer to ITU.

Treatment of choice
Amphotericin/fluocytosine IV
Fluconazole can be given in milder cases (better tolerated).

Your Notes:

---

135. An anxious mother called you to say that her son's best friend in school has caught meningitis.

Diagnosis: Immediate 'contact' of meningitis.

Clinchers
Meningitis prophylaxis:
Talk to your consultant in community disease control. Offer prophylaxis is:
- Household/nurser contacts (i.e. within droplet range)
- Those who have kissed the patient's mouth.

CONFUSA
If the student suffering from meningitis is just a classmate and the best friend of her son, then there is no need of any chemoprophylaxis.

Investigation of choice
None required except screening the skin for any nonblanching petechiae.

Immediate management
Reassure mother

Treatment of choice
Rifampicin prophylaxis
- 600 mg/12 h PO for 2 days
- Children   > 1 yr 10 mg/kg/12 h
              < 1 yr 10 mg/kg/12 h

or
Ciprofloxacin
- 500 mg PO, 1 dose, adult only

Your Notes:

136. Uncomplicated urinary tract infection (UTI)

Diagnosis: Stated as the question itself.

Clinchers
In acute uncomplicated cases, more than 80% of infections are due to *E. coli* and although resistance patterns vary geographically, most strains are sensitive to many antibiotics. Single doses of trimethoprim-sulfamethoxazole (four single strength tablets), trimethoprim alone (400 mg), sulfa alone (2.0 g), and most fluoroquinolones (norfloxacin, ciprofloxacin, ofloxacin) have been used successfully to treat acute uncomplicated episodes.

CONFUSA
The advantages of single dose therapy include less expense, ensured compliance, fever side effects and perhaps less intense pressure following the selection of resistant organisms in the intestinal, vaginal or perianal flora.

Investigation of choice
MSU culture

Immediate management
Exclude STD

Treatment of choice
Trimethoprim.

Your Notes:

137. Pseudomembranous colitis (Patient allergic to vancomycin).

Diagnosis: Stated as the question itself

Clinchers
All suspected antibiotics should be discontinued and this alone may result in the diarrhea stopping. Vancomycin 125 mg orally, QID for 10 days are often used but metronidazole is also effective, considerably it is less expensive and used in cases of vancomycin allergy.

CONFUSA
Relapses are common and toxic dilatation can rarely occur. There is no evidence that changing chemotherapy helps. Patients should be isolated to try to prevent spread to other susceptible individuals. Essentially any antibiotics can cause this syndrome, even metronidazole and vancomycin, which are used to treat the dsiease.

Investigation of choice
Stool culture

Immediate management
Isolation of patient in ward

Treatment of choice

Metronidazole (Since patient is allergic to vancomycin).

Your Notes:

138. Sinusitis in patient allergic to penicillin

Diagnosis: Stated as the question itself

Clinchers
Treatment of sinusitis is always with antibiotics. Many strains of H.influenzae are resistant to amoxycillin so co-amoxiclav or cofactor are preferred. Erythromycin is an alternative for those with penicillin allergy.

> **CONFUSA**
> In addition, nasal treatment with decongestants such as xylometazoline or anti-inflammatory therapy with topical corticosteroids such as fluticasone proprionate nasal spray should be given to reduce swelling of the mucosa and unblock the sinus openings.

Investigation of choice
Clinical diagnosis

Immediate management
Rule out liver disease before starting erythromycin treatment

Treatment of choice
Erythromycin.

Your Notes:

139. Acute otitis media.

Diagnosis: Stated as the question itself

Clinchers
Treatment with antibacterials is indicated in all cases with fever and severe earache. As the most common organisms and strep. pneumonia and H.influenzae, the drugs which are effective in acute otitis media are ampicillin (50 mg/kg/day in 4 divided doses), amoxicillin (40 mg/kg/day) in 3 divided doses). It must be continued for a minimum of 10 days, till tympanic membrane regains normal appearance and hearing returns to normal.

> **CONFUSA**
> Those allergic to penicillins can be given cofactor, cotrimoxaole or erythromycin. In cases where beta-lactamase producing H.influenzae or moraxella catarrhalis are isolated antibiotics like amoxicillin-clavulnate (Augmentin), cefuroxime axetil or cefixime may be used. Early discontinuance of therapy with relief of earache and fever, or therapy given in inadequate doses may lead to secretory otitis medial and residual hearing loss.

Investigation of choice
Bacteriology

Immediate management
Ear toilet + analgesia

Treatment of choice
Amoxicillin.

Your Notes:

140. Acute streptococcal sore throat (patient allergic to penicillin).

Diagnosis: Stated as the question itself

Clinchers
Streptococcal pharyngitis (Group A, beta-hemolytic) is treated with penicillin G, 200,000 to 250,000 units orally four times a day for 10 days or benzathine penicillin G 600,000 units once i.m. for patient less than 60 lb in weight and 1.2 million units once i.m for patient > 60 lb.

> **CONFUSA**
> In penicillin-sensitive individuals, erythromycin, 20 to 40 mg/kg body weight daily in divided oral doses for 10 days is equally effective.

Investigation of choice
Culture of throat swab

Immediate management
Exclude liver disease before starting erythromycin treatment
+
Advise warm saline gargles

Treatment of choice
Erythromycin.

Your Notes:

---

141. A patient in her third pregnancy presents to her GP at 12 weeks gestation. She was mildly hypertensive in both of her previous pregnancies. Her BP is 150/100 mm Hg. Two weeks later at the hospital antenatal clinic her BP is 150/95 mm Hg.

Diagnosis: Essential hypertension (EH)

Clinchers
- *Third pregnancy:* EH is common in older multiparas, and present before pregnancy or in first trimester (in this case 12 weeks).
- *Mildly hypertensive in both of her previous pregnancies:* Those with EH are five times more likely to develop pre-eclampsia. Also increased BP is a positive risk factor for PIH.
- *BP is 150/100 mmHg, two weeks later 150/95 mmHg:* Isolated BP measurements are never reliable in pregnancy. So BP has to be recorded on at least two occasions (at least >4 hrs apart) to make a diagnosis. In this case the BP is more of less the smae on two occasions (two weeks apart). Also the diastolic BP is > 90 mmHg on both occasions.

> **CONFUSA**
> If the symptoms are episodic, think of phaeochromocytoma. PIH by definition does not present before 20 weeks for the first-time.

Investigation of choice
24 hours urinary proteins (to screen for pre-eclampsia).

Immediate management
BP monitoring (biweekly).

Treatment of choice
Oral antihypertensive (as BP should be kept < 140/90 mmHg).

Your Notes:

142. A 22-year-old Nigerian woman has an uneventful first pregnancy to 30 weeks. She is then admitted with epigastric pain. During the first two hours her BP rises from 150/105 to 170/120 mmHg. On dipstick test she is found to have 3+ proteinuria. The fetal cardiotocogram (CTG) is normal.

Diagnosis: Fulminating PIH.

Clinchers

- *First pregnancy:* 70% cases of pre-eclampsia occur in primigravidas. A recurrence rate of 20% is present for multigravidas (with same partner). With a new partner the incidence of recurrence increases.
- *30 weeks:* By definition PIH present for the first-time after 20 weeks.
- *Epigastric pain:* It is due to stretching of liver capsule.
- *PB rises from 150/105 to 170/120 mmHg in two hours:* A rapid rise in BP is a characteristic feature of fulminant PIH and require immediate IV antihypertensives.
- *3 + proteinuria:* It signifies significant proteinuria and hence qualifies for the diagnosis of fulminant PIH.
  CTG is normal: Abnormal CTG signifies fetal distress and warrants an immediate caesarean section. In this case it is not required as CTG is normal. Still regular CTG monitoring (1 to 2 per day of one hour each) must be done.

CONFUSA

In severe (fulminating) PIH, delivery is the only definitive treatment (Note: PIH regress by delivery of placenta and not only fetus). The delivery is often vaginal, except in conditions given below where a caesarian section is preferred (A B C D E)
 A—Abruption
 B—BP unctrollable; breech
 C—Cervix unfavourable
 D—Distress of fetus
 E—Error in induction of delivery (failed induction)
Note: Delivery criteria in PIH
 Mild PIH—can continue till 40 weeks
 Moderate PIH—can continue till 37 weeks
 Severe PIH—as soon as possible
 and eclampsia

Investigation of choice
CTG (already done in this case).

Immediate management
IV hydralazine/Labetalol.

Treatment of choice
Intravenous antihypertensive (hydralazine/labetalol) immediately + Regular monitoring.

143. At an antenatal clinic visit at 38 weeks gestation, a 36-year-old multiparous woman has a BP of 140/90 mmHg. She has no proteinuria and is otherwise well.

Diagnosis: Normal.

Clinchers

- *38 weeks gestation:* PIH usually present in the second trimester and not this late.
- *36-year-old:* Age > 35 years (or < 20 years) is a positive risk factor for PIH/eclampsia).
- *Multiparous:* Usually multiparous females are not affected by PIH if there is no history of it in the previous pregnancies.
- *BP 140/90 mmHg:* By definition the diastolic BP has to cross 90 to qualify for a diagnosis of PIH. The classification criteria of PIH are given in next question (Q 189). This BP does not classify as a criteria for diagnosis.
- *No proteinuria:* Excludes pre-eclampsia/severe PIH.
- *Otherwise well:* Excludes other medical disorders.

CONFUSA

In cases of PIH (pregnancy induced hypertension), admit if
- BP rises by >30/20 mmHg over booking BP
- BP reaches
  - 160/100 without proteinuria
  - 140/90 with proteinuria

PIH can be diagnosed only with BP elevation above in criteria on at least 2 occasions (> 4 hours apart).

Investigation of choice
Biweekly BP monitoring.

Immediate management
Take second BP measurement after four hours.

Treatment of choice
A period of observation for blood pressure.

Your Notes:

144. At 32 weeks, a 22-year-old primigravida is found to have a BP of 145/100 mmHg. She has no proteinuria but is found to have edema of her knees.

Diagnosis: Pregnancy induced hypertension (PIH).

Clinchers
- *32 weeks:* By definition PIH called so only if it appears for first-time after 20 weeks. Hypertension occurring before is usually due to an existing and non-pregnancy induced condition.
- *Primigravida:* PIH is an almost exclusive disease of primigravidas.
- *BP of 145/100 mmHg with no proteinuria:* PIH is classified according to BP and proteinuria.
  Mild PIH—BP upto 140/100 without proteinuria
  Moderate PIH—BP upto 160/110 without proteinuria
  Severe PIH—BP more than 160/110 with proteinuria
  (Proteinuria is > 300 mg excretion of proteins in urine in 24 hours).
- *Oedema of her knees:* Peripheral edema in pregnancy has little significance if it occurs as an isolated finding. But it signifies severe PIH if it occurs along with hypertension and proteinuria.

CONFUSA
PIH is almost exclusively seen in primigravidas. But in multiparous women its risk is increased if the existing pregnancy is with a new partner. Other risk factors for PIH in multigravidas are: history of first pregnancy, H. mole, multiple pregnancy, gestational diabetes mellitus.

Investigation of choice
Fetal USG.

Immediate management
Admit in first instance for assessment and monitoring.

Treatment of choice
Since the disease in question is a moderate PIH, its management is:
- Care in day assessment until/hospital
- Oral antihypertensives if—BP > 160/100 (sustained)
  Note: It is > 170/110 according to OHCS.
- Can continue upto 37 weeks with regular monitoring of:
  Daily—urinary proteins
  Bi-weekly—LFT
  Weekly—Plasma U and E, plasma urate, total urinary proteins.

Indications of delivery in moderate disease
- Progression to pre-eclampsia
- Declining maternal renal function
- Fetal distress
  - Abnormal CTG (cardiotocogram)
  - Absence of end diastolic flow in doppler of umbilical circulation
- Placental abruption.

Your Notes:

145. At 34 weeks, an 86 kg woman complains of persistent headaches and 'flashing lights'. There is no hyper-reflexia and her BP is 150/100 mmHg. Urinalysis is negative but she has finger edema.

Diagnosis: Pre-eclampsia

Clinchers
Preclampsia is a syndrome of sings and when the symptoms occurs, it is usually too late.
- *34 weeks:* It develops after 20 weeks and usually resolves within 10 days of delivery.
- *86 kg woman:* Predisposing factors of pre-eclampsia are

Maternal	Fetal
• Primiparity	• H mole
• History of severe pre-eclampsia	• Multiple pregnancy
• Positive family history	• Placental hydrops
• Height <155 cm	(e.g. Rh disease)
• Overweight	
• Age < 20 or > 35 yrs	
• Pre-existing migraine	
• BP ↑ or renal disease	

- *Persisting headaches:* Frontal>occipital, reason is cerebral edema. It is of dragging/throbbing type
  - Worsen on
    - Supine position
    - Morning
  - Resolves on—mobility
- *Flashing lights:* Visual symptoms are common in pre-eclampsia. They are due to edema of neural layer in retina.
  The most common visual symptoms are
  - Black holes
  - Double vision
  - Flashing lights
- *No hyperreflexia:* Hyperreflexia is said to be present when a reflex can be obtained away from the tendon that usually causes it, e.g. knee reflex by tapping anterior surface of tibia (rather than the tendon). It is an important sign of impending eclampsia.
- *BP is 150/100:* A diastolic BP exceeding 90 mmHg on at least two occasions in the second half of pregnancy, where the blood pressure was previously normal, accompanied by significant proteinuria (> 300 mg/24 h) qualifies for a diagnosis of pre-eclampsia.
- *Urinalysis negative:* It means no proteinuria. Proteinuria is the last feature of pre-eclampsia to appear. It may be trace or at times coupious. There may be few hyaline casts, epithelial cells or even few red cells. It is considered significant only when >300 mg/24 h. Proteinuria may also be missed in an isolated urinary examination, so do a 24 hours total urinary protein excretion measurement to rule it out.
- *Finger edema:* Traditionally the presence of peripheral oedema has been included in the definition, however, this is a common finding in otherwise normal pregnancy and its absence does not preclude the diagnosis (nor does its presence makes the diagnosis). However, tightness of the ring on the finger (finger oedema) is an early manifestation of pre-eclampsia oedema. Gradually the swelling may extend to face, abdominal wall, vulva and even the whole body.

CONFUSA
In the UK, high quality antenatal care has reduced the problems of pre-eclamptic toxaemia to such an extent that 75% of cases of eclampsia now occur in the post-partum period and a similar proportion occur without pre-existing hypertension.

Investigation of choice
24 hours urinary protein.

Immediate management
BP control by IB hydralazine/Labetalol if there is an acute or progressive increase in BP.

Treatment of choice
Oral antihypertensive are given in case of sustained rise of BP till > 160/100 mmHg or at lower levels if cerebral edema is present (i.e. in this case). Antihypertensives that can be uses are;
- Methyldopa—contraindicated in liver disease
- Labetalol—contraindicated in asthma
- Magnesium sulfate—(preferred drug in USA)

Your Notes:

146. A 42-year-old woman complains of excessive thirst, polyuria, polydipsia and constipation. She admits to losing weight. Her fasting blood glucose is 5.4 mmol/L.

Diagnosis: Hypercalcemia

Clinchers
- *Excessive thirst, polyuria, polydipsia and constipation:* All these along with abdominal pain, vomiting, depressions, anorexia, weight loss, tiredness, weakness, BP ↑, confusion, pyrexia, renal stones, corneal calcification and cardiac arrest are the symptoms of hypercalcaemia.
- *Admits to losing weight:* Already discussed above, weight loss is also seen in hypercalcaemia.
- *Fasting glucose of 5.4 mmol/L:* This is normal. Normal range of fasting glucose ranges between 3.5 to 5.5 mmol/L. Fasting glucose of ≥ 7 mmol/L, is diagnostic of diabetes mellitus. A glucose of 6-7 mmol/L implies impaired fasting glucose.

CONFUSA
Since fasting blood glucose level of this patient is 5.4 mmol/L, (i.e. well within normal limits) these signs and symptoms should not be confused with diabetes mellitus.

Investigation of choice
- Blood tests: U & E, Mg^{2+}, Ca^{2+}, PO_4^{3-}
- ECG: Q-T interval ↓

Immediate management
Monitor U & E
Aim to reduce serum calcium as follows:
- Rehydrate with 0.9% salive (IVI) as needed
- Correct hypokalemia/hypomagnesemia, as this will reduce symptoms and ↑ renal Ca^{2+} loss.

Treatment of choice
Once rehydrated
- Give diuretics (Frusemide) avoid thiazide
- Bisphosphate: acts over 2-3 day. Maximum effect is at 1 week. It lowers serum Ca^{2+}.

Your Notes:

---

147. A 23-year-old man being treated for myeloma is brought to the A and E Department, confused. This followed an hour history of severe abdominal pain, vomiting. Prior to this, the patient had complained of polyuria, polydipsia and constipation.

Diagnosis: Hypercalcemia

Clinchers
- *Being treated for myeloma:* Most common cause of hypercalcaemia is malignancy (myeloma, bone metastases, PTH - P↑) and 1° hyperparathyroidism.
- *Brought to A & E department, confused:* Confusion, pyreixa, depression are the important presenting symptoms of hypercalcaemia.
- *History of severe abdominal pain, vomiting:* These along with constipation, polyuria, polydipsia, weight loss, are important signs and symptoms of hypercalcemia.

CONFUSA
Malignancy and 1° hyperparathyroidism are the most common cause of hypercalcemia. Always rule out DM.

Investigation of choice
- Serum calcium (normal — 2.12-2.65 mmol/L)
- Blood sugar
- ECG.

Immediate management
- Monitor U & E
- Aim to reduce serum (Ca^{2+} as follow
  - Rehydrate with 0.9% saline (IVI) as needed
  - Correct hypokalaemia/hypomagnesemia as this will reduce symptoms and ↑ serum Ca^{2+} loss.

Treatment of choice
Once rehydrated:
- Give diuretics (frusemide) avoid thiazides
- Bisphonoate: acts over 2-3 days. Maximum effect is at 1 week. It lowers serum Ca^{2+}.

Your Notes:

148. A 16-year-old frail girl coplains of constipation. Her Body Mass Index (BMI) is found to be 17. She is extremely afraid of eating and admits to sticking a finger down her throat to induce vomiting after meals. She is unusually sensitive to cold.

Diagnosis: Anorexia noervosa

Clinchers

- *16-year-old girl:* Anorexia mainly affects females (sex ratio 10 : 1). The average age of onset is 15-16 years. The prevalence in the UK is about 1% in females aged 12-18.
- *Frail:* It signifies the weight loss.
- *Constipation:* It is due to reduced food intake and not due to any other pathology.
- *BMI 17:* BMI < 17.5 is diagnostic of anorexia in this typical clinical profile.
- *Extremely afraid of eating:* This is found as there is a profound fear of getting fat.
- *Admits to sticking a finger down her throat to induce vomiting after meals:* It social circumstances or binge eating causes more intake than usual, vomiting induced as soon as possible, often in a public rest room.
- *Unusually sensitive to cold:* Cold intolerance is presumable due to a defect in regulatory thermogenesis secondary to hypothalamic dysfunction.

CONFUSA
Patients with anorexia nervosa are vulnerable to sudden death from ventricular tachyarrhythmias. ECG shows prolonged QT intervals. The risk of death becomes high when weight declines 35% below ideal, probably because of protein deficiency.

Investigation of choice
Clinical diagnosis

Immediate management
Admit

Treatment of choice
Cognitive-behaviour therapy.

Your Notes:

---

149. A 60-year-old man with a history of weight loss, presents with bleeding per rectum. He also reports a history of diarrhoea which seems to alternate with constipation. His haemoglobin is 10g/dl.

Diagnosis: Carcinoma of the colon

Clinchers

- *60-year-old man:* Females are affected more than males (carcinoma colon). More common in elderly females.
- *History of weight loss:* Sign of malignancy.
- *Bleeding per rectum:* Diarrhoea in colonic carcinoma is accompanied by mucus (produced by the excessive secretion of mucus from the tumor), or bleeding which may be bright, melaena, or occult.
- *Diarrhoea alternative with constipation:* This is the most common local effect, produced by carcinoma of colon (local effect).

CONFUSA
The most important differential diagnosis is from diverticulosis of colon. It is impossible to be certain of this differentiation clinically or even on special investigations unless a positive biopsy is obtained by flexible sigmoidoscopy or colonoscopy. Ulcerative colitis should also be kept in mind.

Investigation of choice
- Sigmoidoscopy/colonoscopy
- U and E, barium enema (look for filling defect (apple core appearance).

Immediate management
Monitor U and E

Treatment of choice
Principle of operative treatment is wide resection of the growth together with it regional lymphatics.

Your Notes:

150. A 65-year-old woman presents with constipation, and reports difficulty in starting or stopping to walk. She has dysarthria and dribbling.

Diagnosis: Parkinsonism (Shy-Drager syndrome)

Clinchers
- *65-year-old woman:* It generally commences in middle or late life and leads to progressive disability with time. The disease occurs in all ethnic groups, has an equal sex distribution and is common, with a prevalence of 1 to 2 per 1000 of general population and 1 per 100 among people older than 64 years.
- *Constipation + drabbling:* Disturbances of bladder and bowel control characteristic shy-drager syndrome.
- *Difficult in starting or stopping to walk:* Walking is often difficult to initiate and patients may have to lean forward increasingly until they can advance. They walk with small, shuffling steps, have no arm swing and they are unsteady (especially on tuning) and may have difficulty in stopping.
- *Dysarthria:* The voice is hypophasic and poorly modulated.

CONFUSA
Shy-Drager syndrome is a well-characterized severe form of multi-system atrophy that is accompanied by autonomic failure. Most patients present with autonomic dysfunction alone and other neurologic manifestations usually develop within 5 years. Patients with the stiatonigral variant exhibit a form of Parkinsonism in which bradykinesia and rigidity are more prominent that tremor.

Investigation of choice
Clinical diagnosis

Immediate management
Exclude other similar disease + specialist evaluation

Treatment of choice
Levodopa
 +
Speech therapy.

151. A 23-year-old woman has been using heroin (IV) for 4-years. She is not willing to stop using the heroin.

Diagnosis: Risk for HIV and hepatitis B

Clinchers
- *23-year-old woman:* Highest incidence and prevalence of drug abuse is in teens and twenties.
- *IV heroin for 4 years:* She is at high risk of acquiring serious communicable disease like HIV and hepatitis B.
- *Not willing to stop using the heroin:* Although it is the duty of the doctor to counsel the patient for deaddiction, but he can not force it. For patients unwilling to stop drug abuse, the doctor should arrange for enrolment in the local needle exchange programme. The heatlh office maintain a confidential register for that purpose.

CONFUSA
The practice of sharing needles and syringes for IV drug use continues to be a major route for transmission of HIV in both developed countries and parts of Southeast Asia and latin America. In some areas successful education and needle exchange schemes have reduced the rate of transmission by this route. Needle exchange is successful as the drug abusers often do not have enough money to spend on needles and thus extremely share and reuse them.

Investigation of choice
HIV screening after consent

Immediate management
Needle exchange

Treatment of choice
De-addiction counselling and enrolment.

Your Notes:

152. A third-year medical student was drawing blood from a known HIV positive patient gets a needle stick injury.

Diagnosis: HIV and hepatitis B risk

Clinchers
- *Third year medical student:* Most of the needle stick injuries occur due to inexperience and faulty specimen collection techniques.
- *Known HIV positive:* HIV risk is less than 0.5% from an accidental percutaneous exposure from a known HIV positive patient.
- *Needle stick injury:* Seroconversion rate following neeld stick injury is about 0.4% for HIV and 30% for hepatitis B if HBeAg positive. The rates are comparatively higher for hollow fore needles.

CONFUSA
UK guidelines for needle stick injuries are:
- Wash well; encourage bleeding; do not suck or immerse in bleach.
- Note name, address and clinical details of 'donor'.
- Report incidence to occupational health and fill in an accident form.
- Store blood from both parties. If possible, ascertain HIV and HBsAg of both. Immunize (active + passive) against hepatitis B at once, if needed. Counsel and test recipient at 3,6 and 8 months (seroconversion may take this long).
- Give 4 weeks of drugs, if possible within 1 hour of exposure:
  - Low risk—no antiviral medication
  - Higher risk—Zidovudine 300 mg/12 h (AZT).
     +
     Lamivudine 150 mg/12 h
  - Worst episodes (i.e. deep) puncture from wide-bore needle cause bleeding)—add indinavir 800 mg/8 h.

Note:
- All drugs to be given PO
- If female, do a pregnancy test before prophylaxis
- Drug choice may change as evidence accrues

Investigation of choice
HIV antigen testing of recipient.

Immediate management
Sought prompt expert advise + store blood from both parties.

Treatment of choice
Prophylactic AZT (see confusa).

153. A healthy 20-year-old pregnant woman whose partner is a hemophiliac.

Diagnosis: Risk of HIV and haemophilia to both woman and her unborn child

Clinchers
Hemophiliacs, especially those diagnosed and treated before mid1980's, have a high-risk of having HIV infection because of the absence of HIV testing for transfusion factors

CONFUSA
It is advisable to motivate every pregnant woman to go for HIV screening as prophylactic AZT and delivery by caesarian section considerably reduce the incidence of vertical transmission from mother to child.

Investigation of choice
HIV screening (after consent).

Immediate management
Counselling.

Treatment of choice
As per the test results (see confusa also).

Your Notes:

November—2001

154. A 28-year-old haemophiliac with a history of 20 previous blood transfusions presents with a dry cough and fever. His chest X-ray shows widespread mottling.

Diagnosis: Pneumocystitis carinii pneumonia

Clinchers
- *28-year-old haemophiliac with a history of 20 previous blood transfusions:* It suggest a high-risk of acquisition of HIV infection as he must have been diagnosed before 80's (he is 28 now) and must have received a few transfusions before compulsory HIV screening for transfused blood come in vogue.
- *Dry cough and fever:* Suggestive of a fungal pneunomia.
- *Widspread mottling:* In early infection the CXR is normal but the typical appearances are of bilateral perihilar interstitial infiltrates which can progress to confluent alveolar shadowsn through out the lungs.

CONFUSA
After treatment of PCP, long-term secondary prophylaxis is required to prevent relapse, the usual regimen being co-trimoxazole 960 mg thrice-weekly. Patients sensitive to sulphonamide are given either dapsone and pyrimethamine or nebulized pentamidine. The latter only protects the lungs and does not penetrate the upper lobes particularly efficiently; hence if relapses occur on this regimen they may be either atypical or may be extrapulmonary.

Investigation of choice
- *Screening:* CXR
- *Definitive:* Bronchoalveolar lavage.

Immediate management
HIV testing

Treatment of choice
Co-trimoxazole.

Your Notes:

155. A 20-year-old sexually active woman who is going to Thailand for a holiday.

Diagnosis: Risk of HIV

Clinchers
Thailand is a country with high rates of HIV positivity. It is advisable for any sexually active traveller to carry his or her own supply of condoms whenever travelling outside the country.

CONFUSA
The practice of safe sex is the most effective way for sexually active uninfected individuals to avoid contracting HIV infection and for infected individuals to avoid spreading infection. Abstinence from sexual relations is the only absolute way to prevent sexual transmission of HIV infection, but it is not practical. Use of condoms, preferably together with the HIV-inhibiting spermicide nonoxynol-9, can markedly decrease the chance of HIV transmission. It should be remembered that condoms are not 100% effective in preventing transmission of HIV infection, and there is an approximately 10 percent failure rate of condoms used for contraceptive purposes. Latex condoms are preferable, since virus has been shown to leak through natural skin condoms. Petroleum--based gels should never be used for lubrication of the condom, since they increase the likelihood of condom rupture.

Investigation of choice
None required

Immediate management
Counselling

Treatment of choice
Advice to carry condoms and practice safe sex.

Your Notes:

156. A 30-year-old man with AIDS presented in shock. Serum biochemistry reveals: potassium 6.7 mmol/L, bicarbonate 20 mmol/L, chloride 84 mmol/L, creatinine 160 μmol/L

Diagnosis: Acute adrenal insufficiency

Clinchers
- *30-year-old man with AIDS:* Various endocrine abnormalities have been reported with AIDS, including reduced levels of testosterone and abnormal adrenal function. The latter may assume clinical significance in more advanced disease. When intercurrent infection superimposed upon borderline adrenal function may precipitate clear adrenal insufficiency requiring replacement doses of cortico- and mineralo-corticoid CMV is also implicated in adrenal-deficient states.
- *Presents in shock:* Acute adrenal insufficiency typically present in shock (but not always).
- *Potassium 6.7 mmol/L:* Increases as always in this condition.
- *Bicarbonate 20 mmol/L:* Mild acidosis is characteristic.
- *Chloride 84 mmol/L:* Low along with hyponatraemia.
- *Creatinine 160 μmol/L:* Slightly increased.

CONFUSA
Acute adrenal insufficiency or Addisonian crisis can occur in any one with a known Addison's disease, or someone or long-term steroids who has forgotten to take their tablets. Typically it presents with shock but an alternative presentation can be with hypoglycaemia.

Investigation of choice
Blood for cortisol and ACTH (if possible).

Immediate management
Start treating before biochemical results.

Treatment of choice
Hydrocortisone sodium succinate 100 mg IV stat plasma expander followed by 0.9% saline.

---

157. A 41-year-old Londoner developed a temperature of 41°C, 5 weeks after cadaveric renal transplantation. WBC is 2.1 × 1,000,000,000/L, Hb is 8.8 g/dl, creatinine 177 μmol/L. Aspartate aminotransferase (AST) 82 U/L. Alanine aminotransferase (ALT) 132 U/L.

Diagnosis: Cytomegalovirus (CMV) disease.

Clinchers
- *41-year-old Londoner:* CMV has worldwide distribution with London being no exception.
- *Temperature of 41°C:* In transplant recipients on post bone marrow transplantation, CMV present with: fever > pneumonitis > colitis > hepatitis > retinitis. In AIDS, it presents with: retinitis > colitis > CNS defects.
- *After cadavaric renal transplantation:* CMV can be acquired by direct contact, blood transfusion or organ transplantation. Transmission following organs transplantation or blood transfusion is due to silent infection in these tissues. It can well be a CMV reactivation syndrome, developed when T cell (lymphocyte) mediated immunity is compromised after organ transplantation, or in association with lymphoid neoplasms and certain acquired immunodeficiencies (in particular: HIV).
- *WBC is 2.1 × 1000,000,000/L:* Normal range is between 4-11 × 1000,000,000/L. Leukopenia is commonly seen with CMV infection in immunocompromised.
- *Aspartate transaminase (AST) of 82 IU/L:* Normal range of AST is 3-35 IU/L. This show the LFT is deranged. Hepatitis is a common syndrome associated with CMV.
- *Alanine aminotransferase (ALT) of 132 IU/L:* Normal range of ALT is 3-35 IU/L. This shows LFT is deranged. Hepatitis is a common syndrome associated with CMV.

Variety of syndromes associated with CMV are fever, and leukopenia, hepatitis, pneumonitis, esophagitis, gastritis, colitis and retinitis.

CONFUSA
Most primary CNV infections in organ transplant recipients result from transmission of the virus in the graft itself.

Investigation of choice
Isolation of the virus together with rise in antibody titers a fourfold and greater.

Immediate management
Retinoscopy to exclude CMV retinitis.

Treatment of choice: Ganciclovir IV

158. A 36-year-old woman with leukaemia has been treated with amphotericin B for a fungal pneumonia. She presents with muscle weakness. Sodium 137 mmol/L, potassium 2.7 mmol/L, bicarbonate 19 mmol/L, Chloride 110 mmol/L, creatinine 84 μmol/L, urine pH 6.8 mmol/L

Diagnosis: Type I renal tubular acidosis (Distal RTA).

Clinchers
- *36-year-old woman with leukaemia:* Adult onset leukaemia usually affect patients in 30's and 40's. Distal RTA may occur in association with a systemic illness such as Sjögren's syndrome, multiple myeloma or rarely leukemias.
- *Treated with amphotericin B for a fungal pneumonia:* Amphotericin B poisoning can cause distal RTA due to an ability to maintain a pH gradient across the collecting duct.
- *Muscle weakness:* It is due to hypokalemia
- *Sodium 137 mmol/L:* Normal
- *Potassium 2-7 mmol/L:* Low, and is characteristic
- HCO_3^- *19 mmol/L:* Low as alkali is lost from kidneys.
- *Chloride 110 mmol/L:* high, RTA is hyperchloremic acidosis.
- *Creatinine 84 μmol/L:* Normal
- *Urine pH 6.8 mmol/L:* Inappropriately high. Such patients are unable to acidify urine below pH = 5.5.

CONFUSA

These abnormalities suggest that one or both of the active proton pumps present in the collecting duct (the H^+-ATPase or the H^+, K^+-ATPase is defective. In addition, excretory rates of NH_4^+ are uniformly low when the degree of systemic acidosis is taken into account, indicating that the kidney is responsible for the metabolic acidosis. Ammonium excretion is low because of failure to trap NH_4^+ in the medullary collecting duct, as a result of higher than normal tubular fluid pH in this segment and the urine pH is high because of impaired H^+ secretion

Investigation of choice
Urinary pH + serum electrolytes.

Immediate management
Discontinue amphotericin is still taking.

Treatment of choice
Oral alkali (Shohl's solution).

Note: Potassium supplements are not required in distal RTA as correction of acidosis resolves hypokalaemia.

159. An 83-year-old man with small cell lung cancer presents with ankle oedema and is found to have 8 g/day, urine proteinuria. He is started on frusemide. 10 days later his blood pressure is 115/75 mmHg lying and 85/65 mmHg standing. Serum biochemistry was; Sodium 121 mmol/L, bicarbonate 24 mmol/L, potassium 3.6 mmol/L, Creatinine 113 μmol/L, chloride 95 mmol/L, Urea 11.5 mmol/L, Glucose 5.7 mmol/L, albumin 27g, osmolality 263 mOs m/L, urine osmolality 417 mOs m/L

Diagnosis: Dilutional hyponatremia with nephrotic syndrome

Clinchers
- *83-year-old woman:* Incidence of most of the malignancies increases with increasing age.
- *Small cell lung cancer:* SIADH is mostly associated with four malignancies, i.e.
  - Small cell lung carcinoma
  - Pancreas
  - Prostate
  - Lymphoma
- *Ankle oedema + 8g/day urine proteinuria:* Daily urinary protein excretion is < 150 mg in normal persons. This massive proteinuria along with ankle oedema is characteristic of nephrotic syndrome.
- *Frusemide:* Excess diuretics administration can produce a dilutional hyponatremia with electrolyte profile similar to SIADH.
- *10 days later:* Dilutional hyponatraemia develops after repeated administration of the offending diuretic over days.
- *Sodium 121 mmol/L:* Low, as it is dilutional hyponatraemia.
- *BP 115/75 mmHg lying and 85/65 mmHg standing:* Orthostatic hypotension is present in nephrotic syndrome usually.
- *Bicarbonate 24 mmol/L:* Normal.
- *Potassium 3.6 mmol/L:* Normal.
- *Creatinine 113 μmol/L:* Normal.
- *Chloride 95 mmol/L:* Normal.
- *Urea 11.5 mmol/L:* Increased owing to nephrotic syndrome.
- *Glucose 5.7 mmol/L:* Normal.
- *Albumin 27 g:* Low, owing to nephrotic syndrome.
- *Serum osmolality 263 mOsm/L:* Low (normal 278-305) but do not quality for SIADH which is < 260 osmol/L. It is low because of dilutional hyponatremia.
- *Urine osmolality 417 mOsm/L:* It suggest concentrated urine but not > 500 mOsm/L to suggest SIADH.

> **CONFUSA**
> SIADH is an important, but overdiagnosed, caused of hyponatraemia. The diagnosis of SIADH requires, the absence of hypovolemia oedema, or diuretics. SIADH must always be distinguished from dilutional hyponatremia.

Investigation of choice
Serum electrolytes.

Immediate management
Stop diuretics or reset their dose.

Treatment of choice
Treat the cause + fluid restriction.

Your Notes:

160. A fit 50-year-old man is prescribed oral acetazolamide by an ophthalmologist for suspected glaucoma. He presents with lethargy and shortness of breath on exertion. Sodium 140 mmol/L, potassium 3.2 mmol/L, bicarbonate 18 mmol/L, chloride 115 mmol/L, urea 6.7 mmol/L, creatinine 114 μmol/L.

Diagnosis: Type II renal tubular acidosis (Proximal RTA).

Clinchers
- *Fit 50-year-old man:* Excludes any pre-existing pathology to be the cause of this condition.
- *Oral acetazolamide:* Acetazolamide causes increased renal bicarbonate losses. Hence it is the most probable cause in this case.
- *Lethargy and shortness of breath on exertion:* These are due to hypokalemia and acidosis respectively.
- *Sodium 140 mmol/L:* Normal.
- *Potassium 3.5 mmol/L:* Low, as hypokalaemia is a feature.
- *Bicarbonate 18 mmol/L:* Low as acetazolamide ↑ renal losses.
- *Urea 6.7 mmol/L:* Normal, but still on higher side (range 2.5-6.7 mmol/L).
- *Creatinine 114 μmol/L:* Normal.

> **CONFUSA**
> Renal tubular acidosis generally may be secondary to immunological drug-induced or structural damage to the tubular cells, an inherited abnormality, or an isolated (primary) abnormality. As with most disorders which are not well-understood, the nomenclature is confusing.

Investigation of choice
Urinary pH and serum electrolytes.

Immediate management
Discontinue acetazolamide if still taking.

Treatment of choice
Sodium bicarbonate (massive doses may be required to overcome the renal 'leak').

Your Notes:

161. A 60-year-old man presents with malaise and back pain which has been present for three months. He is found to have significant proteinuria.

Diagnosis: Multiple myeloma (MM)

Clinchers
- *Malaise and back pain:* Bone pain or tenderness is common, and often postural, e.g. back, ribs, long bones, and shoulder. Lassitude is from anaemia, renal failure or dehydration is a proximal tuble dysfunction, from light chain precipitation.
- *Significant proteinuria:* as Bence-Jones proteins are passed in urine. In MM proteinuria is not accompanied by hypertension, and the protien is nearly all light chains. Generally there is very little albumin in the urine because glomerular function is usually normal.

CONFUSA

Bone pain in multiple myeloma never occurs in the extremities. If such a symptom is present, myeloma can be safely excluded as a diagnosis.

Investigation of choice
Serum gel electrophoresis from `M' protein spike.

Immediate management
Correct dehydration, if present.

Treatment of choice
Supportive + Melphalan chemotherapy.

Your Notes:

162. A 30-year-old woman presents with a three month history of amenorrhoea.

Diagnosis: Pregnancy

Clinchers
- 30 year old woman: Since pregnancy is the first thing to be excluded as a cause of amenorrhoea in women of the fertile age group.

CONFUSA

Pregnancy produces a physiological hypercoagulable state inspite of the haemodilution effect it produces. In the late pregnancy limited mobility and prolonged bed-rest can precipitate deep vein thrombosis.

Investigation of choice
Urine pregnancy test

Immediate management
Refer to a physiotherapist to teach her the required exercises

Treatment of choice
Regular exercises.

Your Notes:

163. A 60-year-old man with a plethoric appearance presents with pleuritic chest pain. He has palpable splenomegaly.

Diagnosis: Polycythemia rubra vera (PCRV)

Clinchers
- *60-year-old:* It spares no age group amongst adults. Peak age is 45-60 years.
- *Man:* A slight overall male predominance has been observed.
- *Plethoric appearance:* Most often PCRV is first recognised by discovery of a high haemoglobin or haematocrit of plethoric facies.
- *Pleuritic chest pain:* It could be due to pulmonary thromboembolism-a frequent complication of PCRV. But to be sure, one needs more history.
- *Palpable splenomegaly:* Massive splenomegaly is the most common finding on clinical examination on presentation.

CONFUSA
With the exception of aquagenic pruritus (generalized itching after bathing), no symptoms can distinguish polycythaemia vera from other causes of erythrocytosis.

Investigation of choice
Screening—↑PCV
Definitive—^{51}Cr studies to determine RBC mass (> 125% of predicted).

Immediate management
PaO2 mearsurement (as raised RBC mass and splenomegaly in the presence of normal PaO_2 provide a diagnosis).
 +
Refer to haematologist

Treatment of choice
IV 32p/Busulfan

(Note: The treatment is different for younger patients and is based on hydroxyurea).

Your Notes:

164. A 70-year-old man presents with back pain and jaundice.

Diagnosis: Malignancy

Clinchers
- *70-year-old man:* Incidence of malignancy cotinually increases with age. If any old person present with some suggestive symptoms, a malignancy has to be ruled out first.
- *Back pain and jaundice:* Most probably it is carcinoma prostate as it usually presents with metastases to liver (thus producing jaundice) and spine (back pain).

CONFUSA
It should always be kept in mind that only an extensive involvement of liver by metastases can produce jaundice. Usually the presence of liver metastases causing jaundice suggest inoperability and a grage prognosis.

Investigation of choice
Pelvic USG

Immediate management
Take micturition history

Treatment of choice
Palliative.

Your Notes:

165. A 25-year-old woman with a family history of deep vein thrombosis was prescribed a combined oral contraceptive pill six months ago and has not missed any tablets.

Diagnosis: Inherited clotting abnormality

Clinchers

➢ The oral contraceptive pill is contraindicated in those with a tendency of deep vein thrombosis, as suggested in this case by a family history of DVT.

CONFUSA
Contraindications to the pill
— any disorder predisposing to venous or arterial problems
  • abnormal lipids
  • prothrombotic disorders
    — APC resistance
— Many cardiovascular problems
  Except:
  • Mild non-pill related hypertension
  • Varicose veins
— Liver disease
— Migraine
  • Status migranosus
  • Requiring ergotamine
— Gross obesity
— Immobility
— Undiagnosed uterine bleeding

Investigation of choice
PT and aPTT

Immediate management
Discontinue OCP

Treatment of choice
Prescribe alternative methods of contraception, i.e. condoms by male partner.

Your Notes:

166. A 29-year-old man with known arthritis presented with a painful red eye and a brownish rash on his feet. He has recently been treated for dysentery.

Diagnosis: Reiter's syndrome

Clinchers

➢ *29-year-old man:* The sex ratio following enteric infection is 1:1, but genitourinary acquired reactive arthritis is predominantly seen in young males.

➢ *Known arthritis + painful red eye:* Reiter's syndrome describes the triad of arthritis, conjunctivitis, and non-gonococcal urethritis or enteritis (mnemonic: cannot see, cannot pree, cannot climb a tree).

➢ *Brownish rash on his feet:* Mucocutaneous lesions are seen in approximately one-third of patients. These are cutaneous vesicles that become hyperkeratotic, most common on soles and palms.

➢ *Recently been treated for dysentery:* In individuals with appropriate genetic background (HLA-B27 positivity), reactive arthritis, *Shigella, Salmonella, Yersinia* and *Campylobacter enteritis*.

CONFUSA
Differential diagnosis is from septic arthritis (gram +/-) gonococcal arthritis, crystalline arthritis, psoriatic arthritis.

Investigation of choice
Stool cultures.

Immediate management
HIV screening (required in all patients).

Treatment of choice
Symptomatic.

Your Notes:

167. A 30-year-old woman presented to the family GP complaining of difficulty in lifting her arms up. She also reported having difficulty getting up and down stairs. A scaly, erythematous rash was noticed on the dorsum of the hand, and knuckles. She had earlier complained dysphagia.

Diagnosis: Dermatomyositis.

Clinchers
- *30-year-old woman:* The disease may develop at any age. Affected females outnumber males by 2:1.
- *Difficulty in lifting her arms up:* Patient first become aware of weakness of the proximal limb muscles. When shoulder girdle muscles are involved, placing an object on a high shelf or combing the hair becomes difficult.
- *Difficulty getting up and down stairs:* Hip girdle weakness causes difficulty in arising from the squatting or kneeling position and in climbing or descending stairs.
- *Scaly, erythematous rash was noticed on dorsum of hand and knuckles:* The classic iliac-coloured (heliotrope) rash is on the eyelids, bridge of nose, cheeks (butterfly distribution) forehead, chest elbows, knees and knuckles, and around the nail beds.
- *Dysphagia:* At presentation 25% of patients have dysphagia.

CONFUSA
Dermatomyositis and polymyositis are conditions of presumed autoimmune etiology in which the skeletal muscle is damaged by a nonsuppurative inflammatory process dominated by lymphocytic infiltration. The term polymyositis is applied when the condition spares the skin, and the term dermatomyositis when polymyositis is associated with a characteristic skin rash.

Investigation of choice
- *Screening:* Muscle enzyme (CK) levels
- *Definitive:* Muscle biopsy.

Immediate management
Exclude retinitis (cotton wool patches).

Treatment of choice
Rest + prednisolone.

168. A mother brought her 10-year-old son to the GP, with a history of joint pains and recurrent oral ulcers. On examination the boy had hypopyon and mild conjuctivitis.

Diagnosis: Behcet's syndrome.

Clinchers
- *10-year-old son:* It predominantly presents in adolescent males.
- *Joint pains and recurrent oral ulcers:* Behcet's syndrome represents a triad of arthritis, ocular symptoms (pain, visual loss, floaters, irits, hpopyon, retinal vein occlusion) and painful ulcers in mouth, scrotum or labia (Mnemonic: Cannot see, cannot pee, cannot eat spicy curry).
- *Hypopyon and mild conjunctivitis:* Confirms our suspicion of Behcet's syndrome.

CONFUSA
Apart from above mentioned symptoms, GIT involvement as colitis may be present. CNS manifestations can be meningoencephalitis, ↑ IVP, brainstem signs, dementia, myelopathy, encephalopathy, cerebral vein thrombosis, etc.

Investigation of choice
HLA-B5/51 screening.

Immediate management
Specialist referral.

Treatment of choice
Colchicine, steroids (topical ± oral), ciclosporin, and chlorambucil have been used.

Your Notes:

169. A 40-year-old sheep farmer from Kent presented to her GP complaining of muscle and joint pain with an associated chronic headache, which has been present for 3 weeks. On examination, she had an erythematous annular rash with a central clear area, on her abdomen.

Diagnosis: Lyme's disease.

Clinchers

- *40-year-old sheep farmer from kent:* It was originally described in Lyme, connecticut (USA), but is now known to occur in UK (new forest-kent). It spreads by deer or sheep ticks (bite).
- *Muscle and joint pain + headache for 3 weeks:* Headache, fever, malaise, myalgia, arthralgia and lymphadenopathy are the common accompaniments of the first stage of the disease.
- *Erythematous annular rash with a central clear area on her abdomen:* It is the characteristic rash of Lyme's disease and is known as erythema chronicum migrans. It heralds the first stage of disease as a small papule which develops into a spreading large erythematous ring with central fading. It lasts from 48 hr- 3 months and may be multiple.

CONFUSA
The 'agent' causing human granulocyte erlichiosis is also transmitted by the same ticks. It produces a similar clinical picture and can be co-transmitted.

Investigation of choice
Clinical ± serology (if negative, PCR).

Immediate management
Exclude CNS and CVS involvement.

Treatment of choice
Doxycycline 100 mg/12 h PO for 10-21 days (Amoxicillin or penicillin V if < 12 years).

Your Notes:

---

170. A 30-year-old woman presented with tender, red nodules on both lower limbs and forearms. She had painful joints and was febrile. She had a month history of a productive cough and investigations revealed raised, angiotensin converting enzyme levels.

Diagnosis: Sarcoidosis.

Clinchers

- *30-year-old woman:* The peak incidence is in the third and fourth decade with a female preponderance.
- *Tender, red nodules on both lower limbs and forearms:* This is erythema nodosum of which sarcoidosis is the most common cause:
- *Painful joints:* Arthralgia is common in it and can be presenting feature.
- *Was febrile:* 4% of patients present with fever (in UK).
- *Month's history of productive cough:* Dry or productive cough (an secondary infection) with progressive dyspnoea and chest pain are the most common pulmonary manifestations.
- *Raised ACE levels:* This is characteristic and is two standard deviations above the normal mean value in over 75% of patients with untreated sarcoidosis.

CONFUSA
The Kveim test, which involved as intradermal injection of sarcoid tissue, was regularly used for confirmation of the diagnosis. It should not be used because of the risk of transmission of infection. It is less sensitive and less specific than transbronchial biopsy which has superceded it. Patients with bilateral hilar lymphadenopathy alone do not require treatment.

Investigation of choice
- *Screening:*
  CXR
  Serum ACE levels (↑)
- *Definitive:* Transbronchial biopsy.

Immediate management
Lung function tests

Treatment of choice
Acute sarcoidosis: Bed-rest + NSAIDs + corticosteroids.

Note: Corticosteroids should be given only if needed, i.e. in
- Parenchymal lung disease
- Uveitis
- Hypercalcaemia
- Neurological or cardiac involvement.

171. A fit 55-year-old gentleman, complains of recurrent episodes of 'seeing visible veins on his body', which are tender. He has started to lose weight and attributes this to his diarrhoea. The consultant dermatologist thinks he has thrombophlebitis migrans.

Diagnosis: Carcinoma of tail of pancreas.

Clinchers
- *Fit 55-year-old gentleman:* Incidence of neoplasia increases with age.
- *Recurrent episodes of 'seeing visible veins on his body':* Local findings of thrombophlebitis migrans consist of induration of redness and tenderness along the course of a vein. Long saphenous vein is most commonly involved. This is Trousseau's syndrome.
- *Started to lose weight:* It is for any unobvious reason, then in this age it is mostly due to malignancy.
- *Diarrhoea:* This suggest carcinoma pancreas which is characteristically associated with thrombophlebitis migrans.
- *Thrombophlebitis migrans:* It strongly indicates our suspicion.

CONFUSA
Thrombophlebitis migrans is successive crops of tender nodular affecting blood vessels throughout the body, associated with carcinoma of the pancreas (especially body and tail tumors).

Investigation of choice
CT scan

Immediate management
Exclude DVT as it frequently accompanies.

Treatment of choice
Symptomatic.

Your Notes:

---

172. A 49-year-old woman complains of itchy blisters, which are occurring in groups on her knees and elbows. The itch is becoming unbearable and she is contemplating suicide. She responds to 180 mg of Dapsone within 48 hours of treatment.

Diagnosis: Coeliac disease (Gluten sensitive enteropathy).

Clinchers
- *49-year-old female:* It can present at any age. The peak incidence in adults is in the third and fourth decades with a females preponderance.
- *Itchy blisters which are occurring in group on her knees and elbows:* This is an uncommon blistering subepidermal eruption of the skin associated with gluten sensitive enteropathy. The clinical term for it is gluten sensitive enteropathy.
- *Itch is becoming unbearable and she is contemplating suicide:* This disease can produce severe depression in females and can lead to suicide.
- *Responds to 180 mg of dapsone within 48 hours of treatment:* This confirms our diagnosis.

CONFUSA
The skin condition (dermatitis herpetiformis) responds to dapsone but both the gut and the skin will improve only on a gluten free diet in this disease.

Investigation of choice
Endomysial antibodies (IgA).

Immediate management
Psychiatric referral (as she is contemplating suicide)

Treatment of choice
Gluten free diet
+
Dapsone.

Your Notes:

173. A Welsh farmer with malaise and arthralgia is increasingly anxious about a skin lesion which started as a papule (Diameter approx 1 mm) which has progressed to a red ring (Diameter approx 50 mm) with central fading.

Diagnosis: Borrelia burgdorferi infection (Lyme disease).

Clinchers

- *Welsh farmer:* Ticks (on deer and sheep) spreading this infection are widespread in the UK, particularly in forests, and woodlands.
- *Malaise and arthralgia:* These are nonspecific symptoms of Lyme diseases are headache, fever, malaise, myalgia, arthralgia and lymphadenopathy.
- *Skin lesion which started as a papule.... progressed to a red ring with central fading:* This is the typical description of erythema chronicum migrans which heralds this disease and is virtually pathognomic.

CONFUSA
Lyme disease is caused by Borrelia burgdorferi sensu lato. The disease is transmitted by Ixodes dammini or related ixodid ticks (Ixodes ricinus in Europe). In the UK, 300-500 cases are reported annually. Prompt removal of any tick is essential as infection is unlikely to take place until the tick begins to engorge. Ticks should be removed by grasping them with forceps near to the point of attachment to the skin and then withdrawn by gentle traction.

Investigation of choice
Clinical ± serology (if negative, PCR).

Immediate management
Rule out CNS and CVS involvement

Treatment of choice
Doxycycline
(amoxicillin or penicillin V if < 12 years).

Your Notes:

---

174. A 42-year-old woman who reports a loss in weight, presents with a shiny erythematous lesion on her shin. It's centre appear yellowish and edges are beginning to ulcerate with undermining. (Fasting blood glucose is 5.3 mmol/L).

Diagnosis: Necrobiosis lipoidica (NL).

Clinchers

- *42-year-old:* NIDDM may be present in subclinical form for years before diagnosis and the incidence increases markedly with age and degree of obesity.
- *Loss of weight:* This due to fluid depletion and the accelerated breakdown of fat and muscle secondary to insulin deficiency.
- *Shiny, erythematous lesion on her shin:* NL is a shiny plaque like lesion with erythematous margins. It is usually found over the anterior surfaces of the legs (Shins).
- *Centre appears yellwish and edges are begining to ulcerate with undermining:* This is an almost "dictionary description" of the lesion of NL.
- *Fasting blood glucose in 5.3 mmol/L":* Although skin manifestations in diabetes can occur in well-controlled but long-standing diabetes (as in this case), majority of them only present along with glycosuria and hyperglycaemia.

CONFUSA
Diabetic dermopathy ("Shin spots") is a similar but different clinical entity. Its lesions are also located over the anterior tibial surface. The lesions are small, rounded plaques with a raised border. They many crust at the edges and ulcerate centrally (opposite to what is seen in NL).

Investigation of choice
Complete blood sugar profile

Immediate management
Take family history of DM + rule out any malignancy.

Treatment of choice
Strict glycaemic control if diabetes is proven.

Your Notes:

175. A 32-year-old woman complains of palpitations and is found to have red oedematous swellings above both lateral malleoli, which she says are beginning to affect her feet. She is found to have digital clubbing and periorbital puffiness.

Diagnosis: Hyperthyroidism (Graves' disease).

Clinchers
- *32-year-old:* It most often occurs between ages 20 and 40 years.
- *Woman:* Hyperthyroidism affects perhaps 2-5% of all females at sometime and with a sex ratio of 5:1.
- *Red oedematous swellings above both lateral malleoli which she says are beginning to affect her feet:* This is pretibial myxoedema and is characteristic of hyperthyroidism state.
- *Palpitations:* This may be due to atrial fibrillation or other tachycardias, commonly found with hyperthyroidism.
- *Digital clubbing:* This is the rare thyroid acropachy and consists of clubbing, swollen fingers and periosteal new bone formation.
- *Periorbital puffing:* It is due to a specific immune response that causes inflammation and hence focal oedema and glycosaminoglycan deposition followed by fibrosis.

CONFUSA
The eye signs pretibial myxoedema and thyroid acropachy occur only in Graves' disease. Pretibial myxoedema is an infiltration on the skin, essential occurring only with eye disease. In Graves' disease eventually become hypothyroid.

Investigation of choice
TSH receptor antibodies.

Immediate management
Exclude associated disease like IDDM and pernicious anaemia.

Treatment of choice
Carbamizole
(Side effects: drug rash; fever; arthropathy; lymphadenopathy; agranulocytosis).

Your Notes:

---

176. The time span over which a percentage of women with cervical intraepithelial neoplasia (CIN) untreated will develop cancer.

Diagnosis (Answer): 3-10 years

Clinchers
The proportion of severe dysplasia and carcinoma *in situ* that progresses to invasive cancer is uncertain, and such an assessment becomes difficult as recognized cases are treated promptly. It is probable that about 10-30% of cases ultimately progress to cancer in 3-10 years time.

CONFUSA
Initially it was believed that CIN III tended to develop from CIN I and II and only CIN III lesions would progress to invasive cancer. Most authors now believe that CIN III lesions probably arise as such. Apparent progression from CIN I to CIN III is explained on the basis of a smaller area of CIN III only becoming apparent with time as the lesions enlarge. The risk of invasion of CIN I and II abnormalities has not been clearly defined.

Investigation of choice
- *Screening:* Pap smear
- *Definitive:* Colposcopic directed biopsy

Immediate management
Seek specialist advise

Treatment of choice
Completely removing abnormal epithelium of CIN and yearly follow up smears for five years.

Your Notes:

177. The age at which the peak incidence of cervical carcinoma occurs.

Diagnosis (Answer): 30 years

Clinchers
Cervical carcinoma was once a disease of the over-50s it is now seen in under 40s (OHCS, page 34, 5th edn). Cervical cancer occurs almost exclusively among women who are, or have been, sexually active. There is increasing evidence that infection by certain strains of human papilloma virus (HPV) is a factor. Studies have shown that between 10 and 30 percent of sexually active women have acquired HPV infection of the genital tract by the age of 30 years. The proportion of women infected is higher if the woman or her partner have had several sexual partners.

CONFUSA
There is a bit of confusion about age of peak incidence according to various books, e.g.
   Lecture notes (Gyn and Obs) 45-55 years
   OHCS   under 40s
   Ten teachers (Gyn)   younger women
But since the latest evidence points towards younger women in their 30s, we can safely mark this option.

178. The interval for cervical smears to be taken in a woman treated one year previously for cervical intraepithelial neoplasia.

Diagnosis (Answer): 12 months

Clinchers
The follow-up of patients treated for CIN is controversial. In some areas one or two follow-up colposcopies are offered but in others follow-up is entirely by cytology. Women who have undergone treatment for CIN III have approximately a three-fold incidence of invasive carcinoma compared with the background population. Whether this justifies more intensive screening programmes in the long-term has not been clearly defined. Certainly for the first five years women should be offered smears every year and possibly for longer than this.

CONFUSA
Cervical cytological screening is designed to detect over 90 per cent of cytological abnormalities. In theory cervical screening fulfils many of the criteria of a successful screening procedure. The cervical smear test will diagnose the vast majority of cytological abnormalities and the treatment of precancer is simple, safe, non-destructive and usually curative. As a result of women having regular cervical screening the incidence of cervical carcinoma has fallen.

Investigation of choice
Yearly pap smears.

Immediate management
Counselling.

Your Notes:

179. The age at which screening stops for women with a normal smear history.

Diagnosis (Answer): 65 years

Clinchers
- The cervical screening programme includes:
  - Start with 2 smears in the first year of sexual activity
    - Then 3 yearly smears
    - Stop at 65 years age if smear history is normal.

CONFUSA

A successful cervical screening programme can reduce the incidence of invasive carcinoma by 90%. The trouble is those most at risk are the hardest to trace and persuade to have screening, e.g.
- Older woman
- Smoking
- Inner cities

Papanicolaou test (Pap smear) is used for cervical screenings. Positive test require further investigations like:
- Colposcopy
- Cervical biopsy
- Fractional curettage

A pap test can detect about 98% of the cancer cervix, and about 80% of endometrial cancer.

Your Notes:

180. The time scale within which the 50% of patients with recurrent disease will present, following treatment for stage 1B cervical cancer.

Diagnosis (Answer): 12 months.

Clinchers
- In stages IB and IIA there is little difference between the results of surgery and radiotherapy. When the disease recurs it does so:
  - Within one year in 50 percent of patients
  - Within two years in 75 percent
  - Within five years in 90 percent

(Source: Ten teachers (Gyn), 18th edn)

CONFUSA

The prognosis of invasive cervical carcinoma varies depending on the method of treatment chosen, the experience of the radiotherapist or surgeon, and on the country. Expectation of five years survival is:
- Stage I   > 85%
- Stage II   50%
- Stage III 25%
- Stage IV   5%

Your Notes:

181. A 15-year-old boy has very poor grades at school despite being very attentive and hard working. His mother reckons its because he is teased at school because his breasts look like a girl's. On further examination he is found to have small firm testes. He is mildly asthmatic.

Diagnosis: Klinefelter's syndrome.

Clinchers

> *15-year-old:* Patient usually present in adolescence with poor sexual development
> *Poor grades despite being very attentive and hard working:* Patients are occasionally mentally retarded.
> *Breasts look like a girls and small firm testes:* Gynaecomastia and small peanut size but firm testes are signs of androgen deficiency found in Klinefelter's.
> *Mildly asthmatic:* Obesity and varicose veins occur in one-third to one-half and abnormalities of thyroid function, diabetes mellitus, and pulmonary disease may be present in Klinefelter's.

CONFUSA
Gynaecomastia ordinarily develops during adolescence, is generally bilateral and painless, and may become disfiguring. The risk of breast cancer is 20 times that of normal men, but only about a fifth that in women. Most have male psychosexual orientation and function sexually as normal men.

Investigation of choice
Karyotyping

Immediate management
Genetic counselling.

Treatment of choice
Androgen replacement therapy (if patient is mentally subnormal, use it carefully).

Your Notes:

182. A 5-year-old South African boy is brought to the accident and emergency department deeply jaundiced. He is found to have mildly swollen, tender feet and hands. His mucosae are pale.

Diagnosis: Sickle cell disease.

Clinchers

> *5-year-old:* The condition may present in childhood with anaemia and mild jaundice. The hand and food syndrome due to infarcts of small bones is quite common in children and may result in digits of varying lengths.
> *South African:* The disease occurs mainly in Africans and about 25% carry the gene. It is also common in India, middle east and southern Europe.
> *Mildly swollen, tender test and hands:* It is bone pain which is the most common symptom and is due to infarcts of small bones.
> *Mucosae are pale:* Due to anaemia.

CONFUSA
In a given patient the degree of anaemia is usually stable, and during a crisis Hb does not fall unless there is one or more of the following:
- Aplasia
- Acute sequestration
- Hemolysis

Investigation of choice
- *Screening:* Sodium metabisulphite test
- *Definitive:* Hb electrophoresis (No HbA, 80-95% HbSS and 2-20% HbF).

Immediate management
IV fluids + oxygen + adequate analgesia.

Treatment of choice
Exchange transfusion is severe
Penicillin prophylaxis in children
Seek advice from nearest NHS sickle cell and Thalassemia counselling centre.

183. A 6-year-old Asian boy gets regular blood transfusion for his haematological abnormality. His mucosae are pale and skull is grossly bossed. Haematological investigations were done and showed; MCHC 25g/dl, Hb 8g/dl , MCV 74fl.

Diagnosis: Beta thalassemia.

Clinchers
- *6-year-old:* Children affected by severe β-thalassemia present during the first year of life.
- *Regular blood transfusion for his haematological abnormality:* Regular transfusion may be required every 4-6 weeks and are given to keep the Hb above 10 g/dL.
- *Mucosae are pale:* Because of anaemia.
- *Skull is greatly bossed:* It is due to expansion of the bone marrow due to extramedullary haematopoiesis, giving rise to characteristic thalassemic facies.
- *MCHC 25 g/dL:* It is always reduced (normal 30-36 g/dL) as is MCV and MCH.
- *Hb 8 g/dL:* It suggest β-thalassemia major.
- *MCV 74 FL:* It is always M 75 FL in this condition.

CONFUSA
Iron overload caused by repeated transfusions (transfusion haemosiderosis) may lead to damage to the endocrine glands, liver, pancreas and the myocardium by the time patients reach adolescence. The type in question is β-thalassemia because of severity and early age of onset. In β-thalassemia minor, Hb is > 9 g/dL, so this is β-thalassemia major.

Investigation of choice
Hb electrophoresis.

Immediate management
Transfusion to keep Hb > 9 g/dL.

Treatment of choice
Bone marrow transplantation in young patients with HLA matched siblings.

Your Notes:

---

184. A 10-year-old boy is brought to the accident and emergency department with a swollen right arm. His temperature is 38.5°C and is unable to move his arm due to severe pain. Blood culture confirms *Salmonella typhi* osteomyelitis. This is his second presentation this month and earlier presented with an acute onset hepatosplenomegaly associated with severe pallor. The SHO does a Sodium Metabisulphite test on the patient's blood which turns out to be positive.

Diagnosis: Sickle cell disease (SCD).

Clinchers
- *10-year-old:* The complications of sickle cell disease are common around adolescence.
- *Swollen right arm + 38.5°C + severe pain + Salmonella typhi osteomyelitis:* Osteomyelitis can occur in SCD in necrotic bone and is often due to Salmonella.
- *Second presentation this month:* This suggest a recurrent "crises" state which is common in SCD.
- *Sodium metabisulphite test positive:* Red cells assume their characteristic morphologic form when the haemoglobin is deoxygenated, as by treatment with a reducing agent like sodium metabisulphite.

CONFUSA
Salmonella osteomyelitis is rarely seen in normal population. Although the spleen may be enlarged in small children with sickle cell disease, repeated episodes of splenic infarction cause the spleen to be reduced to a small calcified remnant (autosplenectomy). Concurrent α-thalassemia seems to protect on the average against the clinical manifestations of sickle disease.

Investigation of choice
Hb electrophoresis.

Immediate management
Transfusion to keep Hb > 9 g/dL.

Treatment of choice
Bone marrow transplantation in young patients with HLA matched siblings.

Your Notes:

185. A 39-year-old male is getting progressively forgetful and is later found to have Alzheimer's disease. He has small ears and an IQ score of 67.

Diagnosis: Down's syndrome

Clinchers
- *39-year old male ..... Alzheimer's disease:* Alzheimer's dementia usually manifest in late forties or in fifties. Early onset of it is commonly seen in Down's syndrome which predisposes one to it.
- *Small ears:* Facial profile of Down's syndrome is flat with oblique palpebral fissures and epicanthic folds with small ears.
- *IQ score of 67:* Severe mental retardation is a characteristic feature of Down's syndrome.

CONFUSA
Trisomy 21 (Down's syndrome) is observed with a frequency of 1 in 700 like births regardless of geography or ethnic background. Apart from Alzheimer's dementia it predisposes one to all. (Mnemonic: we **all** will go **down** together)

Investigation of choice
Karyotyping.

Immediate management
Genetic counselling.

Treatment of choice
Rehabilitation.

Your Notes:

---

186. A tall young woman developed sharp pain on one side of his chest two days ago. Since then he has been short of breath on exertion.

Diagnosis: Pneumothorax after spontaneous primary rupture

Clinchers
- *Tall:* It increases the risk of having apical bullae became of increased negative intrathoracic pressure.
- *Young:* Spontaneous pneumothorax is predominantly seen in "tens and twenties".
- *Man:* Incidence of spontaneous pneumothorax is more in males.
- *Sharp pain:* It is the characteristic pleuritic pain of pneumothorax.
- *Unilateral:* It is characteristic of pneumothorax as there are two pleural cavities.
- *Shortens of breath on exertion:* It confirms the diagnosis of pneumothorax.
- *2 days ago:* Spontaneous primary rupture of bullae is usually mild.

CONFUSA
Insertion of large guage open bore cannula (16-17 G) is only done for tension pneumothoraces. All other pneumothoraces are treated with water seal.

Investigation of choice
CXR

Immediate management
Serial radiographic observation.

Treatment of choice
Aspiration or underwater seal drainage if necessary.

Your Notes:

187. After a heavy bout of drinking a 56-year-old man vomits several times and develops chest pain. When you examine him, he has a crackling feeling under the skin around his neck.

Diagnosis: Pneumomediastinum after oesophageal rupture.

Clinchers
- *Heavy bout of drinking*: It is a risk factor for Boerhaare's syndrome (oesophageal rupture)
- *56 years old*: Older age cames weakness of oesophageal musculature and hence increases the chances of rupture.
- *Vomits several times*: Recurrent vomiting, especially against a closed glottis (common after a heavy bout of drinking) can produce oesophageal rupture
- *Chest pain*: Always suspect oesophageal perforation of chest pain follows vomiting.
- *Cracklin feeling*: This is subcutaneous emphysema which is characteristically present in suprasternal region after oesophageal rupture. It confirms our diagnosis.

CONFUSA
On more examination Hamman's sign can be found in this patient, i.e.
- Crunching/clicking noise synchronous with heart beat.
- Best heard in left lateral decubitus.
  Drinking is also associated with Mallory Weiss syndrome (MWS). It can be differentiated from Boerhaave's syndrome as:
- MWS has gastric tear in 90% cases (Below squamocolumnar junction) and oesophageal tear in 10% cases
- MWS present with haemetemesis which is not mentioned here.
- Complete tear (perforation) is very rare in MWS
- MWS—forceful vomiting in a chronic alcoholic BS—Recurrent vomiting after bout of alcohol drinking

NOTE:
- Weakest portion of oesophagus is its lower third
- If it is only pneumomediastinum without oesophageal rupture, high flow oxygen (100%) can help in early resorption of air. No surgery is required then.

Investigation of choice: CXR

Immediate management: Crossmatch blood and inform surgeons.

Treatment of choice: Surgical repair (Though oesophageal rupture can also be managed in Boerhaave's syndrome because of high septic load).

188. A 23-year-old woman on the oral contraceptive pill suddenly gets tightness in her chest and becomes very breathlessness.

Diagnosis: Pulmonary venous thromboembolism (PE).

Clinchers
- *23-year-old woman:* She belongs to the typical OCP user age group.
- *OCP*: They increase the risk of pulmonary embolism by producing a hypercoagulable state.
- *Sudden tightness and breathlessness*: Chest pain and shortness of breath are the two most usual symptoms in PE. The pain is most often pleuritic in nature; sharp and worse with deep inspiration and couphing. There may be haemoptysis.

CONFUSA
Sometimes collapse is the presenting symptom. A sudden urge to defaecate may hearald the onset of symptoms. Signs are very variable and often absent. There may be tachycardia and tachypnoea. Areas of crepitus or a pleural rub are sometimes heard, as is a pulmonary flow murmur. Thrombosis of the deep veins is rarely clinically apparent.

Investigation of choice
V/Q scan

Immediate management
High flow O_2 + 10 mg IV morphine + anticoagulation

Treatment of choice
Heparin (loading dose of 5000-10000 units of standard heparin IV followed by a continuous infusion of 1000-2000 units per hour).

Your Notes:

189. A 30-year-old man with Marfan's syndrome has sudden central chest pain going through to the back.

Diagnosis: Aortic dissection (acute).

Clinchers
- *30-year-old*: In patients with Marfan's syndrome aortic dissection tends to present in a relatively younger age.
- *Marfan's syndrome*: It increases the risk of ascending aortic dissection. In fact it is the major cause of mortality in it.
- *Sudden central chest pain going to back*: Sudden onset of pain, localised to front or back of chest, often intersapular region and typically migrates with propapation of dissection.

CONFUSA
Aortic dissection is a potentially life-threatening condition in which disruption of aortic intima allows dissection of blood into vessel wall, may involves ascending aorta (type II) descending aorta (type III), or both (type I). Alternative classification type A –ascending aortic dissection, type B—limited to descending aorta. Involvement of the ascending aorta is most lethal form.

Investigation of choice
Screening/CXR, Definitive/CT/MRI/USG (TOE).

Immediate management
Crossmatch and inform surgeons.

Treatment of choice
Emegent surgical repair/always required in ascending aortic dissection.

Your Notes:

190. A 57-year-old man develops crushing pain in the chest associated with nausea and profuse sweating. The pain is still present when he arrives in hospital an hour later.

Diagnosis: Acute myocardial infarction (AMI).

Clinchers
- *57-year-old*: Incidence of MI increases with age as age is a nonmodifiable risk factor.
- *Man*: Male sex is also a nonmodifiable risk factor
- *Crushing pain*: There is acute central chest pain and is classically described as crushing or heavy. Some patients say it feels like a tight band around their chest; others describe it as like someone sitting on them. It is common for the patient to clench his or her first as an aid to description.
- *Associated with nausea and profuse sweating*: Accompanying symptoms such as sweating, pallor, nausea or general malaise are almost helpful in making a diagnosis as the character of pain.
- *Still present when he arrives in hospital an hour later*: The pain usually lasts longer than 30 minutes (20 minutes according to OHCM). This feature differentiates it form angina.

CONFUSA
Be aware of the middle-aged man with 'indigestion' especially if he has no past dyspeptic history of significance. A few days of vague retrosternal pain is not a history of dyspepsia. It is much more likely to be the warning pain which often predate as MI. Recurrent belching is a sign of autonomic disturbance and as such may accompany as infarction. Even symptomatic relief from antacids should not be relived upon to relied upon to point away from the heart. Some patients present with very atypicaly pain, both in site and character. Examples of this would be pain localized to the abdomen or to the left shoulder or arm alone.

Investigation of choice
ECG (hyperacute T waves, ST elevation or new LBBB)

Immediate management
High flow O_2 + 10 mg IV morphine + anticoagulation.

Treatment of choice
Thrombolysis.

Your Notes:

191. Tuberculosis.

Diagnosis: Sputum culture.

Clinchers
- Tuberculosis is caused by bacteria belonging to Myobacterium tuberclosis complex. Usually affects lungs, though in one-third cases other organs may be involved.
- Tuberculous spinal disease in Egyptian mummies proves, that it is one of the oldest diseases known to affect humanity.
- The key to diagnosis of tuberculosis is high index of suspicion. Go for CXR, followed by AFB microscopy and mycobacterial culture.

CONFUSA
Though in suspected tuberculosis, the first investigation to be done is CxR (shows upper lobe infiltrates with cavitations), sputum culture is the most definitive investigation, where the organism can be isolated and cultured.

Investigation of choice
Sputum culture.
— Sputum microscopy
— CXR

Immediate management
If sputum positive, isolate the patient, and start Antitubercular therapy (ATT) immediately.

Treatment of choice
Five major drugs are considered the first line agents for treatment of tuberculosis.
- Isoniazid (5 mg/kg), max 300 mg daily
- Rifampicin (10 mg/kg), max 600 mg daily
- Pyrazinamide (15-30 mg/kg) max 2 g daily
- Ethambutol (15-25 mg/kg)
- Streptomycin (15 mg/kg) in max 1 gm daily.

Your Notes:

192. Carcinoma of the right main bronchus.

Diagnosis: Fiberoptic bronchoscopy

Clinchers
- Fiberoptic bronchoscopy in the procedure of choice for visualizing an endobronchial tumor and collecting cytologic and histologic specimens. Inspection of the tracheobronchiol mucosa can demonstrate and endobronchial granulomas often seen in sarcoidosis, and endobronchial biopsy of such lesions or transbronchial biopsy of the lung interstition can confirm the diagnosis.
- Inspection of the airway mucosa by bronchoscopy can also demonstrate the characteristic appearance of endobronchial Kaposi's sarcoma in patient with AIDS.
- Symptoms of bronchial carcinoma are cough (80%), haemoptysis (70%), dyspnoea (60%), chest pain (40%), anorexia, weight loss.

CONFUSA
Bronchoscopy gives histological diagnosis and assess operatility. CT stages the tumor, CxR for bony secondaries can be seen besides peripheral circular opacity, hilar enlargement, consolidation and pleural effusion.

Investigation of choice
Fiberoptic bronchoscopy.

Immediate management
Look for complications (local metastatic, endocrine) and treat.

Treatment of choice
Nonsmall cell tumor: Excision for peripheral tumors, with no metastatic spread.

Small cell tumor: These are almost always disseminated at presentation. May respond to chemotherapy.

Your Notes:

193. Pulmonary embolism.

Diagnosis: Already stated as the question.

Clinchers

Since the question, has not given any clinical profile, let us see the most common 'clinchers', that GMC uses in their exams for this condition.
- *Precipitants:* Air travel, recent operation, pregnancy, OCP, hormone replacement therapy, disseminated malignancy, DVT.
- *Symptoms:* Acute breathlessness, pleuritic chest pain, haemoptysis.
- *Signs:* Tachypnoea, tachycardia, hypotension, raised JVP, pleural rub.
- *CXR:* Usually normal (in GMC questions).
- *ECG:* Usually normal (in GMC questions), $S_I Q_{III} T_{III}$ pattern, sinus tachycardia, right bundle branch block.

CONFUSA
Pulmonary embolism produces central cyanosis due to decreased oxygen saturation. Which is produced by only three other common conditions, i.e.
- Pulmonary oedema
- Severe respiratory disease
- Congenital cyanotic heart disease.

Investigation of choice
Investigation of pulmonary embolism is a point of major confusion in PLAB examination. Consider following points while choosing the investigation for PE:
- *Screening*
  - V/Q scan—only if the patient is stable and not severely breathless
  - Spiral CT with contrast—if facilities are available patient's general state do not allow a V/Q scan to be done
- *Definitive:* Pulmonary angiogram—but not usually done because of risk of complications and it being an invasive test.

Note: Always look in the "instructions" to the theme about the type of investigation being asked for, i.e. is it "definitive" or "screening". It is important as the answer is usually different for both and you will end up losing marks for something you know.

Immediate management
Anticoagulation with LMW heparin (Dalteparin 200 U/kg/24 hr SC; max dose 18,000 IU/24h)
- Stop when INR > 2

Treatment of choice
Oral warfarin 10 mg for minimum 3 months

194. Bronchiectasis.

Diagnosis: Already stated as the question.

Clinchers
Bronchiectasis is a frequent question in PLAB exam. The most frequent 'clinchers' used by GMC to describe this condition are:
- *Secondary to:* Cystic fibrosis, kartageneger's syndrome, pertussis in the childhood, allergic bronchopulmonary aspergillosis.

  "Non-GMC" conditions—Young's syndrome (primary ciliary dyskinesia), measles, bronchiolitis, pneumonia, TB, HIV, bronchial obstruction (tumour, foreign body), hypogammaglobulinaemia, rheumatoid arthritis, ulcerative colitis, idiopathic.
- *Symptoms:* Persistent cough, copious purulent sputum, intermittent hemoptysis.
- *Signs:* Finger clubbing, coarse inspiratory, crackles, wheeze.
- *Complications:* Pneumonia, pleural effusion, pneumothorax, hemoptysis, cerebral abscess, amyloidosis.

CONFUSA
Spirometry is bronchiectasis shows an obstructive pattern. Reversability should be assessed to differentiate from asthma.

Investigation of choice
- *Screening:* CXR—Tramline and ring shadows.
- *Definitive:* High resolution CT chest—to assess extent and distribution.

Immediate management
Antibiotics if infection (usually pseudomonas) is present.

Treatment of choice
Postural drainage + bronchodilators (if asthma, COPD, cystic fibrosis, ABPA present) + steroids (if ABPA present).

Indications for surgery are:
- Localized bronchiectasis
- To control severe hemoptysis.

Your notes:

195. Bronchial carcinoid.

Diagnosis: Already stated as the question.

Clinchers
Questions about bronchial carcinoids are a rarity in PLAB exam. Still let us review some salient features of them.
- Usually follow a benign course
- May secrete other hormones, effects of whom constitute the common presenting complaints of this condition. They can secrete
  - ACTH
  - Arginine vasopressin
- Carcinoid syndrome is only produced when any carcinoid has liver metastases. It is characterised by:
  - Cutaneous flush
  - Bronchoconstriction
  - Diarrhoea.

CONFUSA
Bronchial carcinoids and small cell carcinoma both develops from the same cells (kulchitsky cell in bronchial epithelium). But carcinoid can be differentiated by presence of carcinoid syndrome (only in presence of liver metastases) and cardiac valvular lesions—both of these are absent in small cell carcinoma of lung. Paraneoplastic syndromes are not a criteria for differentiation as both can cause them (especially ACTH).

Investigation of choice
- *Screening:* 24 hour urine 5HIAA increase.
- *Definitive:* CXR/CT—usually done only if liver metastases are absent as only then a curative resection is possible.

Immediate management
High dose octreotide for crises + careful fluid balance.

Treatment of choice
- Crises—Octreotide
- Flushing—Ketanserin
- Diarrhoea—Loperamide/cyproheptadine
- Hepatic metastases—embolisation
- Bronchial obstruction—surgical debulking

Your notes:

196. 3 gm sachet of amoxicillin one hour before the procedure.

Answer: Dental treatment of cardiac patients.

Clinchers
Endocarditis prophylaxis before dental procedures:
Local or no anaesthetic.
- Amoxicillin 3g PO, 1 hour before the procedure
- Clindamycin 600 mg PO if: allergic to penicillin, > 1 dose of penicillin in previous month

General anaesthetic, no special risk:
- Amoxicillin 1g IV at induction, followed by 500 mg PO 6 hours later.
- OR amoxicillin 3g PO 4 hours before induction, followed by 3g PO as soon as possible after procedure.

General anaesthetic, special risk patients:
(NOTE: Special risk signify = prosthetic valves
                              = previous endocarditis)
- Amoxicillin 1g IV + gentamicin 120 mg IV at induction followed by Amoxicillin 500 mg PO 6 hours later.
- Consider alternatives if,
  = history of penicillin allergy
  = > 1 dose of penicillin in previous month
- Alternatives are
  - Vancomycin 1g IV over 100 min
    +
    Gentamicin 120 mg IV at induction
  - Teicoplanin 400 mg IV
    +
    Gentamicin 120 mg IV at induction
  - Clindamycin 300 mg IV over 10 min at induction followed by clindamycin 150 mg IV 6 hour later.

CONFUSA
The principal of prophylaxis is to treat before contamination occurs, and this is particularly important with antibiotics, where as adequate antibiotic concentration needs to be present in the blood at the time of exposure of infection. Anyone with congenital heart disease, acquired valve disease or prosthetic valve is at risk of infective endocarditis and should take prophylactic antibiotics before procedures which may result in bacteraemia. The dental procedures considered fit for prophylaxis include extractions, scaling, polishing or gingival surgery.

Investigation of choice
Echocardiography to rule out congenital and often heart diseases if suspected.

Immediate management: Prophylactic antibiotics.

Treatment of choice: Stated as the question itself.

197. Three days of intravenous broad spectrum antibiotics beginning with induction of anaesthesia.

Diagnosis (Answer): Heart valve replacement

Clinchers
- The required prophylactic regimen is Amoxicillin 1g IV + gentamicin 120 mg IV
- First dose is given at induction of anaesthesia and is continued upto 3 days.

CONFUSA
Infection of valve postoperatively is a situation akin to infective endocarditis of a native valve. For more detailed notes on chemoprophylaxis in various disease states refer to British national formularly or www.bnf.org.

Investigation of choice
As per the requirements of the operation.

Immediate management
Antimicrobial chemoprophylaxis.

Treatment of choice
Stated as the question itself.

198. Clear fluids by mouth and two sachets of sodium picosulphate on the day before the operation plus broad spectrum intravenous antibiotics at induction.

Diagnosis(Answer): Sigmoid colectomy.

Clinchers
- *Sodium picosulfate*: Before any colorectal surgery, give 1 sachet of picolax (sodium picosulfate 10 mg + magnesium citrate) each, at:
  - On the morning before surgery
  - During the afternoon before surgery
- *Broad spectrum IV antibiotics at induction*: Cefuroxime 1.5 g 18 h, 3 doses IV/IM + Metronidazole 500 mg/ 8 h, 3 doses IV.

CONFUSA
Sodium picosulfate should be used with care if there is any risk of bowel perforation. Otherwise bowel preparation is of utmost importance before colorectal surgery. Antibiotics used should kill anaerobes and coliforms especially.

Investigation of choice
As per the requirements for the operation.

Immediate management
Meticulous bowel preparation.

Treatment of choice
States as the question itself.

Your Notes:

199. Long-term oral penicillin and immunisation against pneumococcal infection.

Diagnosis (Answer): Splenectomy

Clinchers
- Removal of the spleen predisposes the patient, especially the child, to infection with organisms such as the pneumococcus. The clinical course is of a fulminant bacterial infection, with shock and circulatory collapse, termed overwhelming post splenectomy sepsis (OPSS).
- Prophylactic immunization with
  = pneumococcal
  = meningococcal
  = *Haemophilus influenzae* type of vaccine should be administered, preoperatively where possible. In addition, children should have prophylactive daily low dose oral penicillin until they reach adulthood.

CONFUSA
The major aim of antibiotic prophylaxis in splenectomy is to present serious pneumococcal sepsis. Regarding oral penicillin, the duration of treatment is,
- Children—till adult hood
- Adult—for first year after splenectomy
- Immunosuppressed—life-long.

Investigation of choice
Usually none

Immediate management
Vaccination (if possible preoperatively).

Treatment of choice
Stated as the question itself. Preoperatively also phenoxymethyl penicillin is given (500 mg/12 hourly).

Your Notes:

200. One dose of metronidazole at induction of anaesthesia.

Diagnosis (Answer): Emergency appendicectomy.

Clinchers
- The prophylactive antibiotic regimen for as emergency appendicectomy is:
  Metronidazole 1g 18 h + Cefuroxime 1.5 g/8 h
- These are given in 3 doses IV, the first dose is given 1 hour preoperatively or at the induction of anaesthesia.

CONFUSA
If it is an elective appendicectomy, then give+ 3 dose regimen of metronidazole suppositories 1g/8 h + Cefuroxime 1.5/8 h IV or Gentamicin IV

Investigation of choice
None required usually.

Immediate management
Shift patient to OT.

Treatment of choice
Stated as the question itself.

Your Notes:

September—2001

RxPG Analysis

Total themes:	40
Repeat themes:	7
Repeat themes with a different header:	16

September—2001

THEME 1: INVESTIGATION OF RED EYE

OPTIONS

a. Eye washing
b. Intraocular pressure
c. Flourescein stain
d. Eye secretion swap culture
e. Acrocyst drainage
f. X-ray of orbit
g. Conjunctival cytology
h. MRI
i. Gonioscopy
j. CT
k. None required

*For each presentation below, choose the **most appropriate** investigation from the above list of OPTIONS. Each option may be used once, more than once, or not at all.*

QUESTIONS

1. A 69-year-old patient presented to his GP with sudden onset of redness in the right eye. There was no pain and vision was unaffected.

2. A patient presents with metal pieces to his eyes.

3. A mother brings her 2-year-old child with a squint. On examination a leucokoric right pupil is seen with an absent red reflex.

4. A 12-year-old Libyan boy gave a two weeks history of discomfort, redness and mucopurulent discharge affecting both eyes. His two siblings have a similar problem.

5. A 23-year-old man has a history of recurrent attacks of blurring of vision associated with redness, pain and photophobia. Both eyes have been affected in the past. His brother is currently being investigated for bowel disease and a severe backache.

THEME 2: MANAGEMENT OF SUDDEN VISUAL LOSS

OPTIONS

a. Do nothing
b. Steroids
c. Laser photocoagulation
d. Pilocarpine
e. Lens transplantation
f. Eye surgery
g. Admit for specialist neurosurgical evaluation
h. IV mannitol
i. 1 percent atropine sulphate ointment
j. LASIK
k. Cataract surgery

*For each presentation below, choose the **most appropriate** management from the above list of OPTIONS. Each option may be used once, more than once, or not at all.*

QUESTIONS

6. A 78-year-old man has had a painful scalp and headache for three weeks, and is generally unwell, complains of acute onset of blindness in his right eye.

7. A 50-year-old woman complains of sudden loss of vision in one eye. She describes the incident, like a curtain coming down.

8. An 84-year-old woman notices sudden increased visual impairment. She is found to have homonymous hemianopia.

9. A 68-year-old smoker suddenly notices markedly reduced vision in one eye. He cannot read any letter on visual acuity chart but can count fingers. The fundus is pale.

10. A 30-year-old man has recurrent episodes of an acutely painful red eye with reduced vision.

THEME 3: DIAGNOSIS OF HEAD INJURY

OPTIONS
a. Diffuse brain damage
b. Cerebral haematoma
c. Extradural haematoma
d. Subdural haematoma
e. Temporal linear fracture
f. Subarachnoid haematoma
g. Epilepsy
h. Depression
i. Superficial head injury
j. Insignificant head injury
k. Vasogenic cerebral oedema

For each presentation below, choose the single most likely diagnosis from the above list of OPTIONS. Each option may be used once, more than once, or not at all.

QUESTIONS

11. Following an alcoholic binge a 36-year-old male falls and comes to casualty with a cut in his temporal region his Glasgow Coma Scale is ormal and his neck is cleared by the orthopedic SHO.

12. An 8-year-old boy falls off a swing at his school. He is brought to casualty by one of his teachers. He has a bruise over his right eye but the examination is otherwise normal. He is fully conscious with no history of blackouts since the accident. A skull X-ray is performed, which is normal.

13. A young woman is involved in an RTA and is brought in with a Glasgow Coma Scale of 6. A CT scan shows evidence of diffuse cerebral oedema but no evidence of haemorrhage. She has bilateral papilledema.

14. A young man is involved in a fight and suffers a blow to the back of the head. A skull X-ray reveals a depressed fracture of the occiput. His Glasgow Coma Scale on admission is 14 but falls rapidly within an hour.

15. A 24-year-old patient presents with RTA. The pupil on the left side is dilated and the patient is obtunded. CT scan of the head reveals a biconvex hyperdense lesion on the temporal region.

THEME 4: POISONING MANAGEMENT

OPTIONS
a. Carbon monooxide
b. Warfarin
c. Heparin
d. Ethyl alcohol
e. Quinine
f. Paracetamol
g. Carbamazepine
h. Tricyclic antidepressants
i. Cyanide
j. Aspirin
k. Ecstacy

For each presentation below, choose the single most likely diagnosis management from the above list of OPTIONS. Each option may be used once, more than once, or not at all.

QUESTIONS

16. Condition in which patient was found with nasal involvement and nasal hairs sighing. He presents with myalgia, malaise and headache.

17. Condition in which vitamin K is given to improve patient.

18. A 7-year-old boy accidentally swallowed some unknown white tablets and now complaining of right hypochondrial pain after 12 hours.

19. The side effect is urinary retention, heart block and ringing of ear.

20. A patient who has overdosed on an unknown medication presents with palpitations. What is the most likely cause?

September—2001

THEME 5: DRUGS

OPTIONS
a. Opioid overdose
b. Opioid withdrawal
c. Tricyclic intoxication
d. Carbamazepine
e. Lithium
f. Haloperidol
g. Clozapine
h. Naloxone
i. Natrexone
j. Paracetamol
k. Aspirin

For each presentation below, choose the single most likely cause from the above list of OPTIONS. Each option may be used once, more than once, or not at all.

QUESTIONS

21. Schizophrenic patient under treatment presents with fever, increased WBC, increased muscle creatinine kinase levels.

22. A homeless patient presents to A and E with drowsiness. On examination, abrasions and puncture marks were found on his arm. He has pin point pupil. What would you give?

23. Schizophrenic patient under treatment presents with sore throat, decreased WBC, agranulocytosis.

24. Patient on treatment for bipolar disorder, hypothyroidism features.

25. A patient who has overdosed on an unknown medication presents with palpitations. What is the most likely cause?

THEME 6: INVESTIGATION IN GASTRO-INTESTINAL DISEASE

OPTIONS
a. Chest X-Ray
b. Abdominal USG
c. Amylase level
d. Brain CT
e. Barium enema
f. Laparotomy
g. Stool culture
h. Blood culture
i. Bulk laxatives
j. Stimulant laxatives
k. Colonoscopy
l. Sigmoidoscopy

For each presentation below, choose the most appropriate investigation from the above list of OPTIONS. Each option may be used once, more than once, or not at all.

QUESTIONS

26. For the past two weeks a middle-aged railway engineer has complained of acute constipation. His stools are dark, but not apparently blood stained. Abdominal palpation detects a mass with moderate tenderness.

27. A 43-year-old man says he cannot finish his stool and that what he does pass is streaked with blood. He says he has always been regular. He wants to know if a laxative will help.

28. A 49-year-old lawyer complains of blood and diarrhoea. She is also suffering from abdominal pain, fever, and general ill-health. On palpation you find tenderness in the lower abdomen.

29. A young woman presents with recurrent abdominal pain, episodic diarrhoea, malaise, and fever. Over the past few years she has felt her health to be declining. At presentation she complains of severe abdominal pain and constipation.

30. A young woman complains of cramp like abdominal pain, and difficulties with bowel movements. Acute abdominal pain is frequently relieved by embarrassing flatulence. Barium studies and sigmoidoscopy have proved inconclusive.

THEME 7: DIFFERENTIAL DIAGNOSIS OF DYSPHAGIA

OPTIONS
a. Candidiasis
b. Ebstein-Barr
c. Diffuse oesophageal spasm
d. Achalasia
e. Oesophageal carcinoma
f. Pharyngeal pouch
g. Barret's oesophagus
h. Carcinoma stomach
i. Gastrectomy
j. Sialadenitis
k. Schatzki's rings

*For each presentation below, choose the **most likely** diagnosis from the above list of OPTIONS. Each option may be used once, more than once, or not at all.*

QUESTIONS

31. A known HIV (+) patient presents with pain in swallowing and some lesion in the mouth. The underlying tissue is red when the lesion is taken off.

32. A patient comes with dysphagia for solids for 5 years and now presents with regurgitation when he eats, it relieves a few hours after meal.

33. 65-year-old male presents with weight loss, difficulty in swallowing solid. Dysphagia is getting worse.

34. A patient presents with intermittent dysphagia for both solids and liquids and chest pain. No weight loss.

35. A patient with difficulty in swallowing, filling defect. He has a long standing history of Barret's oesophagus.

THEME 8: DIAGNOSIS OF HEPATOBILIARY DISEASE

OPTIONS
a. Chronic pancreatitis
b. Acute pancreatitis
c. Duodenal ulcer
d. Gastric ulcer
e. Gallstones
f. Hepatitis B
g. CBD obstruction
h. Hereditary haemochromatosis (HHC)
i. Acute cholecystitis
j. Primary biliary cirrhosis (PBC)
k. Hepatoma

*For each presentation below, choose the **single most likely** diagnosis from the above list of OPTIONS. Each option may be used once, more than once, or not at all.*

QUESTIONS

36. Man returned from trip to Asia, complains of anorexia, malaise, dark urine, pale stools.

37. An 80-year-old man has never been out of UK, one month history of epigastric pain, dark urine, pale stools, jaundice.

38. Female with fever, rigors, right upper quadrant pain, jaundice, ultrasound is normal.

39. Female, 50-year-old, 5 years history of mild pruritus. History of pale stools, dark urine, jaundice.

40. Man with history of hemochromatosis and alcohol addiction presents with jaundice, ascites, variceal bleed. USG is unequivocal, high ferritin level.

THEME 9: DIAGNOSIS OF SCROTAL PAIN

OPTIONS
a. Acute epidydimo-orchitis
b. Chronic epididimo-orchitis
c. Hydrocoele
d. Varicocoele
e. Teratoma
f. Seminoma
g. Testicular torsion
h. Lymphoma
i. UTI
j. Sebaceous cyst
k. Seminoma or teratoma

*For each presentation below, choose the **single most likely** diagnosis from the above list of OPTIONS. Each option may be used once, more than once, or not at all.*

QUESTIONS

41. Man after trip to Asia presents with red, swollen scrotum.

42. Man with painful red scrotum and vomiting.

43. Man with painless testicular swelling since 2 months.

44. Man with a swelling of scrotum since 3 years.

45. Man with no history of unsafe sex presents with dysuria and urinary frequency.

THEME 10: MANAGEMENT OF DIABETIC COMPLICATIONS

OPTIONS
a. Hyperglycemia
b. Hypoglycemia
c. Urinary tract infection
d. Somatic neuropathy
e. Autonomic neuropathy
f. Intermittent claudication
g. Atherosclerosis
h. Possible infection
i. Lactic acidosis
j. Ketoacidosis
k. Amyotrophy

INSTRUCTIONS
*For each of the patients listed below, choose the **most likely** complication from the list of options above. Each option may be used once, more than once, or not at all.*

QUESTIONS

46. A 48-year-old female, insulin dependent diabetic, who has been on treatment for 20-year presents with a history of three episodes of severe hypoglycemia. She has not changed her insulin requirement, diet or exercise pattern.

47. A 48-year-old female, insulin dependent diabetic, who has been on treatment for 20-years, presents with urinary frequency but no dysuria or urgency. Her blood glucose is 17.5 mmol/L.

48. A 30-year-old female, insulin dependent diabetic, presents with failure to pass urine.

49. A 68-year-old diabetic on treatment for the last 5-year presents with calf pain exacerbated by movement.

50. A 70-year-old diabetic on treatment with metformin presents with severe epigastric pain, drowsiness and confusion.

THEME 11: INVESTIGATION OF THYROID DISORDERS

OPTIONS
a. Serum TSH levels
b. Serum T₄ levels
c. Skull X-ray
d. Serum T₃ levels
e. Contrast radiographs
f. FNAC
g. USG
h. MRI
i. Biopsy
j. Thyroglobulin autoantibodies
k. TSH receptor autoantibodies

*For each presentation below, choose the **most appropriate investigation** from the above list of OPTIONS. Each option may be used once, more than once, or not at all.*

QUESTIONS

51. Female, 41-year-old, presents with hard, irregular fixed swelling, stridor, dysphagia since 3 months.

52. Old lady with smooth neck swelling, bradycardia, spare coarse hair, macrocytic anemia.

53. Female on treatment for supraventricular tachycardia complains of seeing dots and glare on driving at night, exophthalmos, no goitre.

54. Female, swelling in the neck, tremor irritability, diarrhoea, bruit.

55. A 35-year-old woman who was diagnosed as having coelic disease at the age of 12 years has had good control of her abdominal symptoms for a number of years. She presents with a recent history of weight loss, tiredness, diarrhoea and abdominal pain.

THEME 12: INVESTIGATION OF ABDOMINAL PAIN IN A WOMAN

OPTIONS
a. Transvaginal USG
b. Cervical os exam
c. Laparotomy
d. Colposcopic examination
e. Abdominal USG + high vaginal swab
f. Lupus factor
g. Fibroid study
h. Flexible sigmoidoscopy
i. Laparoscopy
j. None required
k. Endocervical swab

*For each presentation below, choose the **single most appropriate investigation** from the above list of OPTIONS. Each option may be used once, more than once, or not at all.*

QUESTIONS

56. A 35-year-old woman complains of abdominal discomfort relieved by passing flatus or defecation. Over the last 6 months she has had episodes of diarrhoea and constipation, but denied she had lost weight.

57. A 37-year-old woman presents with a sudden onset of severe left iliac fossa pain. On vaginal USG, 2 cm echogenic masses are seen in the broad ligament. She says this pain seems to come on every month.

58. A 23-year-old woman just had an intrauterine device fitted. She complains of a watery brown vaginal discharge and abdominal pain.

59. An 18 weeks pregnant female presents with lower abdominal pain and tenderness, with offensive vaginal discharge. She has high grade fever since last two days.

60. A 32-year-old woman who conscientiously uses the oral contraceptive pill, has experienced monthly vaginal bleeding. On abdominal examination she is uncomfortable. Her temperature is 37°C. She is otherwise healthy.

September—2001

THEME 13: MANAGEMENT OF RENAL DISEASE

OPTIONS
a. IV hydrocortisone
b. Oral prednisolone
c. Indinavir
d. Frusemide
e. Sodium bicarbonate
f. Fluid restriction
g. Potassium supplements
h. Acetazolamide
i. Amphotericin
j. Ganciclovir IV
k. Shohl's solution

*For each presentation below, choose the **most appropriate** management from the above list of OPTIONS. Each option may be used once, more than once, or not at all.*

QUESTIONS

61. A 30-year-old man with AIDS presented in shock. Serum biochemistry reveals: Potassium 6.7 mmol/L, bicarbonate 20 mmol/L, chloride 84 mmol/L, creatinine 160µmol/L.

62. A 41-year-old Londoner developed a temperature of 41°C, 5 weeks after cadaveric renal transplantation. WBC is 2.1 × 1,000,000,000/L, Hb is 8.8 g/dl, creatinine 177µmol/L. Aspartate aminotransferase (AST) 82 U/L. Alanine aminotransferase (ALT) 132 U/L.

63. A 36-year-old woman with leukemia has been treated with Amphotericin B for a fungal pneumonia. She presents with muscle weakness. Sodium 137 mmol/L, potassium 2.7 mmol/L, bicarbonate 19 mmol/L, chloride 110 mmol/L, creatinine 84µmol/L, urine pH 6.8 mmol/L.

64. An 83-year-old woman with small cell lung cancer presents with ankle oedema and is found to have 8 g/day, urine proteinuria. He is started on frusemide. 10 days later his blood pressure is 115/75 mmHg lying and 85/65 mmHg standing. Serum biochemistry was; sodium 121 mmol/L, bicarbonate 24 mmol/L, potassium 3.6 mmol/L, creatinine 113 µmol/L, chloride 95 mmol/L, urea 11.5 mmol/L, glucose 5.7 mmol/L, albumin 27g, osmolality 263 mOsm/L, urine osmolality 417 mOsm/L.

65. A fit 50-year-old man is prescribed oral acetazolamide by an opthalmologist for suspected glaucoma. He presents with lethargy and shortness of breath on exertion. Sodium 140 mmol/L, potassium 3.2 mmol/L, bicarbonate 18 mmol/L, chloride 115 mmol/L, urea 6.7 mmol/L, creatinine 114 mmol/L

THEME 14: IIMMEDIATE MANAGEMENT OF ELECTROLYTE DISTURBANCES

OPTIONS
a. ACE inhibitors
b. Decrease insulin dose
c. Increase insulin dose
d. Thiazides
e. Beta-blockers
f. Frusemide
g. Potassium supplements
h. $NaHCO_3$
i. $NaCl + K^+$ supplements
j. 5% dextrose solution
k. Calcium resonium

*For each presentation below, choose the **most important step in immediate management** from the above list of OPTIONS. Each option may be used once, more than once, or not at all.*

QUESTIONS

66. Man with pyloric stenosis, profuse vomiting, hypokalaemia and increased bicarbonate.

67. Man who is not able to pass urine, tired, complains of hiccups.

68. Man with villous adenoma, profuse diarrhoea.

69. Female, 24 hours after hysterectomy complains of breathlessness, increased JVP.

70. A patient in severe renal failure has potassium level of 2.5 mmol/L.

First Aid for PLAB

THEME 15: INVESTIGATION OF PULMONARY DISEASES

OPTIONS
a. Pleural biopsy
b. V/Q scan
c. Chest X-ray
d. Echocardiography
e. Mediastinoscopy
f. Bronchoscopy
g. Sputum culture and microscopy
h. ECG
i. Brochial lavage
j. Pulmonary function tests
k. Exercise ECG

*For each presentation below, choose the **most descriptive investigations** from the above list of OPTIONS. Each option may be used once, more than once, or not at all.*

QUESTIONS

71. A man who has been worked as boiler worker for 20 years presents with dyspnoea and pleurisy.

72. Female with cough, copious blood tinged sputum for more than a month. She is from south-east Asia.

73. A middle-aged women develops a purulent cough with some haemoptysis. A chest X-ray reveals right upper lobe shadows.

74. Female presents with acute pleuritic chest pain, hemoptysis after undergoing hysterectomy.

75. A patient with an area of consolidation and fever on his chest X-ray is treated with antibiotics. His fever resolves but four weeks later he still has a large area of consolidation.

THEME 16: DIAGNOSIS OF PULMONARY DISEASES

OPTIONS
a. Sarcoidosis
b. COPD
c. Allergic rhinitis
d. Anxiety
e. Pulmonary oedema
f. Mitral stenosis
g. Pulmonary embolism
h. Pneumothorax-spontaneous
i. Pneumothorax-tension
j. Aspiration pneumonitis
k. Asthma

*For each presentation below, choose the **single most likely diagnosis** from the above list of OPTIONS. Each option may be used once, more than once, or not at all.*

QUESTIONS

76. Patient with acute shortness of breath, wheeze. chest X-ray—normal, low oxygen, low $PaCO_2$. PEFR-120 ml/minute.

77. Bilateral hilar opacities, ACE is high.

78. A 20-year-old woman attends A and E complaining of sudden breathlessness and anxiety. She describes palpitations and paresthesiae of her hands, feet and lips. ECG shows sinus tachycardia and O_2 saturation is normal.

79. An alcoholic admitted semi-comatose. ABG shows low oxygen saturation.

80. Patient with recent MI, develops acute breathlessness with hemoptysis. CxR shows dilated pulmonary artery and wedge-shaped area of infarction. Decreased PaO_2 and $PaCO_2$.

THEME 17: MANAGEMENT OF ACUTE CHEST PAIN

OPTIONS
a. Glyceryl trinitrate (0.5 mg) sublingually
b. IV 50 ml of 50% dextrose
c. High flow O_2 and ramipril 2.5 mg/12 hr PO
d. High flow O_2, 10 mg IV morphine + anticoagulation
e. Crossmatch blood and inform surgeons
f. Insert a 16 G cannula in second intercostal space
g. IV heparin 5000-10,000 iu over 5 min
h. Underwater seal drainage
i. 10 mg IV diamorphine
j. Nifedine
k. Ramipril

*For each presentation below, choose the **best management** from the above list of OPTIONS. Each option may be used once, more than once, or not at all.*

QUESTIONS

81. A tall young man developed sharp pain on one side of his chest two days ago. Since then he has been short of breath on exertion.

82. After a heavy bout of drinking a 56-year-old man vomits several times and develops chest pain. When you examine him, he has a crackling feeling under the skin around his neck.

83. A 23-year-old woman on the oral contraceptive pill suddenly gets tightness in her chest and becomes very breathless.

84. A 30-year-old man with Marfan's syndrome has sudden central chest pain going through to the back.

85. A 57-year-old man develops crushing pain in the chest associated with nausea and profuse sweating. The pain is still present when he arrives in hospital an hour later.

THEME 18: COMPLICATIONS OF BREAST CARCINOMA

OPTIONS
a. Pathological fracture
b. Cerebral metastases
c. Hypocalcemia
d. Lymphedema
e. Spinal cord compression
f. Hypercalcemia
g. Hyperparathyroidism

*For each presentation below, choose the **most common complication** from the above list of options. Each option may be used once, more than once, or not at all.*

QUESTIONS

86. Female with breast carcinoma 3 years back, was treated with mastectomy and lymph node clearance on the left side, presents with a swollen limb and decreased hand movements.

87. Presents with thirst, confusion, constipation.

88. Presents with weakness of both legs, difficulty walking, urine retention.

89. Presents with headache, confusion. On examination, papilledema present.

90. Presents with features of fracture femur.

THEME 19: THE DIAGNOSIS OF NON-ACCIDENTAL INJURY

OPTIONS
a. Accidental injury
b. Emotional abuse
c. Physical abuse
d. Sexual abuse
e. Child neglect
f. Osteogenesis imperfecta
g. ITP
h. Normally present in a child.
i. Elderly abuse
j. Henoch-Schönlein purpura
k. Immune thrombocytopenia purpura

For each presentation below, choose the **single most likely diagnosis** from the above list of options. Each option may be used once, more than once, or not at all.

QUESTIONS

91. A 16-year-old mother brings her baby for immunization. The nurse notices the baby has multiple bruises along both arms and legs. The baby is crying excessively. The house officer notices multiple fractures and that the baby has blue sclerae.

92. A 70-year-old man is receiving treatment for Alzheimer's disease. He is looked after by a 23-year-old grand daughter. He has recently developed fecal incontinence. The SHO notices bruises on both wrists and back.

93. An anxious mother brings her 6-year-old daughter who is bleeding per vaginum. Six months prior to this presentation the girl had a confirmed streptococcal sore-throat infection. She is otherwise normal.

94. A 4-day-old girl is brought to casualty by the maternal grandparent who is worried about two dark bluish patches on the child's buttocks. Child's mother is white and the father is black.

95. An 8-year-old girl is noted to have fresh bloody staining of her pants. She also suffers from enuresis. She has recently started horse-riding lessons.

THEME 20: INVESTIGATION OF NECK LUMPS

OPTIONS
a. USG
b. Technetium scan
c. Aspiration and microscopy
d. CT scan
e. MRI scan
f. Chest X-ray
g. Digital substraction angiography
h. FNAC
i. Transillumination test
j. Biopsy

For each presentation below, choose the **single most appropriate investgation** from the above list of OPTIONS. Each option may be used once, more than once, or not at all.

QUESTIONS

96. Patient with a pulsatile hard mass fixed under the upper one-third of the sternomastoid muscle.

97. A 40 year old male has a lump in the supero-posterior area of the anterior triangle.

98. A 16-year-old female has a midline lump in the neck which moves on protrusion of the tongue and is below the hyoid bone.

99. A 19-year-old male has a cystic mass under the anterior border of sternomastoid at the junction of upper one-third and middle one-third of the muscle. Aspiration revealed fluid containing cholesterol crystals.

100. An infant present with a transilluminant swelling in the lower third of neck.

September—2001

THEME 21: IMMEDIATE MANAGEMENT OF BURNS

OPTIONS
a. IV fluids
b. Escharotomy
c. Admit to hospital
d. Carboxyhemoglobin level
e. IV blood transfusion
f. Deroof blister
g. Aspirate blister
h. Blood transfusion
i. Skin grafting
j. Antibiotics
k. Fasciotomy
l. Reassure

*For each presentation below, choose the **most appropriate** immediate management from the above list of OPTIONS. Each option may be used once, more than once, or not at all.*

QUESTIONS
101. Patient after escaping from fire in a building has singed nostrils.

102. Patient has a large tense blister.

1033. An adult patient has partial thickness burns on the anterior chest and upper thighs.

104. An adult patient has full thickness circumferential burns from the elbow to the fingers, covering them completely.

105. Man, slept while sunbathing comes with redness, pain? all over his body. otherwise well.

THEME 22: DEVELOPMENTAL MILESTONES

OPTIONS
a. One week
b. 2 weeks
c. 6 weeks
d. 2 months
e. 6 months
f. 9 months
g. 1 year
h. 2 years
i. 3 years
j. 4 years
k. 4½ years

*For each presentation below, choose the **most appropriate** answer from the above list of OPTIONS. Each option may be used once, more than once, or not at all.*

QUESTIONS
106. Copies circle, can say 4 words,

107. Smiles responsively, Head lags

108. Can walk 4 steps upstairs

109. Holds head up at 45° when prone, vocalise

110. Pincer grip; can say "Mummy" ± "Daddy"

THEME 23: ANATOMICAL LOCALISATION OF MULTIPLE SCLEROSIS

OPTIONS
a. Cerebrum
b. Optic disc
c. Optic nerve
d. Optic radiation
e. Cerebral cortex
f. Brainstem and its cerebellar connections
g. Cervical spinal cord
h. Thoracic spinal cord
i. Facial nerve
j. Trigeminal nerve
k. Fascial nucleus

*For each presentation below, choose the **best answer** from the above list of OPTIONS. Each option may be used once, more than once, or not at all.*

QUESTIONS

111. Known patient of multiple sclerosis now with complaint of urinary incontinence, weakness in all 4 limbs and difficulty walking.

122. Patient has nystagmus, diplopia, and positive past-pointing.

113. Patient has repeated attacks of multiple sclerosis, and now has pale temporal disc.

114. Patient with complaint of blurring of vision, papilledema, pain in eye.

115. A known patient of multiple sclerosis with unilateral facial paralysis with no loss of taste.

THEME 24: ROLE OF IMMUNIZATION AND PREVENTION IN LIVER DISEASES

OPTIONS
a. Hepatitis A immunisation
b. Hepatitis B immunoglobulin
c. Hepatitis B vaccine
d. Leptospirosis
e. Hepatitis A infection
f. Hepatocellular carcinoma
g. Schistosomiasis
h. Lyme disease
i. Cirrhosis
j. Haemangioma
k. Chronic active hepatitis

*For each presentation below, choose the **single most appropriate** from the above list of OPTIONS. Each option may be used once, more than once, or not at all.*

QUESTIONS

116. Not eating sea shell products prevents.

117. Immunization of sewage workers.

118. Not swimming in foreign lakes prevents.

119. Immunization of health workers who are in contact with body fluid.

120. Mass immunization of hepatitis B, besides preventing hepatitis B also prevents.

THEME 25: DIAGNOSIS OF HEARING LOSS

OPTIONS
a. Acoustic neuroma
b. Blast injury
c. petrous temporal bone fracture
d. wax impaction
e. Acute otitis media
f. Ototoxicity
g. Fracture base of skull
h. CSOM
i. Glue ear
j. Herpes Zoster
k. Foreign body

*For each presentation below, choose the **most likely dianosis** from the above list of options. Each option may be used once, more than once, or not at all.*

QUESTIONS

121. Man treated with gentamicin for peritonitis for 10 days presents with deafness.

122. A patient with poor hygenic condition presents with hearing loss after taking a shower.

123. Woman presents with deafness and corneal anaesthesia. On MRI, a widened internal auditory meatus is seen.

124. Male, 20 years, with history of head injury, bruising on the side of head complains of hearing loss.

125. A 54-year-old female develops mild fever, malaise and ear pain. 3 days later she developed multiple painful vesicles over her early canal and external meatus.

THEME 26: INVESTIGATION OF PAINFUL JOINTS IN CHILDREN

OPTIONS
a. Serology for autoantibodies
b. Diagnostic aspiration for WBC demonstration
c. MRI
d. Diagnostic aspiration for culture
e. CT scan
f. Diagnostic aspiration for RBC
g. Serum urate
h. X-ray knee joint
i. Therapeutic aspiration of joint
j. AP X-ray—hip joint
k. Lateral X-ray—hip joint

*For each presentation below, choose the **single most appropriate** from the above list of OPTIONS. Each option may be used once, more than once, or not at all.*

QUESTIONS

126. A six-year-old boy complains of intermittent hip pain for several months. Hematological investigations are normal. X-rays show flattening of the femoral head.

127. A two-year-old girl with one day history of increasing hip pain has become unable to weight bear. Her WCC is 21/fl, with an ESR of 89 mm/hr and a CRP of 300 mg/l. A radiograph of the hip shows a widened jaoint space.

128. A 12-year-old boy with left groin pain for 6 weeks is noticed to stand with the left leg externally rotated. Examination reveals negligible internal rotation of the hip.

129. A four-year-old boy complains of right hip pain a few days following an upper respiratory tract infection. Blood tests are as follows: WCC 12/fl, ESR 10 mm/hr and CRP 2 mg/l

130. A five-year-old girl complains of progressively increasing severe pain in her left hip and upper leg for 6 days. She is able to walk but limps visibly. Blood tests are as follows: WCC 19/fl, ESR 72 mm/hr and CRP 94 mg/l. X-rays and ultrasound scans of the hip are normal.

THEME 27: ETIOLOGY OF ANAEMIA

OPTIONS
a. Chronic blood loss
b. Rheumatoid arthritis
c. Pernicious anaemia
d. Haemolysis
e. Beta-thalassemia
f. Alcoholism
g. Sickle cell anaemia
h. B_{12} deficiency
i. Scurvy
j. Nutritional deficit
k. Malabsorption

*For each presentation below, choose the **single most likely cause of the given profile** from the above list of OPTIONS. Each option may be used once, more than once, or not at all.*

QUESTIONS

131. Patient with atrophic gastritis has megaloblastic anaemia.

132. Patient who is a strict vegetarian has an MCV of 110.

133. Patient has both Iron and Folate deficiency Radiology and sigmoidoscospy—normal, has pale stools which is difficult to flush away.

134. Elderly patient with complaint of anaemia and has bleeding gum.

135. Elderly patient in residential home stay with complaint of tiredness.

THEME 28: MANAGEMENT OF EPISTAXIS

OPTIONS
a. Anterior pack
b. Posterior pack
c. Anterior pack and posterior pack
d. Electrocautery
e. Surgery
f. Review anticoagulation
g. Antihypertensives
h. Embolization of feeding vessel
i. Cocaine spray
j. Ice pack
k. Cryotherapy

*For each presentation below, choose the **most appropriate step in management** from the above list of OPTIONS. Each option may be used once, more than once, or not at all.*

QUESTIONS

136. There is just blood clotting in the nostrils bleeding has stopped.

137. A patient with nose bleeding, on exam vascular damage is found, there is still some leakage.

138. Man with prosthetic heart valve presents with epistaxis.

139. Man who is involved in furniture making presents with recurrent epistaxis and anaesthesia of right cheek.

140. An 80-year-old man with history of epistaxis since 2 hours.

September—2001

THEME 29: IMMEDIATE MANAGEMENT OF COMMON HAEMATOLOGICAL COMPLICATIONS

OPTIONS
a. Central venous line
b. Intraosseous fluid injection
c. Fresh frozen plasma
d. Blood transfusion
e. Blood and platelet transfusion
f. Chemotherapy
g. CT scan skull
h. Hydroxyurea
i. Systemic steroids
j. Anticoagulation
k. Allogenic transplantation

*For each presentation below, choose the **most appropriate first step** from the above list of OPTIONS. Each option may be used once, more than once, or not at all.*

QUESTIONS

141. A 51-year-old is lethargic and found to be anemic. his blood picture is found to have a granulocytic tendency with an increase in the platelet count.

142. A 5-year-old with generalised lymphadenopathy develops fever and neck stiffness and headache. he is found to have a lot of lymphoblasts in the blood picture.

143. 55-year-old man with history of hypertension untreated presents with hemiparesis.

144. A 72-year-old is having a routine examination. he is found to have a mild lymphocytosis and splenomegaly.

145. A 38-year-old woman presents with cervical lymphadenopahty. Mature lymphoblasts are seen on the blood film. Examination reveals a mild splenomegaly. She is on phenytoin for epilepsy.

THEME 30: FIRST INVESTIGATION OF POSSIBLE THROMBOEMBOLIC DISEASE

OPTIONS
a. Muscle biopsy
b. Carotid doppler
c. Retinoscopy
d. MRI
e. ESR
f. Lumbar puncture
g. Peripheral smear
h. CT scan
i. INR
j. Carotid angiography
k. Routine screen

*For each presentation below, choose the **most appropriate first investigation** from the above list of OPTIONS. Each option may be used once, more than once, or not at all.*

QUESTIONS

146. A 27-year-old woman has a long-standing history of headaches associated with nausea and vomiting. On this occasion she present with sudden loss of vision in the right half of the visual field. By the time you see her it has improved considerably.

147. An 82-year-old woman complains of increasing weakness and muscle pain to the point where she is finding it difficulty to brush her hair and get out of a chair. She now presents with sudden loss of vision in her left eye.

148. A woman previously in good health, presents with sudden onset of severe occipital headache and vomiting. Her only physical sign on examination is a stiff neck.

149. A 74-year-old woman had a fall two weeks ago. She is brought into the A and E department with slowly increasing drowsiness. On examination you find mild hemiparesis and unequal pupils.

150. A 73-year-old man presents with hemianopia, hemi-sensory loss, hemiparesis and aphasia of 16 hour duration.

THEME 31: INVESTIGATION OF COMPLICATIONS OF PROSTATIC CARCINOMA

OPTIONS
a. PSA
b. Serum acid phosphatase
c. Serum alkaline phosphatase
d. Transrectal ultrasound
e. Abdominal ultrasound
f. Serum calcium
g. Gallium scan
h. Technitium scan
i. Thallium scan
j. Transrectal biopsy
k. HLA status
l. Urodynamic studies

For each presentation below, choose the **most appropriate investigation** from the above list of options. Each option may be used once, more than once, or not at all.

QUESTIONS

151. 80-year-old with prostatic carcinoma comes with 4 month history of low backache.

152. Patient with prostatic cancer has been treated, now complains of confusion, thirst, bodyaches, constipation.

153. Man on GnRH's for prostate cancer comes after 2 months for a follow up.

154. Man with prostate carcinoma which has extended outside the capsule presenting with features of renal failure.

155. A man having adenocarcinoma prostate which has already spread to pelvic side walls has to be given chemotherapy.

THEME 32: ANALGESIA

OPTIONS
a. IV opiate
b. Subcutaneous opiate infusion
c. Acupuncture
d. Carbamazepine
e. Hypnotherapy
f. NSAIDs IM
g. Oral NSAIDs
h. Oral opiates
i. Proton pump inhibitors
j. SSRI e.g. fluoxetine

For each presentation below, choose the **single most appropriate method of pain relief** from the above list of OPTIONS. Each option may be used once, more than once, or not at all.

QUESTIONS

156. A 65-year-old man presents with severe, retrosternal chest pain and sweating. An ECG shows an acute antero lateral myocardial infarction.

157. A 70-year-old man inoperable gastric cancer causing obstruction, and multiple liver metastases, is taking a large dose of oral analgesia. Despite this, his pain is currently unrelieved.

158. A 25-year-old woman has just been diagnosed a having rheumatoid arthritis and her rheumatologists has begun giving her gold injections. She continues to complain of joint pain and stiffnesss, particularly for the first two hours of each day.

159. A 50-year-old obese man with a known hiatus hernia, presents with recurrent, severe, burning retrosternal chest pain associated with acid regurgitation and increased oral flatulence.

160. A 67-year-old woman reports severe paroxysms of knife-like or electric shock-like pain, lasting secons in the lower part of the right side of her face.

THEME 33: DIAGNOSIS OF GYNAECOLOGICAL CONDITIONS

OPTIONS
a. Crohn's disease
b. Ulcerative colitis
c. Chlamydia
d. E. coli
e. Genital prolapse
f. Procidentia
g. Herpes labialis
h. Chancre
i. Atrophic vaginitis
j. Chancroid
k. Cervicitis

*For each presentation below, choose the **best diagnosis** from the above list of OPTIONS. Each option may be used once, more than once, or not at all.*

QUESTIONS

161. 85-year-old with 14 children, severe heart failure, complains of dysuria, feeling of pressure in lower abdomen.

162. Female with well-controlled diabetes mellitus type 2 with recurrent UTI.

163. A young female with long-standing irregular bowel habit and persistent UTI.

164. An 80-year-old sexually active woman with dyspareunia and recurrent dysuria.

165. A middle-aged woman with a vaginal discharge is found to have several ulcers at the vaginal introitus.

THEME 34: VAGINAL BLEEDING—MEDICAL TRAETMENT

OPTIONS
a. Medroxyprogesterone (depot form)
b. Combined oral contraceptive pill
c. Danazol
d. GNRH
e. Antifibrinolytics
f. Prostaglandin synthetase antagonist
g. Optional hormone replacement therapy
h. Minipill
i. Total hysterectomy ± Radiotherapy
j. Uterine curettage
k. None required

*For each presentation below, choose the **most appropriate treatment modality** from the above list of OPTIONS. Each option may be used once, more than once, or not at all.*

QUESTIONS

166. A 20-year-old woman who has been on oral contraceptive develops bright red postcoital bleeding (PCB).

167. A 55-year-old female develops a single episode of PMB. She stopped menstruation 7 years ago. ultrasound shows endometrial thickness.

168. A 49-year-old woman with complaint of hot flushes, vaginal dryness and her menstruation become irregular 5 months ago.

169. A 14-year-old woman with painless vaginal bleeding.

170. A woman with painful vaginal bleeding with brown clots. She feels embarrassed goint to parties and wants a solution to her problem. Normal remedies over the counter did not help her.

THEME 35: DIAGNOSIS OF VISUAL IMPAIRMENT

OPTIONS
a. Conjunctivitis
b. Blepharitis
c. Dacryocystitis
d. Giant cell arteritis
e. Chronic simple glaucoma
f. Closed angle glaucoma
g. Vitreous haemorrhage
h. Cataract
i. Retinal detachment
j. Cerebral haemorrhage
k. Senile macular degeneration

*For each presentation below, choose the **single most likely** diagnosis from the above list of OPTIONS. Each option may be used once, more than once, or not at all.*

QUESTIONS
171. A 73-year-old complains of a severe right-sided headache associated with an acute loss of right-sided vision. Urgent treatment is needed to prevent left sided vision loss.

172. A 75-year-old has difficulty watching television complaining of a peripheral constriction of vision. On examination, there is cupping of both optical discs.

173. A 50-year-old with a history of SLE complains of loss of vision. On examination, he is found to have multiple opacity in the lens of his eyes.

174. A diabetic on oral hypoglycemics complains of sudden deterioration in vision of his right eye. On examination, he is found to have bilateral proliferative retinopathy with retinal hemorrhage on the right side.

175. An 80-year-old has markedly decreased visual acuity. On fundoscopy, she is found to have bilateral macular pigmentation.

THEME 36: RHEUMATOLOGY—DIAGONSIS

OPTIONS
a. Perthes disease
b. Slipped femoral epiphysis
c. Septic arthritis
d. Osteomyeltis
e. Pelvic fracture
f. Pseudogout
g. Osteoarthritis
h. Fracture femur—intertrochanteric
i. Fracture neck of femur
j. Rheumatoid arthritis
k. Gout

*For each presentation below, choose the **single most likely** diagnosis from the above list of OPTIONS. Each option may be used once, more than once, or not at all.*

QUESTIONS
176. A middle-aged woman with a history of rheumatoid arthritis develops sudden swelling in one of her knees. This knee is swollen and hot to touch.

177. An elderly man with recently diagnosed heart failure has been treated with diuretics. He now develops severe joint pain in his left ankle with swelling and redness.

178. A 78-year-old woman complains of a stiff left hip joint after walking some distance. This is most evident when she attempts to abduct the hip joint with limited abduction.

179. A 34-year-old woman complains of bilateral stiff and painful joints in her hands and feet.

180. A 67-year-old woman complains of right hip pain. On examination the right hip is adducted, externally rotated and flexed.

THEME 37: FIRST STEP IN MANAGEMENT OF MI COMPLICATIONS

OPTIONS
a. Tissue plasminogen activation
b. Heparin
c. Heparin and DC cardioversion
d. Streptokinase
e. Warfarin
f. IV atropine
g. IV digoxin
h. Intraaortic balloon counter pulsation
i. IV fluids
j. Surgery
k. NSAIDs

*For each presentation below, choose the **most appropriate first step in management** from the above list of OPTIONS. Each option may be used once, more than once, or not at all.*

QUESTIONS

181. Patient, 12 hours after MI presents with recurrent chest pain, breathlessness, heart rate—40/min.

182. Patient with pulmonary edema features presents with irregular pulse, heart rate—140/bpm.

183. A woman 10 days following hysterectomy complaints of severe left sided chest pain and breathlessness. Chest X-ray and ECG failed to relieve any abnormality.

184. 10 days after MI, female presents with chest pain on inspiration, persistently elevated ST segment on ECG.

185. Patient after MI found to have a harsh pansystolic murmur at the apex.

THEME 38: FLUID RESUSCITATION IN CHILDREN

OPTIONS
a. Do not do anything
b. IV saline 0.9%
c. IV saline 9%
d. IV Dextrose 5%
e. Water to sip
f. ORS 90 Na mEq/L
g. ORS 150 mEq of Na
h. Haemaccel
i. Ringer lactate
j. Intraosseous infusion
k. Oral opiates

*For each presentation below, choose the **most appropriate resuscitation modality** from the above list of OPTIONS. Each option may be used once, more than once, or not at all.*

QUESTIONS

186. 24-month-old child, brought with a history of having been accidentally locked up in a car for about 3 hours. On examination in the A&E child is crying but his vitals are stable. What is the next step.

187. Female child from Ghana, brought to the A&E with a history of nausea and vomiting. On investigations Ketone 1+, Na 148 meq, Glucose 18 mmol/L.

188. Mother comes to the A&E with her child of 3yrs, history of D&V. On examination the child appears mildly dehydrated.

189. Boy has been brought to the A&E following a traffic accident. He has suffered from moderate blood loss. What is the most optimum method of fluid resuscitation.

190. A 2-year-old child with history of diarrhoea for 18 hours present and A to E. He is drowsy with cold extremities.

THEME 39: ANTIBIOTIC PROPHYLAXIS FOR SURGICAL PATIENTS

OPTIONS

a. Angiography
b. Bronchoscopy
c. Colle's fracture
d. Dental treatment of a cardiac patient
e. Dislocated shoulder
f. Emergency appendicectomy
g. Heart valve replacement
h. Sigmoid colectomy
i. Splenectomy
j. Thyroidectomy

INSTRUCTIONS

For each prophylactic regimen given below, choose the single most likely indication from the above list of options. Each option may be used once, more than once or not at all.

QUESTIONS

191. 3 gm sachet of amoxicillin one hour before the procedure.

192. Three days of intravenous broad spectrum antibiotics beginning with induction of anaesthesia.

193. Clear fluids by mouth and two sachets of sodium picosulphate on the day before the operation plus broad spectrum intravenous antibiotics at induction.

194. Long-term oral penicillin and immunisation against pneumococcal infection.

195. One dose of metronidazole at induction of anaesthesia.

THEME 40: IMMUNIZATION IN CHILDREN

OPTIONS

a. Delay by 2 weeks
b. Omit pertussis and meningitis
c. Give vaccine in hospital
d. Continue as per schedule
e. Give inactivated vaccines
f. Omit pertussis, Hib, measles
g. Don't give any vaccines
h. Omit pertussis only
i. Omit meningitis only
j. Omit measles only
k. Delay by 2 months

*For each presentation below, choose the **correct answer** from the above list of options. Each option may be used once, more than once, or not at all.*

QUESTIONS

196. Child who is HIV+ is due for MMR.

197. Child due for Hib, DPT, etc suffering from acute febrile illness.

198. Child cried for 2 hours after Hib, DPT, etc.

199. Family history of egg allergy. Child due for MMR.

200. History of convulsions. Child due for HiB, DPT, etc.

September—2001

General Medical Council PLAB Test Part 1

Full Name
Test Centre/Date

- Use pencil only • Make heavy makrs that fill the lozenge completely
- Write your candidate number in the top row of the box to the right **AND** fill in the appropriate lozenge below each number
- Give **ONE** answer only for each question

DO NOT WRITE IN THIS SPACE

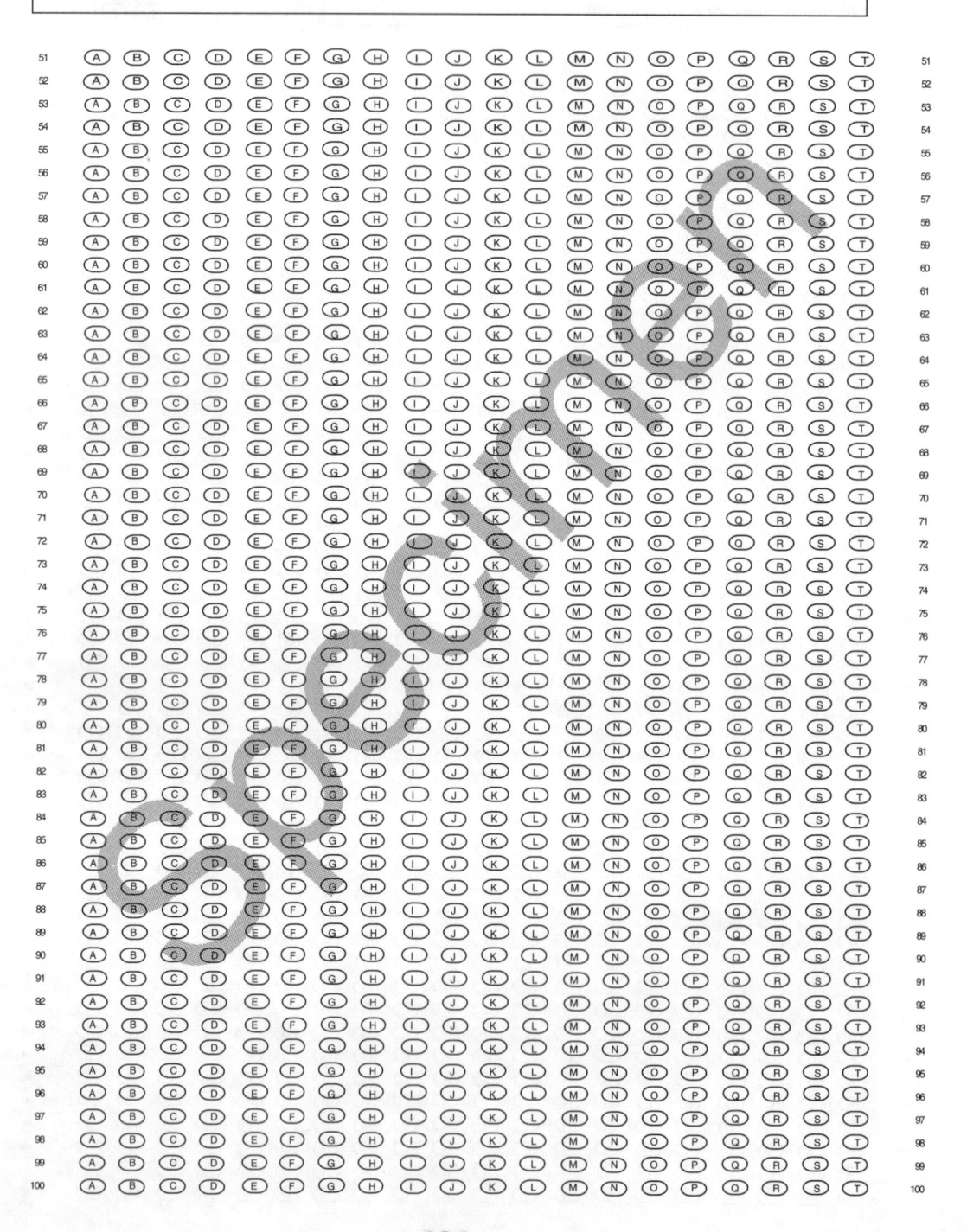

September—2001

DO NOT WRITE IN THIS SPACE

- 485 -

DO NOT WRITE IN THIS SPACE

September—2001

Answers

1	k	None required
2	f	X-ray orbit
3	f	X-ray orbit
4	g	Conjunctival cytology
5	h	MRI
6	b	Steroids
7	c	Laser photocoagulation
8	g	Admit for...........
9	h	IV mannitol
10	i	Atropine sulphate
11	i	Superficial head injury
12	j	Insignificant head injury
13	k	Vasogenic cerebral oedema
14	d	Subdural haematoma
15	c	Extradural haematoma
16	a	Carbon monoxide
17	b	Warfarim
18	f	Paracetamol
19	e	Quinine
20	h	Tricyclic antidepressants
21	f	Haloperidol
22	a	Opioid overdose
23	g	Clozapine
24	e	Lithium
25	c	Tricyclic in toxication
26	k	Colonoscopy
27	l	Sigmoidoscopy
28	e	Barium enema
29	e	Barium enema
30	g	Stool culture

31	a	Candidiasis
32	d	Achalasia
33	e	Oesophageal carcinoma
34	c	Diffuse oesophageal spasm
35	e	Oesophageal carcinoma
36	f	Hepatitis B
37	g	CBD obstruction
38	i	Acute cholecystitis
39	j	PBC
40	h	HHC
41	a	Acute epididimo-orchitis
42	g	Testicular torsion
43	k	Seminoma or teratoma
44	j	Sebaceous cyst
45	i	UTI
46	h	Possible infection
47	a	Hyperglycaemia
48	e	Autonomic neuropathy
49	f	Intermittent Claudication
50	i	Lactic acidosis
51	i	Biopsy
52	j	Thyroglobulin autoantibodies
53	g	Dry induced thyrotoxiosis
54	k	TSH receptor autoantibodies
55	e	Contrast radiographs
56	h	Flexible sigmoidoscopy
57	i	Laparoscopy
58	k	Endocervical swab
59	e	Abdominal USG + High vaginal swab
60	j	None required

61	a	IV hydrocortisone
62	j	Ganciclovir IV
63	k	Shohl's solution
64	f	Fluid restriction
65	e	Sodium bicarbonate
66	i	NaCl+K$^+$ supplements
67	h	NaHCO$_3$
68	g	Potassium supplements
69	f	Frusemide
70	e	Hypokalaemia
71	a	Pleural biopsy
72	c	Chest X-ray
73	g	Sputum culture and microscopy
74	b	V/Q scan
75	f	Bronchoscopy
76	k	Asthma
77	a	Sarcoidosis
78	d	Anxiety
79	j	Aspiration pneumonitis
80	g	Pulmonary embolism
81	h	Underwater seal drainage
82	e	Cross match blood and inform surgeons
83	d	High flow O$_2$ + 10 mg IV morphine + anticoagulation
84	e	Cross match blood and inform surgeons
85	d	High flow O$_2$ + 10 mg IV morphine + Anticoagulation
86	d	Lymphoedema
87	f	Hypercalcaemia
88	e	Spinal cord compression
89	b	Cerebral metastases
90	a	Pathological fracture

91	f	Osteogenesis imperfecta
92	i	Elderly abuse
93	d	Sexual abuse
94	c	Physical abuse
95	a	Accidental injury
96	g	Digital substraction angiography
97	j	Biopsy
98	a	USG
99	c	Aspiration and microscopy
100	i	Transillumination test
101	d	Carboxyhaemoglobin level
102	g	Aspirate blister
103	a	IV fluids
104	b	Escharotomy
105	l	Discharge after dressing
106	i	3 years
107	c	6 weeks
108	h	2 years
109	d	2 months
110	g	1 year
111	g	Cervical spinal cord
112	f	Brain stem and its cerebellar connections
113	c	Optic nerve
114	c	Optic nerve
115	i	Facial nerve
116	e	Hepatitis A infection
117	a	Hepatitis A immunization
118	g	Schistosomiasis
119	c	Hepatitis B vaccine
120	f	Hepatocellular carcinoma
121	f	Ototoxicity
122	d	Wax impaction

123	a	Acoustic neuroma
124	c	Petrous temporal bone fracture
125	j	Herpes zoster
126	k	Lateral X-ray-Hip joint
127	d	Diagnostic aspiration for culture
128	k	Lateral X-ray –Hip joint
129	b	Diagnostic aspiration for WBC demonstration
130	c	MRI
131	c	Pernicious anaemia
132	h	B_{12} deficiency
133	k	Malabsorption
134	i	Scurvy
135	j	Nutritional deficit
136	a	Anterior pack
137	d	Electrocautery
138	f	Review anticoagulation
139	h	Embolization
140	g	Antihypertensives
141	d	Blood transfusion
142	e	Blood and platelet transfusion
143	g	CT scan skull
144	h	Hydroxyurea
145	i	Systemic steroids
146	b	Carotid doppler
147	e	ESR
148	h	CT scan
149	h	CT scan
150	k	Routine screen
151	h	Technitium scan
152	f	Serum calcium
153	a	PSA
154	l	Urodynamic studies

155	d	Transrectal USG
156	a	IV opiate
157	b	SC opiate infusion
158	g	Oral NSAIDs
159	i	Proton pump inhibitors
160	d	Carbamazepine
161	e	Genital prolapse
162	c	Chlamydia
163	a	Crohn's disease
164	i	Atrophic vaginitis
165	g	Herpes labialis
166	k	None required
167	i	Total hysterectomy ± radiotherapy
168	g	Optional hormone replacement therapy
169	k	None required
170	i	Total hysterectomy ± radiotherapy
171	d	Giant cell arteritis
172	e	Chronic simple glaucoma
173	h	Cataract
174	g	Vitreous haemorrhage
175	k	Senile macular degeneration
176	f	Pseudogout
177	k	Gout
178	g	Osteoarthritis
179	j	Rheumatoid arthritis
180	i	Fracture neck femur
181	f	IV Atropine
182	g	IV digoxin
183	b	Heparin
184	k	NSAIDs
185	h	Aortic balloon counter pulsation
186	e	Water to sip

187	b	IV saline 0.9%
188	f	ORS 90 Na MEq/L
189	h	Haemaccel
190	i	Ringer lactate
191	d	Dental treatment of a cardiac patient
192	g	Heart valve replacement
193	h	Sigmoid colectomy

194	I	Splenectomy
195	f	Emergency appendicectomy
196	d	Continue as per schedule
197	a	Delay by 2 weeks
198	d	Continue as per schedule
199	d	Continue as per schedule
200	d	Continue as per schedule

September—2001

EXPLANATIONS

1. A 69-year-old patient presented to his GP with sudden onset of redness in the right eye. There was no pain and vision was unaffected.

Diagnosis: Subconjunctival haemorrhage

Most appropriate management: No treatment.

Clinchers
Red eye may be due to variety of conditions, but here since there is no pain and the vision is unaffected, no active intervention is required. Though in this case we must check the blood pressure of the patient. No need to go for coagulation studies, as one of the options in this questions suggests.

Subconjunctival haemorrhage may be due to rupture of conjunctival capillaries, due to raised pressure, e.g. in whooping cough, strangulation, epileptic fits, etc. May also be seen in vascular diseases such as arteriosclerosis, hypertension and diabetes mellitus.

> **CONFUSA**
> Checking the blood pressure and observation are the main line of treatment in this patient. If any underlying cause is established or suspected, it should be investigated and managed.

Investigation of choice
Not required.

Immediate management
No treatment.

Treatment of choice
Treat the cause when discovered. Assurance to the patient is must. No other active intervention required. Cold compresses can be given in the beginning if bleeding.

Your Notes:

2. A patient presents with metal pieces to his eyes.

Diagnosis: Intraocular foreign bodies (IOFB)

Clinchers
> *Metal pieces to his eyes:* A careful history about of mode of injury may give a clue about the type of IOFB. A thorough ocular examination with slit-lamp including gonioscopy should be carried out. The signs which may give some indication about IOFB are:
- Subconjunctival haemorrhage
- Corneal scar
- Holes in the iris
- Opaque track through the lens

With clear media, sometimes IOFB may be seen on ophthalmoscopy in the vitreous or on the retina. IFOB lodged in the angle of anterior chamber may be visualized by gonioscopy.

> **CONFUSA**
> Anteroposterior and lateral X-rays of the orbit are indispensable for the location of IOFB, as metallic foreign body are radiopaque. Its exact localization is mandatory to plan proper removal.

Investigation of choice
Plain X-rays of orbit

Immediate management
Ophthalmology referral

Treatment of choice
Magnetic foreign body is removed with a hand held magnet.

Nonmagnetic foreign body is picked up with a toothless forceps.

Your notes:

3. A mother brings her 2-year-old child with a squint. On examination a leucokoric right pupil is seen with an absent red reflex.

Diagnosis: Retinoblastoma

Most appropriate management: Enucleation

Clinchers
- *2-year-old child:* Retinoblastoma is the most common intraocular tumor of childhood. Though congenital, it is not recognised at birth, and is usually seen between 1-2 years of age, with no sex predisposition.
- *Squint:* Usually convergent may develop in retinoblastoma.
- *Leucokoric right pupil:* Conditions other than retinoblastoma that present as leucocoria are: congenital cataract, inflammatory deposits in vitreous following a plastic cyclitis or choroiditis, coloboma of the choroid, retrolental fibroplasia, toxocara endophthalmitis and exudative retinopathy of coats.

CONFUSA
Retinoblastoma should be differentiated from other conditions that present as leukocoria.

Investigation of choice
Fundus examination and ophthalmoscopy
Plain X-ray orbit shows calcification
USG and CT are very useful

Treatment of choice
Enucleation (excision of the eyeball)
Absolute indications of enucleation are:
- retinoblastoma, and
- malignant melanoma
  Indications of evisceration (removal of the contents of the eyeball leaving behind the sclera) are
- panophthalmitis
- expulsive choroidal haemorrhage, and
- bleeding anterior staphyloma.

Your Notes:

4. A 12-year-old Libyan boy gave a two-week history of discomfort, redness and mucopurulent discharge affecting both eyes. His two siblings have a similar problem.

Diagnosis: Acute mucopurulent conjunctivitis

Most appropriate management: Immediate antibiotic therapy

Clinchers
- *12-year-old Libyan boy:* Infective conjunctivitis is still common in developing countries.
- *Discomfort, redness, mucopurulent discharge:* There are the symptoms of acute mucopurulent conjunctivitis. Discomfort and foreign body sensation due to engorgement of vessels.
- *Time siblings have similar problem:* Mucopurulent conjunctivitis may be caused by *Staphylococcus aureus* Koch-Weeks bacillus, Pneumococcus or streptococcus. It is infective in nature.

CONFUSA
Conjunctival congestion is more marked in palpebral conjunctiva, fornices and peripheral part of bulbar conjunctiva. Circumcorneal congestion is seen in iridocyclitis.

Investigation of choice
Conjunctival cytology and bacterial examination of secretions and scrapings.

Immediate management
Topical broad spectrum antibiotics to control the infection.

Treatment of choice
Topical antibiotics
- Irrigation of conjunctival sac with sterile warm saline once or twice a day
- Dark goggles
- No bandage
- No steroids (infection may flare up).

Your Notes:

5. A 23-year-old woman has a history of recurrent attacks of blurring of vision associated with redness, pain and photophobia. Both eyes have been affected in the past. She is currently being investigated for bowel disease and a severe backache.

Diagnosis: Multiple sclerosis

Most appropriate management: 0.5% prednisolone drops 2 hrly and cyclopentolate drops

Clinchers
- *23-year-old man:* Multiple sclerosis has female preponderance. Mean age of onset is 30 years.
- *Recurrent attacks of blurring of vision:* Early picture of multiple sclerosis is usually one of relapses followed by remissions become incomplete. In multiple sclerosis, plaques of demyelination are seen at the sites through at the CNS.
- *Bowel disease of severe backache:* Bowel (constipation), fatigue, motor weakness, optic neuritis, incontinence, numbness, tingling in limbs, cerebellar symptoms may be seen in multiple sclerosis.

CONFUSA
Isolated neurological deficits are never diagnostic, but may become so, if a careful history reveals previous episodes.

Investigation of choice
MRI is sensitive

Immediate management
Treat the complication

Treatment of choice
No cure but following may help
- Methylprednisolone (shortens relapses), use sparingly. It does no alter overall prognosis.
- β-*interferon:* ↓ relapse rate by 1/3.

Your Notes:

6. A 78-year-old man has had a painful scalp and headache for three weeks, and is generally unwell, complains of acute onset of blindness in his right eye.

Diagnosis: Temporal arteritis

Clinchers
- *Painful scalp and headache:* Interruption of blood flow to visual cortex causes sudden greying of vision, and other symptoms that mimic migraine.
  Transient monoocular blindness usually occurs from a retinal embolus or severe ipsilateral carotid stenosis.
- *Acute onset blindness in right eye:* Anterior ischaemic optic neuropathy (AION) is an infarction of the optic nerve head due to inadequate perfusion via the posterior ciliary arteries. Patient has sudden loss, often upon awakening, and painless swelling of the optic disc. Arteric AION is caused by *temporal arteritis.*

CONFUSA
Malignant hypertension can cause visual loss from exudates, haemorrhages, cotton wool spots (focal nerve fibre layer infarct) and optic disc edema.

Investigation of choice
Visual field mapping
Ophthalmoscopy
ESR

Immediate management
Immediate glucocorticoid therapy

Treatment of choice
Glucocorticoid therapy for at least 2 years.

Your Notes:

7. **A 50-year-old woman complains of sudden loss of vision in one eye. She describes the incident, like a curtain coming down.**

Diagnosis: Retinal detachment

Clinchers
- *50-year-old woman:* Retinal detachment is most common between 40 and 60 years, though it may occur at any age. F:M (3:2) ratio.
- *Sudden painless loss of vision:* Causes of sudden painless loss of vision are:
  - Retinal detachment
  - Central retinal artery/vein occlusion
  - Vitreous haemorrhage
  - Central serous retinopathy
  - Optic neuritis
  - Methyl alcohol amblyopia
- *Curtain coming down (in one eye):* Appearance of dark cloud, or veil like curtain in front of eye suddenly is the sign of retinal detachment (large and central).

CONFUSA
Retinal detachment should be differentiated from the other causes of sudden painless loss of vision (given above). In early cases of retinal detachment patient notices a localised relative loss in the field of vision (of detached retina) which progresses as detachment proceeds towards the macular area.

Investigation of choice
- *Ophthalmoscopy:* Detached retina gives grey reflex instead of normal pink reflex
- *Visual field charting*
- USG confirms the diagnosis.

Treatment of choice
- Sealing of retinal breaks
- Bring the sclerochoroid and detached retina near to each other

High risk factors for retinal detachment: Myopia, aphakia, retinal detachment in fellow eye, history of retinal detachment in family.

Your Notes:

8. **An 84-year-old woman notices sudden increased visual impairment. She is found to have homonymous hemianopia.**

Diagnosis: Cerebral haemorrhage

Clinchers
- *84-year-old woman:* Incidence of rupture of cerebral vessel aneurysms increases with age. These aneurysms are common in females.
- *Sudden increased visual impairment:* Since the defect is of sudden onset, it rules out tumors or other chronic disease processes as a causation. There is no given history of trauma cerebral embolism can be ruled out as it usually do not produce permanent changes.
- *Homonymous hemianopia:* Most commonly it results from lesions in optic tract (tumours pressing it), geniculate body and optic radiations (cerebral haemorrhage). Since we have ruled out tumors to be cause, cerebral haemorrhage is a safe answer.

CONFUSA
Hemianopia denotes loss of half of the field of vision. The most common clinical form is homonymous hemianopia, in which the right of left half of the binocular field of vision is lost, owing to loss of the temporal half of one field and the nasal half of the other, a condition due to a lesion situated in any part of the visual paths from the chiasma to the occipital lobe. Right hemianopia is more quickly discovered than left owing to the fact that reading is impossible; left hemianopia is often discovered when the patient does not see food on the left side of the plate.

Investigation of choice
MRI/CT

Immediate management
Admit and specialist evaluation

Treatment of choice
Symptomatic + as per radiological findings.

Your Notes:

9. **A 68-year-old smoker suddenly notices markedly reduced vision in one eye. He cannot read any letter on visual acuity chart but can count fingers. The fundus is pale.**

Diagnosis: Central retinal artery occlusion (CRAO)

Clinchers
- *68-year-old smoker:* These are the risk factors for CRAO. More commonly seen in patients suffering from hypertension and other cardiovascular diseases. It is usually unilateral, but rarely be bilateral (1-2% cases).
- *Notices reduced vision in one eye:* CRAO is usually unilateral. Sudden painless loss of vision is suggestive of central retinal artery occlusion.
- *Fundus is pale:* Retina becomes milky white due to oedema. Retinal arteries are markedly narrowed. Fundus is pale.

> **CONFUSA**
> Sudden painless loss of vision occur in central retinal artery occlusion, vitreous haemorrhage, retinal detachment, central retinal vein occlusion, central serous retinopathy, optic neuritis and methyl alcohol amblyopia.

Investigation of choice
Investigate for the cause.

Immediate management
- Immediate lowering of IOP (IV mannitol)
- Vasodilators and inhalation of a mixture of 5% CO_2 and 95% O_2 (may help in relieving angiospasm)
- Anticoagulants
- Intravenous steroids

Treatment of choice
Treatment is unsatisfactory as retinal tissue cannot survive ischaemia for more than a few hours. Emergency treatment (as above) should be followed.

Your Notes:

10. **A 30-year-old man has recurrent episodes of an acutely painful red eye with reduced vision.**

Diagnosis: Uveitis

Clinchers
- *Acutely painful red eye reduced vision:* These symptoms are suggestive of anterior uveitis (iridocyclitis).
- *Pain:* It is a dominating symptom of anterior uveitis, typically worsen at right.
- *Redness:* It is due to circumcorneal congestion, which is a result of active hyperaemia of anterior ciliary, vessels.
- *Reduces vision:* Defective vision in patient with iridocyclitis may vary from slight blur in early phase to marked deterioration in late phase.
- Look for corneal edema and keratic precipitates (KP) at back of cornea.

> **CONFUSA**
> Acute congestive glaucoma and acute conjunctivitis should be kept in mind here, and should be differentiated from iridocyclitis. Other conditions that may cause sudden painful visual loss are chemical or mechanical injuries to the eyeball.

Investigation of choice
Includes battery of tests due to its varied etiology.

Immediate management
1 per cent atropine sulphate eye ointment or drops 2-3 times day. In case of atropine allergy other cycloplegics should be used

Treatment of choice
Local treatment with mydriatic-cycloplegic drugs and corticosteroids (reduce inflammation).

Systemic therapy with corticosteroids (especially in non-granulomatous iridocyclitis). NSAIDs where steroids contraindicated. Adrenocorticotrophic hormone where steroids fail to act.

Finally treat the cause.

Your Notes:

11. **Following an alcoholic binge a 36-year-old male falls and comes to casualty with a cut in his temporal region his Glasgow Coma Scale is normal and his neck is cleared by the orthopedic SHO.**

Diagnosis: Superficial head injury.

Clinchers
- *Following an alcoholic binge*: Alcoholics warrants overnight admission in the hospital as they cannot be assessed properly on presentation for head injury. This is applicable even if the GCS is normal. Other patients warranting admission in spite of normal GCS are children and postictal (confused) patients.
- *Falls:* Most probably it is the reason for the cut in the temporal region. Note that alcoholics are more prone to develop subdural hematomas due to weakening of bridging veins because of repeated falls.
- *A cut in his temporal region:* It must be a simple laceration if there is no associated fracture of temporal bone. It requires prompt suturing to maintain hemostasis.
- *Glasgow Coma Scale is normal:* Rules out any immediate brain damage/hematoma. But not that it is difficult or even misleading in an alcoholic.
- *His neck is cleared by the orthopedic SHO:* It rules out any spinal injury.

CONFUSA
The main confusion is about whom to admit or discharge in a case of head injury. The criteria are:

Criteria for admission in a case of head injury
- Difficult to assess
  - *Child*
  - *Postictal*
  - *Alcohol intoxication*
- CNS signs
- Severe headache or vomiting
- Fracture
- Smelling of alcohol with GCS < 15

Criteria for discharge with written advise (all criteria must be fulfilled)
- Fully conscious on presentation
- No abnormal neurological signs
- Loss of consciousness < 5 min
- Post-traumatic amnesia < 5 min
- No severe headache
- No vomiting
- No skull fracture
- No bleeding disorder
- Good home conditions

Note: Get an X-ray skull in all suspected medicolegal cases (like this one) even if you suspect no bony injury.

Other main confusion is about anterograde and retrograde amnesia. Note the only the extent of anterograte amnesia correlates with severity of injury (admit if > 5 min). Retrograde amnesia does not correlate well with severity. Also retrograde amnesia never occurs without anterograde amnesia. Anterograde amnesia (also known as post-traumatic amnesia—PTA) if under one hour, means mild injury whereas > 24 years denotes severe injury. OHCM has stated on the contrary and thus created this confusion. But refer Kumar and Clark, pg 1084, 4th edn and lecture notes in emergency medicine, pg 36 second edition.

Investigation of choice
X-ray skull (CT in an alcoholic is only indicated if GCS falls).

Immediate management
Suturing of laceration.

Treatment of choice
Monitoring and discharge with written advise after a time period.

Your notes:

12. An 8-year-old boy falls off a swing at his school. He is brought to Casualty by one of his teachers. He has a bruise over his right eye but the examination is otherwise normal. He is fully conscious with no history of blackouts since the accident. A skull X-ray is performed, which is normal.

Diagnosis: Insignificant head injury.

Clinchers

➤ *8-year-old boy:* Children are difficult to assess for head injury and their admission for monitoring is indicated.
➤ *Falls off a swing at his school:* A common mode of injury to a school going child. But the most common head injury is by RTA.
➤ *Brought to casualty by one of his teachers:* That means that no adult member of family is with him—a contraindication for discharge.
➤ *Bruise over his right eye:* Usually children do not suffer from fracture of skull bones as these are more pliable.
➤ *Examination is otherwise normal:* Rules out any cerebral injury GCS scoring should be done on adult scale and children. GCS if for < 5 years.
➤ *Fully conscious:* Also in favour of any cerebral injury but not that young children lose consciousness less readily that adults. Significant brain injury can occur without a history of loss of consciousness.
➤ *No history of blackouts since the accident:* Also a good prognostic sign.
➤ *Skull X-ray is normal:* Rules out any fracture which commands admission. But one should be aware of suture lines and normal anatomical variants while interpreting the X-rays.

CONFUSA
Assessment of consciousness in a child can be difficult. The best judge for minor alteration in consciousness in children are their parents.

Investigation of choice
Skull X-ray (already done in this case).

Immediate management
Antiseptic dressing of the bruise.

Treatment of choice
Admit and monitor.

Your notes:

13. A young woman is involved in an RTA and is brought in with a Glasgow Coma Scale of 6. A CT scan shows evidence of diffuse cerebral oedema but no evidence of haemorrhage. She has bilateral papilledema.

Diagnosis: Vasogenic cerebral edema

Clinchers

➤ *Involved in an RTA:* RTA usually produces vasogenic cerebral edema (i.e. increased capillary permeability).
➤ *Glasgow Coma Scale of 6:* Because cranium defines a fixed volume, brain swelling quickly results in increased ICP which may produce a sudden clinical deterioration. If untreated the GCS may fall further and the patient may be in a risk of brain herniation.
➤ *CT scan shows evidence of diffuse cerebral oedema but no evidence of haemorrhage:* This rules out any focal pathology which might be responsible for increased ICT and hence rules out any surgical intervention (craniotomy/burr hole).
➤ *Bilateral papilledema:* It signifies raised ICT.

CONFUSA
Papilloedema is an unreliable sign, but venous pulsation at the disc may be absent (Note: it is absent in about 50% of normal people, but loss of it is a useful sign).

Investigation of choice
ICT monitoring (as cerebral edema peaks in two-three days).

Immediate management
IV dexamethasone (controversial).

Treatment of choice
IV mannitol + restriction of free water.

Your Notes:

14. A young man is involved in a fight and suffers a blow to the back of the head. A skull X-ray reveals a depressed fracture of the occiput. His Glasgow Coma Scale on admission is 14 but falls rapidly within an hour.

Diagnosis: Subdural hematoma.

Clinchers
- *Is involved in a fight:* This makes it a medicolegal case and thereby warrant at least a skull X-ray (in UK).
- *Suffers a blow to the back of the head:* A blow to the back of head, if strong enough to produce a fracture in skull, will be invariably associated with neck injury. So exclude any cervical spine injury.
- *Skull X-ray reveals a depressed fracture of the occiput:* The principle local complications of skull fractures are:
  - Meningeal artery rupture, causing an extradural hematoma
  - Dural vein tears, leading to subdural hematoma.
- *Glasgow Coma Scale on admission is 14 but falls rapidly within an hour:* Since there is no lucid interval, the suspicion is more towards a subdural hematoma (Note: *Subdural* hematomas often have *subdued* onset, i.e. after sometime—hours to days).

CONFUSA
Linear skull fractures usually do not need any surgical intervention but depressed fractures almost always need surgical elevation and debridement. Cerebral contusions may result in a similar clinical picture to subdural hematoma, with a delayed recovery from trauma.

Investigation of choice
CT scan (since GCS is falling).

Immediate management
Inform neurosurgery after starting resuscitation.

Treatment of choice
Surgical elevation of fracture and evacuation of clot.

Your notes:

15. A 24-year-old patient presents with RTA. The pupil on the left side is dilated and the patient is obtunded. CT scan of the head reveals a binconvex hyperdense lesion on the temporal region.

Diagnosis: Extradural hemorrhage.

Clinchers
- *History of RTA:* Road traffic accidents produces maximum mortality due to head injuries.
- *Pupil on left side is dilated:* In cases of intracranial hematomas localising neurological symptoms (e.g. ipsilateral pupil dilatation, hemiparesis) occurs late (average 63 days in case of subdural hematoma). So the patient is in a critical stage warranting urgent surgical decompression).
- *Obtunded:* Deteriorating level of consciousness is caused by a rising ICP (due to the expanding hematoma).
- *Biconvex hyperdense lesion on the temporal region:* Fresh bleed on CT appears hyperdense. A binconvex hematoma is characterisitc of an extradural hematoma (lens-shaped). Its most common site is temporal region.

CONFUSA
In subdural hematoma, the CT appearance is usually concave on the inner side, most commonly in parietal region. Midline shift may be present.

Investigation of choice
CT scan (already done in this patient).

Immediate management
Urgent evacuation of the clot through multiple burr holes (as the patient is very critical and there is no spare time for transfer to a neurosurgical unit/centre).

Treatment of choice
Identification and ligation of the bleeding vessel (usually middle meningeal vessels).

Your notes:

16. Condition in which patient was found with nasal involvement and nasal hairs sighing. He presents with myalgia, malaise and headache.

Diagnosis: Carbon monoxide poisoning.

Clinchers
> *Nasal involvement and nasal hairs sighing:* This may signify smoke inhalation.

Carbon monoxide poisoning may occur due to:
- Deliberate self-harm (45%)
- Faulty domestic heating (33%)
- Smoke inhalation in fires (20%)

Symptoms of CO poisoning include myalgia, malaise and headache. There may be confusion, coma, dysphagia, hypotension, LVF, metabolic acidosis, hypokalemia.

CONFUSA
This under-recognized condition causes about 1800 deaths every year in the UK. Acidosis in CO poisoning will resolve with oxygenation. It should never be treated with bicarbonate.

Investigation of choice
- Blood gases: metabolic acidosis
- ECG (ischaemia)
- Plasma electrolytes and
- Carboxy hemoglobin levels

Immediate management
High concentration oxygen therapy for 120 minutes, given via an endotracheal tube or tight fitting mask.

Treatment of choice
- High concentration oxygen.
- Consider the need for hyperbaric oxygen therapy
- Unresponsive patients should be intubated and ventilated.
- Acidosis will resolve with oxygenation and should not be treated with bicarbonates.

Your notes:

17. Condition in which vitamin K is given to improve patient.

Diagnosis: Warfarin

Clinchers
Warfarin has a narrow therapeutic range, that varies with the condition being treated. Warfarin inhibits the reductase enzyme responsible for regenerating the active form of vitamin K, thus producing a state analogous to vitamin K deficiency.

If major bleed, treat with IV vitamin K, or FFP.

CONFUSA
If normally on warfarin and not bleeding, but INR dangerously high, give either vitamin K or FFP.

Investigation of choice
Measure INR (a ratio of warfarin compared with a standard prothrombin time).
Vitamin K levels.

Immediate management
If bleeding, treat with vitamin K or FFP. DEFIX® if life threatening (it has factors II, IX, X).
Cholestyramine 4 g/6h PO aids elimination. Warfarin can normally be restarted within 2-3 days but take expert help.

Your notes:

18. A 7-year-old boy accidentally swallowed some unknown white tablets and now complaining of right hypochondrial pain after 12 hours.

Diagnosis: Paracetamol poisoning.

Clinchers
- *Swallowed white tablets, now complaining of right hypochondrial pain:* In this question, tablet was taken accidentally, even otherwise paracetamol is the most common drug involved in self-poisoning. Only early feature of poisoning are nausea and vomiting.
- *Right hypochodrial pain:* Following paracetamol intake, usually signifies the development of hepatocellular necrosis, or there may be renal tubular necrosis.
- Paracetamol 150 mg/kg (12 g or 24 standard tablets for adults) constitutes a significant ingestion of the drug.

CONFUSA
Patient presenting 12 hours or longer after ingestion tend to be more severely poisoned and at a greater risk of serious liver damage.

Investigation of choice
- Plasma paracetamol concentration
- Simultaneously measure plasma salicylates
- LFT

Immediate management
Depends upon the presentation, and time of ingestion. Here let us discuss the management of patient who presents 8-15 hours after ingestion.
- Measure plasma paracetamol concentration
- Consider gastric decontamination with charcoal if the timing is in doubt or if other drugs may be involved.
- Give IV N-acetylcysteine (NAC) while waiting for paracetamol concentration results. The efficacy of the antidote declines from 8 hours after ingestion.
- Assess the possibility of liver damage.
- Arrange medical admission of psychiatric referral.

Your notes:

19. The side effect is urinary retention, heart block and ringing of ear.

Diagnosis: Quinine overdose

Clinchers
Toxicity of quinine is high and dose related 8-10 g taken in a single dose may be fatal. Large single dose or higher therapeutic doses taken for few days produce a clinical syndrome called cinchonism (ringing of ear, nausea, headache, mental confusion, vertigo, visual defects, etc).

Higher doses may cause respiratory depression, hypotension, cardiac arrhythmias.

Quinine occasionally causes haemolysis specially in pregnant women, resulting in haemoglobinuria (black water fever), and kidney damage.

CONFUSA
During pregnancy quinine should be used only for life threatening infection, with special care to prevent hypoglycaemia.

Investigation of choice
U and E, ECG, plasma quinine levels.

Immediate management
Foleys catheterization

Treatment of choice
Stop quinine and manage the complications.

Your notes:

20. A patient who has overdosed on an unknown medication presents with palpitations. What is the most likely cause?

Diagnosis: Tricyclic antidepressants overdose.

Clinchers
Acute poisoning due to overdose of tricyclic antidepressant is not infrequent and it may endanger life. It is usually self-attempted by the depressed patients.

Manifestations include ECG changes, ventricular arrhythmia, tachycardia.

Excitement, delirium and other anticholinergic symptom as seen in atropine poisoning along with respiratory depression with low BP may be present.

CONFUSA
Atropine poisoning should be kept in mind, as it also presents with anticholinergic symptoms.

Investigation of choice
Blood tests
ECG

Immediate management
Physostigmine (0.5-2 mg IV), reversed central and peripheral anticholinergic effects.

Treatment of choice
Treatment is primary supportive
- Correct acidosis by bicarbonate infusion
- Physostigmine
- Propranolol/lidocaine (for arrhythmias)
- Diazepam IV (for convulsions and delirium).

Your Notes:

21. Schizophrenic patient under treatment presents with fever, increased WCC, increased muscle creatinine kinase levels.

Diagnosis: Neuroleptic malignant syndrome (NMS).

Clinchers
- *Schizophrenic patient under treatment:* Most probably he is taking some high potency antipsychotics with whom this syndrome is common.
- *Fever:* Pyrexia is pathognomonic of this condition.
- *Increased WCC:* Investigations invariably show increased WCC.
- *Increased muscle creatinine kinase levels:* Increased creatinine phosphokinase and myoglobin may be present in blood. It lasts 5-10 days after drug withdrawal and may be fatal.

CONFUSA
NMS occurs in 0.2% of patients on antipsychotics (particularly with high potency drugs i.e. Haloperidol). Its symptoms appear a few days to a few weeks after initiation of therapy. Its main presenting symptoms are:
- Hyperthermia
- Muscle rigidity
- Autonomic instability (tachycardia, labila BP, pallor)
- Fluctuating level of consciousness.

Investigation of choice
CPK (↑); WCC (↑); LFT (deranged)

Immediate management
Stop drug immediately and give symptomatic treatment (e.g. temperature reduction)

Treatment of choice
Bromocriptine (to enhance dopaminergic activity)
    +
Dantrolene (to reduce muscle tone)

Your Notes:

22.
A homeless patient presents to A and E with drowsiness. On examination, abrasions and puncture marks were found on his arm. He has pin-point pupil.

Diagnosis: Opioid poisoning

Antidote: Naloxone

Clinchers
- *Homeless patient:* Risk factor for drug addiction.
- *Drowsiness:* Stupor, coma, fall in BP, shallow and occasional breathing are all signs of acute opioid poisoning.
- *Abrasions and puncture marks:* Further support the diagnosis of drug injection.
- *Pin-point pupil:* This confirms the diagnosis of opioid poisoning.

CONFUSA
Drowsiness, coma can be caused by benzodiazepines, alcohol, opiates, tricyclic or barbiturates. Constricted pupils are seen opiates or insecticides (organophosphates). On the other hand dilated pupils are seen in amphetamines, cocaine, quinine or tricyclic.

Investigation of choice
Take blood. Always check for paracetamol and salicylate levels. Diagnosis is mainly from history.

Immediate management
Naloxone e.g. 0.8-2 mg IV repeat every 2 minutes, until breathing adequate.

Treatment of choice
Advocate supportive measures
Start the antidote
Referral to psychiatrist.

Your Notes:

23.
Schizophrenic patient under treatment presents with sore throat, decreased WBC, agranulocytosis.

Diagnosis: Clozapine side effects.

Clinchers
- *Schizophrenic patient:* Clozapine is an atypical antipsychotic and is pharmacologically distinct from other in that it has only weak D_2 blocking action and produces few extrapyramidal symptoms; tardive dyskinesia is also rare with it. It suppresses both positive and negative symptoms of schizophrenia and many patients refractory to typical neuroleptics respond.
- *Sore throat:* It is due to infections secondary to agranulocytosis.
- *Decreased WBC and agranulocytosis:* The major limitation of clozapine is higher incidence of agranulocytosis and other blood dyscrasias.

CONFUSA
Clozapine is used only as a reserve drug in resistant schizophrenia (who have not responded to, or are intolerant of, two other antipsychotics). In UK it is given on a named patient basis and weekly white cell counts are mandatory. It is very expensive (~£ 3000 per year in UK)—though cost benefit analyses are favourable as in-patient care is reduced.

Investigation of choice
Weekly white cell counts.

Immediate management
Stop drug.

Treatment of choice
Change clozapine with new antipsychotics, i.e. risperidone, olanzapine and questiapine which do not have EPS like clozapine but do not need blood tests.

Your Notes:

24. Patient on treatment for bipolar disorder, hypothyroidism features.

Diagnosis: Lithium side effects.

Clinchers
- *Bipolar disorder treatment:* Its first line prophylactic treatment is lithium. Majority of patients stabilizes on lithium and usually do not need alternative or second line drugs.
- *Weight gain and loss of appetite:* This suggests hypothyroidism which is infact a prominent yet rare side effects of lithium. It is due to interference with iodination of tyrosine—decreased thyroxine synthesis.

CONFUSA
Lithium induced hypothyroidism is seen in 20% women. In men it is rare. Other main side effect of lithium on long-term usage is renal diabetes insipidus. Lithium induces granulocytosis and infact sometimes used to treat agranulocytosis (e.g. chemotherapy induced leukopenia and agranulocytosis).

Investigation of choice
TSH.

Immediate management
Rule out primary thyroid disease.

Treatment of choice
Thyroxine administration.

Your Notes:

25. A patient who has overdosed on an unknown medication presents with palpitations. What is the most likely cause?

Diagnosis: Tricyclic antidepressants overdose.

Clinchers
Acute poisoning due to overdose of tricyclic antidepressant is not infrequent and it may endanger life. It is usually self-attempted by the depressed patients.

Manifestations include ECG changes, ventricular arrhythmia, tachycardia.

Excitement, delirium and other anticholinergic symptom as seen in atropine poisoning along with respiratory depression with low BP may be present.

CONFUSA
Atropine poisoning should be kept in mind, as it also presents with anticholinergic symptoms.

Investigation of choice
Blood tests
ECG

Immediate management
Physostigmine (0.5-2 mg IV), reversed central and peripheral anticholinergic effects.

Treatment of choice
Treatment is primary supportive
- Correct acidosis by bicarbonate infusion
- Physostigmine
- Propranolol/lidocaine (for arrhythmias)
- Diazepam IV (for convulsions and delirium).

Your Notes:

26. For the past two weeks a middle aged railway engineer has complained of acute constipation. His stools are dark, but not apparently blood stained. Abdominal palpation detects a mass with moderate tenderness.

Diagnosis: Colonic cancer (left side)

Clinchers
- *Middle aged railway engineer:* Colon cancer may occur at any age, but it more common after 40.
- *Acute constipation for past two weeks:* In it, typically an adult with presiously regular bowel habit suddenly develops irregularity. There may be increasing difficulty in getting the bowels to move, requiring laxatives. The episodes of constipation may be followed by attacks of diarrhoea.
- *Stools are dark, but not apparently blood stained:* This is malaena, signifying blood loss high in the colon. Otherwise bleed may be bright, malaena or occult.
- *Mass with moderate tenderness:* This confirms our suspicious as there is usually a mass palpable either per abdomen or per rectum.

CONFUSA
Tumors of the left side of the colon, where the contained stool is solid, are typically constricting growths, so obstructive features predominate. In contrast, tumors of the right side tend to be proliferative and here the stools are semi-liquid therefore obstructive symptoms are relatively uncommon and the patient with a carcinoma of the caecum or ascending colon often presents with anaemia and loss of weight. In carcinoma of left side of colon, the lump that is felt on abdominal, rectal or bimanual palpation is sometimes not the tumor itself, but impacted faeces above it. When the tumor is situated in a pendulous pelvic colon, a hard movable swelling may be felt in the rectovesical pouch on rectal examination.

Investigation of choice
Colonoscopy

Immediate management
Laxatives for constipation

Treatment of choice
Surgery

27. A 43-year-old man says he cannot finish his stool and that what he does pass is streaked with blood. He says he has always been regular. He wants to know if a laxative will help.

Diagnosis: Rectal carcinoma

Clinchers
- *43-year-old man:* The sexes are equally affected and it occurs in any age group from the twenties onwards, but is particularly common in age range 50-70 years.
- *He cannot finish his stool:* The patients bowels open but there is a sensation that there are more faeces to be passed. This sense of incomplete defecation is typical of rectal carcinoma.
- *What he does pass is streaked with blood:* The patient may endeavour to empty the rectum several times a day (spurious diarrhoea), often with the passage of flatus and a little blood stained mucus (blood slime).
- *He says he has always been regular:* This signify that the alteration in bowel habits is of recent onset and excludes any pre-existing pathology.
- *Wants to know if a laxative will help:* The patient may find it necessary to start taking an aperient, or to supplement the usual dose and as a result the tendency towards diarrhoea ensues.

CONFUSA
Sence of incomplete defecation results in tenesmus which is a painful straining to empty the bowels without resultant evacuation. This "sense" is a very important early symptom and is almost invariably present in tumours of the lower half of the rectum. Pain is a late symptom. Weight loss is suggestive of hepatic metastases. In approximately 90% of cases the neoplasm can be felt digitally.

Investigation of choice
- *Screening:* Proctosigmoidoscopy
- *Definitive:* Biopsy

Immediate management
Laxatives

Treatment of choice
Surgery —upper 1/3—Anterior resection
—middle 1/3—± Anterior resection
—lower 1/3—Abdominoperineal resection

September—2001

28. A 49-year-old lawyer complains of blood and diarrhoea. She is also suffering from abdominal pain, fever, and general ill health. On palpation you find tenderness in the lower abdomen.

Diagnosis: Severe ulcerative colitis (UC)

Clinchers

- *49-year-old lawyer (she):* The sex ratio is equal. It is uncommon before the age of 10 and most patients are between the ages of 20 and 40 at diagnosis.
- *Blood and diarrhoea:* The first symptom is watery or bloody diarrhoea. There may be a rectal discharge of mucus which is either blood-stained or purulent.
- *Abdominal pain, fever, general ill health:* Pain as an early symptom is unusual and suggest severe disease. Other indicators of severe diseases are:
  - more than four motions a day, together with
  - one or more signs of systemic illness, i.e
    - fever over 37.5°C
    - tachycardia > 90/m
    - hypoalbuminemia < 30 g/l
    - weight loss > 3 kg
- *Tenderness in lower abdomen:* May or may not be present in UC.

CONFUSA
Diarrhoea usually implies that there is active disease proximal to the rectum. In 95 percent of cases the disease starts in the rectum and spreads proximally. Bad prognosis is indicated by:
- a severe initial attack
- disease involving whole colon
- increasing age, especially after 60 years

If the disease remains confined to the left colon, the out look is better.

Investigation of choice
- *Screening:* Barium enema
  (findings: • loss of haustrations, • granularity, • pseudopolyps)
- *Definitive:* Colonoscopy and biopsy

Immediate management
Examine for extraintestinal manifestations i.e. arthritis/ skin lesions/eye problems/liver and bile duct diseases).
   +
Admit (this case is a medical emergency since this is a severe attack, 1040, Bailey, 23 edn).

Treatment of choice
IV hydrocortisone 100-200 mg QID + rectal infusion of prednisolone + sulfasalazine maintenance/surgery

29. A young woman presents with recurrent abdominal pain, episodic diarrhoea, malaise, and fever. Over the past few years she has felt her health to be declining. At presentation she complains of severe abdominal pain and constipation.

Diagnosis: Crohn's disease (CD)

Clinchers

- *Young woman:* It is slightly more common in females than in males but is more commonly diagnosed in young patients between the ages of 25 and 40. There does seem to be a second peak of incidence around the age of 17.
- *Recurrent abdominal pain, episodic diarrhoea, malaise, and fever:* There is often a history of mild diarrhoea extending over many months occurring in bouts accompanied by intestinal colic. Patients may complain of pain, particularly in the right iliac fossa and there may be a tender mass palpable. Intermittent fevers, secondary anaemia and weight loss are common.
- *Over the past few years she has felt her health to be declining:* It is due to generalised systemic nonspecific effects like loss of appetite, weight loss, anaemia, etc.
- *Severe abdominal pain and constipation:* This could be due to intestinal obstruction after formation of adhesions. Constipation is otherwise rare in this disease.

CONFUSA
Constipation in CD is rare and can be due to:
- After months of repeated attacks with acute inflammation of the affected area of intestine begins to narrow, with fibrosis causing abdominal pain on eating, giving rise to 'food fear' which leads to no formation of stools.
- Delay and dilatation of small intestine causing partial obstruction
- Intestinal adhesions or strictures.

Investigation of choice
Small bowel enema
   ±
Technetium labelled leucocyte scan

Immediate management
Pain relief

Treatment of choice
Mesalazine (for acute attack like this)

30. A young woman complains of cramp-like abdominal pain, and difficulties with bowel movements. Acute abdominal pain is frequently relieved by embarrassing flatulence. Barium studies and sigmoidoscopy have proved inconclusive.

Diagnosis: Irritable bowel syndrome (IBS).

Clinchers
- *Young woman:* Symptoms of IBS typically begin young adulthood (esp females) and the prevalence of IBS is similar in elderly and young adults.
- *Cramp-like abdominal pain and difficulties with bowel movements:* Abdominal pain and altered bowel habits are non-specific symptoms found in patients with a wide variety of illnesses including IBS.
- *Acute abdominal pain is frequently relieved by embarrassing flatulence:* "Manning criteria" for IBS include abdominal pain or discomfort that is relieved by defecation or associated with a change in stool frequency or consistency, abdominal distension, the sensation of incomplete evacuation, and the passage of mucus.
- *Barium studies and sigmoidoscopy have proved inconclusive:* A diagnosis of IBS is based on a careful history to identify characteristic symptoms (e.g. Manning criteria), physical examination, selected laboratory tests, and if necessary, further testing to exclude other disorders.

CONFUSA
Patients presenting with abdominal pain in the absence of abdominal pain may be considered to have IBS if no alternative explanation for the symptoms is found. However, patients with otherwise unexplained chronic constipation in the absence of abdominal pain are generally considered to have a distinct disorder.

Investigation of choice
All required to exclude other diseases (but not always).

Immediate management
Reassurance + counselling.

Treatment of choice
Symptomatic.

Your Notes:

---

31. A known HIV positive patient presents with pain in swallowing and some lesion in the mouth. The underlying tissue is red when the lesion is taken off.

Diagnosis: Candidiasis

Clinchers
- *Known HIV positive patient:* Let us first get familiar with complications of HIV infection. These are *Pneumocystis carinii* (this is the most common life-threatening opportunistic infection in AIDS). Infection by *M. tuberculosis, M. avium intracellulare, candidiasis, toxoplasma gondii* (a chief CNS pathogen), *Cryptococcus neoformans* (causes incidious meningitis). CMV retinitis, leishmaniasis, Kaposi's sarcoma.
- *Pain in swallowing:* Oesophageal involvement causes dysphagia ± retrosternal discomfort. Oropharyngeal candidiasis in an apparently fit patients suggests underlying HIV infection.
- *Some lesions in mouth:* These with oral pain and discomfort may be caused by candidiasis.
- *Underlying tissue is red when lesion is taken off:* Candidiasis causes white patches or erythema of the buccal mucosa. The patches are hard to remove and bleed if scraped.

CONFUSA
Causes of oral pain/discomfort in HIV positive patient are candidiasis, HSV or aphthous ulceration or tumours.

Investigation of choice
Demonstration of pseudohyphae on wet smear with confirmation by culture is procedure of choice for superficial candidiasis. Deeper lesions due to Candida may be diagnosed by histologic section of biopsy specimen or by blood culture.

Treatment of choice
- *Local treatment:* Nystatin suspension/amphotericin lozenges 4-6 times/day.
- *Systemic treatment:* Fluconazole 50-200 mg/day PO (may cause nausea, hepatitis), ketoconazole 200 mg/day PO (may cause nausea, hepatitis, rash, low platelets)

Your notes:

32. A patient comes with dysphagia for solids for 5 years and now presents with regurgitation when he eats, it relieves a few hours after meal.

Diagnosis: Achalasia

Clinchers
- *Dysphagia for solids for 5 years:* Overall course of achalasia is usually chronic, with progressive dysphagia and weight loss over months to years. Word 'solid' here signifies oesophageal cause and liquids signify pharyngeal cause.
- *Regurgitation:* Dysphagia, chest pain and regurgitation are the main symptoms of achalasia. Dysphagia occurs early, worsened by emotional stress and hurried eating.
- *Relieves a few hours after meal:* Achalasia is a motor disorder of the esophageal smooth muscle in which the LES does not relax properly with swallowing, and the normal peristalsis of esophageal body is replaced by abnormal contractions.

CONFUSA

Achalasia associated with carcinoma is characterized by severe weight loss and a rapid down hill course if untreated.

The presence of gastroesophageal reflux argues against achalasia, and in patients with long standing heartburn, cessation of heart burn and appearance of dysphagia suggest development of achalasia in a patient with reflux esophagitis.

Investigation of choice
- *Chest X-ray:* Absence of gastric air bubble, air fluid level in mediastinum in upright position represents retained food in esophagus.
- *Barium swallow:* Shows oesophageal dilatation or sigmoid shape of oesophagus in advanced cases.
- *Fluoroscopy.*

Immediate management
Depends upon the complications (like aspiration can occur due to regurgitation therefore mange that first).

Treatment of choice
Endoscopic balloon dilatation of Heller's Cardiomyotomy.

Your notes:

33. 65-year-old male presents with weight loss, difficulty in swallowing solid. Dysphagia is getting worse.

Diagnosis: Carcinoma oesophagus.

Clinchers
- *65-year-old male:* Risk factors for Ca oesophagus are tobacco, alcohol, achalasia, old age, Barrets oesophagus, Plummer-Vinson syndrome.
- *Weight loss:* Suspect malignancy.
- *Difficulty in swallowing solid:* Acute or progressive dysphagia requires investigation to exclude malignancy in oesophagus. If dysphagia is predominantly for solids, then suspect oesophageal cause.

Dysphagia, weight loss, retrosternal chest pain, rarely lymphadenopathy are signs of carcinoma of the oesophagus. If uppper 1/3rd of oesophagus is involved it may present with hoarseness and cough.

CONFUSA

Keep in mind the differential diagnosis of dysphagia (refer to page 196, OHCM, 5th edn).

Investigation of choice
Barium swallow, CXR
Oesophagoscopy with biopsy/brushings.

Immediate management
Treat the complications

Treatment of choice
Radiotherapy and surgery complete for dismal statistics (6% vs 4% 5 year survival).

Your notes:

34. A patient presents with intermittent dysphagia for both solids and liquids and chest pain. No weight loss.

Diagnosis: Diffuse oesophageal spasm

Clinchers
- *Intermittent dysphagia for both solids and liquids:* Dysphagia for both solids and liquids is seen in oesophageal spasm, correlated particularly with simultaneous-onset contractions.
- *Chest pain:* Chest pain is particularly marked in patients with esophageal contractions of large amplitude and long duration. It usually occurs at rest, may radiate to back and arms. May mimic the pain of myocardial ischemia.

> **CONFUSA**
> Diffuse oesophageal spasm must be differentiated from other causes of chest pain, particularly ischaemic heart disease with atypical angina. Always go for complete cardiac work up and also carefully distinguish it from reflux oesophagitis.

Investigation of choice
Barium swallow: Shows uncoordinated simultaneous contractions, that produce the appearance of curling or multiple ripples in the wall, sacculations and pseudodiverticula—the "cork screw" oesophagus.

Your notes:

35. A patient with difficulty in swallowing, filling defect, he has a long standing history of Barret's oesophagus.

Diagnosis: Oesophageal carcinoma.

Clinchers (Note: See Q 33 of this theme also)
- *Difficulty in swallowing:* Dysphagia is a hallmark of oesophageal carcinoma but it is often an indication of inoperable lesion.
- *Filling defect:* A filling defect evident on radiograph after barium swallow can be produced by carcinoma oesophagus, pharyngeal pouch and achalasia (in the given list of options).
- *Long-standing history of Barret's oesophagus:* It is a recognized risk factor for development of adenocarcinoma in lower 1/3 of the oesophagus. Other definitive risk factors are: spices, alcohol, tobacco, achalasia, tylosis and Plummer-Vinson syndrome.

> **CONFUSA**
> Plummer-Vinson syndrome is seen mostly in post-menopausal females. Most common site of occurrence of oesophageal carcinoma is middle 1/3 of oesophagus for squamous cell carcinoma and lower 1/3 of oesophagus for adenocarcinoma.

Investigation of choice
Barium swallow, CXR
Oesophagoscopy with biopsy/brushings.

Immediate management
Treat the complications.

Treatment of choice
Radiotherapy and surgery complete for dismal statistics (6% vs 4% 5 year survival).

Your notes:

September—2001

36. Man returned from trip to Asia, complains of anorexia, malaise, dark urine, pale stools.

Diagnosis: Hepatitis B (most probably)

Clinchers
- *Trip to Asia:* Hepatitis A is the most common type of viral hepatitis worldwide, often in epidemics. The disease is commonly seen in autumn and affects children and young adults. Spread of infection is mainly by the faecal-oral route and arises from the ingestion of contaminated food or water (e.g. shellfish). Overcrowding and poor sanitation facilitate spread. It is common in developing countries in Asia.
- *Anorexia malaise:* The viraemia causes the patient to feel unwell with nonspecific symptoms that includes nausea, anorexia and a distaste for cigarettes. Jaundice develops after one or two weeks.
  Note: Many recover at this stage and remain anicetric.
- *Dark urine, pale stools:* As the jaundice deepens, the urine becomes dark and stools pale owing to intra-hepatic cholelithiasis.

CONFUSA
Clinically the differential diagnosis is from all other causes of jaundice—but in particular from other types of viral and drug induced hepatitis. Common cause of jaundice in travellers are:
- Viral hepatitis
- Cholangitis
- Liver abscess
- Leptospirosis
- Typhoid
- Malaria
- Dengue fever
- Yellow fever
- Haemoglobinopathies

Investigation of choice
Viral serology and LFT
- Serum transaminases rise 22-40 days after exposure
- IgM rises from day 25 and signifies recent infection
- IgG remains detectable for life.

Immediate management
Symptomatic and advise to avoid alcohol
Notify health authorities as it is a notifiable disease in UK

Treatment of choice
Supportive
If fulminant hepatitis—interferon α

37. An 80-year-old man has never been out of UK, one month history of epigastric pain, dark urine, pale stools, jaundice.

Diagnosis: Common bile duct obstruction (CBD obstruction).

Clinchers
- *80-year-old man:* The age point more towards malignancy than a stone as the cause of obstruction of CBD.
- *Never been out of UK:* Rules out infective causes like cholangitis or hepatitis.
- *One month history:* It signify that the symptomatology is chronic and rules out infective causes and acute cholecystitis.
- *Epigastric pain:* Gallbladder pathologies produce continuous picture of any obstructive jaundice. Dark urine is due to bilirubinuria and pale stools due to decreased bile pigments.

CONFUSA
A young person is more likely to have hepatitis, so questions should be asked about drug and alcohol se, and sexual behaviour. An elderly person with gross weight loss is more likely to have a carcinoma. All patients may complain of malaise. Abdominal pain occurs in patients with biliary obstruction by gallstones and sometimes with an enlarged liver there is pain resulting from distension of the capsule.

Investigation of choice
ERCP

Immediate management
Heme test of stools (if positive, suspect malignancy)

Treatment of choice
Depends on diagnosis
- Stones—cholecystectomy
- Malignancy—surgery/palliation

Your Notes:

38. Female with fever, rigors, right upper quadrant pain, jaundice, USG is normal.

Diagnosis: Acute cholecystitis.

Clinchers
- *Female:* Female sex is a risk factor for cholesterol stones in gallbladder, which is the usual cause for acute cholecystitis. The disease can occur at any age.
- *Fever, rigors:* The patient is usually ill with a fever and shallow respirations.
- *Right upper quadrant (RUQ) pain:* The main symptoms are severe pain in the epigastrium and right hypochondrium. The pain is continuous, increasing in intensity over 24 hours. It can radiate to back and shoulder. It may be accompanied by nausea and vomiting. Right hypochondrium tenderness is present, being worse on inspiration (Murphy's sign). There is guarding and rebound tenderness.
- *Jaundice:* Mild jaundice occurs in 20% of cases owing to accompanying common duct stones or to surrounding oedema occluding the CBD.
- *USG is normal:* Although can accurately diagnose stones as small as 2 mm, it may be false negative in 2-4 percent of cases.

CONFUSA
A less severe case of acute pancreatitis simulates acute cholecystitis. The fever in acute cholecystitis is more marked than pancreatitis and is in range of 38-39° C with marked toxaemia and leucocytosis. Rigors are almost nerve seen in acute pancreatitis.

Investigation of choice
Oral cholecystography (OCG)
OCG is a useful procedure for diagnosis of gallstones but has been diagnosis replaced by USG. However, OCG is still useful for
- Selection of patients for nonsurgical therapy of gallstone disease such as
  - Lithotripsy
  - Bile duct dissolution therapy
- When USG is inconclusive

Immediate management
Nil by mouth + analgesia

Treatment of choice
Cefuroxime 1.5 g/8 h IV
In suitable candidates do cholecystectomy (laparoscopic if no question of GB perforation).

39. Female 50-year-old, 5 year history of mild pruritus history of pale stools, dark urine, jaundice.

Diagnosis: Primary biliary cirrhosis (PBC).

Clinchers
- *50-year-old female:* Ninety percent of those affected are women in the age range 40-50 years. It used to be rare but now being diagnosed more frequently in its milder forms.
- *5 years history of mild pruritus:* Pruritus is often the earliest symptom, preceding jaundice by a few years.
- *Pale stools, dark urine, jaundice:* This is a characteristic picture of obstructive jaundice. It signifies a late stage of PBC—the patient is jaundiced with severe pruritus. Pigmented xanthelasma on eyelids or other deposits of cholesterol in the creases of the hands may be seen. Hepatosplenomegaly may be present.

CONFUSA
PBC is usually associated with:
- Autoimmune disorders
  - Sjögren's syndrome
  - Scleroderma
  - Rheumatoid arthritis
- Keratoconjunctivitis sicca (dry eyes and mouth) is seen in 70% of cases
- Renal tubular acidosis
- Membranous glomerulonephritis

Mitochondrial antibodies (measured routinely by ELISA—in titres more than 1:160) are present in over 95% of patients. M2 antibody is specific. Other nonspecific antibodies (e.g. ANA and SMA) may also be present.

Investigation of choice
- *Screening:* ELSIA for mitochondrial antibodies
- *Definitive:* Liver biopsy

Immediate management
USG (in a jaundiced patient, extrahepatic biliary obstruction should be excluded)

Treatment of choice
Symptomatic:
- Pruritus: colestyramine
- Diarrhoea: codeine phosphate
- Malabsorption: prophylactic fat soluble vitamin supplements
  - In case serum bilirubin > 100 µmol/L—consider liver transplantation.

40. Man with history of hemochromatosis and alcohol addiction presents with jaundice, ascites, variceal bleed. USG is unequivocal, high ferritin level.

Diagnosis: Hereditary haemochromatosis (HHC)

Clinchers
- *Mass:* Middle-aged males are more frequently and severely affected than women.
- *Haemochromatosis:* HHC is one of the most common inherited (autosomal recessive) single gene disorders in northern Europeans.
- *Alcohol addiction:* The course of the disease depends on a number of factors including sex, dietary iron intake, presence of associated hepatoxins (especially alcohol) and genotype.
- *USG unequivocal:* USG will not demonstrate anything significant. A liver biopsy is definitive (with Perl's stain).
- *High ferritin level:* Serum ferritin is elevated, usually >500μg/L or 240 nmol/L.

CONFUSA
Haemochromatosis tend to present about 10 years later in females than males on the menstrual blood loss is protective. So while in males, its peak incidence is in middle-ages, in case of females it is usually postmenopausal. Iron overload may be present in alcoholics, but alcohol excess per se does not cause HHC. There is a history of excess alcohol intake in 25% of patients.

Investigation of choice
- *Screening:*
  - Homozygotes
    - Serum iron (↑↑)
    - Serum ferritin (↑↑)
  - Heterozygotes
    - Serum ferritin (↑)
    - Transferrin saturation (↑)
- *Definitive*
  - Liver biopsy/MRI

Immediate management
Manage cirrhotic symptoms

Treatment of choice
Venesection routinely
If venesection not tolerated, chelation therapy.

41. Man after trip to Asia presents with red, swollen scrotum.

Diagnosis: Epididymo-orchitis

Clinchers
- *Trip to Asia:* He might have caught gonococcal infection from sex workers in Thailand. Or it could be TB also but that needs a primary infection somewhere else.
Chlamydia can also cause epididymo orchitis in < 35 years old.
- *Red, swollen scrotum:* The patient will have a very painful swelling of the epididymis, often with a secondary hydrocele and constitutional effects (pyrexia, headaches and leucocytosis). There may be a history of dysuri suggesting a UTI, or urethral discharge suggesting a sexually transmitted organism.

CONFUSA
Examination of urine may reveal the presence of organisms and pus cells, but the urine need not be abnormal. Rectal examination of the prostate may reveal coexistent prostatitis. Always look for urethral discharge in a patient of epididymo-orchitis. A 'first-catch' is more likely to show abnormalities than MSU.

Investigation of choice
Urethral swab for culture

Immediate management
Rule out torsion of testis which usually present like epididymo-orchitis
- It the patient is in his teens, torsion is more likely; if he is in his twenties and sexually active, epidymitis is more likely.
- In torsion the testes like high in scrotum and pain is a bit relieved by lifting testes (worsens in epididymo-orchitis).

Treatment of choice
Erythromycin for chlamydia
For others—ciprofloxacin.

Your Notes:

42. Man with painful red scrotum and vomiting.

Diagnosis: Torsion of testis.

Clinchers
- *Painful red scrotum:* The differential diagnoses are:
  - Mumps orchitis
  - Epididymo-orchitis
  - Torsion of testes
  - Torsion of testicular appendage
- *Vomiting:* Of all the above conditions, only torsion produces a pain severe enough to produce vomiting. There may be associated abdominal pain also which is because the nerve supply of the testis is mainly from T_{10} sympathetic pathway.

CONFUSA
Torsion of the testis can also present as a pain in lower abdomen (can mimic appendicitis if on right side) torsion of appendicular appendage can present in similar way but on examination the testis does not lie high in scrotum and a dark blue pea like swelling may be visible through the scrotal skin. Torsion may also mimic a strangulated inguinal hernia.

Investigation of choice
The diagnosis is entirely clinical. The only investigation is to see whether the testis is still viable or not and that is possible only on surgical exploration (usually viability maintained till 6 hours).

Immediate management
Inform surgeons.

Treatment of choice
Urgent surgical exploration.

Your Notes:

43. Man with painless testicular swelling since 2 months.

Diagnosis: Suspected testicular tumor.

Clinchers
- *Painless testicular swelling:* Tumors of the testes usually present as a painless, swollen testicle or lump on a testicle which is hard and may be associated with an overlying secondary hydrocele, which sometimes contains blood stained fluid.
- *Since two months:* Tumors usually become noticeably in a considerable time and one to two months after appearance are taken by the patient to realise that it is abnormal. Age of the man is not specified in this question otherwise a clinical differentiation between suspected seminoma (30-40 years) and teratoma (20-30 years) might have been possible.

CONFUSA
Tumors of testes may present with a misleading history of recent trauma, and rarely it may present having undergone torsion. Occasionally gynaecomastia may be a presenting feature, due to production of paraneoplastic hormones.

Investigation of choice
Scrotal USG may reveal a solid tumor in a hydrocele but a negative finding can not exclude malignancy. Also
- Seminomas—β hCG
- Teratomas—AFP

Immediate management
Staging is essential. Conduct all necessary investigations. (CXR, CT and excision biopsy).

Treatment of choice
Orchidectomy.

Your Notes:

44. Man with a swelling of scrotum since 3 years.

Diagnosis: Sebaceous cyst (most probably)

Clinchers

> *Swelling of scrotum:* Since the question is not about testicular swelling but only a scrotal swelling, we are left with a handful of diagnosis, i.e.
> - *Filarial elephantiasis of the scrotum:* It is due to obstruction of pelvic lymphatics by *Wuchereria bancrofti.* But it is rarely seen in UK and is associated with penile swelling also. So it can be safely excluded as a diagnosis.
> - *Sebaceous cysts:* These are common in scrotal area. Although they are often multiple, a solitary scrotal sebaceous cyst is not an infrequent finding.

CONFUSA
A sebaceous cyst can remain as it is (i.e. with no increase in size) for many years. In scrotal area, they are often small (unlike-skull) and thus do not produce any problem to the patient (except cosmetic). They are painful only when they are infected.

Investigation of choice
The diagnosis of a sebaceous cyst is entirely clinical.

Immediate management
None

Treatment of choice
Complete excision along with cyst wall if:
- Patient ask for it
- Cosmetic reasons
- Infected
- Producing discomfort.

Your Notes:

45. Man with no history of unsafe sex presents with dysuria and urinary frequency.

Diagnosis: Urinary tract infection (UTI)

Clinchers

> *History of unsafe sex:* It is the main risk factor for acquisition of UTI in sexually active population. Exposure to commercial sex workers increases the risk much more.
> *Dysuria:* It is a feature of cystitis. Other features of cystitis are:
> - Frequency
> - Urgency
> - Strangury
> - Haematuria
> - Suprapubic pain
>
> *Urinary frequency:* Also a feature of cystitis in UTI.

CONFUSA
The most common organism causing UTI is *E. coli.* (>70% in community but ≤ 41% in hospital). Among sexually transmitted diseases (like this one) *Chlamydia* is the main culprit (in < 35 years).

Investigation of choice
MSU—send it for lab culture if urine dipsticks show leucocytes, nitrite, proteinuria or haematuria.

Immediate management
Take a detailed history.
If this is not the first UTI of his life, try to differentiate between:
- Recurrent UTI: further infection with new organisms
- Relapse of UTI: further infection with same organisms

Treatment of choice
Trimethoprim 200 mg/12 h PO × 3 days is the DOC for cystitis.
Alternative: cephalexin.

Your Notes:

46. A 48-year-old female, insulin dependent diabetic, who has been on treatment for 20-year presents with a history of three episodes of severe hypoglycemia. She has not changed her insulin requirement, diet or exercise pattern.

Diagnosis: Possible infection

Clinchers
- *48-year-old female with IDDM:* As IDDM usually have an onset at a younger age, she must be having a long history of diabetes.
- *Three episodes of severe hypoglycaemia:* Non compliance to therapy or diet and exercise changes can induce such attacks. But since these have been specifically ruled out in this question, a possible systemic infection seems to be most probable.

CONFUSA
Infections in persons with diabetes may not occur more frequently than in nondiabetics, but they tend to be more severe, possibly because of imparied leukocyte function. In addition to common infections of the skin, urinary tract, lungs and blood stream infections like malignant external otitis, Rhinocerebral mucormycosis, emphysematous cholecystitis and emphysematous pyelonephritis, appear to have a specific relationship with diabetes.

Investigation of choice
Blood culture

Immediate management
Detailed history

Treatment of choice
Treat the infection if present, with broad spectrum antibiotics

Your Notes:

47. A 48-year-old female, insulin dependent diabetic, who has been on treatment for 20 years, presents with urinary frequency but no dysuria or urgency. Her blood glucose is 17.5 mmol/L.

Diagnosis: Hyperglycaemia

Clinchers
- *48 year old female + IDDM:* IDDM patients prone to insulin resistance after a few years and require a greater dose of insulin else they get hyperglycemic
- *Urinary frequency but no dysuria or urgency:* Urinary frequency alone is feature of diabetes mellitus as polyuria would be reported as incresed urinary frequency.
- *17.5 mmol/L blood glucose:* Significant hyperglycaemia.

CONFUSA
Among the given list of options, the confusion can be with—Urinary tract infection, but absence of dysuria and urgency go less in its favour.

Investigation of choice
- Blood sugar fasting.
- Urine culture and sensitivity to rule out concomitant infection since blood glucose has already been done.

Immediate management
Increase dose of insulin.

Treatment of choice
Better diabetic control.

Your Notes:

48. A 30-year-old female, insulin-dependent diabetic, presents with failure to pass urine.

Diagnosis: Autonomic neuropathy

Clinchers
- *IDDM patient:* Such patients are more prone to autonomic neuropathy.
- *Failure to pass urine:* Retention of urine is suggestive of autonomic involvement of the bladder. That occurs with a long-standing history of diabetes. Since the patient is now 30-year-old and IDDM usually have a juvenile onset, one must be having a long history to substantiate our diagnosis.

CONFUSA
Diabetic neuropathy may affect every part of the nervous system, with the possibel exception of brain. While rarely a direct cause of death, neuropathy is a major cause of morbidity. Most common picture is that of a peripheral polyneuropathy.

Investigation of choice
Pelvic USG.

Immediate management
Urinary catheterisation.

Treatment of choice
Chronic catheter drainage.

Your Notes:

49. A 68-year-old diabetic on treatment for the last 5-year presents with calf pain exacerbated by movement.

Diagnosis: Intermittent claudication

Clinchers
- *Calf pain exacerbated by movement:* This is a typical history of intermittent claudication. The pain is initially relieved by rest.
- *68-year-old diabetic:* this female has a high chances of having atherosclerosis secondary to diabetes or as a primary disease. This produces the vascular disease with diminished blood supply which cause intermittent claudication and foot ulcers.

CONFUSA
Hypertriglyceridaemia is common in diabetes and is due both to overproduction of VLDL in the liver and to a disposal defect in the periphery.

Investigation of choice
Doppler USG lower limb (or Duplex USG)

Immediate management
Instruction about proper foot care in an attempt to prevent ulcers.

Treatment of choice
Maintain diabetic control properly to keep hypertriglyceridaemia under control
+
Symptomatic management.

Your Notes:

50. A 70-year-old diabetic on treatment with metformin presents with severe epigastric pain, drowsiness and confusion.

Diagnosis: Lactic acidosis

Clinchers
- *Metformin:* Lactic acidosis is a common side effect of metformin.
- *Severe epigastric pain + drowsiness + confusion:* The usual side effects of metformin are abdominal discomfort, anorexia, nausea, metallic taste, mild diarrhoea and tiredness. Lactic acidosis is the most serious complication of metformin intake.

CONFUSA
Ketoacidosis can be a confusing option, but ketoacidosis is very uncommon in NIDDM patients. Alcohol intake in a patient or metformin therapy precipitates severe lactic acidosis.

Investigation of choice
Arterial blood gases.

Immediate management
IV Fluids.

Treatment of choice
$NaHCO_3$.

Your Notes:

51. Female, 41-year-old, presents with hard, irregular fixed swelling, stridor, dysphagia since 3 months.

Diagnosis: Anaplastic carcinoma thyroid

Clinchers
- *Female:* ♀ : ♂ ≈ 3:1
- *41-year-old:* Its risk and incidence increases with age and mainly occurs in elderly women.
- *Hard, irregular fixed swelling:* It is a typical presentation from anaplastic carcinoma. It needs to be differentiated from sarcoma or lymphoma. Multinodular goitre can also present like this.
  Note: Anaplastic carcinoma tissues do not concentrate iodine.
- *Stridor:* Due to tracheal compression by the rapid internal growth of the tumor. It may also invade the trachea.
- *Dysphagia:* Due to oesophageal compression due to mass effect of the tumor.
- *Since 3 months:* Anaplastic carcinomas are very fast growing and highly malignant.

CONFUSA
Usually the more malignant tumors of thyroid occur in younger age and tumors occurring in elderly patients are usually benign. But anaplastic carcinoma is an exception to this state of affairs as it occurs more in the elderly and is highly malignant (both locally and hematogeneously). Always make it a point to rule out thyroid lymphoma and sarcoma because their presentation is very similar.

Investigation of choice
Biopsy.

Immediate management
Tracheostomy for stridor (if it worsens).

Treatment of choice
- Radical thyroidectomy
- Inoperable tumors
  palliative radiotherapy.

Your Notes:

52. Old lady with smooth neck swelling, bradycardia, spare coarse hair, macrocytic anemia.

Diagnosis: Hashimoto's thyroiditis.

Clinchers
- *Old lady:* It usually occurs in women aged 60-70 years.
- *Smooth neck swelling:* The gland is usually uniformly enlarged and firm, although it may occasionally be a symmetrical and irregular.
- *Bradycardia:* It is due to hypothyroidism which may be a feature of Hashimoto's thyroiditis (although the patient is mostly euthyroid).
- *Sparse coarse hair:* The patients of hypothyroidism have a slow, deep voice and are usually overweight and apathetic, with a dry, coarse skin and thin hair, especially in the lateral third of the eyebrows.
- *Macrocytic anemia:* Hypothyroid patients often have normochromic macrocytic anemia.

CONFUSA
It is important to diagnose the condition correctly by demonstrating the presence of thyroid antibodies and if necessary, by biopsy, because thyroidectomy will precipitate severe hypothyroidism in these cases. Occasionally lymphoma occurs in such glands. Note that in
- Graves' disease—TSH autoantibody ↑
- Hashimoto's thyroiditis—thyroglobulin autoantibody increased

Investigation of choice
Autoantibody titres (thyroglobulin)

Immediate management
Exclude lymphoma in thyroid and other autoimmune diseases.

Treatment of choice
T_4 replacement therapy upto 0.3 mg/day will shrink the gland and the symptoms of myxoedema should disappear.

Your Notes:

53. Female on treatment for supraventricular tachycardia complains of seeing dots and glare on driving at night, exophthalmos, no goitre.

Diagnosis: Drug induced thyrotoxicosis.

Clinchers
- *Female:* Thyroid disorders are overall more prevalent in females, however drug induced thyrotoxicosis have an equal incidence in both sexes:
- *On treatment for SVT:* Given her existing clinical profile, she must be on treatment with amiodarone. Amiodarone is used in a wide range of ventricular and supraventricular arrhythmias. However, because of its toxic potential, its use is limited to resistant VT and recurrent VF. It is also used to maintain sinus rhythm in AF when other drugs here failed. Rapid termination of ventricular and supraventricular arrhythmias can be obtained by IV injection. WPW tachyarrhythmia is obtained can be obtained by suppression of both normal and aberrant pathways. Its long duration of action make it suitable for long-term prophylactic use; but close monitoring is required.
- *Complains of seeing dots and glare on driving at night:* This is due to corneal oedema occurring due to inflammatory reaction in thyrotoxicosis. Otherwise also it can be due to corneal microdeposits occurring due to long-term use of amiodarone.
- *Exophthalmos, no goitre:* Absence of goitre excludes a primary thyroid abnormality. Exophthalmos is due to retro orbital inflammatory and oedema characteristically seen in thyrotoxicosis.

CONFUSA
Had she not been taking drugs for SVT, this clinical profile would have qualified for a diagnosis of Graves' disease. Amiodarone is an iodine containing highly lipophilic long acting antiarrhythmic drug. It interferes with thyroid function in many ways including inhibition of peripheral conversion of T_4 to T_3.

Investigation of choice
Serum T_4.

Immediate management
Review SVT treatment by a cardiologist.

Treatment of choice
Discontinue amiodarone

Your Notes:

54. Female, swelling in the neck, tremor irritability, diarrhoea, bruit.

Diagnosis: Graves' disease

Clinchers
- *Female:* Graves' disease is more prevalent in females, especially in women aged 30-50 years (♀: ♂ ≈ 9:1)
- *Swelling in neck:* The thyroid gland is usually smoothly enlarged but not invariably so.
- *Tremor:* Fine tremor of the outstretched hands is present and reflects the increased sympathetic activity.
- *Irritability:* It is due to the emotional lability commonly seen in hyperthyroidism. Frank psychosis may also develop.
- *Diarrhoea:* It is due to increased sympathetic activity.
- *Bruit:* The thyroid may have a bruit because of its increased vascularity in this condition.

CONFUSA
Additional signs in Graves' disease which differentiate it from other hyperthyroid conditions are:
- Bulging eyes (exophthalmos)
- Thyroid bruit
- Ophthalmoplegia
- Vitiligo
- Pretibial myxedema
- Thyroid acropachy

Investigation of choice
TSH receptor autoantibodies.

Immediate management
Rule out IDDM and pernicious anemia as these are usually associated with Graves' disease.

Treatment of choice
Graves' disease may be treated with antithyroid drugs or radioiodine treatment; subtotal thyroidectomy is rarely indicated.
DOC—carbimazole.

Your Notes:

55. A 35-year-old woman who was diagnosed as having coeliac disease at the age of 12 years has had good control of her abdominal symptoms for a number of years. She presents with a recent history of weight loss, tiredness, diarrhoea and abdominal pain.

Diagnosis: Small bowel lymphoma (probable).

Clinchers
- *35-year-old:* Incidence of lymphomas peak after 30 years
- *Coeliac disease:* The risk of small bowel lymphoma is increased in patients with a prior history of:
  - Malabsorption conditions (e.g. celiac sprue)
  - Regional enteritis
  - Depressed immune function
    - Congenital immunodeficiencies
    - Prior organ transplantation
    - Autoimmune disorders
    - AIDS
- *Good control of abdominal symptoms for a number of years:* Coeliac disease symptoms are very amenable to diet control and since the symptoms are in control in this patient for many years, there is no reason that they should relapse. Considering her age and high risk, lymphoma should be ruled out.
- *Weight loss, tiredness, diarrhoea and abdominal pain:* Characteristic of any malabsorption syndrome (in this case induced by lymphoma).

CONFUSA
Primary intestinal lymphoma accounts for 20% of malignancies of small bowel. Essentially all these neoplasms are non-Hodgkin's lymphoma. Its incidence is: Ileum > jejunum > duodenum (mirrors the relative amount of normal lymphoid cells in these anatomic areas).

Investigation of choice
- *Screening:* Contrast radiographs (infiltration and thickening of mucosal folds, mucosal nodules, ulcerations)
- *Definitive:* Surgical exploration and resection for tissue diagnosis.

Immediate management
Rule out ethnic relation (Jews and Arabs) which produce a nonresectable immunoproliferative small intestinal disease and any non-compliance on gluten free diet.

Treatment of choice
Surgical exploration +
Postresection radio/chemotherapy.

56. A 35-year-old woman complains of abdominal discomfort relieved by passing flatus or- defecation. Over the last 6 months she has had episodes of diarrhoea and constipation, but denied she had lost weight. Her mother died of bowel carcinoma.

Diagnosis: Irritable bowel syndrome (IBS).

Clinchers

- *35 years old woman:* Patients of IBS are usually between 20-40 years and females are more frequently affected.
- *Abdominal discomfort relieved by flatus or defecation:* This is a very important point. This supports the diagnosis of IBS. Other important history is the sensation of incomplete evacuation and the passage of mucus.
- *Episode of diarrhoea and constipation:* Altered bowel habits (constipation alternating with diarrhoea) present in IBS.
- *Since last 6 months:* These symptoms must be present for atleast 3 months, before the diagnose of IBS could be established.
- *No history of weight loss:* Helps to exclude carcinoma.

Investigation of choice

Flexible sigmoidscopy: In over 48 years to exclude colonic neoplasm. In younger patients exclude inflammatory bowel disease.

Treatment of choice

Though there is no treatment for IBS, focus on dietary modification with fiber supplements. Treatment should be directed to the predominant symptom.

Your Notes:

57. A 37-year-old woman presents with a sudden onset of severe left iliac fossa pain. On vaginal USG, 2 cm echogenic masses are seen in the broad ligament. She says this pain seems to come every month.

Diagnosis: Endometriosis

Clinchers

- *37-year-old woman:* Endometriosis is typically seen in those with postmenstrual exposure, common in fourth decade of life.
- *Severe left iliac fossa pain (comes every month):* Pelvic pain classically cyclical at the time if periods is the most common symptoms. Periods are usually heavy and frequent.
- *On USG, 2 cm echogenic masses seen in broad ligament:* Foci if endometrial tissue may be found on an ovary, rectovaginal pouch, uterosacral ligaments, surface if pelvic peritoneum, broad ligament and sometimes in distant organs like lungs.
- *On vaginal examination*
  - Fixed retroverted uterus
  - Nodules in uterosacral ligament
  - General tenderness.

Investigation of choice

Laproscopy shows
- Types cysts
- Peritoneal deposits

Treatment of choice

- Danazol 400-800 mg OD
- Gestrinone 2.5-5 mg PO twice weekly
- Buserelin/goserelin (LHRH analyses)

Surgical local exicision or diathermy of endometriotic tissue or hysterectomy may depend upon site of lesion and women's with for future fertility.

Your Notes:

58. A 23-year-old woman just had an intrauterine device fitted. She complains of a watery brown vaginal discharge and abdominal pain.

Diagnosis: Pelvic inflammatory disease (PID).

Clinchers
- *Intrauterine device fitted:* 10% of cases of PID follow childbirth or instrumentation (insertion of IUCD, TOP) though 90% are sexually acquired (mostly due to *Chlamydia*).
- *Watery brown vaginal discharge:* PID present with abdominal pain and vaginal discharge. Discharge is come times profuse and purulent, or it may be bloody. These is spasm of lower abdominal muscles.
  In chronic cases abdominal mass may also be palpated because the inflammation leads to fibrosis, so adhesions develop between pelvic organs.

Investigation of choice
Endocervical and urethral swabs if practicable. Always check for chlamydia. Go for blood culture if febrile.

Immediate management
Admit for blood culture and IV antibiotics if very unwell.

Treatment of choice
Page 50 (OHCS), 5th edn.

Your Notes:

---

59. An 18 weeks pregnant female presents with lower abdominal pain and tenderness, with offensive vaginal discharge. She has high grade fever since last two days.

Diagnosis: Septic abortion

Clinchers
- *Lower abdominal pain:* In this question this pain may be due to pelvic infection.
- *Offensive vaginal discharge with high grade fever:* This point towards the infection (probably uterus). To support the diagnosis of septic abortion, fever more than 38°C for more than 24 hours (with or withour chills and rigors) should be present. Offensive and purulent vaginal discharge support the diagnosis of infection.
  Majority of infection occurs following illegal induced abortion (rare in UK) in developing Countries.
  Any abortion associated with clinical evidence of infection of the uterus and it content is called septic abortion.

Investigation of choice
Cervical or high vaginal swab for culture. Ultrasonography.

Treatment of choice
Hospitalization. Aim at
- To control sepsis
- Remove source of infection
- Supportive therapy

Go for analgesia, sedatives and antibiotics.

Your Notes:

60. A 32-year-old who conscientiously uses the oral contraceptive pill, has experienced monthly vaginal bleeding. On abdominal examination she is comfortable. Her temperature is 37°C. She is otherwise healthy.

Diagnosis: Break through bleeding.

Clinchers

- *Conscientiously uses—OCP:* It means she is a regular in taking the pills.
- *Monthly vaginal bleeding:* Menstruation is initiated by the withdrawal of oestrogen and progesterone. Such as effect is produced in women receiving oestrogens and progestogens in the form of the combined contraceptive pill or hormone replcement therapy—withdrawal bleeding on completion of a pack.
- *On abdominal examination she is comfortable:* This rules out any pelvic inflammatory disease. Otherwise also OCP use decreases the risk of PID. The only infection whose incidence is increased by using OCP is monoilial vaginitis (candidiasis).

CONFUSA
Intermenstrual spotting is common in the first three months of the start of the pills, but it gradaully disappears. Heavy spotting can be stopped by increasing the dose for a few months.

Investigation of choice
None required.

Immediate management
Reassurance.

Treatment of choice
None required.

Your Notes:

---

61. A 30-year-old man with AIDS presented in shock. Serum biochemistry reveals: potassium 6.7 mmol/L, bicarbonate 20 mmol/L, chloride 84 mmol/L, creatinine 160 µmol/L

Diagnosis: Acute adrenal insufficiency

Clinchers

- *30-year-old man with AIDS:* Various endocrine abnormalities have been reported with AIDS, including reduced levels of testosterone and abnormal adrenal function. The latter may assume clinical significance in more advanced disease. When intercurrent infection superimposed upon borderline adrenal function may precipitate clear adrenal insufficiency requiring replacement doses of cortico- and mineralo-corticoid CMV is also implicated in adrenal-deficient states.
- *Presents in shock:* Acute adrenal insufficiency typically present in shock (but not always).
- *Potassium 6.7 mmol/L:* Increases as always in this condition.
- *Bicarbonate 20 mmol/L:* Mild acidosis is characteristic.
- *Chloride 84 mmol/L:* Low along with hyponatraemia.
- *Creatinine 160 µmol/L:* Slightly increased.

CONFUSA
Acute adrenal insufficiency or Addisonian crisis can occur in any one with a known Addison's disease, or someone or long-term steroids who has forgotten to take their tablets. Typically it presents with shock but an alternative presentation can be with hypoglycaemia.

Investigation of choice
Blood for cortisol and ACTH (if possible).

Immediate management
Start treating before biochemical results.

Treatment of choice
Hydrocortisone sodium succinate 100 mg IV stat plasma expander followed by 0.9% saline.

62. A 41-year-old Londoner developed a temperature of 41°C, 5 weeks after cadaveric renal transplantation. WBC is 2.1 × 1,000,000,000/L, Hb is 8.8 g/dl, creatinine 177 μmol/L. Aspartate aminotransferase (AST) 82 U/L. Alanine aminotransferase (ALT) 132 U/L.

Diagnosis: Cytomegalovirus (CMV) disease.

Clinchers

- *41-year-old Londoner:* CMV has worldwide distribution with London being no exception.
- *Temperature of 41°C:* In transplant recipients on post bone marrow transplantation, CMV present with: fever > pneumonitis > colitis > hepatitis > retinitis. In AIDS, it presents with: retinitis > colitis > CNS defects.
- *After cadavaric renal transplantation:* CMV can be acquired by direct contact, blood transfusion or organ transplantation. Transmission following organs transplantation or blood transfusion is due to silent infection in these tissues. It can well be a CMV reactivation syndrome, developed when T cell (lymphocyte) mediated immunity is compromised after organ transplantation, or in association with lymphoid neoplasms and certain acquired immunodeficiencies (in particular: HIV).
- *WBC is 2.1 × 1000,000,000/L:* Normal range is between 4-11 × 1000,000,000/L. Leukopenia is commonly seen with CMV infection in immunocompromised.
- *Aspartate transaminase (AST) of 82 IU/L:* Normal range of AST is 3-35 IU/L. This show the LFT is deranged. Hepatitis is a common syndrome associated with CMV.
- *Alanine aminotransferase (ALT) of 132 IU/L:* Normal range of ALT is 3-35 IU/L. This shows LFT is deranged. Hepatitis is a common syndrome associated with CMV.
  Variety of syndromes associated with CMV are fever, and leukopenia, hepatitis, pneumonitis, esophagitis, gastritis, colitis and retinitis.

CONFUSA
Most primary CNV infections in organ transplant recipients result from transmission of the virus in the graft itself.

Investigation of choice
Isolation of the virus together with rise in antibody titers a fourfold and greater.

Immediate management
Retinoscopy to exclude CMV retinitis.

Treatment of choice: Ganciclovir IV

63. A 36-year-old woman with leukaemia has been treated with amphotericin B for a fungal pneumonia. She presents with muscle weakness. Sodium 137 mmol/L, potassium 2.7 mmol/L, bicarbonate 19 mmol/L, Chloride 110 mmol/L, creatinine 84 μmol/L, urine pH 6.8 mmol/L

Diagnosis: Type I renal tubular acidosis (Distal RTA).

Clinchers

- *36-year-old woman with leukaemia:* Adult onset leukaemia usually affect patients in 30's and 40's. Distal RTA may occur in association with a systemic illness such as Sjögren's syndrome, multiple myeloma or rarely leukemias.
- *Treated with amphotericin B for a fungal pneumonia:* Amphotericin B poisoning can cause distal RTA due to an ability to maintain a pH gradient across the collecting duct.
- *Muscle weakness:* It is due to hypokalemia
- *Sodium 137 mmol/L:* Normal
- *Potassium 2-7 mmol/L:* Low, and is characteristic
- HCO_3^- *19 mmol/L:* Low as alkali is lost from kidneys.
- *Chloride 110 mmol/L:* high, RTA is hyperchloremic acidosis.
- *Creatinine 84 μmol/L:* Normal
- *Urine pH 6.8 mmol/L:* Inappropriately high. Such patients are unable to acidify urine below pH = 5.5.

CONFUSA
These abnormalities suggest that one or both of the active proton pumps present in the collecting duct (the H^+-ATPase or the H^+, K^+-ATPase is defective. In addition, excretory rates of NH_4^+ are uniformly low when the degree of systemic acidosis is taken into account, indicating that the kidney is responsible for the metabolic acidosis. Ammonium excretion is low because of failure to trap NH_4^+ in the medullary collecting duct, as a result of higher than normal tubular fluid pH in this segment and the urine pH is high because of impaired H^+ secretion

Investigation of choice
Urinary pH + serum electrolytes.

Immediate management
Discontinue amphotericin is still taking.

Treatment of choice
Oral alkali (Shohl's solution).

Note: Potassium supplements are not required in distal RTA as correction of acidosis resolves hypokalaemia.

64. An 83-year-old man with small cell lung cancer presents with ankle oedema and is found to have 8 g/day, urine proteinuria. He is started on frusemide. 10 days later his blood pressure is 115/75 mmHg lying and 85/65 mmHg standing. Serum biochemistry was; Sodium 121 mmol/L, bicarbonate 24 mmol/L, potassium 3.6 mmol/L, Creatinine 113 µmol/L, chloride 95 mmol/L, Urea 11.5 mmol/L, Glucose 5.7 mmol/L, albumin 27g, osmolality 263 mOs m/L, urine osmolality 417 mOs m/L

Diagnosis: Dilutional hyponatremia with nephrotic syndrome

Clinchers

- *83-year-old woman:* Incidence of most of the malignancies increases with increasing age.
- *Small cell lung cancer:* SIADH is mostly associated with four malignancies, i.e.
  - Small cell lung carcinoma
  - Pancreas
  - Prostate
  - Lymphoma
- *Ankle oedema + 8g/day urine proteinuria:* Daily urinary protein excretion is < 150 mg in normal persons. This massive proteinuria along with ankle oedema is characteristic of nephrotic syndrome.
- *Frusemide:* Excess diuretics administration can produce a dilutional hyponatremia with electrolyte profile similar to SIADH.
- *10 days later:* Dilutional hyponatraemia develops after repeated administration of the offending diuretic over days.
- *Sodium 121 mmol/L:* Low, as it is dilutional hyponatraemia.
- *BP 115/75 mmHg lying and 85/65 mmHg standing:* Orthostatic hypotension is present in nephrotic syndrome usually.
- *Bicarbonate 24 mmol/L:* Normal.
- *Potassium 3.6 mmol/L:* Normal.
- *Creatinine 113 µmol/L:* Normal.
- *Chloride 95 mmol/L:* Normal.
- *Urea 11.5 mmol/L:* Increased owing to nephrotic syndrome.
- *Glucose 5.7 mmol/L:* Normal.
- *Albumin 27 g:* Low, owing to nephrotic syndrome.
- *Serum osmolality 263 mOsm/L:* Low (normal 278-305) but do not quality for SIADH which is < 260 osmol/L. It is low because of dilutional hyponatremia.
- *Urine osmolality 417 mOsm/L:* It suggest concentrated urine but not > 500 mOsm/L to suggest SIADH.

CONFUSA
SIADH is an important, but overdiagnosed, caused of hyponatraemia. The diagnosis of SIADH requires, the absence of hypovolemia oedema, or diuretics. SIADH must always be distinguished from dilutional hyponatremia.

Investigation of choice
Serum electrolytes.

Immediate management
Stop diuretics or reset their dose.

Treatment of choice
Treat the cause + fluid restriction.

Your Notes:

65. A fit 50-year-old man is prescribed oral acetazolamide by an ophthalmologist for suspected glaucoma. He presents with lethargy and shortness of breath on exertion. Sodium 140 mmol/L, potassium 3.2 mmol/L, bicarbonate 18 mmol/L, chloride 115 mmol/L, urea 6.7 mmol/L, creatinine 114 μmol/L.

Diagnosis: Type II renal tubular acidosis (Proximal RTA).

Clinchers
- *Fit 50-year-old man:* Excludes any pre-existing pathology to be the cause of this condition.
- *Oral acetazolamide:* Acetazolamide causes increased renal bicarbonate losses. Hence it is the most probable cause in this case.
- *Lethargy and shortness of breath on exertion:* These are due to hypokalemia and acidosis respectively.
- *Sodium 140 mmol/L:* Normal.
- *Potassium 3.5 mmol/L:* Low, as hypokalaemia is a feature.
- *Bicarbonate 18 mmol/L:* Low as acetazolamide ↑ renal losses.
- *Urea 6.7 mmol/L:* Normal, but still on higher side (range 2.5-6.7 mmol/L).
- *Creatinine 114 μmol/L:* Normal.

CONFUSA
Renal tubular acidosis generally may be secondary to immunological drug-induced or structural damage to the tubular cells, an inherited abnormality, or an isolated (primary) abnormality. As with most disorders which are not well-understood, the nomenclature is confusing.

Investigation of choice
Urinary pH and serum electrolytes.

Immediate management
Discontinue acetazolamide if still taking.

Treatment of choice
Sodium bicarbonate (massive doses may be required to overcome the renal 'leak').

Your Notes:

66. Man with pyloric stenosis, profuse vomiting, hypokalemia and increased bicarbonate.

Diagnosis: Metabolic alkalosis.

Clinchers
- *Pyloric stenosis:* Presents with vomiting of large amounts of food some hours after meal. Metabolic alkalosis develops as a result of net gain of (HCO_3^-) or loss of nonvotile acid (usually HCl by vomiting) from extracellular flush.
- *Profuse vomiting:* Which is a sign of pyloric stenosis will lead to loss of acid (HCl). Vomiting/pyloric stenosis is an important cause of hypokalaemia..
  The combination of hypokalemia and alkalosis in a normotensive, nonedematous patient can be due to Bartter's syndrome, magnesium deficiency, vomiting, evogenosis alkali or diuretic ingestion.
  Gastrointestinal loss of H^+ results in retention of HCO_3^-. Increased H^+ loss through gastric secretions can be caused by vomiting, gastric aspiration, or gastric fistula. This loss of fluid and NaCl in vomitus, results in contraction of extracellular fluid volume (ECFV) and increased in secretion of renin and aldosterone. Volume contraction causes a reduction in GFR and an enhanced capacity of the renal tubule to reabsorb HCO_3^-. Thus during active vomiting, there is continued addition of HCO_3^- to plasma in exchange for Cl^-.

CONFUSA
Presence of hypertension and hypokalemia in an alkalotic patient suggests either mineralocorticoid excess or a hypertensive patient receiving diuretics.

Investigation of choice
ABG and serum electrolytes (already done in the patient).

Immediate management
Correct contracted extracellular fluid volume (ECFV) with NaCl, along with K^+ supplements.

Your Notes:

67. Man who is not able to pass urine, tired, complains of hiccups.

Diagnosis: Renal failure.

Clinchers
- *Not able to pass urine:* Oliguria (urine output < 400 mL/d) is a frequent but not invariable feature of acute renal failure.
- *Complains of hiccups:* Hiccups occur when there is increased retention of nitrogenous waste products. In renal failure, there is increase in plasma urea and creatine concentration.

Features suggestive of chronic renal failure include anaemia, neuropathy, radiological evidence of renal osteodystrophy or small scared kidney.

CONFUSA
Renal failure may cause high anion gap acidosis, poor filtration and reabsorption of organic onions contribute to the pathogenesis. In this question the answer could have been metabolic acidosis, if renal failure was not amongst the options.

Investigation of choice
- Blood urea and S creatinine
- Arterial blood gas (ABG) analysis
- S electrolyte

Immediate management
In case of acidosis, replace alkali ($NaHCO_3$), to maintain (CHO_3^-) between 20 and 24 mmol/L.

Treatment of choice
- Identify the cause of ARF
- Eliminate triggering insult (e.g. nephrotoxin) and/or institute disease specific therapy.
- Prevent and manage uremic complications
- Metabolic acidosis is not treated unless, serum bicarbonate concentration falls below 15 mmol/L or arterial pH falls below 7.2.

Your Notes:

68. Man with villous adenoma, profuse diarrhoea.

Diagnosis: Hypokalemia.

Clinchers
Diarrhoea may be associated with villous adenoma (usually with large tumors, more than 3-4 cm in diameter). Here hypokalemia due to potassium loss is common.

Acute diarrhoea is generally infectious. Chronic diarrhoea can be inflammatory, osmotic (malabsorption) or secretory due to intestinal dysmotility.

In cases of villous adenoma, diarrhoea is secretory in nature, caused by abnormal fluid and electrolyte transport not necessarily related to ingestion of food.

Vomiting, diarrhoea, villous adenoma rectum, pyloric stenosis, diuretics, Cushing's syndrome, alkalosis, all are important causes of hypokalaemia. Normal potassium levels in serum: 3.5-5 mmol/L.

CONFUSA
Metabolic alkalosis has been described in cases of villous adenoma, but this is most likely the result of potassium depletion.

Investigation of choice
Serum electrolytes.

Immediate management
In mild cases (>2.5 mmol/L, no symptoms) give oral K^+ supplement. If no thiazide diuretic, hypokalaemia > 3.0 mmol/L rarely needs treating. In severe cases (< 2.5 mmol/L, dangerous symptoms) give IV potassium cautiously, not more that 20 mmol/h, and not more concentrated than 40 mmol/L. Do not give K^+ if oliguric.

Your Notes:

69. Female, 24 hours after hysterectomy complains of breathlessness, increased JVP.

Diagnosis: Fluid overload.

Clinchers
- *24 hours after hysterectomy:* Intravenous fluid and blood components that may have been transfused to this female in this whole process of hysterectomy, may have lead to these signs of fluid overload (breathlessness and increased JVP).

  Blood components are excellent volume expanders and transfusion may quickly lead to volume overload.
- *Breathlessness and increased JVP:* JVP is best indicator of estimating the central venous pressure (CVP), which is no doubt raised in fluid overload. Fluid overload will lead to elevated pulmonary capillary pressure, which may be due to left ventricular dysfunction. This elevation of hydrostatic pressure in the pulmonary vascular bed leads to dyspnoea by multiple mechanisms like pulmonary edema.

Investigation of choice
Central line to measure CVP.

Immediate management
Treatment is aimed by reducing extracellular fluid volume by lowering total body Na$^+$ stores by following mechanisms:
- Reducing dietary intake of Na$^+$
- Increasing its urinary excretion with the aid of diuretics

Treatment of choice
Monitoring the rate and volume of transfusion, along with the use of a diuretic, can minimise this problem of fluid overload.

Your Notes:

70. A patient in severe renal failure has potassium level of 2.5 mmol/L.

Diagnosis: Hypokalemia (Answer: frusemide)

Clinchers
- *Severe renal failure:* May be due to glomerulonephritis, pyelonephritis, interstitial nephritis, DM, hypertension, cystic diseases, etc. In CRF there is usually, irreversible and long-standing loss of renal function. In CRF treatment is aimed at treating reversible causes (relieve obstruction, stop nephrotoxic drugs, treat hypercalcemia). High does of loop diuretics (furosemide) are used to treat edema.
- *Potassium level of 2.5:* Normal range of potassium is 3.5-5 mmol/L. Hypokalaemia is the most significant problem with high ceiling diuretics (frusemide) and thiazides. Usual manifestations of hypokalemia are weakness, fatigue, muscle cramps and cardiac arrhythmias.

CONFUSA
Hypokalemia is less common with standard doses of high ceiling diuretics (frusemide), than with thiazides, possibly because of shorter duration of action of the former which permits intermittent operation of compensatory reflection mechanism.

Investigation of choice
- Blood: FBC, ESR, U and E, Creatinine, S calcium
- Urine: Microscopy, creatinine clearance
- Renal ultrasound

Immediate management
Change furosemid with potassium sparing Diuretics

Treatment of choice
For hypokalaemia: Attempt to maintain serum K$^+$ at or above 3.5 mEq/L, by:
- High dietary K$^+$ intake
- Supplements of KCl (24-72 mEq/day) or
- Concurrent use of K$^+$ sparing diuretics

Your Notes:

71. A man who has been worked as boiler worker for 20 years presents with dyspnoea and pleurisy.

Diagnosis: Asbestosis

Clinchers
- *Boiler worker for 20 years:* Exposure to asbestos occured particularly in naval ship building yards and in power stations, especially boiler workers. There is a considerable time lag between exposures and development of the disease, particularly mesothelioma (20-40 years).
- *Dyspnoea:* It is due to progressive airflow limitation due to fibrosis in this condition.
- *Pleurisy:* It denotes a pleural lesion which is most probably a mesothelioma in this case.

> **CONFUSA**
> Asbestosis is defined as fibrosis of the lungs caused by asbestos dust, which may or may not be associated with fibrosis of the parietal or visceral layers of the pleura. It is a progressive disease characterized by breathlessness and accompanied by finger clubbing and bilateral basal end expiratory crackles. Fibrosis, not detectable on chest X-ray, may be revealed.

Investigation of choice
CXR/CT scan (screening)
Pleural biopsy (definitive)

Immediate management
Legal advise, as he may be entitled for compensation in UK.

Treatment of choice
No treatment is known to alter the progress of the disease, though corticosteroids are often prescribed.

Your notes:

72. Female with cough, copious blood tinged sputum for more than a month. She is from south-east Asia.

Diagnosis: Pulmonary tuberculosis.

Clinchers
- *Cough:* Pulmonary TB may be silent but it causes cough more commonly.
- *Coupious blood tinged sputum:* Coupious sputum is a typical feature of tuberculosis. It may be blood tinged or associated with frank hemoptysis. Other associated presenting features can be:
  - Pneumonia
  - Pleurisy
  - Pleural effusion
- *South-east Asia:* Tuberculosis is most prevent in Indian subcontinent and is mostly seen in UK among immigrants from there (Pakistan, India, Bangladesh).

> **CONFUSA**
> Primary TB is usually asymptomatic, but there may be fever, lassitude, sweats, anorexia, cough, sputum, erythema nodosum or phlyctenular conjunctivitis. The most common nonpulmonary infection is GI, most commonly affecting the ileocaecal junction and associated lymph nodes.

Investigation of choice
- *Screening:* CXR (consolidation, cavitation, fibrosis, calcification)
- *Definitive:* Sputum culture.

Immediate management
Trace family contacts for prophylaxis

Treatment of choice
Directly observed therapy (DOT) with rifampicin, isoniazid, pyrazinamide ± ethambutol x 2 months, and then only with rifampicin and isoniazid for next for months.

Your Notes:

73. A middle-aged woman develops a purulent cough with some haemoptysis. A chest X-ray reveals right upper lobe shadows.

Diagnosis: Pulmonary tuberculosis (PTB)

Clinchers
- *Middle-aged women:* Usually symptomatic primary tuberculosis develops due to reactivation of a primary complex years after the exposure.
- *Purulent cough with some hemoptysis:* Sputum in PTB may be mucoid, purulent or blood-stained.
- *CXR reveals right upper lobe shadows:* The CXR typically shows patchy or nodular shadows in the upper zones, loss of volume, and fibrosis with or without cavitation.

CONFUSA
Reactivation of tuberculosis is usually due to:
- DM
- Malnutrition
- Immunosuppression
- Drugs
  - Cytotoxins
  - Steroids
- Lymphoma
- AIDS

Investigation of choice
- *Screening:* CXR
- *Definitive:* Sputum culture and microscopy.

Immediate management
Find out cause of reactivation (often none found).

Treatment of choice
Directly observed therapy (DOT) x 6 months

Your Notes:

74. Female presents with acute pleuritic chest pain, haemoptysis after undergoing hysterectomy.

Diagnosis: Pulmonary embolism.

Clinchers
- *Acute pleuritic chest pain:* It is the usual presenting feature of pulmonary embolism. Other common associated presenting features can be:
  - Acute breathlessness
  - Haemoptysis
  - Dizziness
  - Syncope
- *Haemoptysis:* Haemoptysis occurs in 30%, often three or more days after the initial event.
- *After undergoing hysterectomy:* Any cause of immobility, i.e. postoperative immobility can increase the risk of pulmonary embolism. This risk is much more in middle-aged females on oral contraceptive pills (it induces hypercoagulability).

CONFUSA
Peluritic chest pain is common with small or medium sized pulmonary embolism. A massive pulmonary embolism give rise to severe central pain because of cardiac ischaemia due to lack of coronary blood flow.

Investigation of choice
- *Screening*
  - If patient stable = V/Q scan
  - If unable to undergo the above test = spiral CT
- *Definitive:* Pulmonary angiogram.

Immediate management
Anticoagulation with LMW heparin

Treatment of choice
Oral warfarin 10 mg PO x 3 months.

Your Notes:

September—2001

75. A 58-year-old man with fever and an area of consolidation on his chest X-ray is treated with antibiotics. His fever resolves but four weeks later but he still has a large area of consolidation.

Diagnosis: Bronchial carcinoma.

Clinchers
- *58-year-old man:* Elderly males with lung symptoms should be investigated to rule out lung cancer especially if they have history of smoking.
- *Fever:* This is because of the secondary pneumonia. Carcinoma causing partial obstruction of a bronchus interrupts the mucociliary escalator, and bacteria are retained within affected lobe.
- *An area of consolidation on his chest X-ray:* Secondary pneumonia due to above described mechanism appears as a lobar consolidation on CXR.
- *Is treated with antibiotics:* Treatment with antibiotics usually clears the pneumonia and resolves the fever within few days.
- *His fever resolves but four weeks later:* Any opacity secondary to inflammation should have been resolved in four weeks.
- *He still has a large area of consolidation:* Any opacity persisting beyound this time should make one strongly suspicious of a neoplastic lesion in this age group.

CONFUSA
The only confusion in this question can exist if one overlook the age of the patient and remain focussed only on the complications of pneumonia.

Investigation of choice
- *Screening:* CXR (already done in this case)
- *Definitive:* Bronchoscopy with biopsy.

Immediate management
Assess operability.

Treatment of choice
- Non-small cell tumors: Surgery (avoided in > 65 yrs with metastatic disease as rate of mortality is more than expected five-year survival)
- Radiotherapy: For bronchial obstruction (as in this case).

Your Notes:

76. Patient with acute shortness of breath, wheeze. Chest X-ray—normal, low oxygen, $PaCO_2$. PEFR-120 ml/minute.

Diagnosis: Asthma.

Clinchers
- *Acute shortness of breath, wheeze:* These are the characteristic of asthma may be associated with cough (often nocturnal) symptoms and sputum.
- *CxR normal:* In asthma CxR may be normal or hyperinflation may be observed. This helps to rule out other chronic lung pathologies.
- *Low oxygen, low $PaCO_2$:* Arterial blood gases (ABG) analysis in asthma usually shows a normal or slightly reduced PaO_2 and low $PaCO_2$ (hyperventilation). If $PaCO_2$ is raised, transfer the patient to ITU for ventilation.
- *PEFR—120 ml/min:* PEFR < 50% of predicted is seen in severe attack of asthma. PEFR < 33% along with silent chest, cyanosis, bradycardia is life-threatening.
  Predicted PEFR: Predicted values of PEFR vary with age, sex and height, and typically 450-600 ml/min in men and 350-500 ml/min in women. Values under 100-200 ml/min indicate severe ventilatory dysfunction.

CONFUSA
Differentiate asthma from the following:
- COPD (often coexists with asthma)
- Pulmonary edema (cardiac asthma)
- Large airway obstruction (e.g. foreign body, tumor)
- SVC obstruction (wheeze/dyspnoea not episodic)
- Pneumothorax
- Pulmonary embolism/bronchiectasis
- Obliterative bronchiolitis (in elderly).

Investigation of choice
- PEFR
- ABG
- Spirometry: obstructive defects ($\downarrow FEV_1$, FVCM $\uparrow$ residual volume).

Immediate management
- Sit patient up and give high dose O_2
- Nebulize with salbutamol 5 mg or terbutaline 10 mg.

Treatment of choice
Once patient starts improving reduce nebulized salbutamol and switch to inhaled β_2-agonists.
- Initiate inhaled steroids and stop oral steroids if possible
- Continue to monitor PEFR.

77. Bilateral hilar opacities, ACE is high.

Diagnosis: Sarcoidosis

Clinchers
- *Bilateral hilar opacities:* Respiratory symptoms are the most common presentation of sarcoidosis, with bilateral hilar opacities (bilateral hilar lymphadenopathy) being characteristic feature. This can be detected on routine chest X-ray.
  Sarcoidosis is a multisystem granulomatous disorder, that presents with bilateral hilar lymphadenopathy, pulmonary infiltration and skin or eye lesions. Diagnosis is confirmed histologically.
- *ACE is high:* In sarcoidosis, serum level of angiotensin converting enzyme is high. Though raised levels of ACE are also seen with patients.

CONFUSA
Differential diagnosis of this bilateral hilar lymphadenopathy includes:
- Lymphoma—though it is rare for this to affect only hilar lymph nodes.
- *Pulmonary tuberculosis:* Though it is rare for the hilar lymph nodes to be symmetrically enlarged.
- *Carcinoma of bronchus with malignant spread to the contralateral hilar lymph nodes:* though rare for this to give rise to typical symmetrical picture.

Investigation of choice
Serum ACE + CXR.

Immediate management
None.

Treatment of choice
Patients with bilateral hilar opacities alone do not require treatment since the majority recover spontaneously.

Your notes:

78. A 20-year-old woman attends A and E complaining of sudden breathlessness and anxiety. She describes palpitations and paresthesiae of her hands, feet and lips. ECG shows sinus tachycardia and O_2 saturation is normal.

Diagnosis: Panic attacks.

Clinchers
- *20-year-old female:* young females are most prone to have panic attacks.
- *Sudden breathlessness and anxiety:* Classically the symptoms begin unexpectedly or 'out-of-the-blue'. Usually there is no apparent precipitating factor. The patient becomes increasingly frightened by an apparent inability to breath adequately. Attempts to breadth rapidly results in dizziness and further anxiety.
- *Palpitations:* It is due to sympathetic overactivity. Other symptoms attributed to sympathetic stimulation are—tachycardia, sweating, flushes, dyspnoea, hyperventilation, dry mouth, frequency and hesitancy of micturition, dizziness, diarrhoea, mydriasis.
- *Paraesthesiae of her hands, feet and lips:* Tachypnoea blows off CO_2 and the resultant respiratory alkalosis causes a fall in ionised calcium. This hypocalcaemia manifest as paraesthesiae in the fingers and perioral area.
- *Sinus tachycycardia:* Due to sympathetic stimulation.
- O_2 *saturation is increased:* due to hyperventilation.

CONFUSA
The most important differential diagnosis in a female is from MVPS (mitral valve prolapse syndrome). This syndrome, more commonly seen in young females (like panic disorder), presents with classical symptoms of panic disorder occurring in episodes. It is caused by prolapse, usually congenital, of the mitral valve into the atrium during ventricular systole. On auscultation, a mid systolic click and a systolic murmur can be heard sometimes. The clininical differentiation between MVPS and panic disorder is difficult. The diagnosis is usually established on echocardiography.

Investigation of choice
To rule out organic respiratory problems (ECG, CXR, ABG).

Immediate management
Confirmation of normality with warm reassurance to the patient.

Treatment of choice
Re-breathing into a closed bag and mask system without oxygen.

79. An alcoholic admitted semi-comatose. ABG shows low oxygen saturation.

Diagnosis: Aspiration pneumonia.

Clinchers

Aspiration of liquid (foreign material), into the tracheobronchial tree results from various disorders that impair normal deglutition, especially disturbances of consciousness and esophageal dysfunction.

➤ *Alcoholic admitted semicomatose:* Consumption of alcohol, cigarette smoking, and use of theophylline are known to relax lower esophageal sphincter. This allows reflux of gastric contents into the esophagus and predisposes to pulmonary aspiration especially at night. But in this question the presentation appears to be acute, and therefore in an alcoholic with disturated consciousness, aspiration of alcohol can be the likely cause, which led to abrupt onset of respiratory distress, thus low oxygen,

CONFUSA

Since the question is incomplete, lefts discuss the differential diagnosis:
- *Alcoholic intoxication:* In severe cases alcohol overdose is marked by respiratory depression, stupor, seizures, shock syndrome, coma and death.
- *Subdural hemorrhage:* Subdural hemorrhage is a common cause of semicomatose presentation in alcoholics, due to fall.
- *Hypoglycaemia:* Alcohol related hypoglycaemia is due to hepatic glycogen depletion combined with alcohol-mediated inhibition of gluconeogenesis.

Investigation of choice
- Arterial blood gases (ABG) analysis.
- Blood sugar.
- CT scan to rule out subdural hemorrhage.

Immediate management
- Maintain airway with high flow oxygen.

Treatment of choice

O_2 to maintain $PaO_2 > 8$ kPa. With aspiration there is risk of aspirating oropharyngeal anaerobes.

Streptococcus pneumonia: Cefuroxime 1.5 g/h IV + Metronidazole 500 mg/8 h IV.

Your Notes

80. Patient with recent MI, develops acute breathlessness and hemoptysis. CxR shows dilated pulmonary artery and wedge shaped area of infarction. Decreased PaO_2 and decreased $PaCO_2$.

Diagnosis: Pulmonary embolism (PE).

Clinchers

➤ *Recent MI:* Though most commonly pulmonary embolism arises from venous thrombosis in pelvis or legs, recent stroke or MI may also lead to PE (right ventricular thrombus).

➤ *Acute breathlessness/hemoptysis:* These are along with pleuritis chest pain, dizziness and family history of thromboembolism are important symptoms of pulmonary embolism.

➤ *CxR:* In pulmonary embolism. CxR may be normal or may show
- Oligemia of affected segment
- Dilated pulmonary artery
- Linear atelectasis
- Small pleural effusion
- Wedge-shaped opacities or cavitations (rare) (wedge-shaped area of infarction).

Decreased PaO_2 and $PaCO_2$

Arterial blood gases (ABG) analysis shows hyperventilation + gas exchange ↓, thereby ↓ PaO_2 and ↓$PaCO_2$.

Investigation of choice
- U and E, ECG
- CT pulmonary angiography (determines emboli in pulmonary arteries
- V/Q scan (ventilation/perfusion scan) may show mismatched defects.

Immediate management
- Oxygen 100%
- Morphine 10 mg IV (if in pain).

Treatment of choice
- Heparin for ≥ 5 days, and until INR > 2.
- If obvious remedial cause, 6 weeks treatment with Warfarin. Otherwise continue for 3-6 months. Patients with recent MI, are at risk of developing DVT and PE and therefore they should be prophylactically heparinized (50000/12 h SC) until fully mobile.

Your Notes

81. A tall young woman developed sharp pain on one side of his chest two days ago. Since then he has been short of breath on exertion.

Diagnosis: Pneumothorax after spontaneous primary rupture

Clinchers
- *Tall*: It increases the risk of having apical bullae became of increased negative intrathoracic pressure.
- *Young*: Spontaneous pneumothorax is predominantly seen in "tens and twenties".
- *Man*: Incidence of spontaneous pneumothorax is more in males.
- *Sharp pain*: It is the characteristic pleuritic pain of pneumothorax.
- *Unilateral*: It is characteristic of pneumothorax as there are two pleural cavities.
- *Shortens of breath on exertion*: It confirms the diagnosis of pneumothorax.
- *2 days ago*: Spontaneous primary rupture of bullae is usually mild.

CONFUSA
Insertion of large guage open pore cannula (16-17 G) is only done for tension pneumothoraces. All other pneumothoraces are treated with water seal.

Investigation of choice
CXR

Immediate management
Serial radiographic observation.

Treatment of choice
Aspiration or underwater seal drainage if necessary.

Your Notes:

82. After a heavy bout of drinking a 56-year-old man vomits several times and develops chest pain. When you examine him, he has a crackling feeling under the skin around his neck.

Diagnosis: Pneumomediastinum after oesophageal rupture.

Clinchers
- *Heavy bout of drinking*: It is a risk factor for Boerhaare's syndrome (oesophageal rupture)
- *56 years old*: Older age cames weakness of oesophageal musculature and hence increases the chances of rupture.
- *Vomits several times*: Recurrent vomiting, especially against a closed glottis (common after a heavy bout of drinking) can produce oesophageal rupture
- *Chest pain*: Always suspect oesophageal perforation of chest pain follows vomiting.
- *Cracklin feeling*: This is subcutaneous emphysema which is characteristically present in suprasternal region after oesophageal rupture. It confirms our diagnosis.

CONFUSA
On more examination Hamman's sign can be found in this patient, i.e.
- Crunching/clicking noise synchronous with heart beat.
- Best heard in left lateral decubitus.
  Drinking is also associated with Mallory Weiss syndrome (MWS). It can be differentiated from Boerhaave's syndrome as:
- MWS has gastric tear in 90% cases (Below squamo-columnar junction) and oesophageal tear in 10% cases
- MWS present with haemetemesis which is not mentioned here.
- Complete tear (perforation) is very rare in MWS
- MWS—forceful vomiting in a chronic alcoholic BS— Recurrent vomiting after bout of alcohol drinking

NOTE:
- Weakest portion of oesophagus is its lower third
- If it is only pneumomediastinum without oesophageal rupture, high flow oxygen (100%) can help in early resorption of air. No surgery is required then.

Investigaation of choice: CXR

Immediate management: Crossmatch blood and inform surgeons.

Treatment of choice: Surgical repair (Though oesophageal rupture can also be managed in Boerhaave's syndrome because of high septic load).

83. A 23-year-old woman on the oral contraceptive pill suddenly gets tightness in her chest and becomes very breathlessness.

Diagnosis: Pulmonary venous thromboembolism (PE).

Clinchers

- *23-year-old woman:* She belongs to the typical OCP user age group.
- *OCP:* They increase the risk of pulmonary embolism by producing a hypercoagulable state.
- *Sudden tightness and breathlessness:* Chest pain and shortness of breath are the two most usual symptoms in PE. The pain is most often pleuritic in nature; sharp and worse with deep inspiration and couphing. There may be haemoptysis.

> **CONFUSA**
> Sometimes collapse is the presenting symptom. A sudden urge to defaecate may hearald the onset of symptoms. Signs are very variable and often absent. There may be tachycardia and tachypnoea. Areas of crepitus or a pleural rub are sometimes heard, as is a pulmonary flow murmur. Thrombosis of the deep veins is rarely clinically apparent.

Investigation of choice
V/Q scan

Immediate management
High flow O_2 + 10 mg IV morphine + anticoagulation

Treatment of choice
Heparin (loading dose of 5000-10000 units of standard heparin IV followed by a continuous infusion of 1000-2000 units per hour).

Your Notes:

84. A 30-year-old man with Marfan's syndrome has sudden central chest pain going through to the back.

Diagnosis: Aortic dissection (acute).

Clinchers

- *30-year-old:* In patients with Marfan's syndrome aortic dissection tends to present in a relatively younger age.
- *Marfan's syndrome:* It increases the risk of ascending aortic dissection. In fact it is the major cause of mortality in it.
- *Sudden central chest pain going to back:* Sudden onset of pain, localised to front or back of chest, often intersapular region and typically migrates with propapation of dissection.

> **CONFUSA**
> Aortic dissection is a potentially life-threatening condition in which disruption of aortic intima allows dissection of blood into vessel wall, may involves ascending aorta (type II) descending aorta (type III), or both (type I). Alternative classification type A —ascending aortic dissection, type B—limited to descending aorta. Involvement of the ascending aorta is most lethal form.

Investigation of choice
Screening/CXR, Definitive/CT/MRI/USG (TOE).

Immediate management
Crossmatch and inform surgeons.

Treatment of choice
Emegent surgical repair/always required in ascending aortic dissection.

Your Notes:

First Aid for PLAB

85. A 57-year-old man develops crushing pain in the chest associated with nausea and profuse sweating. The pain is still present when he arrives in hospital an hour later.

Diagnosis: Acute myocardial infarction (AMI).

Clinchers
- *57-year-old:* Incidence of MI increases with age as age is a nonmodifiable risk factor.
- *Man:* Male sex is also a nonmodifiable risk factor
- *Crushing pain:* There is acute central chest pain and is classically described as crushing or heavy. Some patients say it feels like a tight band around their chest; others describe it as like someone sitting on them. It is common for the patient to clench his or her first as an aid to description.
- *Associated with nausea and profuse sweating:* Accompanying symptoms such as sweating, pallor, nausea or general malaise are almost helpful in making a diagnosis as the character of pain.
- *Still present when he arrives in hospital an hour later:* The pain usually lasts longer than 30 minutes (20 minutes according to OHCM). This feature differentiates it form angina.

CONFUSA
Be aware of the middle-aged man with 'indigestion' especially if he has no past dyspeptic history of significance. A few days of vague retrosternal pain is not a history of dyspepsia. It is much more likely to be the warning pain which often predate as MI. Recurrent belching is a sign of autonomic disturbance and as such may accompany as infarction. Even synptomatic relief from antacids should not be relived upon to relied upon to point away from the heart. Some patients present with very atypicaly pain, both in site and character. Examples of this would be pain localized to the abdomen or to the left shoulder or arm alone.

Investigation of choice
ECG (hyperacute T waves, ST elevation or new LBBB)

Immediate management
High flow O_2 + 10 mg IV morphine + anticoagulation.

Treatment of choice
Thrombolysis.

Your Notes:

86. Female with breast carcinoma 3 years back, was treated with mastectomy and lymph node clearance on the left side, presents with a swollen limb and decreased hand movements.

Diagnosis: Acquired lymphoedema of arm.

Clinchers
- *Breast carcinoma:* The late oedema of the arm is a troublesome complication of breast cancer treatment. It is seen more commonly when radical axillary lymph node dissection and radiotherapy are combined.
- *3 years back:* It usually present late but can occur anytime from months to years after treatment.
- *Mastectomy and lymph node clearance on left side:* It involves massive removal of lymphatics which hampers the lymphatic drainage of arm. Radical axillary dissection is now rarely combined with radiotherapy (radiotherapy produced postradiation fibrosis which when compounded by impaired lymphatic drainage due to block dissection, increases the risk of lymphoedema by several times) because of this complication, but still it does occur with either modality of treatment alone.
- *Swollen arm:* Due to impaired lymphatic drainage.
- *Decreased hand movements:* It is due to compression of the nerves supplying the hand in compartments of arm and forearm.

CONFUSA
There is usually no precipitating cause but recurrent tumor must be excluded as neoplastic infiltration on the axilla can cause arm swelling due to both lymphatic and venous blockage. The differentiating features is that the neoplastic infiltrations are often painful due to nerve involvement. The diagnosis of lymphoedema also depends on exclusion of other causes of oedema, e.g. venous oedema. Lymphoedema cannot be differentiating from venous oedema by "pitting sign" in acute stage (as both will pit on pressure). However, when lymphoedema becomes chronic the subcutaneous tissue become indurated from fibrous tissue replacement, the pitting will not then occur.

Investigation of choice: Lymphangiography using radio-opaque contrast or radioactive isotope will confirm lymphatic obstruction, and contrast lymphangiography may demonstrate megalymphatics.

Immediate management: Rule out recurrence of carcinoma.

Treatment of choice: Treatment of late oedema is difficult but limb-elevation, elastic arm stockings and pneumatic compression devices can be useful.

87. Presents with thirst, confusion, constipation.

Diagnosis: Hypercalcemia of malignancy.

Clinchers
- *Thirst, confusion, constipation:* signs and symptoms of hypercalcemia of malignancy are:
  - Lethargy
  - Anorexia
  - Nausea
  - Polydipsia
  - Polyuria
  - Constipation
  - Dehydration
  - Confusion
  - Weakness

These signs and symptoms are most obvious with serum calcium > 3 mmol/L.

Hypercalcemia of malignancy is the most common paraneoplastic endocrine syndrome and is responsible for about 40% of all hypercalcemia.

CONFUSA
Hypercalcemia of malignancy can occur by one of the two mechanisms:
1. Humoral hypercalcemia—caused by circulating hormones (e.g. PTH)
2. Local osteolytic hypercalcemia—caused by local paracrine factors secreted by cancers within bone. This type occurs in relation with breast carcinoma which produces lytic bone metastases. Other cancers involved are kidney, ovary and skin.

Investigation of choice
Serum calcium.

Immediate management
Rehydrate with 3-4 litres of 0.9% saline IV (over 24 hours).
Note: Avoid diuretics

Treatment of choice
Bisphosphonate pamidronate (60-90 mg IV) decreases osteoclastic bone resorption.

Alteration of mental status (as in this case) is indicated of severe hypercalcemia and require treatment with calcitonin in addition to all of the above measures.

Your Notes:

88. Presents with weakness of both legs, difficulty walking, urine retention.

Diagnosis: Vertebral compression fracture due to metastases.

Clinchers
- *Breast carcinoma:* Bone is a common site for the disposition of secondary tumors usually of epithelial origin. Breast metastases are common in
  - Ribs
  - Thoracic vertebrae
  - Clavicles
- *Weakness of both legs:* Vertebral fractures involving the cord may entrap cord to produce paraplegia below the level of the fracture. Usually legs are involved in fracture of thoracic vertebrae. Upper limbs are also involved if there is cervical vertebral fracture.
- *Difficulty walking:* Due to paraplegia.
- *Urinary retention:* Bladder tone is lost immediately after cord injury. Distension leads to ureteric reflux and renal damage. Later on the bladder may become automatic or neurogenic bladder. Bowel dysfunction will also be present.

CONFUSA
Causes of spinal cord compression can be either extension of tumor from vertebral body (osteoblastic metastases) or crush fracture (osteoclastic metastases). Breast carcinoma commonly produces osteoclastic metastases though it can produce osteoblastic metastases too. Prostatic carcinoma produces osteoblastic metastases.

Investigation of choice
- *Screening:* Urgent plain X-ray spine
- *Definitive:* MRI/myelogram

Immediate management
Get neurosurgery and clinical oncology opinions.

Treatment of choice
Dexamethasone 8-16 mg IV then 4 mg/6h PO
Surgical decompression is the definitive treatment.

Your Notes:

89. Presents with headache, confusion. On examination, papilledema present.

Diagnosis: Raised intracranial pressure (ICP) due to cerebral metastases.

Clinchers
- *Headache:* It is the most common symptom of raised intracranial pressure. It is often worse in the morning and is accompanied by nausea and vomiting. Fits or focal neurological signs may appear as the ICP rises.
- *Confusion:* It is due to cerebral edema secondary to brain metastases.
- *Papilledema:* It is due to edema of retinal nerve layer and a common finding on fundoscopy (in both the eyes) in increased ICP.

CONFUSA
Breast carcinoma commonly metastasizes to brain, bone and liver. Brain metastases are usually solitary and produce reactive cerebral edema.

Investigation of choice
CT scan

Immediate management
Ventilatory support.

Treatment of choice
Dexamethasone 4 mg/6h PO
Radiotherapy/surgery for isolated metastases.

Your Notes:

90. Presents with features of fracture femur.

Diagnosis: Metastatic tumor producing pathological fracture.

Clinchers
- *Fracture femur:* Breast carcinoma (and most other epithelial tumors) commonly metastasizes to bone. Usually it is the local bones which are involved but arterial spread may result in deposition anywhere in the skeleton, particularly the flat bones, vertebrae and proximal ends of femur and humerus. Usually the breast carcinoma produces osteolytic (clastic) metastases which increases the risk of fractures especially in weight bearing bones like femur and vertebrae.

CONFUSA
Presence of bony metastases usually means a poor prognosis for life. So the priority in treating any pathological fracture is not restoration of bone congruity but the improvement of life's quality.

Investigation of choice
- *Screening:* X-ray femur (radiolucency)
- *Definitive:* Whole body bone scan

Immediate management
Splinting and take opinion of an orthopaedician and a clinical oncologist.

Treatment of choice
Pathological fractures are normally best treated by internal fixation to enable the patient to mobilize early. Still the best treatment is to treat the primary. Breast carcinoma may respond to hormone therapy, e.g. oophorectomy, androgen or steroid treatment. Tamoxifen is a common antiestrogen drug used for this purpose.

Your Notes:

91. A 16-year-old mother brings her baby for immunization. The nurse notices the baby has multiple bruises along both arms and legs. The baby is crying excessively. The house officer notices multiple fractures and that the baby has blue sclerae.

Diagnosis: Osteogenesis imperfecta.

Clinchers

- *16-year-old mother:* Not of much significance except the fact that battered baby condition is more prevalent among teenage mothers.
- *Multiple bruises along both arms and legs:* Because of connective tissue involvement, the skin scars extensively.
- *Crying excessively:* Because of pain induced by fractures and generalised illness.
- *Multiple fractures:* It is the hallmark of severe osteogenesis imperfecta. But these are also found in battered baby syndrome (non-accidental injury).
- *Blue sclerae:* It is the differentiating feature from non-accidental injury as blue sclerae are almost pathognomic of osteogenesis imperfecta with this clinical profile.

CONFUSA
Non-accidental injury is the main differential diagnosis in this case. Other thing to be noted is that osteogenesis imperfecta is known by many different names and they can appear in the options as such, i.e. fragilitas ossium, brittle bone syndrome, Adair-Dighton syndrome.

Investigation of choice
Screening: X-ray (decrease in bone density)
Definitive: Absorptiometry (X-ray/photon)

Immediate management
Symptomatic treatment (i.e. fractures—traction followed by light cast).

Treatment of choice
Judicious exercise programme to prevent loss of bone mass secondary to physical inactivity.

Your notes:

92. A 70-year-old man is receiving treatment for Alzheimer's disease. He is looked after by a 23-year-old granddaughters. He has recently developed fecal incontinence. The SHO notices bruises on both wrists and back.

Diagnosis: Elderly abuse.

Clinchers

- *70-year-old:* Proves that he is an elderly person!
- *Alzheimer's disease:* Such patients are usually very difficult to look after and one usually requires the services of a trained nurse to care for such demented persons.
- *Fecal incontinence:* Must have compounded the problems of the young granddaughters who was looking after him.
- *Bruises on both wrists and back:* Bruises on both wrists strongly suggest towards use of handcuffs on him, (which his granddaughter might have used to prevent him from wandering aimlessly and getting lost—a frequent occurrence in dementia). The bruises on the back could result either from direct assaults or from the violent attempts of the patient to get free from the handcuffs (thereby bruising his back against wall/bed/chair).

CONFUSA
This is a straight forward question with only a mild confusion between some terminologies in the options. It can qualify as a physical abuse alos, but elderly abuse is more specific and his children rather than the granddaughter are more responsible for his condition.

Investigation of choice
Detailed history.

Immediate management
Admission in hospital and inform social services.

Treatment of choice
Rehabilitation.

Your notes:

93. An anxious mother brings her 6-year-old daughter who is bleeding per vaginum. Six months prior to this presentation the girl had a confirmed streptococcal sore-throat infection. She is otherwise normal.

Diagnosis: Sexual abuse.

Clinchers
- *6-year-old:* Usually such a young child cannot give a proper history of sexual abuse.
- *Bleeding per vaginum:* A common finding in children's sexual abuse. Other common finding is presence of veneral disease before puberty.
- *Confirmed streptococcal sore throat six months back:* This is important as it can be a precipitating factor of Henoch-Schölein purpura. However, it usually does not occur after so long as six months as it is IgA mediated. It usually presents within 2-6 weeks.
- *Otherwise normal:* Rules out any systemic disease.

CONFUSA
The main differential diagnosis in this case is HSP. However, the main finding in HSP is a purpura on extensor surfaces which is excluded in this question (as the child is otherwise normal). So it is safe to answer as a childhood sexual abuse. (Also do not forget the theme is non-accidental injury).

Investigation of choice
Forensic specimens (pubic hair, vaginal swabs) by an expert.

Immediate management
Inform social services.

Treatment of choice
Follow local guidelines of the region.

Your notes:

94. A 4-day-old girl is brought to casualty by the maternal grandparent who is worried about two dark bluish patches on the child's buttocks. Child's mother is white and the father is black.

Diagnosis: Battered baby.

Clinchers
- *Brought to casualty by the maternal grandparent.* Always suspect abuse if accompanying adult is not a parent.
- *Two dark bluish patches on the child's buttocks.* Injury to buttocks is one of the most common finding in battered baby syndrome.
- *Child's mother is white and the father is black.* Inter-racial marriages are often a risk factor for battered baby syndrome.

CONFUSA
The main differential diagnosis in this case is 'birth marks' or congenital nevus. But they are usually present either at birth or after seven days (Strawberry angioma). Here the socio-cultural history is also raising suspicious of battered baby syndrome.

Investigation of choice
Detailed history from accompanying adult + complete physical examination.

Immediate management
Inform social services.

Treatment of choice
Follow local guidelines of region/hospital.

Your notes:

95. An 8-year-old girl is noted to have fresh bloody staining of her pants. She also suffers from eneuresis. she has recently started horse-riding lessons

Diagnosis: Accidental injury.

Clinchers

- *Fresh bloody staining of her pant:* Most probably from trauma as the history given in question does not potray any illness.
- *She also suffers from eneuresis:* Bedwetting occurs on most nights in 15% of 5-year-olds, and is still a problem in upto 3% of 15-year-olds (usually from delayed maturation of bladder control). So it is probably normal.
- *She has recently started horse-riding lessons:* It can be reason for trauma, most probably rupture of hymen, which is common in horse riding training for adolescent girls.

CONFUSA
GMC has tried to mislead us by putting the history of eneuresis in this question. But eneuresis has nothing to do with bleeding anywhere. So the question is still straight enough.

Investigation of choice
For bleeding: Local examination.

For eneuresis: Test for UTI, GU abnormality and DM.

Immediate management
Reassurance.

Treatment of choice
Desmopressin nasal spray.

Your notes:

---

96. Patient with a pulsatile hard mass fixed under the upper 1/3 of the sternomastoid muscle.

Diagnosis: Chemodectoma

Clinchers

- *Hard mass:* Chemodectomas arise from carotid body and usually firm. Occasionally they are soft and pulsatile. It does not usually cause bruits.
- *Fixed:* These tumors more from side to side but not up and down. Most behave in a benign fashion, in a few patients the tumor becomes locally invasive and may metastasize.
- *Under the upper 1/3 of the sternomastoid muscle:* This tumor must be suspected in masses just anterior or under the upper third of sternomastoid.

CONFUSA
The tumor presents as a slowly growing enlarging mass in a patient over the age of 30 years. Occasionally, pressure on the carotid sinus from the tumor produces attacks of faintness. Extension of the tumour may lead to cranial nerve palsies (VII, IX, X, XI and XII), resulting in dysphagia and hoarseness.

Investigation of choice
Digital substraction angiography

Immediate management
Check the opposite side as the tumor is often bilateral.

Treatment of choice
Extirpation by vascular surgeon.

97. A 40-year-old male has a lump in the superoposterior area of the anterior triangle.

Diagnosis: Parotid tumor.

Clinchers
- *40 years old:* Ninety percent parotid tumors present before the age of 50 although any age may be affected.
- *Male:* Sex distribution is equal.
- *Lump in superoposterior area of anterior triangle:* In a > 40 year old patient, a lump in this area is most likely to be a parotid tumor (498, OHCM, 5th edn). Although the swelling can be anywhere within the parotid gland, but usually in the lower pole and in the region of the angle of the jaw. The lump is well defined, usually firm or hard but sometimes cystic in consistency.

CONFUSA
The facial nerve is never involved in parotid tumors, except by frankly malignant tumors. Its integrity, however, should always be confirmed. Although slow growing, there tumors cannot be considered benign because of the lack of encapsulation, the occasional wide infiltration of the surrounding tissues and the tendency to recur.

Investigation of choice
Biopsy

Immediate management
Check the integrity of facial nerve

Treatment of choice
Superficial parotidectomy

98. A 16-year-old female has a midline lump in the neck which moves on protrusion of the tongue and is below the hyoid bone.

Diagnosis: Thyroglossal cyst

Clinchers
- *16-year-old:* Thyroglossal cyst almost always presents before 20 years of age.
- *Female:* The sex ratio is nondiscriminatory.
- *Midline lump:* It is a fluctuant swelling in the midline of the neck.
- *Moves on protrusion of tongue:* It is diagnosed by its characteristic physical signs:
  - It moves upwards when the patient protrudes the tongue because of its attachment to the tract of the thyroid descent
  - It moves on swallowing because of its attachment to the larynx by the pretracheal fistula
- *Below the hyoid bone:* This is its most common location.

CONFUSA
Thyroglossal cyst may be present in any part of the thyroglossal tract. The common situations, in order of frequency are:
1. Beneath the hyoid
2. In the region of thyroid cartilage
3. Above the hyoid bone

Such a cyst occupies the midline, except in the region of the thyroid cartilage, where the thyroglossal tract is pushed to one side, usually to the left.

Investigation of choice
Entirely clinical diagnosis. USG may help.

Immediate management
Rule out an infected cyst which indicates a delay in surgery.

Treatment of choice
Excision (because infection is inevitable)

99. A 19-year-old male has a cystic mass under the anterior border of sternomastoid at the junction of upper 1/3 and middle 1/3 of the muscle. Aspiration revealed fluid containing cholesterol crystals.

Diagnosis: Branchial cyst (BC).

Clinchers
- *19-year-old:* BC usually presents in early adult life.
- *Male:* The sex ratio is nondiscriminatary.
- *Cystic mass:* BC forms a soft swelling like a "half-filled hot water bottle."
- *Under the anterior border of sternomastoid at the junction of upper 1/3 and middle 1/3 of the muscle:* This is the typical location of the branchial cyst and it bulges forward from beneath the anterior border of sternomastoid.
- *Fluid containing cholesterol crystals:* This confirms the diagnosis of BC as it always contains pus like material, which is in fact cholesterol crystals. These are demonstrated under the microscope.

CONFUSA
BC often presents following an upper respiratory tract infection. Occasionally the cyst may be infected. It signifies the persistence of remnants of the second branchial arch. A rare first branchial arch cyst may present just below the external auditory meatus at the angle of the jaw, with extension closely related to VII nerve.

Investigation of choice
Aspiration and microscopy (already done in this case).

Immediate management
Rule out cyst infection but is an indication for delay in surgery.

Treatment of choice
Surgical excision.

---

100. An infant present with a transilluminant swelling in the lower third of neck.

Diagnosis: Cystic hygroma (CH)

Clinchers
- *Infant:* CH usually manifests itself in the neonate or in early infancy and occasionally may be present at birth and be so large as to obstruct labour.
- *Transilluminant swelling:* The characteristic that distinguishes CH from all other neck swellings is that it is brilliantly transilluminant.
- *Lower third of neck:* Swelling in CH usually occurs in the lower third of the neck and as it enlarges it passes upwards towards the ear. Often the posterior triangle of the neck is mainly involved.

CONFUSA
As a result intercommunication of its many compartments, the swelling of CH is soft and partially compressible. It visibly increases in size when the child coughs or cries. The cheek, axilla, groin and mediastinum are other, although less frequent, sites for a cystic hygroma.

Investigation of choice
Transillumination test

Immediate management
Rule out infection of the cyst

Treatment of choice
Excision of all the cyst at an early stage.

Your notes:

101. Patient after escaping from fire in a building has singed nostrils.

Diagnosis: Inhalation injury

Clinchers
- *After escaping from fire in a building:* Incapacity, which occurs quickly in domestic and industrial fires, is caused by a combination of
  - Hypoxia
  - Carbon monoxide poisoning (caused by incomplete combustion)
  - Hydrogen cyanide poisoning

  Soft furnishing are a particular hazard, producing many topic substances, including highly irritant and lethal hydrogen chloride.
- *Signed nostrils:* Burns around the lips, mouth, throat or nose, including singeing of nasal hairs invariably points towards associated inhalation injury.

CONFUSA
Beware of conventional blood gas analyser readings in patients who may have high carboxy or methemoglobin levels. The oxygen electrode measures oxygen dissolved in plasma only and oxygen saturation is then calculated assuming all hemoglobin to be normal. PaO_2 and oxygen saturation may thus appear to be satisfactory despite very low total blood oxygen content.

Investigation of choice
Carboxy hemoglobin (CoHb).

Immediate management
High concentration O_2 + early intubation.

Treatment of choice
Admit and observation for 24 hours (even if burns appear minimal).

102. Patient has a large tense blister.

Diagnosis: Dermal burns

Clinchers
- *Large tense blister:* Small blisters can be left alone. Large ones can be slit open at the dependent edge to allow drainage. Alternatively they can be aspirated with a needle.

CONFUSA
Complete derooting of any blister is unnecessary and leaves a painful base. So avoid it. Blisters are absent in epidermal burns. Superficial dermal burns with blistering are usually dressed to absorb exudate, prevent desiccation, provide pain relief, encourage epithelialisation and prevent infection.

Investigation of choice
None required.

Immediate management
Drainage of blister/aspirate blister.

Treatment of choice
Regular dressing.

103. An adult patient has partial thickness burns on the anterior chest and upper thighs

Diagnosis: Significant burns requiring admission

Clinchers
- *Partial thickness burns:* They can be managed by clearning the wound and covering with a non adherent dressing such as paraffin gauze or with sliver sulfadiazine (flamazine cream)
- *On anterior chest and upper thighs:* According to Lund and Browder chart anterior chest is 7½ and upper thigh = $4\frac{3}{4}$. So the total area is 7½ + $4\frac{3}{4}$ + 4 = 17%. A burn of more than 15% in adults (>10% in children) require IV fluids and hence an admission to the hospital and treatment in a burns unit.

> **CONFUSA**
> Infection can easily convert a partial thickness burn to a full thickness burn, so ensure proper prevention from infection. For IV fluid resuscitation, the priming fluid can be isotolic saline. Thereafter a colloid is used. The choice of colloid includes synthetic sugars, gelatin and starch, albumin, plasma protein fraction and reconstitute plasma. Whole blood will be required if there is a significant element of full thickness skin loss.

Investigation of choice
Urine output.

Immediate management
Admit and refer to burns unit after starting IV fluids and maintaining airway.

Treatment of choice
- Regular dressing
- Grafting and contracture release after healing.

104. An adult patient has full thickness circumferential burns (from the elbow to the fingers, covering them completely.

Diagnosis: Circumferential full thickness burns over limb.

Clinchers
- *Circumferential full thickness burns:* These can contract and impair blood flow to the hand and forearm. Such contractions must be excised acutely to save the limb (escharotomy).
- *From elbow to fingers:* Face, hands and the joint flexures and priority areas for immediate skin grafting as scanning or contractures at these sites will obviously produce considerable deformity and disability.

> **CONFUSA**
> Eschar is a completely burnt and coagulated skin. Apart from limbs they can cause mechanical obstruction is present around the chest (by restricting chest movements they impair respiration). Moreover, they become a culture medium for bacteria such as *Streptococcus pyogenes* and *Pseudomonas aeruginosa*.

Investigation of choice
Urine output.

Immediate management
Escharotomy

Treatment of choice
Immediate excision and split skin grafting.

105. Man, slept while sunbathing comes with redness, and pain all over his body. Otherwise well.

Diagnosis: Sunburns.

Clinchers

- *Sunbathing:* It can cause sunburns if prolonged, but these are usually not serious.
- *Redness:* It is superficial erythema and is never taken into accounting when calculating the area of burn.
- *Pain:* Simple erythema is extremely painful. Even patients expected to go home after treatment may need parenteral analgesia.
- *Other wise well:* This rules out any other injury or fluid compromise. Since simple erythema do not require active treatment, he can be safely discharged home.

CONFUSA
Unprotected exposure to UV radiation can cause extremely painful, blistering, oedematous skin. In general the treatment is as for any other burn.

Investigation of choice
None required.

Immediate management
Oral analgesia if required.

Treatment of choice
Reassure and discharge
+
Regular application of hydrocortisone 1% cream

Your Notes:

106. Copies circle, can say 4 words.

Answer: 3 years

Clinchers
Apart from these a 3 year child can do:
- Jumps
- Can stand on one foot
- Can build an 8-cube tower
- Knows his first and last name
- Dress with help
- Imitate bridges with cubes
- Imitates vertical line within 30°
- Recognizes 3 colours
- Plays interactive games like TAG

CONFUSA

Copies circle	3 years
Copies cross	4 years
Copies square	5 years

Your notes:

107. Smiles responsively, Head lags.

Answer: 6 weeks

Clinchers
At 6 weeks, an infant can:
- Vocalizes, not crying
- Smiles responsively
- Move eyes 90° to midline
- Regards face

CONFUSA	
Smiles responsively	6 weeks
Smiles spontaneously	4 months

Your notes:

108. Can walk 4 steps upstairs.

Answer: 2 years

Clinchers
Other milestones seen in a 2 years old child
- Dons shoes not tied
- Washes and dries hands
- Jumps in place
- Kicks a ball
- Over arm bowling
- Gets undressed

CONFUSA	
Walks holding on to furniture	9 months
Walks well	12 months
Walks backwards	14 months
Walks up steps	17 months
Heel to toe walk	3½ years

Your notes:

109. Holds head up at 45° when prone, vocalise.

Answer : 2 months

Clinchers

Things that a 2 months old child can do
- Holds head at 45°when prone
- Vocalizes
- Smiles responsively
- Move eyes 90° to midline and past midline
- Laughs
- Hands together

CONFUSA	
Lifts head when prone	1 month
Holds head at 45° when prone	2 months
Holds head at 90° when prone	2½ months
Sits with head steady	4 months

Your notes:

110. Pincer grip; can say "Mummy" ± "Daddy"

Answer: 1 year

Clinchers

Other things that a 1 year old child can do is
- Just stands
- Walks using a table's support
- Clashes cubes
- Plays 'pat a cake'
- Indicates wants (not cry)
- Drinks from cup

CONFUSA	
Dada or mama (nonspecific)	7 months
Dada or mama (Specific)	9 months
2 words other than mama, dada	13 months
Combines 2 different words	19 months
Defines 6 words	4 ½ years

Your notes:

September—2001

111. Known patient of multiple sclerosis now with complaint of urinary incontinence, weakness in all 4 limbs and difficulty walking.

Diagnosis (of anatomical site): Cervical spinal cord.

Clinchers
- *Known patient of multiple sclerosis:* Multiple sclerosis is characterised by chronic inflammation, and selective destruction of CNS myelin: sparing the peripheral nervous system. It presents a recurrent attacks of focal neurologic dysfunction.
- *Difficult walking:* The symptoms of multiple sclerosis often worsen with fatigue, stress, exercise or left.
- *Urinary incontinence:* Sensory system involves urinary urgency or frequency, visual difficulties, abnormalities of gate and coordination.
  Motor involvement presents as heavy, stiff, weak or clumsy limb.
- Difficulty in walking, Lhermitte's sign (paraesthesia in limbs on flexing legs) and urinary symptoms are common in spinal and lesion.
- Paraparesis (weakness of both lower limbs) is characteristically diagnostic (not always) of spinal cord lesion.

CONFUSA
Initial individual plaques of MS (e.g. in optic nerve, brainstem or cord) must be distinguished from compressive, inflammatory, mass or vascular lesions. Other conditions that mimic the pattern of relapsing MS are CNS sarcoidosis, SLE and Behcet's syndrome.

Investigation of choice
MRI of the brain and spinal cord is the first line of investigation.

Immediate management
Refer to neurology.

Treatment of choice
When diagnosed, inform the patient of the diagnosis. There is no cure.
- *Polyunsaturated fats*—may help.
- *Methylprednisolone*—shortens relapses
- β-interferon 1b
  - ↓ relapse rate by 1/3
  - ↓ lesion accumulation on MRI
  - Slow accumulation of disability

112. Patient has nystagmus, diplopia, and positive past pointing.

Diagnosis (of anatomical site): Brainstem and its cerebellar connections

Clinchers
- *Nystagmus:* A rhythmic oscillation of the eye is a sign of disease of either the ocular or the vestibular system and its connection. In the lesions of brainstem and the cerebellum, long lasting horizontal or rotatory jerk and nystagmus are present.
- *Diplopia:* Diplopia in multiple sclerosis is the result of many different lesions—a sixth nerve lesion and the internuclear ophthalmoplegia (INO) are true examples.
- *Positive past pointing:* It is a sign of cerebellar lesion. Others include positive and gate disturbances, nystagmus, dysarthmia, etc.

CONFUSA
A typical picture of sole brainstem demyelination is sudden diplopics and vertigo with nystagmus, but without tinnitus or deafness.

Investigation of choice
MRI (magnetic resonance imaging).

Immediate management
Refer to neurology.

Treatment of choice
When diagnosed, inform the patient of the diagnosis. There is no cure.
- *Polyunsatured fats*—may help
- *Methylprednisolone*—shortens relapses
- β-interferon 1b
  - ↓ relapse rate by 1/3
  - ↓ lesion accumulation on MRI
  - Slow accumulation of disability.

113. Patient has repeated attacks of multiple sclerosis, and now has pale temporal disc.

Diagnosis (of anatomical site): Optic nerve

Clinchers
> *Pale temporal disc:* Disc pallor following an attack of multiple sclerosis is a sign of optic atrophy. It is first seen in temporal region.

The optic disc appearance depends upon the site of the plaque of multiple sclerosis, within the optic nerve. If the lesion is in the nerve head, there is disc swelling (optic neuritis). If the lesion is several millimeters behind the disc, there is generally no ophthalmoscopic feature. Here the doctor sees nothing and the patient sees nothing.

After the attack subsides, usually there is no residual symptom, but small scotoma or defects in colour vision can be demonstrated. Disc pallor is a late sequelae of multiple sclerosis and a sign of optic atrophy.

CONFUSA
Disc swelling from optic neuritis causes early and measurably visual acuity loss, thus distinguishing it from disc swelling from raised intracranial pressure.

Investigation of choice
MRI (magnetic resonance imaging)

Immediate management
Refer to neurology

Treatment of choice
When diagnosed, inform the patient of the diagnosis. There is no cure.
- *Polyunsatured fats*—may help.
- *Methylprednisolone*—shortens relapses
- β-interferon 1b
  - ↓ relapse rate by 1/3
  - ↓ lesion accumulation on MRI
  - Slow accumulation of disability.

114. Patient with complaint of blurring of vision, papilledema and pain in eye.

Diagnosis (of anatomical site): Optic nerve

Clinchers
> *Blurring of vision:* Optic neuritis produces variable loss. It usually begins as blurring of the central visual field, which may remain mild or progress to severe visual loss, or rarely, to complete loss of light perception. In mild cases, the patient may complain only of a subjective loss of brightness in the affected eye. Symptoms are generally monocular, but attacks may be bilateral.
> *Papilledema:* This is due to optic neuritis fundoscopic examination in it may be normal or with swelling of optic disc.
> *Pain in eye:* Pain, localized to the orbit or supraorbital area is frequently present and may precede visual loss. The pain typically worsens with eye movement.

CONFUSA
Visual blurring in MS may result from optic neuritis or diplopia. They are distinguished by asking the patient to cover each eye sequentially and observing whether the visual difficulty clears. Diplopia in MS is often due to an internuclear ophthalmoplegia (INO) or to a sixth nerve palsy; ocular muscle palsies due to involvement of the third or fourth cranial nerve are rare.

Investigation of choice
MRI

Immediate management
Refer to neurology

Treatment of choice
When diagnosed, inform the patient of the diagnosis. There is no cure.
- *Polyunsatured fats*—may help
- *Methylprednisolone*—shortens relapses
- β-interferon 1b
  - ↓ relapse rate by 1/3
  - ↓ lesion accumulation on MRI
  - Slow accumulation of disability.

115. A known patient of multiple sclerosis with unilateral facial paralysis with no loss of taste.

Diagnosis (of anatomical site): Facial nerve

Clinchers
- *Patient of multiple sclerosis with unilateral facial paralysis:* Facial paralysis, resembling idiopathic. Bell's palsy may be due to MS. It is a unilateral weakness of all the muscles of facial expression on the same site.
- *No loss of taste:* In MS, facial palsy is usually not associated with:
  - Ipsilateral loss of taste sensation
  - Retroaural pain at onset

Which are clinical characteristics of Bell's palsy.

> **CONFUSA**
> Chronic flickering contractions of the facial musculature, termed *facial myokymia*, is common in MS; it is thought to arise from involvement of corticobulbar tracts that deafferentation of the facial nucleus.

Investigation of choice
MRI

Immediate management
Refer to neurology

Treatment of choice
When diagnosed, inform the patient of the diagnosis. There is no cure.
- *Polyunsatured fats*—may help
- *Methylprednisolone*—shortens relapses
- β-interferon 1b
  - ↓ relapse rate by 1/3
  - ↓ lesion accumulation on MRI
  - Slow accumulation of disability

116. Not eating sea shell products prevents.

Diagnosis: Hepatitis A

Clinchers
- Sea shell products can transmit the following infections:
- Hepatitis A: because of unhygienic cooking methods employed. This is the most common infection due to their consumption and the cause is contamination with faecal matter.
- Vibrio parahaemolyticus—It is a natural resident of sea foods.

> **CONFUSA**
> Prevention of hepatitis A
> *Passive immunization*—with normal human immunoglobulin (0.02 ml/kg IM) gives < 3 months immunity to those at risk (travellers, household contacts).
> *Active immunization*—Havrix monodose, an inactivated protein derived from hepatitis A virus.

Investigation of choice
IgM (rises from day 25)
+
Serum transaminases
(both tests are done to diagnose recent infection)

Immediate management
Counselling about healthy eating habits, especially for travellers.

Treatment of choice
If infection occurs—symptomatic.

Your notes:

117. Immunization of sewage workers.

Diagnosis: To decrease risk of hepatitis A.

Clinchers
Hepatitis A spreads by faecal-oral route, so sewage workers are at special risk. Active immunization against hepatitis A is available and very effective. It is made from an inactivated protein derived from hepatitis A virus.

Dose: If > 16 years, 1 IM dose (1 mL to deltoid) gives immunity for 1 year (10 years if booster is given at 6 months).

Note: Trade name of hepatitis A vaccine in UK.
- Havrix monodose.

Passive immunization is with normal human Ig. It gives less than 3 months immunity to those at acute risk, i.e.
- Travellers
- Household contacts

CONFUSA
Sewage workers are also at risk of leptospirosis as its spread is by contact with infected rat urine. But there is no effective vaccination against it.

Investigation of choice
IgG antibody (presence signifies previous infection).

Immediate management
Rule out recent exposure. If present give immunoglobulin.

Treatment of choice
Vaccination.

Your notes:

118. Not swimming in foreign lakes prevents.

Diagnosis: Schistosomiasis prevention (S. hematobium).

Clinchers
> *Foreign lakes:* Schistosomiasis is the most prevalent disease causes by flukes, affecting 200 million people worldwide. The snail vectors release cercariae which can penetrate the skin, e.g. during swimming/paddling, may cause on itchy papular rash ('swimmers itch'). It is not so common in UK reservoirs but is very common in sub saharan Africa (particularly in lake Malawi), the middle east and Indian ocean.

CONFUSA
Hematospermia is a rare and interesting sign sometimes found in schistosoma hematobium infections.
- Leptospirosis (Weil's disease) is also avoidable by swimming in reservoirs but it is also common in UK and thus the question will not be specific about foreign lakes only.

Investigation of choice
Finding egg in urine.

Immediate management
Abdominal X-ray to look for bladder calcification characteristic of chronic infection.

Treatment of choice
Praziquantel.

Your notes:

119. Immunization of health workers who are in contact with body fluid.

Diagnosis: Risk of hepatitis B

Clinchers
- *Health workers:* Health workers should be particularly immunised against hepatitis B vaccine as its seroconversion rate after accidental exposure are dangerously high (much more than HIV). Now the protocol is to immunise everyone (and not just health workers) for hepatitis B vaccine in UK. The past strategy of vaccinating at risk gropus—health workers, IV drug abusers, homosexual, hemodialysis patients have been unsuccessful here.
- *Who are in contact with body fluid:* Body fluid can transmit many infections of which hepatitis B, hepatitis C and HIV are of not. Of these hepatitis B has maximum potential of seroconversion but because of its effective screening and immunization, the incidence of hepatitis C is on the rise.

CONFUSA
Older age, smoking and male sex correlates to low antibody levels even after immunization against hepatitis B vaccine. So time boosters with serology. Often there are cases of nonresponders to the vaccine. If the the question is about social worker, then hepatitis A vaccine (Havrix Monodose) would have been the answer.

Investigation of choice
Anti HBs status (positive in vaccinated or after recovery).

Immediate management
Universal precautions.

Treatment of choice
Passive immunization (specific anti HBV immunoglobulin) may be given to nonimmune contacts after high risk exposure).

Your notes:

120. Immunization of hepatitis B, besides preventing hepatitis B also prevents.

Diagnosis: Reduction in risk of hepatocellular carcinoma.

Clinchers
- *Immunization of hepatitis B:* Hepatitis B vaccine (Engerix B) is given as a 1 mL dose into deltoid and is repeated at 1 and 6 months (child: 0.5 mL x 3 into anterolateral thigh). Now it is given to everyone in UK. The immunocompromised may need more boosters.
- *Besides preventing hepatitis B also prevents:* Since chronic viral hepatitis (HBV, HCV) also causes hepatocellular carcinoma in the long run, the hepatitis B vaccine is preventive against it also.

CONFUSA
Anti HBs serology advice in UK is different from rest of the world. Please note:

Anti HBs	Actions and comments
> 1000 IU/L	Retest in 4 years
100-1000 IU/L	Retest in 1 year
< 100 IU/L	Given booster and retest
< 10 IU/L	Non-responder, give booster and retest if still < 10, get consent to check hepatitis B status

Investigation of choice
Anti HBs serology.

Immediate management
See previous question.

Treatment of choice
See previous question.

Your notes:

121. Man treated with gentamicin for peritonitis for 10 days presents with deafness.

Diagnosis: Ototoxicity.

Clinchers
Various drugs and chemicals can damage the inner ear and cause sensorineural deafness and tinnitus.

Symptoms of ototoxicity are—hearing loss, tinnitus, and/or giddiness, may manifest during treatment or after completion of treatment.

Ototoxic drugs: *Aminoglycoside antibiotics*: Gentamicin is the most important of all. Other includes—streptomycin, tobramycin, neomycin, etc.
- *Diuretics*: Furosemide, ethacrinic, etc.
- *Antimalarials*: Quinine, chloroquine.
- *Cytotoxic drugs*: Nitrogen, mustard, cisplatin
- *Analgesics*: Salicylates, indomethacin, ibuprofen.
- *Chemicals*: Alcohol, tobacco, marijuana, carbon monoxide poisoning.

Investigation of choice
Rinne test (positive), i.e. air conduction < bone conduction.

Immediate management
Weber lateralised to better ear.

Treatment of choice
Stop gentamicin at once.

Your Notes:

122. A patient with poor hygenic condition presents with hearing loss after taking a shower.

Diagnosis: Ear wax

Clinchers
- *Poor hygiene*: Normally only small amount of wax is secreted by ceruminous glands, which dries up and is later expelled from the meatus by movement of yaw. In people with poor hygiene wax dries up and forms hard impacted mass.
- *Prevents with hearling loss*: Wax impacted patients generally present with impairment of hearing or sense of blocked ear. Tinnitus of giddiness may result from impaction of wax against the drum head.
- *After taking a shower*: It confirms our diagnosis as wax impaction usually presents in this way (as wax swells up by absorbint water).

> **CONFUSA**
> Some times the onset of symptoms may be sudden. This is when water enters the ear canal during bathing or swimming and wax smells up.

Investigation of choice
Otoscopy.

Immediate management
Removal of wax by syringing or instrumental manipulation.

Treatment of choice
Remove wax by syringing or instrumental manipulation. Hard impacted mass may sometimes require prior softening with wax solvents.

Advice hygiene.

Your Notes:

123. Woman presents with deafness and corneal anaesthesia. On MRI, a widened internal auditory meatus is seen.

Diagnosis: Acoustic neuroma.

Clinchers
- *Woman:* No significance. Acoustic neuroma is present equally in both the sexes. It is mostly seen in age group of 40-60 years.
- *Deafness:* Progressive unilateral sensorineural hearing loss often accompanied by tinnitus is the presenting symptom of acoustic neuroma.
- *Corneal anaesthesia:* Acoustic neuroma may uninvolve V, IX, X and XI cranial nerve as it grows. The earliest cranial nerve to be involved is V cranial nerve, presenting with reduced corneal sensitivity, numbness or paraesthesia of face.
- *Widened internal auditory meatus:* Acoustic neuroma, a benign, slow growing tumor of 8th nerve expands and causes widening and erosion of the internal auditory meatus.

CONFUSA
Acoustic neuroma should be differentiated from the cochlear pathology (i.e. Meniere's disease) and other cerebellopontine angle tumours, e.g. meningioma, primary cholesteatoma and arachnoidal cyst.

Treatment of choice
Surgical removal.

Your Notes:

124. Male, 20 years, with history of head injury, bruising on the side of head complains of hearing loss.

Diagnosis: Petrous temporal bone fracture.

Clinchers
- *Head injury:* Head injury can cause hearing loss due to:
  - Ossicular disruption
  - Haemotympanum
  - CSF otorrhoea
  - VIII cranial nerve palsy

All these can occur in fracture of petrous temporal bone which houses the middle ear and VIII nerve.
- *Bruising on side of head:* This almost confimrs our suspicion of pterous temporal bone.

CONFUSA
A complaint of reduced hearing in one ear after trauma points to a haemotypanum most commonly. Blood in the external auditory meatus after trauma is usually caused by basal fracture but is rarely secondary to temporomandibular joint injury. In such cases direct auroscopic examination of the canal should be avoided as it may introduce infection via torn meninges.

Investigation of choice
Skull X-rays (special views).

Immediate management
GCS + admit

Treatment of choice
Usually conservative. For hearing loss discuss with an ENT surgeon.

Your Notes:

125. A 54-year-old female develops mild fever, malaise and ear pain. 3 days later she developed multiple painful vesicles over her ear canal and external meatus.

Diagnosis: Herpes zoster

Clinchers
- *Mild fever, malaise, ear pain:* Fever, malaise signifies viral infection. Herpes zoster oticus is a viral infection involving geniculate ganglion of facial nerve. There may be anaesthesia of face, giddiness and hearing impairment due to involvement of V and VIII nerves.
- *Multiple painful vesicles;* Herpes zoster infection (oticus) is characterised by appearance of vesicles on the tympanic membrane, deep meatus, concha and reteroauricular sulcus. There may be a vesicular rash in the external auditory canal and pinna.

CONFUSA
Nose tip involvement is virtually diagnostic if present in a case of Herpes zoster. It is known as Hutchinsons signs and means involvement of the nasociliary branch of the trigeminal nerve which also supplies the globe and makes it highly likely that the eye will be affected.

Investigation of choice
Fluoroscent antibody tests and Tzank smears (but both rarely needed as the diagnosis is clinically easy).

Immediate management
Keeping cool may reduce the number of lesions. Tell her to avoid scratching. Give adequate analgesia.

Treatment of choice
Aciclovir 800 mg
- five times a day
- for 7 days

Your Notes:

126. A six-year-old boy complains of intermittent hip pain for several months. Hematological investigations are normal. X-rays show flattening of the femoral head.

Diagnosis: Perthes' disease (Legg-Calve-Perthes disease).

Clinchers
- *Six-year-old boy:* Perthes' disease is commonly present in the 3-11 years age group though the usual presentation is at age 4-7 years.
  It is more common in boys and about 15% cases are bilateral. There is a definite familiar tendency and the condition has been described in identical twins.
- *Intermittent hip pain for several months:* In the initial stages, the symptoms tend to be relatively minor. Pain and a limp are usual presenting features. Pain is often slight and may have been present over several weeks or months.
- *Hematological investigations are normal:* Since the disease is secondary to epiphyseal ischaemia and infarction and not due to inflammation, the hematological investigations are usually normal.
- *X-rays show flattening of the femoral head:* This specific feature is caused by localized osteonecrosis. The X-ray changes are characteristic and it is often obvious that the condition has been present for time prior to presentation.

Radiological progression of perthes disease:

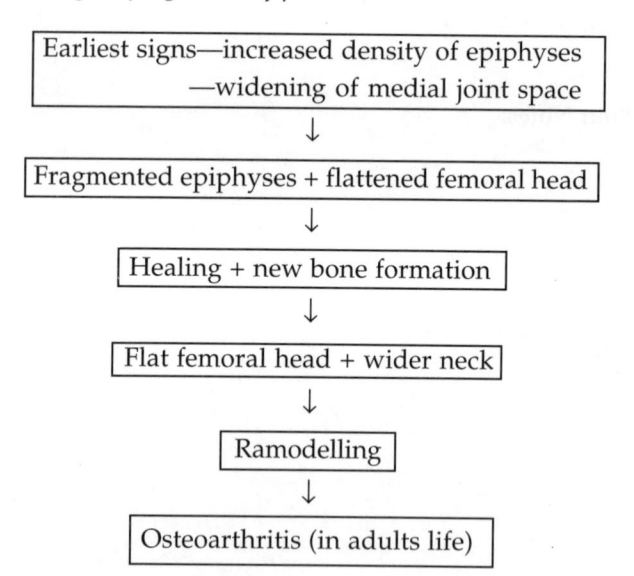

Earliest signs—increased density of epiphyses —widening of medial joint space
↓
Fragmented epiphyses + flattened femoral head
↓
Healing + new bone formation
↓
Flat femoral head + wider neck
↓
Ramodelling
↓
Osteoarthritis (in adults life)

The prognosis is better in
- Younger child
- Partial involvement of head of femur
- Boys.

Investigation of choice
Early X-rays (lateral view)

Immediate management
Admission for observation and rest

Treatment of choice
Depends upon femoral head involvement:
- *<½ of femoral head affected + joint space depth well preserved*—bed rest until pain subsides, followed by X-ray surveillance.
- *>½ of femoral head affected + narrowing of total joint space*—surgery may be considered.

Your Notes:

127. A two-year-old girl with one day history of increasing hip pain has become unable to weight bear. Her WCC is 21/fl, with an ESR of 89 mm/hr and a CRP of 300 mg/l. A radiograph of the hip shows a widened joint space.

Diagnosis: Septic arthritis.

Clinchers
- *Two-year-old girl:* It occurs most commonly below the age of four years. When it occurs in neonates it is known as Smith's arthritis.
- *One day history of increasing hip pain:* In older child it usually presents as an acute fever with extensive pain and spasm in the joint. It is rapid in onset (difference from Perthes' disease).
- *Unable to weight bear:* Child is unable to walk in septic arthritis because of pain (difference from Perthes' disease in which child can walk but with a limb).
- *WCC 21/fl, ESR 89 mm/hr, CRP 300 IU/l:* Normal WCC is 4-11/fl, ESR < 20 mm/hr and CRP < 10 IU/L. Any increase in these inflammatory markers denotes a sepsis somewhere in the body.
- *Radiograph of the hip shows a widened joint space:* Fluid in joint makes the joint space look wide on radiographs. An aspiration will confirm the presence of fluid.

CONFUSA
Differential diagnosis of septic arthritis is from 'irritable hip' and acute onset of Perthes' disease. Rheumatic fever and Still's disease occasionally present initially as a monoarthritis.

Investigation of choice
Diagnostic aspiration and culture of joint.

Immediate management
Joint aspiration, as it releives pain also + Analgesia.

Treatment of choice
Open surgical drainage and appropriate antibiotics.

Your Notes:

128. A 12-year-old boy with left groin pain for 6 weeks is noticed to stand with the left leg externally rotated. Examination reveals negligible internal rotation of the hip.

Diagnosis: Slipped upper femoral epiphyses (SUFE).

Clinchers
- *12-year-old boy:* SUFE is found in older children. The child is frequently overweight and may have delayed sexual development
- *Boys > girls:* It is a bilateral in 24% of patients.
- *Left groin pain for 6 weeks:* Classically symptoms are insiduous in onset, as the displacement is gradual. It is often associated with a limp (like Perthes' disease).
- *Stand with the left leg externally rotated:* External rotation of the limb at rest is pathognomic. Also the limb may be slightly short.
- *Negligible internal rotation of the hip:* Passive internal rotation is characteristically diminished in SUFE.

CONFUSA
The condition may not be apparent in early stages on an AP X-ray, but is detectable on a lateral film. A line drawn through the centre of the femoral neck in any X-ray projection should pass through the centre of the head. If it does not then some displacement has occurred.

Investigation of choice
Special lateral X-ray view
(Findings: Posterior displacement of the upper femoral epiphysis)

Immediate management
Orthopaedics referral.

Treatment of choice
- *Acute symptoms*
  - Traction in internal rotation
  - Alternatively manipulation under GA
- *Chronic symptoms*
  - Pinning
  - If not possible—osteotomy.

Your Notes:

---

129. A four-year-old boy complains of right hip pain a few days following an upper respiratory tract infection. Blood tests are as follows: WCC 12/fl, ESR 10 mm/hr and CRP 2 mg/l.

Diagnosis: Irritable hip syndrome (transient synovitis).

Clinchers
- *Four-year-old boy:* It is essentially a disease of childhood.
- *Right hip pain:* It is because of a sterile effusion in the hip (as it is a type of reactive arthritis).
- *A few days following an upper respiratory tract infection:* It often follows an upper respiratory tract infection.
- *WCC 12/fl, ESR 10 mm/hr and CRP 2 mg/l:* Blood tests are usually normal in irritable hip syndrome. Moreover the children are not systemically ill. Also there are no X-ray changes.

CONFUSA
When there has been unilateral limitation of all hip movements but a spontaneous recovery after bed-rest in the presence of normal X-rays, a retrospective diagnosis of transient synovitis is made. If other joints are involved, consider the diagnosis of juvenile rheumatoid arthritis. Rarely in irritable hip, an X-ray taken several weeks later may show the early changees of Perthes' disease.

Investigation of choice
Microscopy of hip joint aspirate.
(Typical findings: fluid containing WBC but no organisms).

Immediate management
Aspiration of the hip joint (as it reduces pain).

Treatment of choice
Bed-rest + observation.

Your Notes:

130. A five-year-old girl complains of progressively increasing severe pain in her left hip and upper leg for 6 days. She is able to walk but limps visibly. Blood tests are as follows: WCC 19/fl, ESR 72 mm/hr and CRP 94 mg/l. X rays and ultrasound scans of the hip are normal.

Diagnosis: Osteomyelitis (acute).

Clinchers

- *Five-year-old girl:* Acute osteomyelitis occur mainly in children. Poor lining conditions predipose to it, and there may be an obvious primary focus of infection such as a boil, sore throat, etc.
- *Progressively increasing severe pain in her left hip and upper leg for 6 days:* Pain is usually localized to the metaphyseal region of the bone.
- *Able to walk but limps visibly:* There is an unwillingness to move because of pain. There may be a visible limp if area of hip and femur and involved.
- *WCC 19/fl, ESR 72 mm/hr and CRP 94 mg/l:* All the inflammatory markers rise as it is as infective condition.
- *X-rays and ultrasound scans of the hip are normal:* X-ray changes are not apparent for few days but then shows haziness and loss of density of affected bone—subperiosteal reaction—sequestrum and involucrum.

CONFUSA

Osteomyelitis can be difficult to differentiate clinically from septic arthritis. But a typical difference between the two is in walking. In osteomyelitis the child may still be able to walk which is not the case with septic arthritis. Also the pain in osteomyelitis is more chronic in onset and less severe than septic arthritis.

Investigation of choice
MRI.

Immediate management
Send blood culture (positive in 60%).

Treatment of choice
Flucloxacillin 250-500 mg/6hr IVI or IM till sequesterum culture reports are known.

Open surgery to drain abscess and remove sequestera.

Your Notes:

---

131. Patient with atrophic gastritis has megaloblastic anemia.

Diagnosis: Pernicious anemia (PA)

Clinchers

- *Atrophic gastritis:* PA is a condition in which there is atrophy of gastric mucosa with consequent failure of intrinsic factor production and vitamin B_{12} malabsorption.
- *Megaloblastic anemia:* It is characterised by the presence in the bone marrow of erythroblasts with delayed nuclear maturation because of defective DNA synthesis (megaloblasts). Megaloblasts are large (>110 MCV) and have large immature nuclei. The nuclear chromatin is more finely dispensed than normal and has an open stippled appearance. It occurs in:
  - Vitamin B_{12} deficiency or abnormal B_{12} metabolism
  - Folic acid deficiency or abnormal metabolism
  - DNA synthesis defects, i.e.
    - Orotic aciduria
    - Drugs
      - hydroxyurea
      - azathioprine
      - AZT
  - Myelodysplasia due to dyserythropoiesis.

CONFUSA

Beware of diagnosing pernicious anemia in those under 40 years old: look for GI malabsorption with small bowel biopsy in them. Pernicious anemia must always be distinguished from other causes of vitamin B_{12} deficiency. Any disease involving the terminal ileum or bacter overgrowth in the small bowel can produce vitamin B_{12} deficiency. Gastrectomy can lead, in the long term, to vitamin B_{12} deficiency. A careful dietary history should be obtained.

Investigation of choice
Schilling test (expect it to show that < 7% of an oral administered dose of labelled B_{12} is excreted—unless concurrent intrinsic factor is given).

Immediate management
Rule out associated disease i.e.
- Thyroid disease
- Vitiligo
- Addison's disease
- Carcinoma stomach

Treatment of choice
Hydroxycobalamin (B_{12}) IM
- 1 mg alternate days
- For 2 weeks (or, if CNS signs, until improvement stops)
- Maintenance: 1 mg IM every 2 months for life.

132. Patient who is a strict vegetarian has an MCV of 110.

Diagnosis: B_{12} deficiency anaemia

Clinchers
- *Strick vegetarian:* Vitamin B_{12} is synthesized by certain micro-organisms, and humans are ultimately dependent on animal sources. It is found in meat, fish, eggs and milk. No vegetable sources contain B_{12}. Strict vegetarians develop its deficiency if they do not even take milk or milk products.
- *MCV of 110:* This signifies a megaloblastic anemia (criteria: MCV $\geq$ 110). The peripheral blood film shows macrocytes with hypersegmented polymorphs with six or more lobes in the nucleus.

CONFUSA
Causes of vitamin B_{12} deficiency or abnormal metabolism:
I. Low dietary intake
   - Vegans (as is this case)
   - Alcoholics.
II. Impaired absorption
   A. Stomach
      - Pernicious anaemia
      - Gastrectomy
      - Congenital deficiency of IF.
   B. Small bowel
      - Ileal disease or resection
      - Bacterial overgrowth
      - Tropical sprue
      - Fish tapeworm (*Diphyllobrothrium latum*).
   C. Abnormal metabolism
      - Congenital transcobalamin II deficiency
      - Nitrous oxide (inactivates B_{12}).

Note:
- Malabsorption of B_{12} due to pancreatitis, coeliac disease or treatment with metformin is mild and does not usually result in significant vitamin B_{12} deficiency.
- Body stores of vitamin B_{12} are usually sufficient for 3 years.

Investigation of choice
- *Screening:* Deoxyuridine suppression test or Schilling's test.
- *Definitive:* Serum vitamin B_{12} (Normal: 160 ng/L).

Immediate management
Careful and detailed dietary history.

Treatment of choice
Replenish stores with hydroxyocobalamin (B_{12}) (Doses—see previous question).

133. Patient has both Iron and Folate deficiency Radiology sigmoidoscospy—normal, has pale stools which are difficult to flush away.

Diagnosis: Malabsorption (pancreatic insufficiency)

Clinchers
- *Both iron and folate deficiency* Malabsorption produces the signs of following deficiencies:
   - anemia ($\downarrow$Fe, $\downarrow B_{12}$, $\downarrow$folate)
   - bleeding ($\downarrow$vitamin K)
   - edema ($\downarrow$protein).
- *Radiology and sigmoidoscopy normal:* This rules out other causes of malabsorption, e.g. Crohn's disease and coeliac disease.
- *Pale stools which are difficult to flush away:* This suggest pancreatic insufficiency to be the cause.

CONFUSA
Most common cause of malabsorption in UK are:
- Coeliac disease
- Crohn's disease
- Chronic pancreatitis (usually due to alcoholism).

Investigation of choice
USG (dilated biliary tree; stones)

Immediate management
Prescribe low fat diet + take alcohol history

Treatment of choice
As per the causation.

September—2001

134. Elderly patient with complaint of anemia and has bleeding gum.

Diagnosis: Scurvy

Clinchers

- *Elderly:* Vitamin C deficiency is seen mainly in infants fed with boiled milk and in the elderly and single people who cannot be bothered to eat vegetables. It can be seen in UK among Asian countries where people prefer to eat rice and chapatis and also in food faddists.
- *Anemia:* In scurvy the anemia is usually hypochronic but occasionally a normochromic or megaloblastic whether iron deficiency (owing to decreased absorption or loss due to hemorrhage) or folate deficiency (folate being largely found in green vegetables) is present.
- *Bleeding gums:* Swollen, spongy gums with bleeding and super-added infection and loosening of teeth are characteristic of scurvy.

CONFUSA

Humans, along with a few other animals (e.g. primates and the guinea pigs) are unusual in not being able to synthesize ascorbic acid from glucose. Vitamin C is present in all fresh fruits and vegetables. Unfortunately, ascorbic acid is easily leached out of vegetables when they are placed in water and it is also oxidised to dehydroascorbic acid during cooking, exposure to copper or alkalis. Potatoes is a good source and many people eat a lot of them, but vitamin C is lost during storage.

Investigation of choice
Plasma ascorbic acid level (Normal $\geq 11\mu mol/L$)

Immediate management
Detailed dietary history

Treatment of choice
Ascorbic acid
- Initial: 250 mg daily
  - Maintenance: 40 mg daily

135. Elderly patient in residential home a complaints of tiredness.

Diagnosis: Nutritional deficit (most probably)

Clinchers

- *Elderly:* Nutritional deficits in the elderly may be due to many factors such as:
  - Dental problems
  - Lack of cooking skills (particularly in widowers)
  - Depression
  - Lack of motivation
  - Disabilities.
- *Residential home stay:* This will result in vitamin D deficiency. In elderly patients who are confirmed to their houses, vitamin D supplements may be required because often these people do not go into sunlight.
- *Tiredness:* It is a common non-specific symptom of malnutrition.

CONFUSA

The daily energy requirement of elderly people (aged 60 and above, irrespective of age) has been set to approximately $1.5 \times BMR$. The BMR is reduced, owing to a fall in the fat-free mass, from an average of 60 kg to 50 kg in men and from 40 kg to 35 kg in women. The diet should contain the same proportions of nutrients, and essential nutrients are still required. Owing to the high prevalence of osteoporosis in elderly people, daily calcium intake should be 1-1.5 g.

Investigation of choice
Tests for various nutritional deficiencies

Immediate management
A detailed dietary history

Treatment of choice
Prescribe proper diet + treatment of any deficiency.

136. There is minor bleeding from the nose, but the site of bleeding is difficult to localize.

Diagnosis: Epistaxis

Clinchers
In cases of active anterior epistaxis nose is cleared of blood clots by suction, and attempt is made to localise the bleeding sites. In minor bleeds from the accessible sites cauterisation of bleeding area can be done.

When the bleeding is profuse or when site of bleeding is difficult to localise, anterior packing should be done.

CONFUSA
In profuse bleeding and/or when site of bleeding is not localised, anterior packing is the treatment of choice. When the bleeding point has been localised, cauterization is useful in anterior epistaxis.

Investigation of choice
Keep a check on pulse, BP and respiration.

Immediate management
Anterior packing.

Treatment of choice
Investigate and treat the patient for any underlying local or general cause.

Causes of Epistaxis
Local causes:
- Trauma
- Infections
- Foreign body
- Neoplasm of nose of paranasal sinuses
- Atmospheric changes
- Deviated nasal septum

General causes:
- Cardiovascular system (e.g. HT, mitral stenosis, arteriosclerosis).
- Disorder of blood and blood vessels.
- Liver disease (prothrombin deficiency).
- Drugs (Excess salicylates and anticoagulant for heart disease)
- Mediastinal compression
- Vicarious menstruation (epistaxis occurring at time of menstruation.

Your notes:

137. A patient with nose bleeding, on examination vascular damage is found, there is still some leakage.

Diagnosis: Epistaxis

Clinchers
Most of the time bleeding occurs from littles area and can easily be controlled by pinching the nose with thumb and index finger for about 5 minutes. But in this question since on examination, vascular damage is found, this area should be anaesthetised, and bleeding point cauterised with a bead of silver nitrate or coagulated with electrocautery.

It is important to note that whenever the bleeding point is not localised, anterior packing should be done, and when bleeding point is localised, then electrocautery is the better option.

CONFUSA
Anterior packing is preferred when the bleeding point is not localised. Here cauterization is better option.

Investigation of choice
Keep check on pulse, BP and respiration.

Immediate management
Electrocautery

Treatment of choice
Investigate and treat the patient for underlying local or general cause.

Causes of Epistaxis
Refer Q 136.

Your notes:

September—2001

138. Man with prosthetic heart valve presents with epistaxis.

Diagnosis: Anticoagulant overdose.

Clinchers
- *Prosthetic heart valve:* Patients with prosthetic heart valves are treated with anticoagulants, indefinitely.
- *Epistaxis:* Littles area is very prone to bleeding. Here there is convergence of the anterior ethmoidal artery, the septal branches of the sphenopalatine and the superior labial arteries and greater palatine.
  Anticoagulant overdose is an important cause of bleeding tendency (e.g. Warfarin anticoagulation)
  Other causes of epistaxis are degenerative arterial disease and hypertension in older people, and local causes are atrophic rhinitis, hereditary telangiectasia and tumors of the nose of sinuses.

Investigation of choice
INR.

Immediate management
Treat shock and replace blood if necessary.

Treatment of choice
Titrate the dose of anticoagulant for prosthetic heart valve. For epistaxis:
- Apply firm uninterrupted pressure of nostrils f/w finger and thumb for 10 minutes, possibly with ice pack over bridge of nose.
- If still bleeding spray—2.5-10% cocaine solution over mucosa. This will anaesthetize the mucosa and reduce bleeding by constricting vessels. Cauterize any bleeding points.
- Pack the nose.
- If bleeding recurs, further packs.
- Rarely arterial ligation.
- In severe, resistant bleeds, consider embolization of the feeding vessel.

Your Notes:

139. Man who is involved in furniture making presents with recurrent epistaxis and anaesthesia of right cheek.

Diagnosis: Carcinoma of maxillary antrum.

Clinchers
- *Involved in furniture making:* People working in hardwood furniture industry, nickel refining, leather work and manufacture of mustard gas has shown higher incidence of sinunasal cancer.
  Maxillary carcinoma is common in Bantus of South Africa. They use locally made snuff, rich in nickel and chromium.
- *Recurrent epistaxis and anaesthesia of maxillary antrum:* These are the early features of maxillary antrum. Other features are nasal stiffness, blood stained discharge, facial paraesthesia or pain and epiphora.

CONFUSA
Workers of furniture industry develop adenocarcinoma of the ethmoids and upper nasal cavity, while those engaged in nickel refining get squamous cell and anaplastic carcinoma.

Investigation of choice
Radiograph of sinuses. CT scan helps in staging the disease. Biopsy confirm the suspicion of malignancy.

Immediate management
Embolization of feeding vessel as epistaxis of malignancy is not remediable by simple measures.

Treatment of choice
Investigate as above for malignancy. If malignancy proved, histological nature of malignancy is important in deciding the line of treatment, e.g. in squamous cell carcinoma, combination of radiotherapy and surgery gives better result then either alone.

Your Notes:

140. An 80-year-old man with history of epistaxis since 2 hours.

Diagnosis: Hypertension.

Clinchers
- *An 80-year-old man:* Since only age is specified in this question, and no other relevant history is given, we can think of only two important factor, that relate age to epistaxis. They are:
  - Hypertension and
  - Degenerative arterial disease.
- *Since 2 hours:* This further supports our diagnosis of hypertension. Since local causes of epistaxis (atrophic rhinitis, hereditary telangectasia and tumor of nose and sinuses) can be excluded.

Immediate management
Immediate lowering of BP.

Treatment of choice
- For epistaxis refer Q-8 (March 2002)
- For hypertension—hypertension is a major risk factor for stroke and myocardial infarction. Out aim should be for BP < 140/85, but in 130/80 in patients with diabetes.

Your Notes:

141. A 51-year-old man is lethargic and found to be anemic. His blood picture is found to have a granulocytic tendency with an increase in the platelet count.

Diagnosis: Myelofibrosis.

Clinchers
- *51-year-old man:* Usually it occurs in older patients.
- *Lethargic:* The disease presents insidiously with lethargy, weakness and weight loss. Patients often complains of a fullness in the upper abdomen due to splenomegaly.
- *Anemic:* Anemia with leucoerythroblastic features is present. Poikilocytes and red cells with characteristic tear-drop forms are seen. The WBC count may be over 100×10^9/L, and the differential WBC count may be very similar to that seen in CML; later leucopenia may develop.
- *His blood picture is found to have a granulocytic tendency with an increase in the platelet count:* The platelet count may be very high but in later stages, thrombocytopenia occurs. The granulocytic tendency is due to increased WBC counts (see above) with many granulocyte precursors in the peripheral blood.

CONFUSA
The major diagnostic difficulty is the differentiation of myelofibrosis from CML as in both conditions there may be marked splenomegaly and a raised WBC count with many granulocyte precursors in the peripheral blood. The main distinguishing features are the appearance of the bone marrow and the absence of the Philadelphia chromosome in myelofibrosis. Fibrosis of the marrow, often with a leucoerythroblastic anemia, can occur secondarily to leukemia or lymphoma, tuberculosis or malignant infiltration with metastatic carcinoma, or to irradiation.

Investigation of choice
Bone marrow trephine biopsy (show markedly increased fibrosis and megakaryocytes).

Immediate management
Blood transfusion (as he is anemic).

Treatment of choice
- Support blood count + folate + analgesics + allopurinol
- Hydroxyurea/busulfan to reduce high metabolic acitivity and WBC and platelet levels
- Chemotherapy and radiotherapy to reduce slpeen size.

September—2001

142. A 5-year-old boy with generalised lymphadenopathy develops fever and neck stiffness and headache. He is found to have a lot of lymphoblasts in the blood picture.

Diagnosis: Acute lymphoblastic leukemia (ALL)

Clinchers

- *5-year-old boy*
    cALL—2-4 yrs old
    tALL—10-12 yrs old
    ALL is predominantly a disease of children.
- *Generalised lymphadenopathy:* In addition the other usual signs and symptoms are bone pain, arthritis, splenomegaly, thymic enlargement and cranial nerve palsies. Marrow failure produces anemia, infection and bleeding.
- *Fever and neck stiffness and headache:* These are the signs of leukemic meningitis (CNS is also a potential site of relapse ALL, other such sites are testes).
- *Lot of lymphoblasts in the blood picture:* ALL manifests as a neoplastic proliferation of lymphoblasts which is evident in peripheral blood picture.

CONFUSA

Fever per se is absent in ALL (characteristically present in AML). The fever in this case may be due to secondary infections which are usually viral, but Candida, Pneumocystis pneumonia and bacterial septicemia can also occur. Neck stiffness can be feature of subarachnoid haemorrhage and shigella dysentry apart from its most common cause meningitis (leukemic meningitis in this case). But beware of the fact that neck stiffness is usually absent in neonatal meningitis.

Investigation of choice
- *Screening:* Peripheral blood smear.
- *Definitive:* Bone marrow aspiration/biopsy.

Immediate management
- Blood and platelet transfusions
- IV antibiotics at first sign of infection
- Prophylactic neutropenic regimen

Treatment of choice
Chemotherapy (under UK national trials).

Your notes:

---

143. A 55-year-old man with history of hypertension untreated presents with hemiparesis

Diagnosis: Intracerebral haemorrhage.

Clinchers

- *55-year-old man:* Elderly person are more prone to hypertensive complications especially if it is left-untreated. Incidence of hypertension in males is more.
- *History of hypertension untreated:* Intracerebral haemorrhage occurs typically in patients with untreated hypertension. SAH is also associated with hypertension but its association is not so typical and usually present with severe headache and neck stiffness.
- *Presents with hemiparesis:* Focal neurological deficits are more common with intracerebral bleeds (cf SAH) which occurs at well-defined sites (basal ganglia, pons, cerebellum and subcortical white matter) due to rupture of Charcot-Bouchard aneurysms.

CONFUSA

- Hemiplegia/hemiparesis
    - Early—suggests formation of an intracerebral hematoma
    - Late—suggests vasospasm and ischaemia
- Clinically thre is no entirely reliable way of distinguishing between intracerebral hemorrhage and thromboembolic infarction, as both produce a sudden focal deficit. Intracerebral hemorrhage, however, tends to be dramatic and accompanied by a severe headache (but still less severe than that of SAH).

Investigation of choice
Visualized reliably by immediate CT (cf. infarction).

Immediate management
Urgent neurosurgical evacuation of the clot should be considered when an intracerebral hematoma behaves as an expanding mass, causing deepening coma and coning.

Treatment of choice
Unlike thromboembolism antiplatelet drugs are contraindicated. Surgery is indicated if conservative measures fail.

Your notes:

144. A 72-year-old man is having a routine examination. He is found to have a mild lymphocytosis and splenomegaly.

Diagnosis: Chronic myeloid leukemia (CML).

Clinchers
- *72-year-old:* Though it occur most commonly in middle age, old age is no exception for it.
- *Is having a routine examination:* 10% cases of CML are detected by chance. Its symptoms are mostly chronic and insidious, e.g. weight loss, tiredness, gout, fever, sweats, bleeding or abdominal pain.
- *He is found to have a mild lymphocytosis and splenomegaly:* Splenomegaly (often massive) is characteristic of CML (Note: that AML and CML are characterised by early megaly'-spleno and/or hepato-). In the chronic phase of CML, there is only mild lymphocytosis.

CONFUSA
It might be a little difficult to rule out other conditions with such a meagre information but it is safe to diagnose CML. In CLL splenomegaly is a late presentation, i.e. even after the disease can be diagnosed from blood film but in CML the splenomegaly is positive even on presentation.

Investigation of choice
Blood film ± bone marrow aspiration/biopsy.

Immediate management
Hydroxyurea 0.5-2 g/24 h PO.

Treatment of choice
- Allogenic transplantation of bone marrow

Note: But it is attempted only if:
- Patient < 55 years
- Patient is in chronic phase.
- Since the age of this patient is 72 years it will not be attempted.

Your notes:

---

145. A 38-year-old woman presents with cervical lymphadenopathy. Mature lymphoblasts are seen on the blood film. Examination reveals a mild splenomegaly. She is on phenytoin for epilepsy.

Diagnosis: Phenytoin side effects.

Clinchers
- *Cervical lymphadenopathy:* It can occur as a syndrome of hypersensitivity to phenytoin. It includes rashes, DLE and neutropenia. It is rare but requires discontinuation of therapy.
- *Mature lymphoblasts.* It is also a component of the above mentioned hypersensitivity syndrome. It manifest as leukocytosis often with atypical lymphocytes and eosinophils.
- *Mild splenomegaly:* Can occur in phenytoin treatment as a response to various blood dyscrasias phenytoin causes as side effects.

CONFUSA
Acute myeloid leukemia can be excluded as the presenting cells are not myeloblasts. Plus it need bone marrow biopsy for definitive diagnosis. Nevertheless, gum hyperplasia can occur in this condition also in addition to phenytoin therapy. (So even if you are confused, you would not be wrong). Acute lymphoblastic leukemia is characterised by immature lymphoblasts and not mature lymphoblasts (as in this case).
Note: Ciclosporin also causes gum hypertrophy.

Investigation of choice
Phenytoin blood levels (Normal: 40-80 µmol/L).

Immediate management
Systemic steroids to reduce symptoms.

Treatment of choice
Discontinue phenytoin.

Your Notes:

146. A 27-year-old woman has a long-standing history of headaches associated with nausea and vomiting. On this occasion she present with sudden loss of vision in the right half of the visual field. By the time you see her it has improved considerably.

Diagnosis: Migraine

Clinchers

- *27-year-old woman has a long-standing history of headaches:* Onset of migraine is usually in childhood, adolescence or early adulthood; however, initial attack may occur at any age. It is more frequent in women, family history is often positive.
- *Headaches associated with nausea and vomiting:* Classic triad of migraine is:
  1. Premonitoring visual (scotoma or scintillations), sensory or motor symptoms
  2. Unilateral throbbing headache
  3. Nausea and vomiting
- *Sudden loss of vision in the right half of visual field:* Visual symptoms of migraine can be visual chaos (cascading, distortion, melting and jumbling of print lines, dots, spots, zig-zag fortification specta) and hemianopia.
- *By the time you see her it has improved considerably:* Visual symptoms in migraine last for about 15 minutes and then improved. It is generally followed by the headache within one hour.

CONFUSA
TIAs can mimic migraines visual symptoms of migraine.

Investigation of choice
Carotid doppler to rule out TIA.

Immediate management
Dispersible high dose aspirin.

Treatment of choice
Migraine prophylaxis (if attacks > twice/month) with pizotifen.

Note:
- Premenstrual migraine may respond to diuretics or depot oestrogens.
- Contraceptive pill need not be discontinued if migraine is causing no focal pathology.

Your notes:

147. An 82-year-old woman complains of stiffness and muscle pain to the point where she is finding it difficult to brush her hair and get out of a chair. She now presents with sudden loss of vision in her left eye.

Diagnosis: Polymyalgia rheumatica (PMR)

Clinchers

- *82-year-old:* The patient of PMR is always over 50 years.
- *Weakness and muscle pain:* PMR causes a sudden onset of severe pain and stiffness of the shoulders and neck, and of the hips and lumbar spine (a limb girdle pattern).
- *Finding it difficult to brush her hair:* This implies a shoulder girdle weakness as she has difficulty lifting her hand overhead.
- *Difficulty getting out of chair:* This implies a hip girdle weakness.
- *Sudden loss of vision in her left eye:* PMR is associated with temporal arteritis in 25% of people (the patient may have current PMR, a history of rencet PMR, or be on treatment for PMR). Involvement of the ophthalmic arteritis in temporal arteritis causes sudden painless temporary and permanent visual loss.

CONFUSA
It is often difficult to remember the differentiating clinical features of common 'PLAB' myopathies. Here is a refreshes:
Polymyositis—proximal pain and weakness
PMR—Proximal morning stiffness and pain
Myopathy—No pain, no stiffness, only weakness

Investigation of choice
ESR and/or CRP.

Immediate management
Ophthalmology referral urgently.

Treatment of choice
Prednisolone high dose IV immediately.

Your Notes:

148. A woman previously in good health, presents with sudden onset of severe occipital headache and vomiting. Her only physical sign on examination is a shift neck.

Diagnosis: Subarachnoid haemorrhage (SAH)

Clinchers
- *Woman:* Females have a slightly higher incidence of SAH. Lack of estrogen in the postmenopausal females has been cited as a reason.
- *Previously in good health:* Rules out any other medical disorder. Also most of the patient of SAH present with a sudden and spontaneous occurrence with no preceeding disorder. The typical age for SAH is 35-65 years.
- *Sudden onset:* It's onset is sudden (within a few seconds). Some patient may earlier experience a sentinal headache due to small warning leaks from the offending aneurysm.
- *Severe occipital headache:* SAH presents with a devastating headache which the patients usually describe as "the worst headache of my life" or "I thought I had been kicked in the head". It is most commonly occipital. Vomiting may accompany.
- *Stiff neck:* (Kernig's positive). It is a feature of SAH but takes six hours to develop.

CONFUSA
Other differential diagnoses for stiff neck are—Shigella gastroenteritis and meningitis.
- Focal neurology (i.e. hemiplegia) in SAH may give diagnostic clues, e.g.
  - *Early development*—suggests intracerebral hematoma
  - *Late development*—suggests vasospasm and ischaemia

Investigation of choice
Early CT (shows subarachnoid or ventricular blood).

Immediate management
Immediate neurosurgical opinion if
- Consciousness decrease
- Progressive focal deficit
- Suspected cererbellar hematoma

Treatment of choice
Surgical clipping of aneurysms/guglielmi coils
    +
Control hypertension

---

149. A 74-year-old woman had a fall two weeks ago. She is brought into the A and E department with slowly increasing drowsiness. On examination you find mild hemiparesis and unequal pupils.

Diagnosis: Subdural hematoma.

Clinchers
- *74-year-old:* Bridging veins in the skull becomes more prone to rupture in old age. It is due to cortical atrophy producing gradual shrinkage of brain and thereby producing more traction on the veins.
- *Slowly increasing drowsiness:* It means that the hematoma which is now behaving like a SOL (space occupying lesion) is still expanding and there is danger if it is not evacuated urgently.
- *Two weeks ago:* Remember subdural hematomas are usually subdued in appearance i.e. they can occur weeks to months after the initial injury (as the bleeding is from very small veins).
- *Mild hemiparesis and unequal pupils:* Ipsilateral pupillary dilatation is a lagte sign. Focal neurological signs are an indication for urgent intervention.

CONFUSA
Do not rely on absence of ipsilateral pupillary dilatation as it is a late sign. Alteration in the conscious level is the cardinal feature; lateralising signs may be absent or minimal.

Investigation of choice
CT scan is diagnostic, showing a collection with an inner concave border (extradural—binconvex).

Immediate management
Urgent neurological opinion.

Treatment of choice
Surgical evacuation of the hematoma.

Your notes:

150. A 73-year-old man presents with hemianopia, hemisensory loss, hemiparesis and aphasia of 16 hours duration.

Diagnosis: TIA involving the carotids.

Clinchers

- *73-year-old man:* Incidence of TIA increases with age. Most common cause is atherosclerosis.
- *Hemianopia:* Homonymous hemianopia is typical of a carotid territory ischaemia.
- *Hemisensory loss:* Contralateral weakness/numbness is present in *hemiparesis* carotid territory ischaemia.
- *Aphasia:* Dysphasia, aphasia and dysarthria are characteristic pointers for carotid territory ischaemia.
- *Of 16 hours duration:* The sudden onset of focal CNS signs or symptoms due to temporary occlusion, usually by emboli, of part of the cerebral circulation is termed a TIA if symptoms are present for less than 24 hours and fully resolve within this period.

CONFUSA

80% of the TIA are in the carotid territory. Suspect then whenever there is:
- Unilateral paresis
- Unilateral sensory loss
- Aphasia
- Monocular visual loss.

Investigation of choice

CT is usually not indicated in patients over 55 years. Do a routine screen (FBC, ESR, U and E, glucose, ECG, CXR).

Immediate management

Give O_2 + monitor vital signs.

Treatment of choice

Oral aspirin (300 mg) unless contraindicated thereafter 150 mg daily.

Your notes:

---

151. 80-year-old with prostatic carcinoma comes with 4 month history of low backache.

Diagnosis: Metastatic disease.

Clinchers

- *Carcinoma prostate:* Carcinoma of prostate is more usually discovered at a stage when it has already spread beyond its capsule and may have invaded pelvic cellular tissues, bladder base and bone.
- *Low backache for 4 months:* Once the diagnosis of prostate carcinoma has been established, it would be normal to perform a bone scan as part of the staging procedure if the PSA is >20 nmol/mL. If the PSA is < 29 nmol/mL than a bone scan would only be performed on clinical indications (like low backache). So a bone scan is must in this case.

CONFUSA

The bone scan is performed by the injection of technetium-99m, which is then monitored using a gamma camera. It is more sensitive in the diagnosis of metastases than a skeletal survey, but false positives occur in areas of arthritis, osteomyelitis or a healing fracture.

Investigation of choice

Tc^{99} bone scan.

Immediate management

TNM staging of tumor.

Treatment of choice

The main stay of treatment of metastatic prostatic carcinoma is androgen suppression or the use of specific androgen antagonists, which produce symptomatic relief in 75% cases.

Your Notes:

152. Patient with prostatic cancer has been treated, now complains of confusion, thirst, body aches, constipation.

Diagnosis: Hypercalcemia

Clinchers
- *Prostate carcinoma:* It produces osteoblastic metastases to the bone.
- *Has been treated:* The patient might have been operated upon to remove the local disease. The metastases to bone would either have been missed then or have now presented as a recurrence.
- *Confusion, thirst, body aches, constipation:* These all are symptoms of hypercalcemia. Other symptoms and signs can be:
  - Lethargy
  - Anorexia
  - Nausea
  - Polydipsia
  - polyuria
  - Dehydration
  - Weakness.

CONFUSA
Hypercalcemia is produced by following cancers:
- Myeloma (40% cases of hypercalcemia in malignancy)
- Breast
- Prostate
- Bronchus
- Kidney
- Thyroid

Investigation of choice
Serum calcium.

Immediate management
Rehydrate (3-4 litres of 0.9% saline IV over 24 hours)

Treatment of choice
Bisphosphonate IV
- Best treatment is control of underlying malignancy
- Resistant hypercalcemia—calcitonin

Your Notes:

153. Man on GnRH's for prostate cancer comes after 2 months for a follow up.

Diagnosis: Follow-up case of hormone therapy for prostate carcinoma.

Clinchers
- *GnRH for prostate cancer:* GnRH agonists, e.g. buserilin and goserilin, which inhibit the release of luteinizing hormone (LH) from the anterior pituitary, with consequent reduction of testicular production of testosterone. The exact mechanism is

  GnRH agonists
  ↓
  Initially stimulate hypothalamic GnRH receptors
  ↓
  Later down regulation of hypothalamic GnRH receptors
  ↓
  Cessation of pituitary LH production
  ↓
  Decrease in testosterone production to levels akin to castration levels

- *Comes after 2 months for a follow up:* GnRH agonists are usually given in 2-3 month depot injection so the patient has to come every 2 months for follow up. PSA (prostate specific antigen) is the best way to follow the response after hormone therapy.

CONFUSA
Though transrectal USG can also be used for follow up and to measures response to treatment, PSA is the accurate and best way. Transrectal USG will also be used, but as an additional investigation to measure the size and regression.

Investigation of choice
PSA

Immediate management
Check for gynaecomastia or other such side effects of GnRH therapy.

Treatment of choice
Give second depot injection of GnRH agonist.

Your Notes:

September—2001

154. Man with prostate Ca which has extended outside the capsule presenting with features of renal failure.

Diagnosis: Bladder outflow obstruction (BOO).

Clinchers
- *Prostate carcinoma which has extended outside capsule:* It means that it is a locally advanced disease. Bladder base is a frequent site of prostatic metastases. Otherwise also, prostatic enlargement due to carcinomatous growth can produce BOO.
- *Features of renal failure:* The obstruction to outflow of the bladder may result in renal failure with drowsiness, headache and impairment of intellect due to uraemia.

> **CONFUSA**
> Pain is not a symptom of BOO and its presence should prompt the exclusion of acute retention, urinary infection stones carcinoma of the prostate and carcinoma *in situ* of the bladder (1242, Bailey and Love, 23rd edn).

Investigation of choice
Pressure-flow urodynamic studies

Immediate management
Suprapubic catheterisation

Treatment of choice
Prostatectomy.

Your Notes:

155. A man having adenocarcinoma prostate which has already spread to pelvic side walls has to be given chemotherapy.

Diagnosis: Metastatic prostate carcinoma

Clinchers
- *Adenocarcinoma:* This is the most common variety of carcinoma prostate and is usually well-differentiated. Occasionally anaplastic variety is seen.
- *Spread to pelvic side walls:* Carcinoma prostate is more usually discovered at a stage when it has already spread beyond its capsule and may well have involved other organs, particularly the pelvic cellular tissues, bladder base and bone. The mainstay of this disease is androgen suppression or the use of specific androgen antagonists, which will produce symptomatic relief in disseminated prostatic cancer is about 75% of patients.

> **CONFUSA**
> This chemotherapy in this case is most probably stilbesterol, an oestrogen analogue, which is used as primary therapy is majority of cases. It may have feminising side effects such as gynaecomastia, nipple and scrotal pigmentation and testicular atrophy. More importantly, it may result in fluid retention and precipitate congestive cardiac failure, so that in elderly patients with cardiovascular disease bilateral orchidectomy should be performed.

Investigation of choice
Transrectal USG (can assess extracapsular spread)

Immediate management
Rule out heart disease

Treatment of choice
Stilbesterol.

Your Notes:

156. A 65-year-old man presents with severe, retrosternal chest pain and sweating. An ECG shows an acute anterolateral myocardial infarction.

Diagnosis: Acute myocardial infarction (MI).

Clinchers
- *65-year-old man:* The incidence and severity of almost all the risk factors of MI increases with age, hence contributing to increase the risk for MI. Male sex is a definitive risk factor for MI.
- *Severe, retrosternal chest pain:* Pain is the most common presenting complaint. In some instances, the discomfort may be severe enough to be described as the worst pain the patient has even felt. The pain is deep and visceral; adjectives commonly used to describe it are heavy, squeezing and crushing, although occasionally it is described as stabbing or burning. It is similar in character to exertional angina, but usually is more severe and lasts longer (>20 minutes). Typically the pain involves the central portion of the chest and/or the epigastrium, and an occasion it radiates to arms (most commonly), abdomen, back, lower jaw and neck.
- *Severe retrosternal chest pain:* The pain of MI may radiate as high as the occipital area but not below the umbilicus. Painless infarcts also occur especially in:
  - Diabetes mellitus
  - Elderly (present as sudden onset breathlessness, which may progress to pulmonary oedema)
- *Vomiting and sweating:* Due to intense sympathetic stimulation.
- *Anterolateral MI:* If the infarction involves both the anterior and lateral surfaces of heart, a Q wave will be present in V_3 and V_4 and in the leads that look at the lateral surface—I, VL and V_{5-6}.

Investigation of choice
12 lead ECG.

Immediate management
High flow O_2 by face mask (caution, if COPD).

Treatment of choice
IV opiate (5-10 mg), repeated every 5 min.

157. A 70 year old man inoperable gastric cancer causing obstruction, and multiple liver metastases, is taking a large dose of oral analgesia. Despite this, his pain is currently unrelieved.

Diagnosis: Inoperable gastric carcinoma.

Clinchers
- *70-year-old man:* Gastric carcinoma can affect any age but particularly common in 50-70 year age groups (Incidence of most solid organ malignancies increases with age). In general men are more affected.
- *Inoperative gastric cancer:* Unequivocal evidence of incurability are
  - Hematogenous metastases
  - Involvement of distant peritoneum
  - N4 nodal disease
  - Disease beyond N4 nodes
  - Fixation to structures that cannot be removed (It is important to note that the involvement of another organ *per se* does not imply incurability provided it can be removed).
- *Causing obstruction:* The active medial management of malignant bowel obstruction includes:
  - The relief of intestinal colic using an antispasmodic such as hyoscine butylbromide 60-80 mg daily.
  - Treating continuous pain with adequate analgesia such as diamorphine.
  - Treating vomiting if nausea is a problem with a centrally acting antiemetic such as cyclizine 150 mg daily or haloperidol 5-10 mg daily.
- *Multiple liver metastases:* Liver metastases occur hematogenously and hematogenous spread implies inoperability.
- *Taking large dose of oral analgesia but ineffective pain relief:* It can be due to—non-absorption of oral dry due to obstruction

This necessiates the change of mode of administration. For cancer patients, who need long-term analgesia, continuous subcutaneous infusion is the preferred route.

CONFUSA
Diamorphine is preferred for subcutaneous infusion because of its greater solubility). By subcutaneous or intramuscular injection, diamorphine is approximately twice as potent as morphine orally.

Investigation of choice: USG (for obstruction).

Immediate management
Subcutaneous opiate infusion (diamorphine).

Treatment of choice: In patients suffering from significant symptoms of either obstruction or bleeding, palliative resection is appropriate.

158. A 25-year-old woman has just been diagnosed a having rheumatoid arthritis and her rheumatologist has begun giving her gold injections. She continues to complain of joint pain and stiffness, particularly for the first two hours of each day.

Diagnosis: Rheumatoid arthritis (RA).

Clinchers

- *25-year-old:* RA presents from early childhood (rare) to late old age. The most common age of onset is between 30 and 50 years.
- *Woman:* Women before menopause are affected three times more often than men. After the menopause the frequency of onset is similar between the sexes.
- *Gold injections:* gold is a disease modifying antirheumatic drug (DMARD). Usually DMARDs are used after symptomatic treatment, but in seropositive patients with a poor prognosis they should be used early, before the appearance of erosions on X-rays of hands and feet. DMARDs are only prescribed by a rheumatologist in UK. DMARDs exert minimal direct nonspecific anti-inflammatory or analgesic effects, and therefore NSAIDs must be continued during their administration (except in few cases when the true remissions are induced with them).
- *Continues to complain of joint pain and stiffness:* As already explained, DMARDs have very poor analgesic action and NSAIDs have to be given with them. Moreover NSAIDs produce symptomatic improvement in morning stiffness.
- *Particularly in the first two hours of each day:* This is an indirect way to describe the pathognomonic morning stiffness.

CONFUSA

The cheapest and most safe (in terms of propensity to cause GI bleed). NSAID is ibuprofen. Naproxen is an alternative and advantageous in having only twice daily dosage and being more anti-inflammatory. Diclofenac can also be given. NSAIDs should be combined with a gastroprotection agent (proton pump inhibitor or prostaglandin analogue misoprostol) if there is—

- History of
  - peptic ulcer disease
  - dyspepsia.
- Age > 70
- Taking
  - steroids
  - aspirin.

Note: Avoid NSAIDs
- On Warfarin
- Active peptic ulcer disease
- Asthma

Investigation of choice

Rheumatoid factor (often negative initially, if positive at onset, the treatment plan differs—see above).

Immediate management

Physiotherapy referral for exercise programs.

Treatment of choice

Oral NSAIDs

159. A 50-year-old obese man with a known hiatus hernia, presents with recurrent, severe, burning retrosternal chest pain associated with acid regurgitation and increased oral flatulence.

Diagnosis: Gastro-oesophageal reflux disease (GORD)

Clinchers

- *50-year-old:* Hiatus hernia is most common in the elderly, but may occur in young fit people.
- *Obese:* Hiatus hernias probably represent a progressive weakening of the muscles of the hiatus. They occur in obese commonly.
- *Man:* Generally hiatus hernias are four times more common in females than males.
- *Known hiatus hernia:* Incompetence of cardiac sphincter is invariably present in the initial stages of hiatus hernia, but disappear as distortion of the cardia increases. This incompetence leads to GORD.
- *Recurrent, severe, burning retrosternal chest pain:* In GORD there is a burning, retrosternal discomfort that is related to:
  - Meals
  - Lying down
  - Stooping
  - Straining

It is typically relieved by antacids.

- *Acid regurgitation:* This is 'acid brash' and typical of GORD. It can also be due to bile regurgitation. Wather brash is also seen in GORD and is due to excessive salivation.
- *Increased oral flatulence:* This is due to unopposed release of intestinal gas through incomplete lower oesophageal sphincter.

CONFUSA
Gastro-oesophageal reflux occurs as a normal event, and the clinical features of GORD occurs only when the antireflux mechanisms fail sufficiently to allow gastric contents to make prolonged contact with the lower oesophageal mucosa. Hiatus hernia reduce acid clearance of oesophagus owing to trapping of acid within the hernial sac. Moreover a large hiatus hernia can impair the "pinchcork" mechanism of diaphragm. GORD can also occur with hiatus hernia.

Investigation of choice
- *Screening:* Endoscopy ± barium swallow (show hiatus hernia)
- *Definitive:* 24 hr oesophageal pH monitoring + Oesophageal manometry

Immediate management: Proton pump inhibitors

Treatment of choice: Rule out gastric carcinoma (Common at this age)

---

160. A-67-year old woman reports severe paroxysms of knife-like or electric shock-like pain, lasting seconds in the lower part of the right side of her face.

Diagnosis: Trigeminal neuralgia (dic douloureux)

Clinchers

- *67 year old:* It is chiefly a condition of those over 50 years old.
- *Woman:* ♂/♀ > 1
- *Severe paroxysms of knife like or electric shock like pain lasting seconds:* The patient suffers paroxysms of intense, stabbing pain, lasting only seconds in the trigeminal nerve distribution.
- *In the lower part of the right side of her face:* Pain is unilateral, affecting the mandibular and maxillary divisions most often, and the ophthalmic division only rarely. The face may screw up with pain (hence tic douloureux). Pain may recur many times in a day and can often by precipitated by
  - touching the skin of affected area
  - washing
  - shaving
  - eating
  - talking
  - cold wind

CONFUSA
The pain characteristically do not occur at night (contraindication! OHCM, page 335, 5th edn, says it do occur at night—333, 5th edn; Kumar and Clark page 1021, 4th edn. on the contrary—1021, 4th edn). Spontaneous remissions last for months or years before recurrence, which is almost inevitable)

Investigation of choice
Diagnosis is on clinical grounds alone.

Immediate management
Exclude structural causes i.e.
- Multiple sclerosis (suspect when it present in young age)
- Vascular malformation
- Cerebello-pontine angle tumors

Treatment of choice
- Drugs:
  - Carbamazepine
  - Alternatives: Phenytoin, clonazepam
- Surgical: Used when drug therapy fails
  - Radiofrequency ablation of ganglion
  - Neurovascular decompression
  - Sectioning of sensory root
  - Alcohol injection

September—2001

161. An 85-year-old with 14 children, severe heart failure, complains of dysuria, feeling of pressure in lower abdomen.

Diagnosis: Genital prolapse

Clinchers

- *85-year-old:* Prolapse is more evident in older age (i.e. late after menopause) when there is general weakening and shrinking of the supports of the pelvic organs.
- *With 14 children:* Each labour increases the risk of prolapse. It is due to overstretching of the uterine supports during labour.
- *Severe heart failure:* This patient is unfit for operation on medical grounds. So pessary treatment is indicated here.
- *Dysuria:* Urinary symptoms in genital prolapse are:
  - *Frequency of* micturition is common and is often only at day time. Nocturnal frequency may be present if there is added cystitis
  - *Urgency* of micturition due to weakness of the bladder sphincter mechanism and urge incontinence may occur in some cases
  - *Difficulty in emptying:* The bladder completely
  - *Retention of urine* following urethral overstretch
  - *Stress incontinence.*
- *Feeling of pressure in lower abdomen:* A dragging sensation or bearing down in the back or lower abdomen is a common complaint in prolapse. Other associated complaints can be:
  - A feeling of fullness of vagina
  - A lump coming down

CONFUSA
Symptoms similar to those of prolapse may be caused by:
- Varicose veins of the vulva
- Haemorrhoids
- Rectal prolapse
- Cystitis
- Vaginitis with congestion of vulva
- Pressure form a large abdominal tumor

There are a few cases where a ring pessary fails to control prolapse and operation cannot be performed. In these cases use: *Cup and stem pessary.*

Investigation of choice
- Colposcopy
- Urine microscopy and culture if UTI is also suspected

Immediate management
Reassurance that the condition is treatable

Treatment of choice: Plastic ring pessary.

162. Female with well-controlled diabetes mellitus type 2 with recurrent urinary tract infection (UTI).

Diagnosis: Chlamydial UTI

Clinchers

- *Well-controlled diabetes:* Infections in persons with diabetes may not occur more frequently than in non-diabetics but they tend to be more severe, possibly because of impaired leucocyte function, a frequent accompaniment of poor control. But since this case has a well-controlled diabetes, this is also ruled out. Most probably this is a case of recurrent UTI with no identifiable source.
- *Recurrent UTI:* Females have a higher incidence of UTI because of a short urethra which is prone to entry of bacteria during intercourse poor perineal hygiene and the occasional inefficient voiding ability (due to diabetic neuropathy).

CONFUSA
In women with recurrent acute urinary symptoms, pyuria and urine that is sterile (even when obtained by suprapubic aspiration), sexually transmitted urethritis—producing agents such as *Chlamydia trachomatis*, *Neisseria gonorrhoeae*, and herpes simplex virus are etiologically important.

Investigation of choice
- *Screening:* MSU—nitrate stick test
- *Definitive:* MSU—culture (pure growth of more than 10^5 organisms per ml urine).

Immediate management
Rule out diabetic neuropathy (i.e. bladder involvement) and pyelonephritis).

Treatment of choice
Recurrent UTI for which an identifiable source has not been found may be managed by long-term low dose antimicrobial therapy, such as trimethoprim. Ciprofloxacin or norfloxacin can be alternatives.

Your Notes:

163. A young female with long-standing irregular bowel habit and persistent UTI.

Diagnosis: Probable Crohn's disease (CD)

Clinchers
- *Young female:* CD has peak incidence at between 20 and 40 years. It is uncommon before the age of 10 years and both sexes are equally affected.
- *Long-standing irregular bowel habit:* The major symptom of inflammatory bowel disease (including CD) is irregular bowel habit. Mainly it presents as diarrhoea, abdominal pain and weight loss.
- *Persistent UTI:* Fistula formation is common in CD and it may atypically present with symptoms of fistula rather than those of bowel. Although uncommon a persistent UTI in the setting of CD, should be suspected to be due to enterovesical fistula.

CONFUSA
Pneumaturia (air in the urine) present as bubbling while micturition and is a definitive symptom of enterovesicle fistula. Other causes of enterovescile fistula can be malignancy and regional enteritis (chronic). Irritable bowel disease can also cause UTI (due to impaired local hygiene) but that will be recurrent rather than persistent.

Investigation of choice
Small bowel barium enema

Immediate management
High dose urinary antibacterials

Treatment of choice
Surgical closure of fistula

Your Notes:

---

164. An 80-year-old sexually active woman with dyspareunia and recurrent dysuria.

Diagnosis: Atrophic vaginitis

Clinchers
- *80-year-old:* This condition is always seen postmenopausally because of lack of oestrogens.
- *Sexually active women:* Because of vaginal wall dryness and thinning, there can be discomfort during intercourse. If the woman would not have been sexually active, atrophic vaginitis, if mild, would have been asymptomatic.
- *Dyspareunia:* There is *superficial* dyspareunia in this condition.
- *Recurrent dysuria:* Low grade infection can coexist with atrophic vaginitis.

CONFUSA
Hormone replacement therapy postmenopausally produces withdrawal bleeds. Topical estorgens are enough to thicken the epithelium and reduce the pH, but insufficient to produce excessive endometrial stimulation or other causes of bleeding.

Investigation of choice
Urine culture and sensitivity

Immediate management
Advice topical lubrication during coitus.

Treatment of choice
- If there is secondary infection, antibiotics to which the organism is sensitive may be given
- Topical oestrogen creams or pessaries (e.g. dienoestrol or premarin (once or twice a week)

Your Notes:

165. A middle-aged woman with a vaginal discharge is found to have several ulcers at the vaginal introitus.

Diagnosis: Herpes labialis

Clinchers
- *Middle-aged woman:* Herpes labialis is most common in sexually active females, so its incidence is characteristically minimal in children and elderly.
- *Vaginal discharge:* Pain, itching, dysuria, vaginal and urethral discharge, and tender inguinal lymphadenopathy are the predominant local symptoms.
- *Several ulcers of the vaginal introitus:* Widely spaced bilateral lesions of the external genitalia are characteristic. In it painful vesicles develop initially which then coalesce into multiple ulcers.

CONFUSA
First episodes of genital herpes in patients who have had prior HSV-1 infection are associated with less frequent systemic symptoms and faster healing than primary genital herpes. In primary herpes, if the case is seen very early it may only affect a small part of the vulva appearing to be a recurrent episode. It is sensible therefore to routinely prescribe a course of antiviral medication for five days for all patients presenting with first attack, even if the clinical suspicion is of a secondary episode.

Investigation of choice
Culture/electron microscopy.

Immediate management
Rule out any past history of genital herpes.

Treatment of choice
Aciclovir 200 mg, 5 times a day for five days
+ Analgesics
+ bathing in salt water
+ lignocaine gel.

Your Notes:

166. A 20-year-old woman who has been on oral contraceptive develops bright red postcoital bleeding (PCB).

Diagnosis: Cervical ectropion

Clinchers
- *OCP:* Ectocervix contain a transformation zone, where the stratified squamous epithelium of the vagina meets the columnar epithelium of the cervical canal. The anatomical site of this squamocolumnar junction fluctuates under hormonal influence, and the high turnover of this tissue is important in the pathogenesis of cervical carcinoma. The columnar epithelium is normally visible with the speculum during
  - Ovulatory phase of menstrual cycle
  - Pregnancy
  - OCP use
- *Postcoital bleeding:* It may give rise to postcoital bleeding, as fine blood vessels, within the columnar epithelium are easily traumatised.

CONFUSA
Cervical ectropion is sometimes termed as cervical erosion. Usually the main complaint of cervical ectropion is excessive nonpurulent discharge, as the surface area of the columnar epithelium containing mucus glands is increased. It may give rise to spotting during pregnancy in which case it is usually left untreated till after the pregnancy.

Investigation of choice
Per speculum exam (red ring around OS because the endocervical epithelium has extended its territory over the paler epithelium of the ectocervix).

Immediate management
Reassurance about cause and treatment.

Treatment of choice
Usually none required.
If symptoms are distressing
- Thermal cautery (sometimes confusingly called cold coagulation).

Your Notes:

167. A 55-year-old female develops a single episode of postmenopausal bleeding. She stopped menstruation 7 years ago. Ultrasound shows endometrial thickness.

Diagnosis: Endometrial carcinoma

Clinchers
- *55 years old:* It usually presents after the menopause.
- *Single episode of postmenopausal bleeding:* Any postmenopausal vaginal bleeding must be investigated as the cause may be endometrial carcinomas.
- *Stopped menstruation 7 years ago:* Occasional bleeding is common upto 1 year after menopause but not upto 7 years.
- *USG shows endometrial thickness:* This clearly suggest endometrial growth and hence indicate a need to obtain the tissue diagnosis.

> **CONFUSA**
> Postmenopausal bleeding is an early sign and generally leads a woman to see her doctor, but examination is usually normal. Endometrial carcinoma is less common than carcinoma of cervix. Most endometrial tumors are adenocarcinomas and are related to excessive exposure to oestrogens unopposed by progesterone.

Investigation of choice
Uterine sampling or curettage

Immediate management
Take detailed history

Treatment of choice
- Stage I and II—total hysterectomy with bilateral salpingo-oophorectomy
- Inoperable cases—radiotherapy

168. A 49-year-old woman with complaint of hot flushes, vaginal dryness and her menstruation become irregular 5 months ago.

Diagnosis: Menopause

Clinchers
- *49-year-old:* The manopause or cessation of periods, naturally occurs about the age of 45-55 years.
- *Hot flushes, vaginal dryness:* Features of oestrogen deficiency are hot flushes (which occurs in most women and can be disabling), vaginal dryness and atrophy of the breasts. There may also be vague symptoms of loss of libido, loss of self-esteem, nonspecific, aches and pains, irritability, depression, loss of concentration and weight gain.
- *Menstruation become irregular 5 months ago:* Most women notice irregular scanty periods carrying on over a variable period, though in some sudden amenorrhoea or menorrhagia occur.

> **CONFUSA**
> Menopause may also occur surgically with radiotherapy to the ovaries and with ovarian disease (e.g. premature menopause).

Investigation of choice
Urinary FSH concentration (↑)-Just to reassure her that these are not symptoms of some pathology

Immediate management
Reassurance and counselling

Treatment of choice
Option of hormone replacement therapy

169. A 14-year-old women with painless vaginal bleeding.

Diagnosis: Menarche

Clinchers

- *14-year-old:* Menarche usually occurs at age of 11-15 years.
- *Painless vaginal bleeding:* In this age group it most commonly represents menarche though any traumatic bleed must also be excluded.

CONFUSA
In girls events of puberty start age of 9-13 years with breast bud enlargement and continues to 12-18 years. Pubic hair commences at ages 9-14 years and is completed at 12-16 years. Menarche occurs relatively late (11-15 years) but peak height velocity is reached much earlier than in boys (10-13 years). Growth is completed earlier than in boys.

Investigation of choice
None required usually

Immediate management
Exclude traumatic bleed

Treatment of choice
None

---

170. A 55-year-old lady with history of intermittent postmenopausal bleeding. Vaginal and speulum examinations are normal.

Diagnosis: Endometrial carcinoma

Clinchers

- *A 55-year-old:* Mean age of presentation is 56 years. It is rare under the age of 40.
- *Intermittent postmenopausal bleeding:* This symptom should always be assumed to be caused by carcinoma of endometrium until proven otherwise.
- *Vaginal and speculum examination are normal:* This has ruled out any local cause of bleeding (e.g. vaginal trauma) so this warrants examination of the endometrium now.

CONFUSA
Endometrial carcinoma is associated with hyperestrogenic states, i.e.
- Obesity
- Diabetes
- Late menopause
- Prolonged use of unopposed oestrogens
- Oestrogen secreting tumors

Investigation of choice
- *Screening:* Ultrasound (to assess dimensions of any tumor and to show endometrial thickness)
- *Definitive:* Uterine sampling or curettage

Immediate management
Perform staging to decide the line of treatment.

Treatment of choice
Usually surgical

Uterus	Tumor	Surgery
Small	Well differentiated	Total abdominal hysterectomy + bilateral salpingo-oophorectomy + internal iliac node frozen section biopsy
Enlarged	Confined to upper part of corpus	Extended hysterectomy + bilateral salpingo-oophorectomy + removal of a cuff of vagina + lymph node sampling
Cervix invaded		Wertheim's (Removal of upper lost half of the vagina and pelvic lymph node)

- *Radiotherapy*
    - If node is involved
    - If there is deep invasion of myometrium
- *Hormone therapy:* Progestogens inhibit the rate of growth and spread of endometrial carcinoma.

171. A 73-year-old complains of a severe right sided headache associated with an acute loss of right sided vision. Urgent treatment is needed to prevent left sided vision loss

Diagnosis: Giant cell arteritis (GCA).

Clinchers
- *73-year-old:* Cranial arteritis is common after 55 years of age (60 years according to Kumar and Clark).
- *Severe right sided headache:* Headache is almost invariable in GCA. Pain is felt over the inflamed superficial, temporal or occipital arteries. Though the disease process ultimately involves arteries bilaterally, in the initial stages it is usually unilateral.
- *Associated with an acute loss of right sided vision:* Visual loss owing to inflammation and occlusion of the ciliary and/or central retinal artery occurs in 25% of cases and untreated GCA. It is characteristically sudden, painless, partial or complete, uniocular visual loss. Amaurosis fugax may precede total visual loss.
- *Urgent treatment is needed to prevent left sided vision loss:* Urgent GCA patients need to have an ESR and high dose. Oral steroids immediately. However if visual symptoms are present, give higher doses IV as it could be sight saving.

CONFUSA
Other forms of arteritis, such as SLE and PAN, can occasionally present with similar features (but PLAB questions on GCA are usually straight forward). Also note that GCA is closely related to polymyalgia rheumatica and these can occur in the same patient.

Investigation of choice
- *Screening:* ESR.
- *Definitive:* Temporal artery biopsy (skip lesions occur, so repeat any negative biopsy if there are strong clinical pointers)

Immediate management
Two things are to be done immediately"
1. ESR
2. High dose oral steroids (IV if visual symptoms).

Treatment of choice
Prednisolone, 40-60 mg/24h, PO
- Dose is reduced as ESR falls/is increased if symptoms recurs.
- Headache subsides within hours of first large dose.
- Remission in 2 years usually.
- Steroid treatment is the main cause of death in long-term in GCA patients.

172. A 75-year-old has difficulty watching television complaining of a peripheral constriction of vision. On examination there is cupping of both optical discs

Diagnosis: Chronic simple glaucoma (CSG).

Clinchers
- *75-year-old:* CSG risk increases with increasing age.
- *Difficulty watching television:* CSG can produce intermittent blurring of vision or peripheral constriction of visual field, both of which can interfere in sight.
- *Complaining of a peripheral constriction of vision:* Characteristic of CSG. Nasal and superior fields are lost first with the last vision remaining in the temporal field. Since the central field is intact, good acuity is maintained.
- *On examination there is cupping of both optical discs:* Intraocular pressure >21 mmHg causes optic disc cupping ± capillary closure, hence nerve damage, with sausage-shaped field defects (scotomata) near the blind spot, which may then coalesce to form major defects. Normal optic cups are similar in both eyes in shape and occupy < 50% of optic disc. In glaucoma these enlarge (widens and deepens) and optic disc pales (atrophy).

CONFUSA
Simple glaucoma is asympatomatic until visual fields are severely and irreversibly impaired. Some people may get glaucoma with normal intraocular pressure (IOP).

Investigation of choice
IOP measurement + perimetry.

Immediate management
Dorzolamide (if IOP ↑)

Treatment of choice
- Medical reduction of IOP (i.e. timolol)
- Surgery if medical intervention fails (flap valve trabeculectomy)

Note: In older patient (like this case) Argon laser trabeculoplasty is preferred over surgery.

Your notes:

173. A 50-year-old with a history of SLE complains of loss of vision. On examination he is found to have multiple opacities in the lens of his eyes

Diagnosis: Cataract.

Clinchers

- *History of SLE:* SLE is nonorgan specific due to immune disease in which antinuclear antibodies (ANA) occurs. There is no direct relationship between SLE and opacities in the lens. Though retinal exudates are sometimes seen in SLE patients.
- *In this question, since it is a diagnosed case of SLE:* We presume that patient is on treatment. Steroids are the most commonly prescribed drugs in SLE. This question could be explained on this basis (corticosteroid induced cataract).
- *Multiple opacities in the lens of his eyes:* These are associated with the use of topical as well as systemic steroids. Prolonged use of steroids may result in cataract formation.

CONFUSA
Since the patient is 50-year-old, it can well be a senile cataract also.

Immediate management
- Decrease the dose of steroids.
- Low dose steroids have value in chronic disease.

Treatment of choice
For cataract: ECCE with PCIOL.

Your notes:

---

174. A diabetic on oral hypoglycemics complains of sudden deterioration in vision of his right eye. On examination he is found to have bilateral proliferative retinopathy with retinal hemorrhage on the right side.

Diagnosis: Vitreous hemorrhage.

Clinchers

- *Diabetic:* The most common and characteristic form of involvement of eye in diabetes is retinopathy. Diabetes is the leading cause of blindness in UK in those aged 20-65.
- *On oral hypoglycemics:* Oral hypoglycemics does not have any specific visual side effects.
- *Complains of sudden deterioration in vision of his right eye:* The cause of it must be vitreous hemorrhage.
- *Bilateral proliferative retinopathy with retinal hemorrhage on the right side:* High retinal blood flow induces a microangiopathy in capillaries, precapillary arterioles and venules, causing occlusion and leakage. Occlusion causes ischaemia which leads to new vessel formation in the retina, the optic disc and on the iris, i.e. proliferative retinopathy. New vessels can bleed, causing vitreous hemorrhage. Rupture of micro-aneurysms causes retinal hemorrhages, flame hemorrhages when at nerve root level, blot hemorrhage when deep in retina.

CONFUSA
Although retinal detachment (which is also common in diabetic retinopathy) can present with same picture, it will be evident on fundoscopy which has been done in this case.

Investigation of choice
Fundus fluorescein angiography to elucidate areas of neovascularisation, leakage and capillary non-perfusion.

Immediate management
Control of hypertension (usually associated and can deteriorate a case of vitreous hemorrhage) + refer urgently to ophthalmologist.

Treatment of choice
If vitreous hemorrhage is massive and does not clear, surgical vitrectomy may be needed. Otherwise do photocoagulation.

Your notes:

175. An 80-year-old has markedly decreased visual acuity. On fundoscopy she is found to have bilateral macular pigmentation.

Diagnosis: Senile macular degeneration (SMD).

Clinchers
- *80-year-old:* As the name suggests it occurs in elderly people. It is the most common cause of registrable blindness in UK. Usually it occurs above 65 years age.
- *Markedly decreased visual acuity:* Loss of central vision (hence visual acuity) is the main presenting complaint in SMD. Visual fields are unaffected.
- *Bilateral macular pigmentation:* SMD is a bilateral disease. The disc appears normal but there is pigment, fine exudate and hemorrhage at the macula. It is of two types—exudative and nonexudative. Drusen of Bruch's membrane is one of the earliest findings in the macula, varying in size, shape and colour. Drusen need not result in visual loss, and visual impairment may occur associated with a generalised pigmentary granularity and/or with atrophy of retinal pigment epithelium, photoreceptors and choriocapillaries.

CONFUSA
Though it is a bilateral disease, the fellow eye may appear quite different in its fundus appearance. Macula holes are an uncommon type of macula degeneration, which may present with distorted vision as well as visual loss.

Investigation of choice
Fundoscopy by an expert.

Immediate management
None except counselling.

Treatment of choice
For most there is no effective treatment (especially for nonexudative SMD).
Laser photocoagulation is indicated in patients with exudative SMD having foveal choroidal neovascularisation to prevent further loss of vision.

Your notes:

176. A middle-aged woman with a history of rheumatoid arthritis develops sudden swelling in One of her knees. This knee is swollen and hot to touch.

Diagnosis: Pseudogout.

Clinchers
- *Middle-aged:* Though pseudogout occurs more commonly in old age, no age after thirties is exempt from it.
- *Woman:* There is a slight preponderance of female incidence.
- *Sudden swelling in one of her knees:* Knee is the main joint to get involved in it. A minority will have involvement of multiple joints.
- *This knee is swollen and hot to touch:* involved joint is erythematous, swollen, warm and painful.
- *History of rheumatoid arthritis:* Any existing arthritis is a risk factor for pseudogout. Other risk factors are old age, dehydration, intercurrent illness, hyperparathyroidism, myxoedema, diabetes mellitus, phosphate decrease, magnesium deficiency, hemochromatosis, acromegaly, gout, ochronosis, surgery.

CONFUSA
Acute pseudogout is less severe and longer lasting than gout and affects different joints. Pseudogout can even be secondary to gout. It cannot be septic arthritis also as there is no preceding history of joint trauma of presence of fever.

Investigation of choice
- *Screening:* Wrist X-ray (calcium deposition in triangular ligament or chondrocalcinosis)
- *Definitive:* Joint fluid aspiration and microscopy (positively birefringent calcium pyrophosphate crystals in plane polarised light).

Immediate management
Analgesia.

Treatment of choice
NSAIDs ± intra-articular injection of glucocorticoids ± colchicine.

Your Notes:

177. An elderly man with recently diagnosed heart failure has been treated with diuretics. He now develops severe joint pain in his left ankle with swelling and redness.

Diagnosis: Gout (acute attack).

Clinchers
- *Diuretics:* Attacks of gout can be precipitated by:
  - Trauma
  - Surgery/some antibiotics
  - Starvation/purine rich foods (liver, offal, oily fish)
  - Infection
  - Diuretics
  - Alcohol
- *Severe joint pain in his left ankle:* Gout produces an acute inflammatory arthritis which is exquisitely painful monoarthritis (usually) but can be polyarticular also. It is often accompanied by fever. It usually affects the distal joints of the hands and feet and the knees. It particularly (and characteristically) affects the metatarso-phalangeal joints of the great toes.
- *Swelling and redness of ankle:* In acute attacks the affected joints, usually single, become severely painful, swollen, often red and impossible to move. This usually settles in less than three weeks.

CONFUSA
Gout is a chronic disease, but is characterised by acute attacks. Predisposing conditions to gout can be blood dyscrasias such as myeloid leukemia and polycythaemia. Most common extra-articular complication of gout is recurrent renal stones. Paradoxically renal failure can be a cause for gout.

Investigation of choice
Synovial fluid microscopy (urate crystals—negatively birefringent).

Immediate management
Pain relief by NSAID (Ibuprofen/Naproxen)
- If NSAID contraindicated—colchicine
- If cholchicine contraindicated—streroids

Treatment of choice
Allopurinol (but not until 3 weeks after an attack).

Note: Aspirin is absolutely contraindicated in gout.

Your Notes:

178. A 78-year-old woman complains of a stiff left hip joint after walking some distance. This is Most evident when she attempts to abduct the hip joint (limited abduction).

Diagnosis: Osteoarthritis (OA).

Clinchers
- *78-year-old woman:* The mean age of onset of OA is 5 years. OA is sympatomatic three times more in women.
- *Shift hip joint after walking some distance:* Typically in OA, there is pain on movement. It is usually worse at end of day. There may be some background pain at rest.
- *Limited adduction of hip joint:* There can be stiffness of the joint which limits the movements (poor range of movements). There can be associated joint instability.
Joints affected in OA
  - Most commonly: DIP joints, first MCP joint, cervical and lumbar spine
  - Next most common: Hip joint
  - Other most common: Knee joint.

CONFUSA
Lets have a good look at the differentiating features of osteoarthritis and rheumatoid arthritis, the two most common arthritis of elderly females

	OA	RA
Joint stiffness	Late evening	Early evening
Palpable osteophytes	+	-
Skin redness	+/-	+
Swelling	+/-	+
Ligaments stretch	-	+
Age	Usually older	Usually adolescents
Arthrodesis use	Good	Poor
Fibrillation	+	-
Pannus	-	+
Bone arround joint	Sclerotic	Osteoporotic
Joint deformity	Varus	Valgus

Investigation of choice
Joint X-ray (findings: Loss of joint space, Subchondral sclerosis, Subchondral cysts, Marginal osteophytes).

Immediate management: Paracetamol for pain.

Treatment of choice
Reduce weight + walking aid
- Contralateral hand—for hip
- Ipsilateral hand—for knee
- Joint replacement is done for end stage disease.
- If PCM does not bring relief from pain, then give
  - Day pain—NSAID
  - Night pain—TCA in low doses (tricyclic antidepressant)

179. A 34-year-old woman complains of bilateral stiff and painful joints in her hands and feet.

Diagnosis: Rheumatoid arthritis (RA)

Clinchers
- *34-year-old woman:* Although the peak onset of RA is fifth decade, no age is exempt from it. The incidence of RA is three times more in women.
- *Bilateral:* RA is a symmetrical arthropathy, i.e. affect the same joints bilaterally.
- *Stiff and painful joints in her hands and feet:* RA presents typically with swollen, painful and stiff hands and feet, especially in the morning. This gradually gets and feet, especially in the morning. This gradually gets worse and large joints become involved

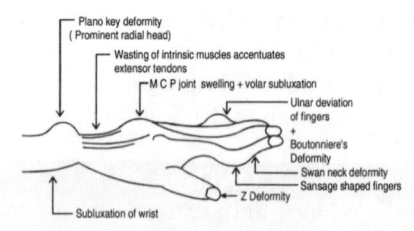

Fig. "Handy" thesaurus for signs of RA

CONFUSA
In the PLAB exams, Felty's syndrome has been indirectly asked on at least a couple of occasions. So always keep an eye open for any mention of splenomegaly in a patient of RA.
(Felty's syndrome: RA + Splenomegaly + WCC ↓)

Investigation of choice
Rheumatoid factor often negative at start, but becomes positive in 80% over the time. But note that it may be false positive in several other chronic diseases.

Immediate management
Analgesia.

Treatment of choice
- Naproxen/Ibuprofen
- Disease modifying drugs if:
  - 12 week trial of 3 NSAIDs do not control pain.
  - Synovitis > 2 months.

Your Notes:

---

180. A 67-year-old woman complains of right hip pain. On examination the right hip is adducted, externally rotated and flexed.

Diagnosis: Fracture neck of femur.

Clinchers
- *67-year-old woman:* Osteoporosis is the main cause of spontaneous fractures of neck of femur in elderlies (as it is a weight bearing joint). Usually females are more prone to fracture neck of femur in old age.
- *Right hip pain:* There is pain in the hip, thigh or knee but may be little to see on local examination.
- *Right hip is adducted, externally rotated and flexed:* The affected leg may be shortened and externally rotated but this classical appearance is dependent on the grade of the fracture. A more valuable sign is pain on gental passive rotation of the extended leg. If the fracture has impacted, other movements may be good with minimal pain including even straight leg raising. Tenderness is most marked posteriorly.

CONFUSA
There are three circumstances in which fracture neck of femur occurs:
1. At any age: Associated with major voilence and multiple injuries
2. In the elderly: After a simple fall.
3. Spontaneously: As a result of osteoporosis or bony secondary deposits.

Investigation of choice
X-ray
- AP view of hips and pelvis
- Lateral view of affected hip.

Immediate management
A box splint to control leg movements + Analgesia.

Treatment of choice
Internal fixation or hemiarthroplasty is usually performed within 24 hours.

Your Notes:

181. Patient, 12 hours after MI presents with recurrent chest pain, breathlessness, heart rate—40/min.

Diagnosis: Heart block with haemodynamic compromise

Clinchers
- *12 hours after MI:* It means that it must be an acute complication of MI. Complication of MI in acute phase (i.e. within first two or three days following MI are—cardiac arrhythmia, cardiac failure and pericarditis. Late complications of MI are post-myocardiac infarction syndrome (Dressler's syndrome), ventricular aneurysm, and recurrent cardiac arrhythmias.
- *Recurrent chest pain and breathlessness:* These are the symptomatologies of the associated haemodynamic compromise.
- *Heart rate—40/min:* It is low as bradycardia is present.

CONFUSA
Condition of heart block in this patient may require pace maker insertion. But it may not be necessary after inferior MI if:
- QRS is narrow and reasonably stable
- And pulse ≥ 40-50 (as in this patient).

A more detailed evaluation is required to consider pacemaker insertion in this patient.

Investigation of choice
ECG monitoring

Immediate management
Atropine IV (0.5 mg initial, upto 2.0 mg total)

Treatment of choice
Persistent bradycardia (<40 bpm) despite atropine is treated with electrical pacing.

Your Notes:

182. Patient with pulmonary edema features presents with irregular pulse, heart rate—140 bpm.

Diagnosis: Acute atrial fibrillation (AF)

Clinchers
- *Pulmonary oedema:* It is indicative of heart failure. Heart failure usually precipitates AF due to atrial irritation.
- *Irregular pulse:* The pulse in AF is characteristically irregularly irregular, the apical pulse rate is greater than radial rate and the first heart sound is of variable intensity.
- *Heart rate—140/bpm:* AF is a chaotic, irregular atrial rhythm at 300-600 bpm. But radial pulse is always lesser. It is so as the AV node responds intermittently producing an irregular ventricular rate.

CONFUSA
Atrial fibrillation is an early complication of myocardial infarction, occurring in about 10% patients. Apart from heart failure, other precipitants of AF can be
- Pericarditis
- Acute ischaemia or infarction

Investigation of choice
ECG (absent P waves; irregular QRS complexes)

Immediate management
IV digoxin or IV amiodarone

Treatment of choice
Treatment of underlying pathology (in this case, heart failure).

Your Notes:

First Aid for PLAB

183. A woman 10 days following hysterectomy complaints of severe left sided chest pain and breathlessness. Chest X-ray and ECG failed to relieve any abnormality.

Diagnosis: Pulmonary embolism.

Clinchers
➤ *10 days following hysterectomy:* Any cause of immobility or hypercoagulability, e.g. recent surgery (in this case hysterectomy), recent stroke or MI, disseminated malignancy, thrombophilia/antiphospholipid syndrome, prolonged bed-rest and pregnancy.
➤ *Severe left chest pain/breathlessness:* Symptoms of pulmonary embolism are—acute breathless, pleuritic chest pain, hemoptysis, dizziness and syncope.
➤ *Chest X-ray and ECG show no abnormality:* Chest X-ray and ECG is generally normal in pulmonary embolism.

Investigation of choice
- *Screening:* V/Q scan or spiral CT.
- *Definitive:* CT pulmonary angiography. This shows clots down to 5th order pulmonary arteries.

Immediate management
Screen for DVT.

Treatment of choice
Anticoagulation.

Your Notes:

---

184. 10 days after MI, female presents with chest pain on inspiration, persistently elevated ST segment on ECG.

Diagnosis: Acute pericarditis

Clinchers
➤ *10 days after MI:* Acute pericarditis is common in the first few days after MI, particularly in anterior wall infarction.
➤ *Chest pain on inspiration:* It is characterised by sharp chest pain, aggravated by
- Movement
- Respiration
- Lying down (characteristic)

➤ *Persistently elevated ST segment:* ECG in acute pericarditis shows generalised ST segment elevation (concave upward) with upright, peaked T waves.

CONFUSA
Sequence of ECG changes in MI are:
1. Normal ECG
2. ST elevation
3. Appearance of Q waves
4. Normalization of ST segments
5. Inversion of T waves

So ST elevation is a normal feature in MI. However, if it remains persistently elevated, always suspect pericarditis, especially with saddle-shaped ST elevation.
Note:
- In pericarditis after MI, anticoagulation is avoided.
- In case of recurrent pericarditis, suspect Dressler's syndrome.

Investigation of choice
ECG (already done in this patient).
Each to check effusions.

Immediate management
Stop anticoagulation if continuing after MI.

Treatment of choice
NSAIDs.

Your Notes:

185. Patient after MI found to have a harsh pansystolic murmur at the apex.

Diagnosis: Papillary muscle rupture.

Clinchers
- *After MI:* Mitral valve papillary muscle rupture is common complication of MI.
- *Harsh pansystolic murmur at apex:* It is due to mitral regurgitation. It can also be a finding in ventricular septal perforation, more common than papillary muscle rupture, after MI. A systolic thrill may be found in both the cases.

CONFUSA
The cardiac rupture syndrome results from the mechanical weakening that occurs in necrotic and subsequently inflamed myocardium and includes:
1. *Rupture of ventricular free wall (**most common**)*—with haemopericardium and cardiac tamponade and usually fatal.
2. *Rupture of ventricular septum (less commonly)*—leading to a left to right shunt.
3. *Papillary muscle rupture (least common)*—resulting in acute onset of severe mitral regurgitation.

Note:
- Pansystolic murmur can be heard in (2) and (3).
- ECG is usually normal in cardiac rupture.

Investigation of choice
Echocardiography (colour flow doppler)

Immediate management
Lowering aortic systolic pressure
- Intraortic balloon counter pulsation
- Nitroglycerin/Nitroprusside

Treatment of choice
Surgical repair/mitral valve repalcement.

Your Notes:

---

186. 24-month-old child, brought with a history of having been accidentally locked up in a car for about 3 hours. On examination in the A&E child is crying but his vitals are stable. What is the next step.

Diagnosis: Insignificant fluid loss

Clinchers
- *24 months of child:* Dehydration in a child, if not corrected, can end up fatally.
- *Accidentally locked up in a car for about 3 hours:* The existence of dehydration in this case depends upon the weather conditions. If it is sunny outside, the child can loose a significant amount of fluid in perspiration. But nothing of that sort has been mentioned in the question.
- *Crying but vitals are stable:* In mild dehydration, the only feature usually is the irritable child. Stable vitals exclude severe dehydration though they can often be deceptive in case of children.

CONFUSA
The body loses about 125 ml of fluids in urine, stools, exhaled air and perspiration and gains 15 ml of fluid endogenously as a metabolic by product for every 100 calories metabolized. In case of accidental locking of a child in car for prolonged periods on a sunny day, sunburns should also be excluded.

Investigation of choice
None required

Immediate management
Check skin turgor and urine output

Treatment of choice
Give water to sip

Your notes:

187. Female child from Ghana, brought to the A&E with a history of nausea and vomiting, on investigations Ketone 1+, Na 148 mEq, Glucose 18 mmol/L.

Diagnosis: Diabetic ketoacidosis (DKA)

Clinchers
- *Female child from Ghana:* Although sickle cell anaemia is more prevalent in Ghana, this information is inconsequential in this question except for the fact that infections like malaria can precipitate DKA.
- *History of nausea and vomiting:* Abdominal pain, nausea and vomiting are common presenting symptoms in DKA.
- *Ketone 1+:* Ketones are usually > 2 mmol/L in DKA. Their presence almost confirms the diagnosis of DKA if blood glucose is elevated.
- *Glucose 18 mmol/L:* The cut off for DKA is glucose > 16 mmol/L.
- *Na 148 mEq:* Hypernatremia in this case is due to severe dehydration.

CONFUSA
In case of DKA in children, dehydration may be so profound as to cause shock. DKA has a mortality rate of 9% in children. The cause of death is cerebral oedema in 50% of cases. To minimize the risk of this, metabolic abnormalities must be corrected slowly.

Investigation of choice
ABG + serum electrolytes + blood culture + blood sugar

Immediate management
Protect the airway and give high concentration O_2
+
Discuss the child with a paediatrician as soon as possible. Arrange intensive care.

Treatment of choice
Commence a normal saline (0.9%) infusion with added potassium (20 mmol/L)
↓
Start an infusion of soluble insulin at a rate of 0.1 units/kg/hour
↓
Once blood sugar has fallen below 10 mmol/L, the IV infusion should be changed to 0.45% saline with dextrose.
↓
According to clinical improvement, can reduce insulin infusion to 0.05 units/kg/hr.

188. Mother comes to the A&E with her child of 3 yrs, history of D&V. On examination the child appears mildly dehydrated.

Diagnosis: Mild dehydration

Clinchers
- *3 years old child:* The key to effective fluid management in childhood diarrhoea is early replacement of fluid losses, starting with the first sign of liquid stool.
- *Diarrhoea and vomiting:* Diarrhoea and vomiting (D & V) are common but potentially serious illnesses in early childhood. In most cases of acute diarrhoea, electrolytes such as chloride and sodium besides water are actively secreted from the gut mucosa and are thus lost in stools.
- *Mild dehydration:* In cases of mild to moderate dehydration, fluid, electrolyte and acid-base homeostasis should be preserved and maintained. Usually if renal function is maintained, such imbalances can not occur.

CONFUSA
A child may lose almost as much water and electrolytes from the body during an episode of diarrhoea as an adult, since the length and surface area of intestinal mucosa of a child, from where the diarrhoeal fluids are secreted, are fairly large. Loss of one litre of fluid from the body of a child weighing 7 kg is much more hazardous compared with a similar depletion from an adult of 70 kg weight.

Investigation of choice
Stool culture and microscopy

Immediate management
Give anti-emetics

Treatment of choice
ORS 90 meE (This is WHO ORS and provides 90 mEq/L of Na^+, 20 mEq/L of K^+, 80 mEq/L of Cl^- and 30 mEq/L of HCO_3 or citrate).

Your notes:

189. Boy has been brought to the A&E following a traffic accident. He has suffered from moderate blood loss. What is the most optimum method of fluid resuscitation.

Diagnosis: Moderate blood loss

Clinchers
- *Boy:* Blood loss in children do not alter the vitals until and unless it is severe.
- *Moderate blood loss:* Even if the vitals are looking stable, the blood loss should be replaced immediately. However tachycardia is a common finding in such cases.

CONFUSA
The assessment of hypovolaemia in the trauma patient is notoriously difficult for the following reasons:
- The interaction of autonomic reflexes, head injury, pain, drugs and blood loss is complex and still not fully elucidated.
- Rapid blood loss may produce a reflex bradycardia.
- Haematocrit is an unreliable index of shock; a nearly normal value does not rule out significant blood loss.

So all abnormalities of colour, pulse, BP and consciousness should be regarded with suspicion in such cases.

Investigation of choice
Urine output

Immediate management
Control external blood loss

Treatment of choice
Commence rapid fluid replacement with a bolus of 20 ml/kg. After reassessment of the patient this can be repeated. In small children, if venous access is not achieved within a few minutes, the intra-osseous route is most suitable (femoral venous access is an alternative). Cross matched blood (whether by urgent or full cross match) is seldom available within 1 hour (even in UK) and is therefore not normally appropriate for unstable hypovolaemic patients (So use plasma expanders like Haemaccel).

Your notes:

190. A 2-year-old child with history of diarrhoea for 18 hours present to A and E. He is drowsy with cold extremities.

Diagnosis: Severe dehydration

Clinchers
- *2-year old child:* Dehydration in a child is a potentially fatal condition and is a medical emergency.
- *Diarrhoea:* It is the main cause of dehydration in children. It can be due to infections or nutritional causes. Rotavirus is the most common infection causing diarrhoea in children.
- *For 18 hours:* It indicates a prolonged diarrhoea and hence is producing the serious state of dehydration, the child is currently in.
- *Drowsy with cold extremities:* A severely dehydrated patient appears drowsy, is apathetic and becomes moribund. As he goes into peripheral circulatory failure, extremities appear cold, though the body may be warm.

CONFUSA
If a child develops severe dehydration, it is prudent to start and IV drip of Ringer's lactate solution, given at a rate of 30 ml/kg of body weight in the first hour. The rate of drip is slowed to 20 ml/kg per hour in the next 2 hours. If the child does not pass urine within three hours of starting IV infusion, acute renal failure must be suspected.

Investigation of choice
Urinary output

Immediate management
Refer to ICU under paediatric supervision

Treatment of choice
Ringer lactate infusion

Your notes:

First Aid for PLAB

191. 3 gm sachet of amoxicillin one hour before the procedure.

Answer: Dental treatment of cardiac patients.

Clinchers
Endocarditis prophylaxis before dental procedures:
Local or no anaesthetic.
- Amoxicillin 3g PO, 1 hour before the procedure
- Clindamycin 600 mg PO if: allergic to penicillin, > 1 dose of penicillin in previous month

General anaesthetic, no special risk:
- Amoxicillin 1g IV at induction, followed by 500 mg PO 6 hours later.
- OR amoxicillin 3g PO 4 hours before induction, followed by 3g PO as soon as possible after procedure.

General anaesthetic, special risk patients:
(NOTE: Special risk signify = prosthetic valves
= previous endocarditis)
- Amoxicillin 1g IV + gentamicin 120 mg IV at induction followed by Amoxicillin 500 mg PO 6 hours later.
- Consider alternatives if,
    = history of penicillin allergy
    = > 1 dose of penicillin in previous month
- Alternatives are
    - Vancomycin 1g IV over 100 min
        +
      Gentamicin 120 mg IV at induction
    - Teicoplanin 400 mg IV
        +
      Gentamicin 120 mg IV at induction
    - Clindamycin 300 mg IV over 10 min at induction followed by clindamycin 150 mg IV 6 hour later.

CONFUSA
The principal of prophylaxis is to treat before contamination occurs, and this is particularly important with antibiotics, where as adequate antibiotic concentration needs to be present in the blood at the time of exposure of infection. Anyone with congenital heart disease, acquired valve disease or prosthetic valve is at risk of infective endocarditis and should take prophylactic antibiotics before procedures which may result in bacteraemia. The dental procedures considered fit for prophylaxis include extractions, scaling, polishing or gingival surgery.

Investigation of choice
Echocardiography to rule out congenital and often heart diseases if suspected.

Immediate management: Prophylactic antibiotics.

Treatment of choice: Stated as the question itself.

192. Three days of intravenous broad spectrum antibiotics beginning with induction of anaesthesia.

Diagnosis (Answer): Heart valve replacement

Clinchers
➤ The required prophylactic regimen is Amoxicillin 1g IV + gentamicin 120 mg IV
➤ First dose is given at induction of anaesthesia and is continued upto 3 days.

CONFUSA
Infection of valve postoperatively is a situation akin to infective endocarditis of a native valve. For more detailed notes on chemoprophylaxis in various disease states refer to British national formulary or www.bnf.org.

Investigation of choice
As per the requirements of the operation.

Immediate management
Antimicrobial chemoprophylaxis.

Treatment of choice
Stated as the question itself.

193. Clear fluids by mouth and two sachets of sodium picosulphate on the day before the operation plus broad spectrum intravenous antibiotics at induction.

Diagnosis(Answer): Sigmoid colectomy.

Clinchers
- *Sodium picosulfate*: Before any colorectal surgery, give 1 sachet of picolax (sodium picosulfate 10 mg + magnesium citrate) each, at:
  - On the morning before surgery
  - During the afternoon before surgery
- *Broad spectrum IV antibiotics at induction*: Cefuroxime 1.5 g 18 h, 3 doses IV/IM + Metronidazole 500 mg/ 8 h, 3 doses IV.

CONFUSA
Sodium picosulfate should be used with care if there is any risk of bowel perforation. Otherwise bowel preparation is of utmost importance before colorectal surgery. Antibiotics used should kill anaerobes and coliforms especially.

Investigation of choice
As per the requirements for the operation.

Immediate management
Meticulous bowel preparation.

Treatment of choice
States as the question itself.

Your Notes:

194. Long-term oral penicillin and immunisation against pneumococcal infection.

Diagnosis (Answer): Splenectomy

Clinchers
- Removal of the spleen predisposes the patient, especially the child, to infection with organisms such as the pneumococcus. The clinical course is of a fulminant bacterial infection, with shock and circulatory collapse, termed overwhelming post splenectomy sepsis (OPSS).
- Prophylactic immunization with
  = pneumococcal
  = meningococcal
  = *Haemophilus influenzae* type of vaccine should be administered, preoperatively where possible. In addition, children should have prophylactive daily low dose oral penicillin until they reach adulthood.

CONFUSA
The major aim of antibiotic prophylaxis in splenectomy is to present serious pneumococcal sepsis. Regarding oral penicillin, the duration of treatment is,
- Children—till adult hood
- Adult—for first year after splenectomy
- Immunosuppressed—life-long.

Investigation of choice
Usually none

Immediate management
Vaccination (if possible preoperatively).

Treatment of choice
Stated as the question itself. Preoperatively also phenoxymethyl penicillin is given (500 mg/12 hourly).

Your Notes:

195. One dose of metronidazole at induction of anaesthesia.

Diagnosis (Answer): Emergency appendicectomy.

Clinchers
- The prophylactive antibiotic regimen for as emergency appendicectomy is:
  Metronidazole 1g 18 h + Cefuroxime 1.5 g/8 h
- These are given in 3 doses IV, the first dose is given 1 hour preoperatively or at the induction of anaesthesia.

CONFUSA
If it is an elective appendicectomy, then give 3 dose regimen of metronidazole suppositories 1g/8 h + Cefuroxime 1.5/8 h IV or Gentamicin IV

Investigation of choice
None required usually.

Immediate management
Shift patient to OT.

Treatment of choice
Stated as the question itself.

Your Notes:

196. Child who is HIV positive is due for MMR.

Diagnosis: Balanced risk.

Clinchers
- *MMR vaccines:* Those age 18 months to 5 years who have not had the vaccine (even if they have had single measles vaccine) may have MMR with the preschool of DPT. There is no upper age limit.
- As per the UK schedule, first dose of MMR (0.5 mL SC) is given between 12-18 months.
- *HIV positive:* Immunodeficiencies are a contraindication for MMR vaccination but these include only primary immunodeficiencies and not HIV or AIDS (208, OHCS, 5th edn).

CONFUSA
Contraindications for MMR vaccination

Condition	Delay for
Fever	till fever resolves
Pregnancy	till one month postpartum
Previous line vaccine	till 3 weeks
Previous Ig	till 3 months
Primary immunodeficiencies (except HIV and AIDS)	not given
Steroid therapy	till 3 months after discontinuation
Leukemia	not given
Lymphoma	not given
Recent radiotherapy	till 6 months to one year
Anaphylaxis history by • egg • neomycin • kanamycin	not given

- Steroid therapy implies prednisolone $\geq$ 2 mg/kg/day from > 1 week (or equivalent doses)
- Neomycin or kanamycin are the vaccine preservatives
- The vaccine is chick embryo based, so a history of anaphylaxis by egg protein (and not egg allergy) is a contraindication

Investigation of choice
None required.

Immediate management
None required.

Treatment of choice
Continue as per schedule.

Your Notes:

197. Child due for HiB, DPT, etc. suffering from acute febrile illness.

Diagnosis: Risk of febrile convulsions.

Clinchers
Note: An acute febrile illness is a contraindication for any vaccine.
- *HiB vaccine:* It is a bacterial polysaccharide protein conjugate vaccine for hemophilus influenza type V strain. It has a few insignificant local effects and no serious reactions.
- *DPT vaccination:* It is a combination vaccine against diphtheria, pertussis and tetanus. In them diphtheria and tetanus are toxoids and pertussis is an a cellular vaccine. According to UK schedule the first dose is given at 2 months of age (in preterm babies—2 month postnatally).
- *Acute febrile illness:* It is a contraindication for DPT vaccination (not so for H:B) as the pertussis component in it produces a post vaccination fever of >39.5°C within 48 hours. Since the child is already febrile, it can compound the problem and can lead to febrile convulsions. Its better to delay the vaccine till the fever resolves or at least 2 weeks.

CONFUSA
The only other contraindication for pertussis vaccination is a past severe reaction to pertussis vaccine—i.e. indurated redness most of the way around the arm, or over most of the anterolateral thigh (depending on the site of injection) or a generalised reaction.
Note: According to BNF (British National Formulary) website, evolving neurological problems are also a contraindication untill the condition is stable.

Investigation of choice
Fever workup.

Immediate management
Paracetamol ± tepid sponging.

Treatment of choice
Delay by 2 weeks.

Your Notes:

---

198. Child cried for 2 hours after Hib, DPT, etc.

Diagnosis: No risk from further vaccination.

Clinchers
- *Cried for 2 hours after Hib, DPT:* Persistent, inconsolable crying lasting ≥ 3 hours within 48 hours after DPT vaccination is a valid *precaution* for further vaccination. Since this child does not meet this criteria, the rest of the immunisation schedule can be safely continued.

CONFUSA
Since the above criterion is only a precaution and not a contraindication, it warrants further vaccination after careful review. The benefits and risk of administering a specific vaccine to an individual under the circumstances are considered. It benefits outweigh the risk, e.g. during on outbreak or foreign travel, the vaccine should be administered.

Investigation of choice
A complete work up to find the cause of inconsolable crying.

Immediate management
A complete work up to find the cause of inconsolable crying.

Treatment of choice
Continue as per schedule.

Your Notes:

199. Family history of egg allergy. Child due for MMR.

Diagnosis: Insignificant risk of anaphylaxis.

Clinchers
- *Family history of egg allergy:* The only contraindication for MMR (a chick embryo based vaccine) is previous history of anaphylaxis by egg intake. History of other egg allergies in the subject to be vaccinated or in his family is a contraindication.

Note: Other vaccine which can produce complications in previous history of egg allergy is HiB vaccine.

CONFUSA
Persons with a history of anaphylactic reactions (and not just history of egg allergy in himself or in family) following egg ingestion be vaccinated only with caution. Protocols have been developed for vaccinating such persons and should be consulted.

Investigation of choice
None.

Immediate management
Cautions vaccination and monitoring thereafter.

Treatment of choice
Continue as per schedule.

Your Notes:

200. History of convulsions. Child due for HiB, DPT, etc.

Diagnosis: Insignificant risk of febrile convulsions.

Clinchers
- *History of convulsions:* The parents of children with a tendency to have convulsions should be counselled on the management of any fever developing after immunization. Febrile convulsions may occur 5-10 days after measles vaccination (or MMR) whereas they may take place in the first 72 hours after pertussis immunization. Suggestion may include paracetamol, sponge with tepid water, give extra fluids, dress in thin clothing and place in a cool room. In high-risk children, an antipyretic drug may be suggested routinely for the first 72 hours after immunization. Where the tendency is severe, the parents may be instructed on rectal diazepam administration (source: BNF website).
- *HiB, DPT*—Only the pertussis component is known to produce a febrile syndrome postvaccination (Hence increase the risk of febrile convulsions)

CONFUSA
Presence of history of convulsions (personal/family) is a special consideration (i.e. require individual care review) and not a contraindication for vaccination. Most children with idiopathic epilepsy, or a family history of epilepsy (sibling or parent) should be vaccinated. If in doubt, seek expert advice rather than withholding the vaccine. Those with special CNS conditions (e.g. cerebral palsy, spina bifida) are *especially recommended* for vaccination.

Investigation of choice
None required.

Immediate management
Counsel and teach the parents about the prevention and management of febrile convulsions.

Treatment of choice
Continue as per schedule.

Your Notes:

July—2001

RxPG Analysis

Total themes:	40
Repeat themes:	5
Repeat themes with a different header:	11

July—2001

THEME 1: PRESCRIPTION AND RENAL FAILURE

OPTIONS
a. Ciclosporin
b. Bendrofluazide
c. Spirinolactone
d. Cyclophosphamide
e. Captopril
f. Gentamicin
g. Calcium
h. Magnesium
i. Acetazolamide
j. Furosemide
k. Paracetamol

*For each presentation below, choose the **most appropriate drug producing the given condition** from the above list of OPTIONS. Each option may be used once, more than once, or not at all.*

QUESTIONS

1. A 60-year-old woman hypertensive was started on antihypertensive 2 weeks ago. Now has a creatinine level of 500 micromol/L

2. A child with recurrent nephrotic syndrome is brought for treatment. 3 weeks after start of treatment, he now has massive haematuria.

3. A patient in severe renal failure has potassium level of 2.5 mmol/L.

4. Patient with complaint of ataxia and tinnitus and mild hearing loss. He has moderate renal failure.

5. A fit 50-year-old man is prescribed oral Acetazolamide by an ophthalmologist for suspected glaucoma. He presents with lethargy and shortness of breath on exertion. Sodium 140 mmol/L, potassium 3.2 mmol/L, bicarbonate 18 mmol/L, chloride 115 mmol/L, Urea 6.7 mmol/L, creatinine 114 mmol/L

THEME 2: INVESTIGATION/ MANAGEMENT OF CYSTITIS

OPTIONS
a. IVU
b. Cystoscopy
c. Ultrasound kidney and bladder
d. MSU after 3 weeks
e. MSU monthly for 6 months
f. MSU culture
g. ^{99}Technetium renography
h. Urine culture and sensitivity
i. Catheter culture
j. Suprapubic aspiration
k. Urethral culture

*For each presentation below, choose the **most appropriate investigation** from the above list of OPTIONS. Each option may be used once, more than once, or not at all.*

QUESTIONS

6. A 3-year-old boy has a first confirmed urinary tract infection. Abdominal ultrasound is normal.

7. A female presents with frequent dysuria. This is the 3rd episode. At this time *E. coli* confirmed.

8. A 70-year-old with prostatic symptoms. Urine culture is negative.

9. A 25-year-old male has a first confirmed urinary tract infection. IVU is normal.

10. A one and half year old girl, was brought with complaint of dysuria. Culture of urine reveals mixed bacteria.

THEME 3: DIFFERENTIAL DIAGNOSIS OF VOMITING IN CHILDREN

OPTIONS
a. Gastro-oesophageal reflux (physiological)
b. Gastroenteritis
c. Pyloric stenosis
d. Intussusception
e. Urinary tract infection
f. Diabetes mellitus
g. Gatro-oesophageal reflux (pathological) (UTI)
h. Meconium ileus
i. Necrotising enterocolitis
j. Poisoning
k. Septicaemia

*For each presentation below, choose the **single most likely diagnosis** from the above list of OPTIONS. Each option may be used once, more than once, or not at all.*

QUESTIONS

11. A 3-week-old presents with projectile vomiting, appearing hungry after each emesis. On examination dehydration is present and there is a mass in abdomen.

12. A 1-year-old child presents with vomiting, crying and lifting her legs. Nappy is stained red. On examination sausage-shaped mass is palpated per abdominally.

13. A 3-month-old child is brought with recurrent vomiting, but is otherwise thriving well and healthy. The symptom seems to subside when the child is strapped in baby's seat.

14. A 6-year-old girl presents with fever, frequency, dysuria and abdominal pain.

15. Child with vomiting and diarrhoea. Brother had a similar problem 2 weeks ago.

THEME 4: DIFFERENTIAL DIAGNOSIS OF ACUTE DYSPNOEA (DATA INTERPRETATION-CO_2, OXYGEN, CHEST X-RAY, ECG)

OPTIONS
a. Panic attacks
b. Asthma
c. Pulmonary embolism
d. Cor pulmonale
e. Aspiration pneumonia
f. Alcohol withdrawal
g. Hypoglycaemia
h. Depression
i. Pulmonary edema
j. Pneumothorax
k. Mitral stenosis

*For each presentation below, choose the **most likely diagnosis** from the above list of OPTIONS. Each option may be used once, more than once, or not at all.*

QUESTIONS

16. Patient had bilateral fluffy opacities and increased interstitial markings. Had low oxygen, normal CO_2.

17. Patient with acute shortness of breath, wheeze. chest X-ray—normal, low oxygen, low $PaCO_2$. PEFR-120 ml/minute.

18. A 20-year-old woman attends A and E complaining of sudden breathlessness and anxiety. She describes palpitations and paresthesiae of her hands, feet and lips. ECG shows sinus tachycardia and O_2 saturation is normal.

19. An alcoholic admitted semi-comatose. ABG shows low oxygen saturation.

20. Patient with recent MI, develops acute breathlessness with hemoptysis. CxR shows dilated pulmonary artery and wedge-shaped area of infarction. Decreased PaO_2 and $PaCO_2$.

THEME 5: MANAGEMENT OF MULTIPLE TRAUMA

OPTIONS
a. Gain IV access + normal saline/haemaccel
b. Gain IV access + blood transfusion
c. Apply external pressure
d. Needle thoracostomy
e. Chest drain
f. Maintain open airway
g. Intubation and ventilation
h. Splint fracture
i. Urgent blood transfusion
j. Chest strapping
k. Analgesics

*For each presentation below, choose the **next most appropriate action** from the above list of OPTIONS. Each option may be used once, more than once, or not at all.*

QUESTIONS

21. Patient involved in road traffic accident (RTA), neck immobilised. Has massive head and facial injuries, together with noisy breathing despite administration of 100% oxygen.

22. Girl in road traffic accident (RTA). Neck is immobilised and line established. Has deformed, swollen thigh, pale.

23. Known asthmatic patient involved in road traffic accident (RTA). Has a right-sided chest pain. On ausculation right side is hyper-resonant. Trachea is deviated to the left.

24. A 19-year-old has fallen off her horse. Neck is immobilised + 100% oxygen. Has left upper abdominal pain, is pale and tachycardiac.

25. A 15-year-old girl has cut her wrist and bled profusely. She is pale, tachycardiac and does not want to live.

THEME 6: DIFFERENTIAL DIAGNOSIS OF ALTERED BOWEL HABIT

OPTIONS
a. Carcinoma rectum
b. Carcinoma caecum
c. IBS with diarrhoea
d. IBS with constipation
e. Faecal impaction
f. Diverticulosis
g. Ulcerative colitis
h. Crohn's disease
i. Fissure in ano
j. Paralytic ileus
k. Hemorrhoids
l. Acute hematoma around anal region

*For each presentation below, choose the **single most likely diagnosis** from the above list of OPTIONS. Each option may be used once, more than once, or not at all.*

QUESTIONS

26. A 19-year-old female with complaint of a 1 year history of bloody diarrhoea and tenesmus. Has pale skin lesions. On examination-sigmoidoscopy shows inflammation and granulomata

27. 65-year-old mal with weight loss, right-sided pain, tenesmus. on examination-mass in the rectum

28. An 18-year-old presents with frequent diarrhoea for about 3/52, relieved by defaecation. Sigmoidoscopy is normal.

29. An 80-year-old with complaint of diarrhoea and urinary retention

30. After an abdominal operation, a patient presents with subfebrile state and abdominal distention. There is associated abdominal tenderness, constipation. On auscultation no bowel sounds are heard.

THEME 7: DIFFERENTIAL DIAGNOSIS OF ACUTE URINARY RETENTION

OPTIONS
a. Ureteric colic
b. Carcinoma prostate
c. BPH
d. Urinary tract infection
e. Stricture
f. Periventricular region lesion
g. Brainstem lesion
h. Spinal cord lesion
i. Antidepressant
j. Urethral valves
k. Ruptured ureters

*For each presentation below, choose the **single most likely diagnosis** from the above list of OPTIONS. Each option may be used once, more than once, or not at all.*

QUESTIONS

31. A patient of multiple sclerosis has had urinary catheterisation for 4 years with intermittent obstruction

32. 60-year-old with complaint of frequency, dysuria. PSA is 120 ng/ml, also has back pain

33. Female patient with complaint of sever flank pain, is restless and the pain radiates to the groin.

34. A 65-year-old man presents with history of ferquency, urgency and decreased urinary flow.

35. A 39-year-old female presents with weakness of both legs, difficulty walking and urinary retention.

THEME 8 INVESTIGATION/MANAGEMENT OF MENINGITIS

OPTIONS
a. ZN staining
b. Serum urate
c. CT skull
d. Parenteral penicillin
e. IV aciclovir
f. Rifampicin
g. IV mannitol
h. Lumbar puncture
i. Blood culture
j. IV fluids
k. Hib vaccine

*For each presentation below, choose the **next most appropriate action** from the above list of OPTIONS. Each option may be used once, more than once, or not at all.*

QUESTIONS

36. A young boy back from holiday in North Africa presents with night fever, weight loss. Began on antibiotics with minimal improvement. CSF shows: protein-960 mg/dL, glucose-2 mmol/L, cells- Lymphocytes

37. An 8-year-old boy with acute leukemia is admitted in a comatose state. He is found to have lymphoblast depletion prevention.

38. A 14-year-old boy presents with drowsiness and generalised headache. He is recovering from a bilateral parotitis. His CT scan is normal.

39. An intravenous drug abuser presents with suspected meningitis. The organism is confirmed in the CSF by India ink preparation.

40. An anxious mother called you to say that her son's best friend in school has caught meningitis.

THEME 9: DIFFERENTIAL DIAGNOSIS OF SHOCK

OPTIONS
a. Anaphylaxis
b. Tension pneumothorax
c. Aortic aneurysm
d. Ruptured ectopic pregnancy
e. Salpingitis
f. Acute pancreatitis
g. Adrenal insufficiency
h. Simple pneumothorax
i. Surgical emphysema
j. Haemoperitoneum
k. Haemothorax

*For each presentation below, choose the **most likely diagnosis** from the above list of OPTIONS. Each option may be used once, more than once, or not at all.*

QUESTIONS

41. Patient stabbed in right chest. ultrasound showed no free fluid per abdominally, patient is breathless, pale.

42. woman history of 8/52 amenorrhoea presents with abdominal pain rigidity and is pale.

43. Patient with history of suggestive of atherosclerosis, now presenting with shock.

44. Patient admitted with suspected tetanus and is given tetanus immunoglobulin and an antibiotic to which he is not allergic. 10 minutes later the patient is breathless with tachycardia

45. A known asthmatic on treatment with inhaled Beta-2-agonist and steroid. Now presents with hypotension.

THEME 10: INVESTIGATION OF AORTIC ANEURYSM

OPTIONS
a. Abdominal ultrasound
b. Spiral CT
c. IVU
d. Coronary angiography
e. Echocardiography
f. Plain abdomen X-ray
g. Chest X-ray
h. MRI
i. Only ECG
j. DTPA scan
k. High resolution CT

*For each presentation below, choose the **most appropriate investigation** from the above list of OPTIONS. Each option may be used once, more than once, or not at all.*

QUESTIONS

46. A 60-year-old attends A and E and it is thought he may have aortic aneurysm.

47. A tall 34-year-old man develops severe central chest pain radiating to his back. He soon develops a dense hemiplegia.

48. A patient is to have a repair of of his aortic aneurysm but also has severe myocardial ischaemia

49. Patient with aortic aneurysm has unstable angina

50. Elderly patient suspected of having aortic dissection with complaint of abdominal pain yesterday, but is now haemodynamically stable.

THEME 11: INVESTIGATION/DIFFERENTIAL DIAGNOSIS OF ABDOMINAL PAIN

OPTIONS
a. Mesenteric angiogram
b. Perforated peptic ulcer
c. Nonulcer dyspepsia
d. Retrocaecal appendicitis
e. Ureteric colic
f. Carcinoma of stomach
g. Oesophagitis
h. Hepatitis
i. Acute pancreatitis
j. Acute cholecystitis
k. Myocardial infarction

*For each presentation below, choose the **single most likely** diagnosis or investigation from the above list of OPTIONS. Each option may be used once, more than once, or not at all.*

QUESTIONS

51. A patient presents with intermittent abdominal Pain for about 30 minutes after meals. Also has history of abdominal pain radiating to the back. on examination-abdominal bruit. Also has intermittent claudication.

52. Patient on antacids for extensive epigastric pain presents with acute abdominal pain, rigidity and is pale.

53. Female patient with 24 hour history of severe abdominal pain and vomiting. She is restless and afebrile. She has a history of chronic alcoholism.

54. Patient with presenting complaint of severe flank pain. He is now restless. He says that the pain is radiating to the groin he is passing reddish urine.

55. A 50-year-old chronic alcoholic presents with a sudden onset difuse abdominal pain. It is radiating to the back. He has generalised abdominal tenderness with vomiting and rigidity.

THEME 12: DIFFERENTIAL DIAGNOSIS OF FRACTURES IN CHILDREN

OPTIONS
a. Green stick fracture
b. Fracture shaft radius
c. Fracture ulna
d. Fracture shaft of femur
e. Pulled elbow
f. Fracture supracondylar
g. Slipped upper femoral epiphysis
h. Fracture neck of femur
i. Fracture scaphoid
j. Colle's fracture
k. Gallezzi fracture.

*For each presentation below, choose the **single most likely** diagnosis from the above list of OPTIONS. Each option may be used once, more than once, or not at all.*

QUESTIONS

56. A 7-day-old baby cries whenever lifted. Labour was difficult.

57. Young girl tripped while holding mother's hand. Now cannot use arm at all.

58. Young boy fell off horse onto his hand. Now with complaint of mild tenderness over the clavicle but able to use forearm.

59. Young child fell on outstretched hand and now has absent radial pulse.

60. A 12-year-old boy with left groin pain for 6 weeks is noticed to stand with the left leg externally rotated. Examination reveals negligible internal rotation of the hip.

July—2001

THEME 13: MULTIPLE SCLEROSIS-ANATOMICAL SITES INVOLVED

OPTIONS
a. Cerebrum
b. Optic disc
c. Optic nerve
d. Optic radiation
e. Cerebral cortex
f. Brainstem and its cerebellar connections
g. Cervical spinal cord
h. Thoracic spinal cord
i. Facial nerve
j. Trigeminal nerve
k. Fascial nucleus

*For each presentation below, choose the **most likely** anatomical site involved from the above list of OPTIONS. Each option may be used once, more than once, or not at all.*

QUESTIONS

61. Known patient of multiple sclerosis now with complaint of urinary incontinence, weakness in all 4 limbs and difficulty walking.

62. Patient has nystagmus, diplopia, and positive past-pointing.

63. Patient has repeated attacks of multiple sclerosis, and now has pale temporal disc.

64. Patient with complaint of blurring of vision, papilledema, pain in eye.

65. A known patient of multiple sclerosis with unilateral facial paralysis with no loss of taste.

THEME 14: DIFFERENTIAL DIAGNOSIS OF CHRONIC NEUROLOGICAL DISEASES

OPTIONS
a. Alzheimer's
b. Multiple sclerosis
c. Myasthaenia gravis
d. Space occuyping lesion
e. Acromegaly
f. Polymyositis
g. Dermatomyositis
h. Polymyalgia rheumatica
i. Parkinsonism
j. Dermatomyositis
k. Fibromyosis

*For each presentation below, choose the **single most likely** diagnosis from the above list of OPTIONS. Each option may be used once, more than once, or not at all.*

QUESTIONS

66. Patient gets diplopia when he works very hard.

67. Patient with attacks of numbness in left hand and right sided headache.

68. This disease is characterised by neurofibrillary tangels and sinel plaques.

123. A 40-year-old female comes with complaints of headache, bitemporal hemianopia, increase in shoe size.

70. A middle-aged woman presents with recurrent nausea, weight loss and fever. She has pain, stiffness and weakness inher hips and shoulders. She does not have a rash, but the skin around the neck and shoulders appears thickened.

THEME 15: IMMEDIATE MANAGEMENT OF BURNS

OPTIONS
a. IV fluids
b. Escharotomy
c. Admit to hospital
d. Carboxyhemoglobin level
e. IV blood transfusion
f. Deroof blister
g. Aspirate blister
h. Blood transfusion
i. Skin grafting
j. Antibiotics
k. Fasciotomy
l. Reassure

*For each presentation below, choose the **most appropriate management** from the above list of OPTIONS. Each option may be used once, more than once, or not at all.*

QUESTIONS

71. Patient after escaping from fire in a building has singed nostrils.

72. Patient has a large tense blister.

73. An adult patient has partial thickness burns on the anterior chest and upper thighs.

74. An adult patient has full thickness circumferential burns from the elbow to the fingers, covering them completely.

75. Man, slept while sunbathing comes with redness, pain all over his body. Otherwise well.

THEME 16: DIFFERENTIAL DIAGNOSIS OF HEARING TESTS

OPTIONS
a. Bilateral sensory neural deafness
b. Bilateral conductive deafness
c. Bilateral total deafness
d. Unilateral sensory neural deafness
e. Unilateral conductive deafness
f. Threshold shift
g. High compliance on tympanogram
h. Absent recruitment
i. Mixed deafness
j. 50% SISI score
k. Cortical pathology

*For each presentation below, choose the **single most likely diagnosis** from the above list of OPTIONS. Each option may be used once, more than once, or not at all.*

QUESTIONS

76. Otosclerosis.

77. Presbycusis.

78. Otitis media with effusion.

79. Acoustic neuroma.

80. Noise-induced hearing loss (NIHL).

July—2001

THEME 17: BIOSTATISTICS

OPTIONS

a. Specificity
b. Sensitivity
c. Mode
d. Mean
e. Median
f. Chi-square
g. Standard deviation
h. Cohort studies
i. Case control studies
j. Range
k. Random deviation

*For each presentation below, choose the **single most appropriate answer** from the above list of OPTIONS. Each option may be used once, more than once, or not at all.*

QUESTIONS

81. The ability of a test to detect people who do have the disease.

82. Measure of dispersion.

83. Relative risk can be obtained from these studies.

84. The best indicator of central value when one or more of the lowest or the highest observations are wide apart or not so evenly distributed.

85. The most frequently occurring observation in a series.

THEME 18: EPIDEMIOLOGY IN CARDIAC CONDITIONS

OPTIONS

a. IHD
b. Atrial fibrillation
c. Warfarin
d. Angina
e. Congenital aortic stenosis
f. Aortic regurgitation
g. Pericarditis
h. Hypertension
i. Rheumatic fever
j. HOCM
k. Aortic stenosis

*For each presentation below, choose the **correct answer** from the above list of OPTIONS. Each option may be used once, more than once, or not at all.*

QUESTIONS

86. The single largest cause of death in adults in the UK.

87. Warfarin decreases the incidence of stroke by about 30%.

88. Inteferes with the function of vitamin K.

89. Probably most important public health problem in developed countries. Its ratio of frequency in women verses men increases from 0.6 to 0.7 at age 30 to 1.1 to 1.2 at age 65.

90. Its incidence in industrialized countries of the world has declined markedly. Peak age-relaged incidence is between 5 and 15 years.

First Aid for PLAB

THEME 19: MANAGEMENT OF MYOCARDIAL INFARCTION

OPTIONS
a. Diuretic
b. Thrombolysis
c. Beta-blockers
d. Nitrates
e. Oxygen
f. Cardiac pacing
g. High flow oxygen and morphine
h. Heparin
i. Digoxin
j. Adrenalin IM
k. Warfarin

*For each presentation below, choose the **most appropriate management** from the above list of OPTIONS. Each option may be used once, more than once, or not at all.*

QUESTIONS

91. A patient who developed myocardial infarction one month ago is now breathless and has basal crackles.

92. Patient presents with one and a half hours of epigastric pain radiating to his arm. ECG shows acute inferior myocardial infarction. Oxygen + analgesia have already been given

93. Patient recovering from myocardial infarction has a heart rate of 36/minute.

94. A 57-year-old man develops crushing pain in the chest associated with nausea and profuse sweating. The pain is still present when he arrives in hospital an hour later.

95. Not given in a chronic asthmatic after a myocardial infarction.

THEME 20: CAUSATION OF DISEASES

OPTIONS
a. Skin-to-skin
b. Close community contact
c. Animal to human
d. Tinea
e. Female mite
f. Immunodeficiency
g. Blood
h. Mosquito bite
i. Deer tick
j. Allergens
k. Rat-flea

*For each presentation below, choose the **most likely route of transmission** from the above list of OPTIONS. Each option may be used once, more than once, or not at all.*

QUESTIONS

96. Scabies.

97. Candidial nappy rash.

98. Impetigo.

99. Toxoplasmosis.

100. A first year university student develops headache, fever, photophobia, in the 1st week of term.

THEME 21: MANAGEMENT AND INVESTIGATIONS OF SPEECH DISORDERS

OPTIONS
a. Hearing test
b. Speech therapy
c. Reassure
d. Refer to ENT
e. Milestone assessment
f. Carotid doppler
g. EEG
h. USG
i. CT
j. Polysomnography
k. Adenoidectomy

*For each presentation below, choose the **most appropriate step in management** from the above list of OPTIONS. Each option may be used once, more than once, or not at all.*

QUESTIONS

101. Male patient has nasal speech, snores at night. Day time he is sleepy.

102. A 2-year-old been developing well, but now has decreased hearing. Motor function is normal.

103. An 18 month old patient can still says a few words, …mother is worried.

104. A 50-year-old male wakes up with a tingling and numbness in his right hand. This is accompanied by slurring of speech which recovers following about four hours.

105. A 3-year-old with a persistent and rough voice.

THEME 22: TRANSMISSION OF DISEASES

OPTIONS
a. Mite
b. Faecal-oral
c. Blood-borne
d. Tick-borne
e. Louse-borne
f. Air-borne
g. Fomites
h. Sexual transmission
i. Animal to man
j. Dog bite
k. Spores

*For each presentation below, choose the **most likely route of transmission** from the above list of OPTIONS. Each option may be used once, more than once, or not at all.*

QUESTIONS

106. Warts.

107. Typhoid fever.

108. Hepatitis C.

109. HIV.

110. Lyme disease.

THEME 23: MANAGEMENT OF ACUTE PSYCHOSES

OPTIONS
a. Hospital hostel
b. Family therapy
c. Supportive
d. Education
e. Rehabilitation
f. Cognitive therapy
g. Oral antipsychotic
h. Risk management strategy
i. Detention under mental health act
j. Electro-convulsive treatment (ECT)
k. Psychiatric general wards
l. Sedation

*For each presentation below, choose the **most appropriate step in management** from the above list of OPTIONS. Each option may be used once, more than once, or not at all.*

QUESTIONS

111. A schizophrenic who stabbed his mother's hand with a screw driver was recently admitted and treated with depot injection antipsychotic. He is now symptom-free and ready for discharge.

112. Patient (schizophrenia) has had about 8 admissions in the last 5 years. He is uncompliant with drugs.

113. Young patient now 25 years was diagnosed with schizophrenia. At 15, but despite different medications has not recovered fully. The family is very supportive.

114. Patient 35-year-old is admitted depressed and has not been eating/drinking for many days. Has lost weight.

115. 40-year-old patient with features of paranoid schizophrenia.

THEME 24: MANAGEMENT OF ANXIETY

OPTIONS
a. Cognitive and behavioural therapy (CBT)
b. Psychoanalysis
c. Desensitisation
d. Supportive therapy
e. Interpersonal therapy
f. Relation therapy
g. Electroconvulsive therapy
h. Alprazolam
i. Amitryptiline
j. MAO inhibitors
k. Lorazepam

*For each presentation below, choose the **most definitive management** from the above list of OPTIONS. Each option may be used once, more than once, or not at all.*

QUESTIONS

116. Arachnophobia

117. Post-traumatic stress disorder (PTSD)

118. Bereavement

119. A female lawyer is becoming increasing anxious when she has to speak in front of people. This is affecting her work as she needs to speak out in court.

120. This treatment is very effective in endogenous anxiety and phobias.

THEME 25: BASICS OF POISONING

OPTIONS
a. CO
b. TCA
c. Paracetamol
d. Digoxin
e. Aspirin
f. Organophosphate
g. Paraquat
h. Ectasy
i. Cyanide
j. Botulinum toxin
k. β-blockers

*For each presentation below, choose the **single most likely cause** from the above list of OPTIONS. Each option may be used once, more than once, or not at all.*

QUESTIONS

121. Interferes with glutathione (reversible by methionine and acetyl cysteine).

122. Interferes with haemoglobin

123. Anticholinergic effects arrhythmias

124. Patient on treatment for atrial fibrillation, now has palpitations.

125. This interferes with metabolism at the mitochondrial level.

THEME 26: INVESTIGATION OF ANAEMIA

OPTIONS
a. Dietary history
b. B_{12} levels
c. Folate
d. FBC
e. Schilling's test
f. Barium meal
g. Barium enema
h. LFT
i. Isotope scan of liver
j. alcohol history
k. Vitamin C levels

*For each presentation below, choose the **most appropriate intial investigation** from the above list of OPTIONS. Each option may be used once, more than once, or not at all.*

QUESTIONS

126. Patient with atrophic gastritis has megaloblastic anaemia.

127. Patient who is a strict vegetarian has an MCV of 110.

128. Patient has both Iron and Folate deficiency radiology and sigmoidoscospy—normal, has pale stools which is difficult to flush away.

129. Elderly patient with complaint of anaemia and has bleeding gum.

130. Elderly patient in residential home stay with complaint of tiredness.

THEME 27: MANAGEMENT OF ASTHMA

OPTIONS
a. Inhaled long acting β_2 agonists
b. Inhaled short acting β_2 agonists
c. Nebulised β_2 agonists
d. Oral theophylline
e. Oral steroid
f. IV hydrocortisone
g. IV aminophylline
h. Inhaled steroid
i. Inhaled cromolyn
j. Reduce steroid dose
k. Aspiration

*For each presentation below, choose the **most appropriate management** from the above list of OPTIONS. Each option may be used once, more than once, or not at all.*

QUESTIONS
131. A 25-year-old patient now has to use inhaled β_2 2-3 times a day.

132. A 35-year-old uses β_2 agonist + lowdose steroid but symptoms still uncontrolled.

133. A 37-year-old female presents with breathlessness, high RR.

134. A patient who was on 1000 microgram of beclomethasone has now developed oral thrush.

135. An asthmatic patient presents to A and E department with sudden onset dyspnoea. On examination there is reduce expansion, and diminished breath sounds on one side of chest. Trachea is deviated towards otherside.

THEME 28: INITIAL MANAGEMENT/INVESTIGATION IN EYE CONDITIONS

OPTIONS
a. ESR
b. CT
c. Intraocular pressure
d. Artificial tears
e. Visual acuity assessment
f. Visual field mapping
g. Pilocarpine
h. Blood sugar
i. Conjunctival cytology
j. Lumbar puncture
k. X-ray orbit

*For each presentation below, choose the **most appropriate answer** from the above list of OPTIONS. Each option may be used once, more than once, or not at all.*

QUESTIONS
136. A 70-year-old with complaint of malaise, weight-loss, anorexia. Then develops sudden left-sided visual loss.

137. A 60-year-old develops tunnel vision, there is enlargement of the optic cup.

138. A 50-year-old woman with history of symmetrical joint pains complains of eye symptoms and Schirmer's test is positive.

139. Woman, 30-year-old with complaint of blurred vision. CT is normal but she has bilateral papilledema.

140. A woman who is a Visual Display Operator develops headache when she works several hours.

July—2001

THEME 29: MANAGEMENT/INVESTIGATION OF HEAD INJURY

OPTIONS
a. Admit to hospital
b. Discharge
c. Discharge with advice after normal skull X-ray
d. CT
e. IV mannitol
f. IV dexamethasone
g. Burr hole
h. MRI
i. Refer to social services
j. Skull X-ray
k. Dipstick glucose test

*For each presentation below, choose the **most appropriate next step in management** from the above list of OPTIONS. Each option may be used once, more than once, or not at all.*

QUESTIONS
141. A 2-year-old boy ran and hit his forehead on the door. No history of loss of consciousness, and since then is playing well. No neurological signs.

142. An 8-year-old boy falls off a swing at his school. He is brought to casualty by one of his teachers. He has a bruise over his right eye but the examination is otherwise normal. He is fully conscious with no history of blackouts since the accident. A skull X-ray is performed, which is normal.

143. A 19-year-old involved in an road traffic accident (RTA). He is talking, responding and smells of alcohol.

144. A 74-year-old woman had a fall two weeks ago. She is brought into the A and E department with slowly increasing drowsiness. On examination you find mild hemiparesis and unequal pupils.

145. A 24-year-old patient presents with RTA. The pupil on the left side is dilated and the patient is obtunded. CT scan of the head reveals a biconvex hyperdense lesion on the temporal region.

THEME 30: DIFFERENTIAL DIAGNOSIS OF JOINT DISEASE

OPTIONS
a. Gout
b. Pseudogout
c. Osteoarthritis (OA)
d. Rheumatoid arthritis
e. Enteropathic arthritis
f. Septic arthritis
g. SUFE
h. Reiter's disease
i. Perthes' disease
j. Congenital dysplasia of hip
k. SLE

*For each presentation below, choose the **single most likely diagnosis** from the above list of OPTIONS. Each option may be used once, more than once, or not at all.*

QUESTIONS
146. A 40-year-old hypertensive male with complaint of left knee pain. Also history of similar attacks. Joint aspirate is cloudy.

147. A patient's ECG shows T wave inversion and ST depression.

148. Three days of intravenous broad spectrum antibiotics beginning with induction of anaesthesia.

149. A middle-aged woman with a history of rheumatoid arthritis develops sudden swelling in one of her knees. This knee is swollen and hot to touch.

150. A 78-year-old woman complains of a stiff left hip joint after walking some distance. This is most evident when she attempts to abduct the hip joint with limited abduction.

THEME 31: CAUSES OF CONFUSION IN THE ELDERLY

OPTIONS
a. Subdura hematoma
b. Infection toxicity
c. Hyperthyroidism
d. Hypothyroidism
e. Acute pancreatitis
f. Hypoglycemia
g. Korsakoff's psychosis
h. Wernikes-Korsakoff's syndrome (WKS)
i. Wernike's encephalopathy
j. Acute psychaitric disturbance
k. Hypopituitarism

*For each presentation below, choose the **single most likely diagnosis** from the above list of OPTIONS. Each option may be used once, more than once, or not at all.*

QUESTIONS

151. A chronic alcoholic presents with increasing confusion and confabulation.

152. A patient presents with weight gain, hypothermia and confusion.

153. Elderly patient with complaint of fever and increasing confusion.

154. A 57-year-old male comes to the A and E with his daughter, in a confused state. The daughter said that her father was started on some medication by his GP.

155. An elderly man found wandering aimlessly, brought to the A and E by neighbours, who inform that his GP had called on him yesterday.

THEME 32: INVESTIGATION OF VAGINAL BLEEDING

OPTIONS
a. Endometrial sampling
b. Urinary FSH
c. Serum LH
d. Vaginal ultrasound
e. Pregnancy test
f. Colposcopy
g. Per speculum examination
h. Laparoscopy
i. None required
j. Estrogen levels
k. Blood culture

*For each presentation below, choose the **most appropriate investigation** from the above list of OPTIONS. Each option may be used once, more than once, or not at all.*

QUESTIONS

156. Female on OCP's complains of postcoital bleeding.

157. A 55-year-old female develops a single episode of PMB. She stopped menstruation 7 years ago. ultrasound shows endometrial thickness.

158. A 49-year-old woman with complaint of hot flushes, vaginal dryness and her menstruation become irregular 5 months ago.

159. A 14-year-old woman with painless vaginal bleeding.

160. A 55-year-old lady with history of intermittent postmenopausal bleeding. Vaginal and speulum examinations are normal.

THEME 33: INVESTIGATION OF THYROID DISEASE

OPTIONS
a. FNAC
b. Ultrasound thyroid
c. Thyroid scan
d. Serum TSH
e. Serum T_3 and T_4
f. Radioactive iodine uptake
g. USG
h. Chest X-ray
i. Isthmusectomy
j. Free T_3 and T_4
k. TSH and T_4

*For each presentation below, choose the **most appropriate next investigation** from the above list of OPTIONS. Each option may be used once, more than once, or not at all.*

QUESTIONS

161. A 39-year-old woman on thyroxine replacement comes for first check-up.

162. A 40-year-old woman, euthyroid (TSH normal) complains of palpitations, weight loss and diarrhoea.

163. A 13-year-old woman, euthyroid has a soft diffuse swelling that moves with swallowing.

164. An elderly woman presents with a hard fixed lump ultrasound shows no cystic spaces.

165. An elderly man presents with hoarse voice. On examination he has dilated chest vessels and engorged neck veins.

THEME 34: DIAGNOSIS OF LUMPS OF THE HEAD AND NECK

OPTIONS
a. Cystic hygroma
b. Carotid body tumour
c. Brachial cyst
d. Lymph node
e. Carotid artery aneurysm
f. Cx rib
g. Subclavian aneurysm
h. Branchial fistula
i. Thyroglossal cyst
j. Thyroglossal fistula
k. Parotid tumour

*For each presentation below, choose the **most appropriate investigation** from the above list of OPTIONS. Each option may be used once, more than once, or not at all.*

QUESTIONS

166. Patient with a pulsatile hard mass fixed under the upper one-third of the sternomastoid muscle.

167. A 40-year-old male has a lump in the supero-posterior area of the anterior triangle.

168. A 16-year-old female has a midline lump in the neck which moves on protrusion of the tongue and is below the hyoid bone.

169. A 19-year-old male has a cystic mass under the anterior border of sternomastoid at the junction of upper one-third and middle one-third of the muscle. Aspiration revealed fluid containing cholesterol crystals.

170. An infant present with a transilluminant swelling in the lower third of neck.

THEME 35: POSTOPERATIVE COMPLICATIONS

OPTIONS
a. DVT
b. Septicaemia
c. Impending wound dehiscence
d. Wound infection
e. Urinary tract infection
f. Myocardial infarction
g. Acute tubular necrosis
h. Transfusion reaction
i. Cardiac failure
j. Pelvic abscess
k. Pulmonary collapse

For each presentation below, choose the **single most likely diagnosis** from the above list of OPTIONS. Each option may be used once, more than once, or not at all.

QUESTIONS

171. A 50-year-old woman underwent an anterior resection for carcinoma of the rectum one week ago. Has low grade fever and with complaint of pain in the calf + tenderness in the calf.

172. A young woman underwent emergency appendicectomy 6 days ago for perforated appendix. She appeared to be making a good recovery but has developed intermittent pyrexia (up to 39 deg. C). On examination—no obvious cause found, but he is tender anteriorly on rectal examination

173. An elderly man underwent an emergency repair of an abdominal aortic aneurysm. Had been severely hypotensive before and during surgery. After surgery, his blood pressure was satisfactory, but urine output only 5 ml/hr in the first 2 hours.

174. An elderly woman underwent emergency laparotomy for peritonitis. Fourth post-operative day she is noted to have sero-sanuinous discharge from the wound, but there is no erythema or tenderness around the wound.

175. A 60-year-old with features of septicaemia (warm peripheries, low BP, etc.).

THEME 36: MODE OF INHERITANCE

OPTIONS
a. X-linked recessive
b. Autosomal dominant
c. Autosomal co-dominance
d. Autosomal recessive
e. Polygenic
f. Single gene defect
g. X-linked dominant
h. Y-linked
i. Mismatch mutation

For each presentation below, choose the **most appropriate answer** from the above list of OPTIONS. Each option may be used once, more than once, or not at all.

QUESTIONS

176. A 4-year-old boy gets haemarthrosis with trivial injury. He had similar episodes before maternal grand father and uncle had a similar problem.

177. A young girl with complaint of prolonged bleeding following dental extraction. Father had a work-up for anaemia and mother had multiple transfusion.

178. A 15-year-old girl with features of diabetes mellitus.

179. An 11-year-old boy presents with increasing difficulty walking, tremor and instability. Father died in his 40's with same disease.

180. An 18-year-old female underwent caries tooth extraction and developed profuse bleeding. On taking history she revealed menorrhagia. Her mother and her grand father had the same disease.

THEME 37: PROGRESSION OF CARCINOMA BREAST

OPTIONS
a. Asthma
b. Axillary recurrence
c. Bone marrow infiltration
d. Bony metastasis
e. Cerebral metastasis
f. Hypercalcaemia
g. Left ventricular failure
h. Liver metastasis
i. Local recurrence
j. Spincal cord compression
k. Pleural effusion

*For each presentation below, choose the **single most like diagnosis** from the above list of OPTIONS. Each option may be used once, more than once, or not at all.*

QUESTIONS
181. A 56-year-old woman who underwent mastectomy for a breast tumor four years ago, now complains of increasing breathlessness. On examination of her respiratory system, she is noted to have decreased movement of the left hemithorax which is dull to percussion and has absent breath sounds.

182. A 60-year-old woman is admitted to the accident and emergency department having fallen in the street. She is complaining of pain in the right hip and the right lower limb is lying in external rotation. She had breast conserving surgery, radiotherapy and chemotherapy eight years also for breast cancer.

183. A 43-year-old woman treated two years ago for a grade 3 axillary node positive breast cancer presents with increasing confusion, headache and vomiting. On examination, she is drowsy but has no focal neurological signs. She does have blurring of the optic disc margins.

184. A 35-year-old woman treated one year ago for a breast cancer with 12/20 nodes positive, presents with a two days history of increasing confusion, She is drowsy and disoriented. Her husband reports that she has been complaining of severe thirst for the past week.

185. A 45-year-old woman treated three years ago for breast cancer is unable to walk. She complains of increasing weakness in her leg for the last seven days. She has been constipated and unable to pass urine for the last 24 hours.

THEME 38: PRESCRIBING FOR PAIN RELIEF

OPTIONS
a. IV opiate
b. Subcutaneous opiate infusion
c. Acupuncture
d. Carbamazepine
e. Hypnotherapy
f. NSAIDs IM
g. Oral NSAIDs
h. Oral opiates
i. Proton pump inhibitors
j. SSRI e.g. fluoxetine

*For each presentation below, choose the **single most appropriate method of pain relief** from the above list of OPTIONS. Each option may be used once, more than once, or not at all.*

QUESTIONS
186. A 65-year-old man presents with severe, retrosternal chest pain and sweating. An ECG shows an acute antero lateral myocardial infarction.

187. A 70-year-old man inoperable gastric cancer causing obstruction, and multiple liver metastases, is taking a large dose of oral analgesia. Despite this, his pain is currently unrelieved.

188. A 25-year-old woman has just been diagnosed a having rheumatoid arthritis and her rheumatologists has begun giving her gold injections. She continues to complain of joint pain and stiffnesss, particularly for the first two hours of each day.

189. A 50-year-old obese man with a known hiatus hernia, presents with recurrent, severe, burning retrosternal chest pain associated with acid regurgitation and increased oral flatulence.

190. A 67-year-old woman reports severe paroxysms of knife-like or electric shock-like pain, lasting secons in the lower part of the right side of her face.

THEME 39: DIFFERENTIAL DIAGNOSIS OF ACUTE ABDOMINAL PAIN IN A YOUNG WOMAN

OPTIONS
a. Acute gastroenteritis
b. Acute pancreatitis
c. Appendicitis
d. Biliary colic
e. Cholecystitis
f. Ectopic pregnancy
g. Mesenteric thrombosis
h. Perforated peptic ulcer
i. Renal colic
j. Salpingitis
k. Strangulated hernia

*For each presentation below, choose the **single most likely diagnosis** from the above list of OPTIONS. Each option may be used once, more than once, or not at all.*

QUESTIONS

191. A 20-year-old married woman presents in the accident and emergency department with the onset of acute lower abdominal pain. Her past menstrual period was six weeks previously. She has pain radiating to the left shoulder.

192. A 15-year-old girl presents with a 24 hours history of central abdominal pain, followed by the right iliac fossa pain, worse on coughing. She has fever and rebound in the right iliac fossa.

193. A 30-year-old woman has severe colic and upper abdominal pain radiating to her right scapula and is vomiting.

194. A 12-year-old girl has central abdominal pain and is vomiting. On examination, her abdomen is found to be distended with no rebound and a tender lump in the right groin.

195. A 31-year-old woman has severe colic and upper abdominal pain. She is febrile and vomiting. Haematological investigations show a moderate leukocytosis.

THEME 40: ETHICAL PRACTICE OF MEDICINE IN UK

OPTIONS
a. Report him to trust managers.
b. Do not do anything, since the actions of your consultant do not seem to be affecting the progress of patient's condition.
c. Call police and inform them at once.
d. Give her the pills after explaining risks to her and disregard her mother completely.
e. Carry out the termination even without the parent's knowledge.
f. Carry out operation to save at least one baby.
g. Repect parents decision and let nature take it's course, even if this means certain death for both babies.
h. Carry out the sterilization.
i. Tell her you cannot give her the pills without mother's consent.
j. Give her pills and phone the mother and tell her about the pills.
k. Tell the parents and only carry out termination, with their consent.
l. Get partners written and informed consent before carrying out sterilization.
m. Inform health minister, as situation is complicated
n. Seek a judicial review

*For each presentation below, choose the **correct answer** from the above list of OPTIONS. Each option may be used once, more than once, or not at all.*

QUESTIONS

196. You are the SHO on the psychiatry ward. Your consultant is having a sexual relationship with a widow. She has been treated for depression. The lady is getting better and is awaiting discharge.

197. A 34-year-old woman wants to have a sterilization. Her last born child has cerebral palsy and her partner strongly objects to the procedure. They are married.

198. A mother has siamese twins. One of the twins has no heart and liver and depends on the other for survival, and as such without an operation to save the one with major organs they will both perish. Since having the operation means certain death of one of the babies, the parents who are staunch christians oppose the operation. What should be done?

199. A 12-year-old girl wants oral contraceptive pills. She does not want her parents to know about this.

200. A 9-year-old girl wants to have a termination of pregnancy. She is 14 weeks pregnant. The procedure to terminate is not without complications. She does not want her mother informed about the termination.

First Aid for PLAB

General Medical Council PLAB Test Part 1

Full Name _____

Test Centre/Date _____

- Use pencil only • Make heavy makrs that fill the lozenge completely
- Write your candidate number in the top row of the box to the right **AND** fill in the appropriate lozenge below each number
- Give **ONE** answer only for each question

[Answer sheet with 50 rows, each having bubbles A through T. Specimen.]

July—2001

DO NOT WRITE IN THIS SPACE

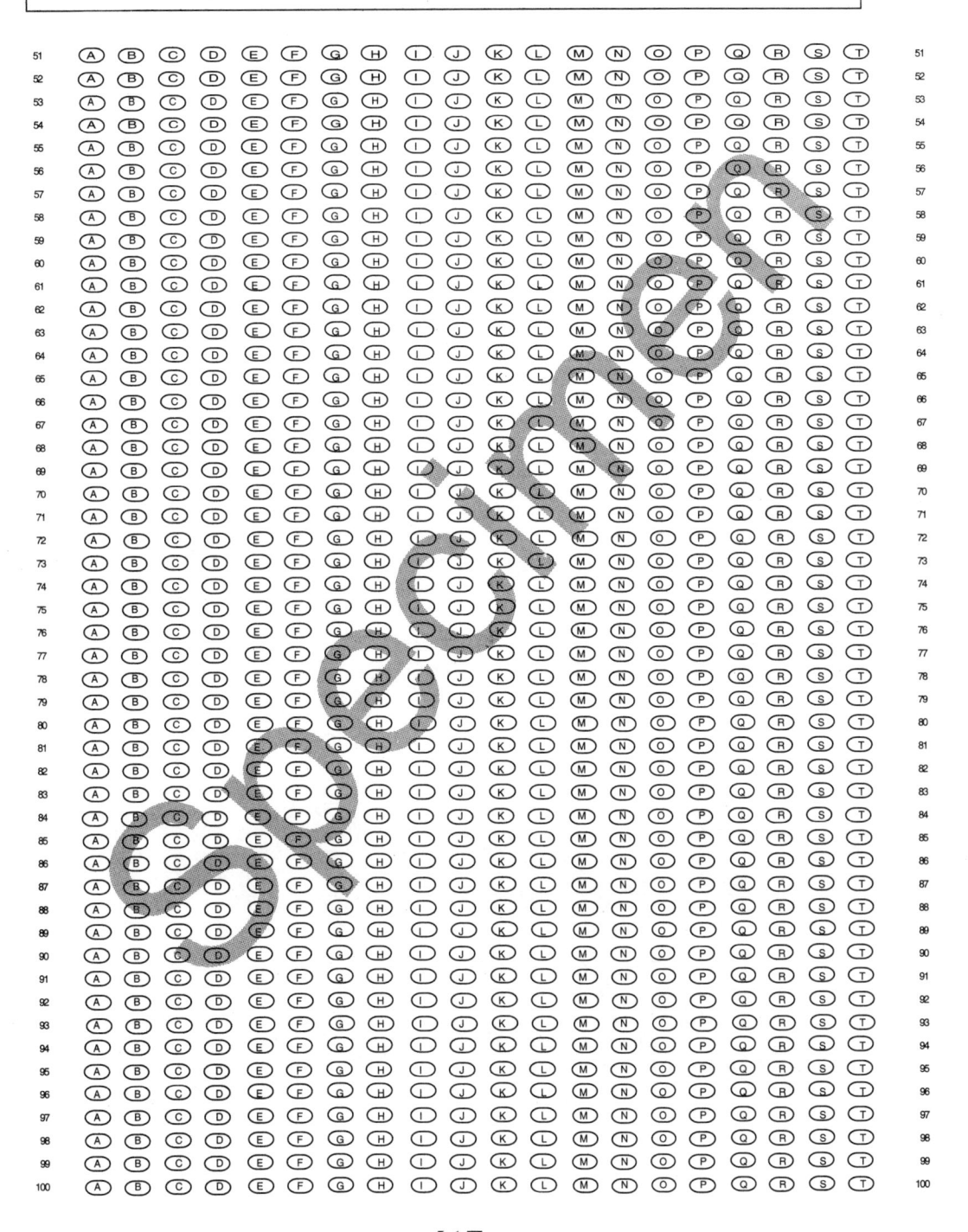

DO NOT WRITE IN THIS SPACE

July—2001

DO NOT WRITE IN THIS SPACE

Answers

1	e	Captopril		31	h	Multiple sclerosis with spinal cord lesion
2	d	Cyclophosphamide		32	b	Carcinoma prostate
3	j	Frusemide		33	a	Ureteric colic
4	f	Genatamicin		34	c	BPH
5	i	Acetazolamide		35	h	Spinal cord lesion
6	d	MSU after 3 weeks		36	a	Zn staining
7	a	IVU		37	b	Serum urate
8	c	USG kidney and bladder		38	h	Lumbar puncture
9	d	MSU after 3 weeks		39	h	Lumbar puncture
10	f	MSU culture		40	f	Rifampicin
11	c	Pyloric stenosis		41	k	Haemothorax
12	d	Intussusception		42	d	Ruptured ectopic pregnancy
13	a	GER (physiological)		43	c	Aprtic aneurysm
14	e	UIL		44	a	Anaphylaxis
15	b	Gastroenteritis		45	b	Tension penumothorax
16	i	Pulmonary edema		46	a	Abdominal USG
17	b	Asthma		47	h	MRI
18	a	Panic attacks		48	d	Coronary angiography
19	e	Aspiration pneumonia		49	d	Coronary angiography
20	c	Pulmonary embolism		50	e	Echocardiography
21	g	Intubation and ventilation		51	a	Mesenteric angiogram
22	i	Urgent blood transfusion		52	b	Perforated peptic ulcer
23	d	Needle thoracostomy		53	i	Acute pancreatitis
24	a	Gain IV access + normal saline/Haemaccel		54	e	Ureteric colic
25	c	Apply external pressure		55	i	Acute pancreatitis
26	g	Ulcerative colitis		56	d	Fracture shaft of femur
27	a	carcinoma rectum		57	e	Pulled elbow
28	c	IBS with diarrhoea		58	a	Green stick fracture
29	e	Faecal impaction		59	f	Supracondylar fracture
30	j	Paralytic ileus		60	g	Slipped upper femoral epiphysis

61	g	Cervical spinal cord
62	f	Brainstem and its cerebellar connections
63	c	Optic nerve
64	c	Optic nerve
65	i	Facial nerve
66	c	Myaesthenia gravis
67	d	Space occupying lesion
68	a	Alzheimer's disease
69	e	Acromegaly
70	f	Polymyositis
71	d	Carboxyhemoglobin level
72	g	Aspirate blister
73	c	Admit to hospital
74	b	Escharotomy
75	l	Reassure
76	b	Bilateral conductive deafness
77	a	Bilateral sensory neural deafness
78	e	Unilateral conductive deafness
79	d	Unilateral sensory neural deafness
80	f	Threshold shift
81	b	Sensitiving
82	g	Sytandard derivation
83	h	Cohort studies
84	e	Median
85	c	Mode
86	a	IHD
87	b	Atrial fibrillation
88	c	Warfarin
89	h	Hypertension
90	i	Rheumatic fever
91	a	Diuretic
92	b	Thrombolysis

93	f	Cardiac pacing
94	g	High flow O_2 and morphine
95	c	B-blockers
96	e	Female mite
97	f	Immunodeficiency
98	b	Close community contact
99	c	Animal to human
100	b	Close community contact
101	j	Polysomnography
102	d	Refer to ENT
103	c	Reassure
104	f	Carotid Doppler
105	d	Refer to ENT
106	h	Sexual transmission
107	b	Faeco-oral
108	c	Blood borne
109	h/c	Sexual transmission or blood borne
110	d	Tick borne
111	b	family therapy
112	f	Cognitive therapy
113	d	Education
114	j	ECT
115	l	Sedation
116	a/j	CBT/MAO inhibitors
117	a	CBT
118	d	Supportive therapy
119	c	Densensitization
120	j	MAO inhibitors
121	c	Paracetamol
122	a	CO
123	b	TCA
124	d	Digoxin

125	-	-		157	a	Endometrial sampling
126	e	Schilling's test		158	b	Urinary FSH
127	b	B_{12} levels		159	i	None required
128	j	Alcohol history		160	d	Vaginal USG
129	k	Vitamin C levels		161	d	Serum TSH
130	a	Dietary history		162	e	Serum T_3 and T_4
131	h	Inhaled steroid		163	k	TSH and T_4
132	a	Inhaled long acting B_2 agonist		164	i	Isthmusectomy
133	c	Nebulized B_2-agonist		165	h	Chest X-ray
134	j	Reduce steroids		166	b	Carotid body tumour
135	k	Aspiration		167	k	Parotid tumour
136	a	ESR		168	i	Thyroglossal cyst
137	f	Visual field mapping		169	c	Brachial cyst
138	d	Artificial tears		170	a	Cystic hygroma
139	j	Lumbar puncture		171	a	DVT
140	e	Visual acuity assessment		172	j	Pelvic abscess
141	b	Discharge		173	g	Acute tubular necrosis
142	j	Skull X-ray		174	c	Impending wound dehiscence
143	a	Admit to hospital		175	b	Septicaemia
144	d	CT		176	a	X-linked recessive
145	g	Burr hole		177	b	Autosomal dominant
146	a	Gout		178	e	Polygenic
147	d	rheumatoid arthritis		179	b	Autosomal dominant
148	f	Septic arthritis		180	d	Autosomal recessive
149	b	Pseudogout		181	k	Pleural effusion
150	c	Osteoarthritis		182	d	Bony metastases
151	h	WKS		183	e	Cerebral metastases
152	d	hypothyroidism		184	f	Hypercalcaemia
153	b	Infection toxicity		185	j	Spinal cord compression
154	f	Hypoglycaemia		186	a	IV opiate
155	j	Acute psychiatric disturbance		187	b	Subcutaneous opiate infusion
156	g	per speculum examination		188	g	Oral NSAID

July—2001

189	i	Proton pump inhibitors
190	d	Carbamazepine
191	f	Ectopic pregnancy
192	c	Appendicitis
193	d	Biliary colic
194	k	Strangulated hernia

195	e	Cholecystitis
196	a	Report him to trust managers
197	n	Seek a judicial review
198	n	Seek a judicial review
199	d	Give her the pills after...
200	e	Carry out...

EXPLANATIONS

1. A 60-year-old woman hypertensive was started on antihypertensive 2 weeks ago. Now has a creatinine level of 500 micromol/L.

Diagnosis: Acute renal failure

Clinchers
- *On antihypertensive 2 week ago:* Angiotensin converting enzyme activity inhibition (ACE inhibitors) and renal prostaglandin biosynthesis (cyclooxygenase inhibitor) inhibitors are the major culprits, leading to renal hypoperfusion, leading to prerenal azotemia.
  Captopril is an ACE inhibitor that lowers the BP.
  Captopril induces hypotension as a result of decrease in total peripheral resistance. Both systolic and diastolic BP falls.
- *Creatinine level of 500 Hmol/L:* Normal value of creatinine in plasma ranges between 70-≤ 150 mmol/L. Recent increase in the plasma urea and creatinine concentration are the biochemical indictors of acute renal failure.

CONFUSA
On captopril, renal blood flow is not compromised even when BP falls substantially, but for him patients with bilateral renal artery stenosis due to dilatation of efferent arterioles and fall in glomerular filtration pressure; contraindicated in such patients.

Investigation of choice
- Blood tests: U and E, FBC, creatinine, blood culture.
- Urine: Microscopy and biochemical tests.
- ECG (hyperkalemia).

Immediate management
- Change in antihypertensive therapy.
- Adjust doses of renally excreted drugs.
  Manage complications, (hyperkalemia, pulmonary edema, bleeding). Seek specialist help sooner rather than later.

Drug producing this condition
Captopril.

Your Notes

---

2. A child with recurrent nephrotic syndrome is brought for treatment. 3 weeks after start of treatment, he now has massive hematuria.

Diagnosis: Hemorrhagic cystitis

Clinchers
- *Child with recurrent nephrotic syndrome:* Minimal change disease accounts for 80% of nephrotic syndrome in children. MCD is highly steroid responsive, but relapses occur in 50% of cases following withdrawal of glucocorticoids. In such patients upto fail to achieve lasting remission, alkylating agents are usual. *Cyclophosphamide* (2 to 3 mg/kg per day) or chlorambucil (0.1 to 0.2 mg/kg per day) is started after steroid induced remission and continued for 8 to 12 weeks.
- *Now develops massive hematuria:* Microscopic hematuria may be present in MCD (in 20-30 percent cases). But massive hematuria here is a sign of cystitis, which may occur with the use of cyclophosphamide.

CONFUSA
The benefits of cyclophosphamide must be balanced against risk of infertility, cystitis, alopecia, infection and secondary malignancies.

Investigation of choice
Cystoscopy.

Immediate management
Stop cyclophospamide.

Treatment of choice
Long-term renal and patient survival is excellent in MCD. Titrate the risk of cyclophosphamide, otherwise MCD is highly steroid.

Drug producing this condition
Cyclophosphamide.

Your Notes

3. A patient in severe renal failure has potassium level of 2.5 mmol/L.

Diagnosis: Hypokalemia (Answer: frusemide)

Clinchers
- *Severe renal failure:* May be due to glomerulonephritis, pyelonephritis, interstitial nephritis, DM, hypertension, cystic diseases, etc. In CRF there is usually, irreversible and long-standing loss of renal function. In CRF treatment is aimed at treating reversible causes (relieve obstruction, stop nephrotoxic drugs, treat hypercalcemia). High does of loop diuretics (furosemide) are used to treat edema.
- *Potassium level of 2.5:* Normal range of potassium is 3.5-5 mmol/L. Hypokalaemia is the most significant problem with high ceiling diuretics (frusemide) and thiazides. Usual manifestations of hypokalemia are weakness, fatigue, muscle cramps and cardiac arrhythmias.

CONFUSA
Hypokalemia is less common with standard doses of high ceiling diuretics (frusemide), than with thiazides, possibly because of shorter duration of action of the former which permits intermittent operation of compensatory reflection mechanism.

Investigation of choice
- Blood: FBC, ESR, U and E, Creatinine, S calcium
- Urine: Microscopy, creatinine clearance
- Renal ultrasound

Immediate management
Change frusemide with potassium sparing Diuretics

Treatment of choice
For hypokalaemia: Attempt to maintain serum K^+ at or above 3.5 mEq/L, by:
- High dietary K^+ intake
- Supplements of KCl (24-72 mEq/day) or
- Concurrent use of K^+ sparing diuretics

Your Notes

4. Patient with complaint of ataxia and tinnitus with mild hearing loss. He has moderate renal failure.

Diagnosis: Ototoxicity (Answer: Gentamicin)

Clinchers
Aminoglycoside antibiotics (gentamicin) have a narrow therapeutic index. Most important side effects being nephrotoxicity and ototoxicity. Rarely respiratory depression may be observed.

Nephrotoxicity is manifested clinically by a gradual rise in serum creatinine levels after a few days of therapy.

Ototoxicity from aminoglycosides therapy presents as either auditory or vestibular damage.

CONFUSA
Fear to toxicity should not prevent the use of aminoglycosides for a legitimate indication, since toxicity is usually mild and reversible.

Investigation of choice
- Serum concentration of gentamicin
- Blood urea and serum creatinine

Immediate management
Stop gentamicin. When serum concentrations are monitored and duration of therapy kept minimum, then adverse effect are unlikely.

Treatment of choice
Stop gentamicin. No other intervention required, since the toxicity is usually mild and reversible.

Your Notes

5. A fit 50-year-old man is prescribed oral acetazolamide by an ophthalmologist for suspected glaucoma. He presents with lethargy and shortness of breath on exertion. Sodium 140 mmol/L, potassium 3.2 mmol/L, bicarbonate 18 mmol/L, chloride 115 mmol/L, urea 6.7 mmol/L, creatinine 114 mmol/L.

Diagnosis: Type II renal tubular acidosis (Proximal RTA).

Clinchers
- *Fit 50-year-old man:* Excludes any pre-existing pathology to be the cause of this condition.
- *Oral acetazolamide:* Acetazolamide causes increased renal bicarbonate losses. Hence it is the most probable cause in this case.
- *Lethargy and shortness of breath on exertion:* These are due to hypokalemia and acidosis respectively.
- *Sodium 140 mmol/L:* Normal.
- *Potassium 3.5 mmol/L:* Low, as hypokalaemia is a feature.
- *Bicarbonate 18 mmol/L:* Low as acetazolamide ↑ renal losses.
- *Urea 6.7 mmol/L:* Normal, but still on higher side (range 2.5-6.7 mmol/L).
- *Creatinine 114 mmol/L:* Normal.

CONFUSA
Renal tubular acidosis generally may be secondary to immunological drug-induced or structural damage to the tubular cells, an inherited abnormality, or an isolated (primary) abnormality. As with most disorders which are not well-understood, the nomenclature is confusing.

Investigation of choice
Urinary pH and serum electrolytes.

Immediate management
Discontinue acetazolamide if still taking.

Treatment of choice
Sodium bicarbonate (massive doses may be required to overcome the renal 'leak').

Your Notes

---

6. A 3-year-old boy has a first confirmed urinary tract infection. Abdominal ultrasound is normal.

Diagnosis: UTI

Clinchers
- *3-year-old:* New renal scars appear in 43% of those less than 1-year-old, 84% of those aged 1-5, and 80% of those less than 5-year-old.
- *Boy:* Annual incidence of UTI in UK is:
    Boys: 0.17-0.23%
    Girls: 0.31-1%
  Sex ratios are reversed in neonates.
- *First confirmed UTI:* This suggest that it is an uncomplicated case of UTI. Also it rules out need for MCU (see confusa).
- *Abdominal USG is normal:* USG is worthwhile even in first UTI. It has 99% specificity and 43% sensitivity. It may miss reflux and scarring.

CONFUSA
Almost all the significant lesions missed by USG either occur in infants < 2 years, or occurs with fever and vomiting, so if these are present and USG is normal, proceed not to IVU, which is radiation rich and unreliable but to:
- ^{99}Technetium renography—static for scarring.
- Isotope cystography—dynamic for obstructive uropathy.
- Isotope cystography—Micturating cystourethrogram (MCU) is still the best way of excluding reflux but it is not done if:
    - Pyelonephritis is unlikely
    - There is no family history of reflux
    - There are not recurrent UTIs

Since this case is just a first episode of UTI, MCU is not indicated.

Investigation of choice
MSU (midstream urine).

Immediate management
Start antibiotics.

Treatment of choice
Trimethoprim 50 mg/5 mL and follow up MSU after 3 week to find response to treatment.

Your Notes

July—2001

7. A female presents with frequent dysuria. This is the 3rd episode. At this time *E. coli* confirmed.

Diagnosis: UTI

Clinchers
- *Female:* The vast majority of acute symptomatic UTI involve young women. Such infections are unusual in men under the age of 50.
- *Frequent dysuria:* Approximately 30% of women with acute dysuria have midstream urine cultures that show either no growth or insignificant bacterial growth.
- *Third episode:* Gross hematuria, suprapubic pain, an abrupt onset of illness, a duration of illness of less than 3 days and a history of previous UTI favour the diagnosis of *E. coli* infection.
- *E. coli confirmed: E. coli* is the most common pathogen in UTI accounting for > 70% cases in community (but ≤ 41% cases in hospitals) frequent relapses suggest P-strain of *E. coli* that infect individuals with P positive erythrocytes.

CONFUSA
Not all strains of E. coli are equally able to infect the intact urinary tract. Only the uropathogenic *E. coli* (with P-pilus and hemolysin secretion) produce persistent infections.

Investigation of choice
IVU (always indicated for relapsing/recurrent UTI).

Immediate management
Blood group P antigen testing (not always required-optional).

Treatment of choice
Trimethoprim.

Your Notes

8. A 70-year-old with prostatic symptoms. Urine culture is negative.

Diagnosis: Bladder outflow obstruction.

Clinchers
- *70-year-old:* This person can have prostatic enlargement either by prostatic carcinoma or benign hyperplasia. *Note:* 70% of the men have benign hyperplasia by the age of 70 years.
- *Prostatic symptoms:* These can hesitancy, terminal dribbling frequency, urgency, nocturia and acute retention.
- *Urine culture negative:* This rules out UTI which can either produce similar symptoms or can be secondary to bladder outflow obstruction.

CONFUSA
USG will demonstrate bladder enlargement, hydronephrosis and hydroureter following voiding it can be used to estimate the amount of residual urine in the bladder. Normally these is none; however, in the presence of bladder outflow obstruction the bladder cannot be completely emptied. USG has replaced the IVU in the routine investigation of patients with outflow obstruction.

Investigation of choice
USG

Immediate management
Exclude carcinoma prostate.

Treatment of choice
- TURP/finasteride + prazosin—if BHP
- Prostatectomy/chemotherapy—if carcinoma.

Your Notes

9. A 25-year-old male has a first confirmed urinary tract infection. IVU is normal.

Diagnosis: Uncomplicated UTI

Clinchers
- *25-year-old male:* Although UTI is unusual in adults males below 50 years of age they may occur in certain conditions, e.g.
  - renal stones
  - instrumentation.
- *First confirmed UTI:* This signify that there is low-risk of resistant infection and trimethoprim will work.
- *IVU is normal:* This rules out any renal tract malformation or abnormality and thus makes the diagnosis of uncomplicated UTI.

CONFUSA
A UTI in a young adult male with normal GU tract should prompt one to initiate investigations for any underlying immunosuppression or diabetes mellitus.

Investigation of choice
None required.

Immediate management
Blood sugar (to rule out diabetes).

Treatment of choice
Trimethoprim
and follow up MSU after 3 weeks.

Your Notes

10. A one and half year old girl, was brought with complaint of dysuria. Culture of urine reveals mixed bacteria.

Diagnosis: UTI

Clinchers
- *One and half year old girl:* Incidence of UTI in girls is more after then neonatal age.
- *Dysuria:* At such age, dysuria suggests only a UTI. It could be secondary to some GU tract abnormality.
- *Culture of urine reveals mixed bacteria:* This suggests contamination of the urine sample. A repeat clean midstream catch should be sent again for culture. Genitals should be washed with water and tap repeatedly (in cycles of 1 min) before the "catch".

CONFUSA
In infants, suprapubic aspiration is definitive and any organisms found in it are significant.

Investigation of choice
MSU culture.

Immediate management
Counsel parents about keeping local hygiene of the child.

Treatment of choice
Trimethoprim.

Your Notes

11.
A 3-week-old week presents with projectile vomiting, appearing hungry after each emesis. On examination dehydration is present and there is a mass in abdomen.

Diagnosis: Pyloric stenosis

Clinchers
- *3-week-old:* Pyloric stenosis is not present at birth, but develops during the first month of life.
- *Projectile vomiting:* Vomiting typically occurs after feeds, and becomes projectile, e.g. vomiting over far end of cot.
- *Appearing hungry after each emesis:* Even though the patient is ill, he is rarely obtunded: he is alert, anxious, and hungry—and possibly malnourished, dehydrated and always hungry.
- *Dehydration:* It is almost invariably present because of the inability to take oral fluids (i.e. milk).
- *Mass in abdomen:* An olive-sized pyloric mass is present in this condition.

CONFUSA
Congenital pyloric stenosis is distinguished from other causes of vomiting (e.g. gastric reflux) by 3 important points:
1. The vomit does not contain bile, as the obstruction, is so high.
2. No diarrhoea: constipation is likely (occasionally starvation stools).
3. Even though patient is ill, he does not look so.

Investigation of choice
USG

Immediate management
Wide bore nasogastric tube

Treatment of choice
Ramstedt's pyloromyotomy

Your Notes

12.
A 1-year-old child presents with vomiting, crying and lifting her legs. Nappy is stained red. On examination sausage-shaped mass is palpated per abdominally.

Diagnosis: Intussusception

Clinchers
- *1-year-old:* Patients may be of any age but usually of 5-12 months.
- *Presents with vomiting, crying and lifting her legs:* Patients usually present with episodic intermittent inconsolable crying with drawing the legs up (colic) ± vomiting.
- *Nappy is stained red:* The child must have passed blood per rectally as it is a feature of this condition. The bleed is like red-currant jam or merely flecks.
- *Sausage-shaped abdominal mass:* It is a characteristic finding in this condition.

CONFUSA
Children older than 4 years present differently with intussusception:
- Rectal bleeding is less common
- More likely to have a long history (> 3 weeks)
- More likely to have some contributing pathology, e.g. HSP, Peutz-Jeghers syndrome, cystic fibrosis, ascariasis, nephrotic syndrome

Investigation of choice
USG

Immediate management
PR examination (always indicated when rectal bleeding is present intussusception).

Treatment of choice
Reduction by air enema
If it fails, reduction at laparoscopy or laparotomy is needed.

Your Notes

13. A 3-month-old child is brought with recurrent vomiting, but is otherwise thriving well and healthy. The symptom seems to subside when the child is strapped in baby's seat.

Diagnosis: Physiological gastro-oesophageal reflux (GFR).

Clinchers
- *3-month-old:* GFR usually presents in the first year of age. GE reflux persisting after that is always pathological.
- *Recurrent vomiting:* Recurrent regurgitation and vomiting is a common symptoms initially.
- *Otherwise thriving well and healthy:* Since it is a physiological condition, the child will have minimal or no effect on its health.
- *Symptom seems to subside when the child is strapped in baby's seat:* The cause of physiologic GER is inadequate development of lower oesophageal pressure regurgitation (dysmotility). This results in spontaneous effortness regurgitation of gastric contents into the oesophagus. Obviously these symptoms can subside if there is a firm strap over the lower chest (baby's seat).

CONFUSA
GER persisting after one year is always pathological. Most such cases are associated with inappropriate transient relaxation of lower oesophageal sphincter. These transient relaxation episodes may occur along with swallowing and pharyngeal contractions. There is also delayed clearance of acid from the distal oesophagus. Such a patient may have complications like:
- Recurrent lower respiratory infections (aspiration)
- GI blood loss (hematemesis)
- Anemia
- Failure to thrive

Investigation of choice
Esophageal pH monitoring but usually none required till one year of age.

Immediate management
Counselling of mother to nurse child in semi-upright position.

Treatment of choice
Observation till one year of age.

Your Notes

---

14. A 6-year-old girl presents with fever, frequency, dysuria and abdominal pain.

Diagnosis: Urinary tract infection (UTI)

Clinchers
- *6-year-old girl:* Prevalence of covert bacteriuria in school going girls in UK is 3%. Recurrence is 35% if more than 2-year-old. Overall the annual incidence of UTI in girls is more in UK (Girls: 0.31-1%, Boys: 0.17-0.23%).
- *Fever, frequency, dysuria and abdominal pain:* Suprapubic tenderness. Occurs in symptomatic bacteriuria unequivocally suggests UTI especially distal GU tract (i.e. cystitis).

CONFUSA
In the newborn period the incidence of UTI is about the same in boys and girls, since:
- The route of infection may be hematogenous.
- Boys have a higher incidence of urinary tract anomalies.

Beyond infancy the incidence of UTI is higher in girls. Asymptomatic bacteriuria is also more frequent in girls.

Investigation of choice
Urinanalysis and culture.

Immediate management
Exclude reflux (with MCU).

Treatment of choice
Trimethoprim.

Your Notes

15. Child with vomiting and diarrhoea. Brother had a similar problem 2 weeks ago.

Diagnosis: Gastroenteritis.

Clinchers

- *Vomiting and diarrhoea:* These are the hallmarks of gastroenterities and can be fatal as they produce dehydration ± urea and electrolyte imbalance.
- *Brother had a similar problem 2 weeks ago:* It suggest an infective etiology. 2 weeks might be the incubation period of this infection. The most common cause in Rotavirus but that has a short incubation period.

CONFUSA
Causes of secretory infective diarrhoea in children are:
- Bacteria
  - *Camphylobacter*
  - *Staphylococcus*
  - *E. coli*
  - *Salmonella*
  - *Shigella*   Where sanitation is poor
  - *Vibrio cholerae*
- Virus
  - Rotavirus
- Protozoan
  - Giardiasis
  - Amoebiasis
- Fungus
  - Cryptosporidium

Investigation of choice
Stool for ova, cysts, parasites, and culture (electron microscopy for rotavirus).

Immediate management
Rehydrate
Educate family about personal hygiene (as incidence of faeco-oral transmission has occurred).

Treatment of choice
As per the cause.

Your Notes

16. Patient had bilateral fluffy opacities and increased interstitial markings. Had low oxygen, normal CO_2.

Diagnosis: Pulmonary oedema.

Clinchers

- *Bilateral fluffy opacities and increased intestinal markings:* These are the chest radiograph findings seen in pulmonary edema. Other findings that may be found on CxR are:
  - Blurring of vascular outlines
  - Butterfly pattern (bat wing appearance) of distribution of alveolar edema
  - Heart may be enlarged or normal.
- *Other features essential for diagnosis of pulmonary edema:*
  - Acute onset or worsening of dyspnoea at rest
  - Tachycardia, cyanosis, pink frothy sputum
  - Pulmonary rales, ronchi, expiratory wheezing
  - Arterial hypoxemia.
- *Causes of pulmonary edema:*
  - Cardiovascular
    - Left ventricular failure—post MI
    - Ischemic heart disease
    - Mitral stenosis/arrhythmias.
  - *ARDS* (lung damage and release of inflammatory mediators) increased capillary permeability cause noncardiogenic pulmonary edema.

CxR findings in left ventricular failure

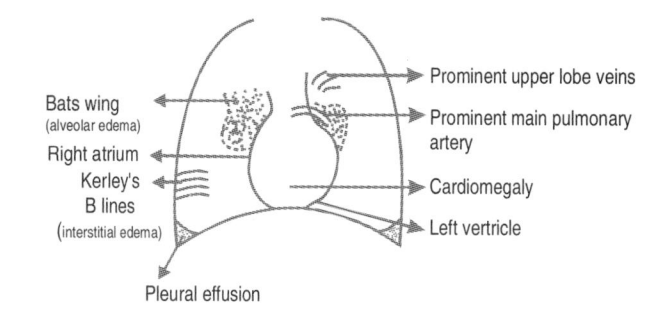

Bats wing (alveolar edema)
Right atrium
Kerley's B lines (interstitial edema)
Pleural effusion
Prominent upper lobe veins
Prominent main pulmonary artery
Cardiomegaly
Left ventricle

Fig

Investigation of choice
- CxR
- ECG (may indicate cause).

Immediate management
- Sit patient upright
- Oxygen (100% if no history of previous lung disease).

Treatment of choice
Investigate while continuing treatment.

17. Patient with acute shortness of breath, wheeze. Chest X-ray—normal, low oxygen, PaCO₂. PEFR-120 ml/minute

Diagnosis: Asthma.

Clinchers
- *Acute shortness of breath, wheeze:* These are the characteristic of asthma may be associated with cough (often nocturnal) symptoms and sputum.
- *CxR normal:* In asthma CxR may be normal or hyperinflation may be observed. This helps to rule out other chronic lung pathologies.
- *Low oxygen, low $PaCO_2$:* Arterial blood gases (ABG) analysis in asthma usually shows a normal or slightly reduced PaO_2 and low $PaCO_2$ (hyperventilation). If $PaCO_2$ is raised, transfer the patient to ITU for ventilation.
- *PEFR—120 ml/min:* PEFR < 50% of predicted is seen in severe attack of asthma. PEFR < 33% along with silent chest, cyanosis, bradycardia is life-threatening. *Predicted PEFR:* Predicted values of PEFR vary with age, sex and height, and typically 450-600 ml/min in men and 350-500 ml/min in women. Values under 100-200 ml/min indicate severe ventilatory dysfunction.

CONFUSA
Differentiate asthma from the following:
- COPD (often coexists with asthma)
- Pulmonary edema (cardiac asthma)
- Large airway obstruction (e.g. foreign body, tumor)
- SVC obstruction (wheeze/dyspnoea not episodic)
- Pneumothorax
- Pulmonary embolism/bronchiectasis
- Obliterative bronchiolitis (in elderly).

Investigation of choice
- PEFR
- ABG
- Spirometry: obstructive defects (↓FEV_1, FVCM ↑ residual volume).

Immediate management
- Sit patient up and give high dose O_2
- Nebulize with salbutamol 5 mg or terbutaline 10 mg.

Treatment of choice
Once patient starts improving reduce nebulized salbutamol and switch to inhaled $β_2$-agonists.
- Initiate inhaled steroids and stop oral steroids if possible
- Continue to monitor PEFR.

18. A 20-year-old woman attends A and E complaining of sudden breathlessness and anxiety. She describes palpitations and paresthesiae of her hands, feet and lips. ECG shows sinus tachycardia and O_2 saturation is normal.

Diagnosis: Panic attacks.

Clinchers
- *20-year-old female:* young females are most prone to have panic attacks.
- *Sudden breathlessness and anxiety:* Classically the symptoms begin unexpectedly or 'out-of-the-blue'. Usually there is no apparent precipitating factor. The patient becomes increasingly frightened by an apparent inability to breath adequately. Attempts to breadth rapidly results in dizziness and further anxiety.
- *Palpitations:* It is due to sympathetic overactivity. Other symptoms attributed to sympathetic stimulation are—tachycardia, sweating, flushes, dyspnoea, hyperventilation, dry mouth, frequency and hesitancy of micturition, dizziness, diarrhoea, mydriasis.
- *Paraesthesiae of her hands, feet and lips:* Tachypnoea blows off CO_2 and the resultant respiratory alkalosis causes a fall in ionised calcium. This hypocalcaemia manifest as paraesthesiae in the fingers and perioral area.
- *Sinus tachycardia:* Due to sympathetic stimulation.
- *O_2 saturation is increased:* due to hyperventilation.

CONFUSA
The most important differential diagnosis in a female is from MVPS (mitral valve prolapse syndrome). This syndrome, more commonly seen in young females (like panic disorder), presents with classical symptoms of panic disorder occurring in episodes. It is caused by prolapse, usually congenital, of the mitral valve into the atrium during ventricular systole. On auscultation, a mid systolic click and a systolic murmur can be heard sometimes. The clininical differentiation between MVPS and panic disorder is difficult. The diagnosis is usually established on echocardiography.

Investigation of choice
To rule out organic respiratory problems (ECG, CXR, ABG).

Immediate management
Confirmation of normality with warm reassurance to the patient.

Treatment of choice
Re-breathing into a closed bag and mask system without oxygen.

July—2001

19. An alcoholic admitted semi-comatose. ABG shows low oxygen saturation.

Diagnosis: Aspiration pneumonia.

Clinchers

Aspiration of liquid (foreign material), into the tracheo-bronchial tree results from various disorders that impair normal deglutition, especially disturbances of consciousness and esophageal dysfunction.

- *Alcoholic admitted semicomatose:* Consumption of alcohol, cigarette smoking, and use of theophylline are known to relax lower esophageal sphincter. This allows reflux of gastric contents into the esophagus and predisposes to pulmonary aspiration especially at night. But in this question the presentation appears to be acute, and therefore in an alcoholic with disturated consciousness, aspiration of alcohol can be the likely cause, which led to abrupt onset of respiratory distress, thus low oxygen,

CONFUSA

Since the question is incomplete, lefts discuss the differential diagnosis:
- *Alcohol intoxication:* In severe cases alcohol overdose is marked by respiratory depression, stupor, seizures, shock syndrome, coma and death.
- *Subdural hemorrhage:* Subdural hemorrhage is a common cause of semicomatose presentation in alcoholics, due to fall.
- *Hypoglycaemia:* Alcohol related hypoglycaemia is due to hepatic glycogen depletion combined with alcohol-mediated inhibition of gluconeogenesis.

Investigation of choice
- Arterial blood gases (ABG) analysis.
- Blood sugar.
- CT scan to rule out subdural hemorrhage.

Immediate management
- Maintain airway with high flow oxygen.

Treatment of choice

O_2 to maintain $PaO_2 > 8$ kPa. With aspiration there is risk of aspirating oropharyngeal anaerobes.

Streptococcus pneumoniae: Cefuroxime 1.5 gh IV + Metronidazole 500 mg/8 h IV.

Your Notes

---

20. Patient with recent MI, develops acute breathlessness and hemoptysis. CxR shows dilated pulmonary artery and wedge shaped area of infarction. Decreased PaO_2 and decreased $PaCO_2$.

Diagnosis: Pulmonary embolism (PE).

Clinchers
- *Recent MI:* Though most commonly pulmonary embolism arises from venous thrombosis in pelvis or legs, recent stroke or MI may also lead to PE (right ventricular thrombus).
- *Acute breathlessness/hemoptysis:* These are along with pleuritis chest pain, dizziness and family history of thromboembolism are important symptoms of pulmonary embolism.
- *CxR:* In pulmonary embolism. CxR may be normal or may show
  - Oligemia of affected segment
  - Dilated pulmonary artery
  - Linear atelectasis
  - Small pleural effusion
  - Wedge-shaped opacities or cavitations (rare) (wedge-shaped area of infarction).

Decreased PaO_2 and $PaCO_2$

Arterial blood gases (ABG) analysis shows hyperventilation + gas exchange ↓, thereby ↓ PaO_2 and ↓$PaCO_2$.

Investigation of choice
- U and E, ECG
- CT pulmonary angiography (determines emboli in pulmonary arteries
- V/Q scan (ventilation/perfusion scan) may show mismatched defects.

Immediate management
- Oxygen 100%
- Morphine 10 mg IV (if in pain).

Treatment of choice
- Heparin for ≥ 5 days, and until INR > 2.
- If obvious remedial cause, 6 weeks treatment with Warfarin. Otherwise continue for 3-6 months. Patients with recent MI, are at risk of developing DVT and PE and therefore they should be prophylactically heparinized (50000/12 h SC) until fully mobile.

Your Notes

21. Patient involved in road traffic accident (RTA), neck immobilised. Has massive head and facial injuries, together with noisy breathing despite administration of 100% oxygen.

Diagnosis: Partial upper airway obstruction.

Clinchers
- *RTA:* It usually causes polytrauma requiring ICU maintenance.
- *Neck immobilised:* It means that cervical spine has been protected.
- *Massive head and facial injuries:* These require continuous observation and monitoring till a definitive diagnosis of any specific injury is made. Facial injuries often produce upper respiratory obstruction due to discontinuing in respiratory tract.
- *Noisy breathing despite 100% oxygen:* High flow 100% oxygen is the second step in primary survey after protecting the neck. Noises from the upper airway indicate airway obstruction. There may be snoring, rattles, stridor or other sounds.

CONFUSA
Any partial upper airway obstruction require urgent intubation as there is high-risk of development of a complete obstruction.

Investigation of choice
Skull and face X-rays.

Immediate management
Intubate and PPV under expert care.

Treatment of choice
As per the diagnosis.

Your Notes

22. Girl in road traffic accident (RTA). Neck is immobilised and IV line established. Has deformed, swollen thigh, pale.

Diagnosis: Fracture shaft of femur and severe blood loss.

Clinchers
- *RTA:* Fracture of long bones is very common in victims of RTA.
- *Neck is immobilised and IV line established:* These suggest that primary survey is over.
- *Deformed, swollen thigh:* This is most probably a fracture of femoral shaft. Such fractures are often associated with massive blood loss (especially if there is concomitant pelvic fractures).
- *Pale:* This confirms the presence of blood loss and indicate urgent blood transfusion.

CONFUSA
In the primary survey the state of the circulation is quickly assessed by observation of:
- Skin colour and temperature
- Pulse rate and volume
- Capillary refill time at a finger pulp or nail bed
- JVP
- BP

Investigation of choice
X-ray thigh.

Immediate management
Blood transfusion and orthopaedic referral.

Treatment of choice
Splinting of the thigh and then evaluation by orthopaedicians. But these has to be done after blood transfusion.

Your Notes

23. Known asthmatic patient involved in road traffic accident (RTA). Has a right-sided chest pain. On auscultation, right side is hyper-resonant. Trachea is deviated to the left.

Diagnosis: Tension pneumothorax (right side).

Clinchers
- *Asthmatic patient:* In patients over 40 years of age, COPD most commonly predisposes to pneumothorax. Rarer causes include bronchial asthma, carcinoma, a lung abscess breaking down and leading to bronchopulmonary fistula and severe pulmonary fibrosis with cyst formation.
- *RTA:* A simple pneumothorax in a patient of trauma may develop into a tension pneumothorax—particularly when the patient receives IPPV.
- *Right sided chest pain:* This is pleuritic pain which is variably in intensity.
- *Hyper-resonance on same side:* This rules out cardiac tamponade and confirms pneumothorax.
- *Trachea is deviated to left:* Signs of tension pneumothorax are:
  - Hypotension
  - Distended neck veins
  - Trachea deviated away from the side of pneumothorax
  - Severe respiratory distress.

> **CONFUSA**
> A CXR should not be performed if a tension pneumothorax is suspected as it will delay immediate necessary treatment. The clinical picture of tension pneumothorax may be mistaken for that of a cardiac tamponade. However, tension pneumothorax is more common and may be differentiated by the hyperresonance over the affected side.

Investigation of choice
CXR but only after needle thoracocentesis.

Immediate management
Needle thoracocentesis urgently.

Treatment of choice
Chest drain (always required in a traumatic pneumothorax irrespective of its size).

Your Notes

---

24. A 19-year-old girl has fallen off her horse. Neck is immobilised + 100% oxygen. Has left upper abdominal pain, is pale and tachycardiac.

Diagnosis: Splenic rupture (hypotensive shock).

Clinchers
- *19-year-old has fallen off her house:* Falls in a young person usually produce polytrauma and blunt injuries.
- *Neck is immobilized + 100% O_2:* This means that the airway and breathing in primary survey is taken care of. Now there is a need to assess the circulation (ABC approach).
- *Left upper abdominal pain:* This could be due to rib fracture or blunt impact over this area. Such a finding should make one strongly suspicious of splenic rupture.
- *Pale and tachycardiac:* This suggest that patient is in hypotensive shock (most probably due to massive blood loss into peritoneum after splenic rupture).

> **CONFUSA**
> In hypotensive shock after massive blood loss, give colloid (Hemaccel) fast IV until BP ↑, pulse ↓, urine flows (> 30 mL/h) and crossmatched blood arrives.

Investigation of choice
USG/peritoneal lavage.

Immediate management
Crossmatch blood and inform surgeons after starting IV fluids.

Treatment of choice
Immediate laparotomy.

Your Notes

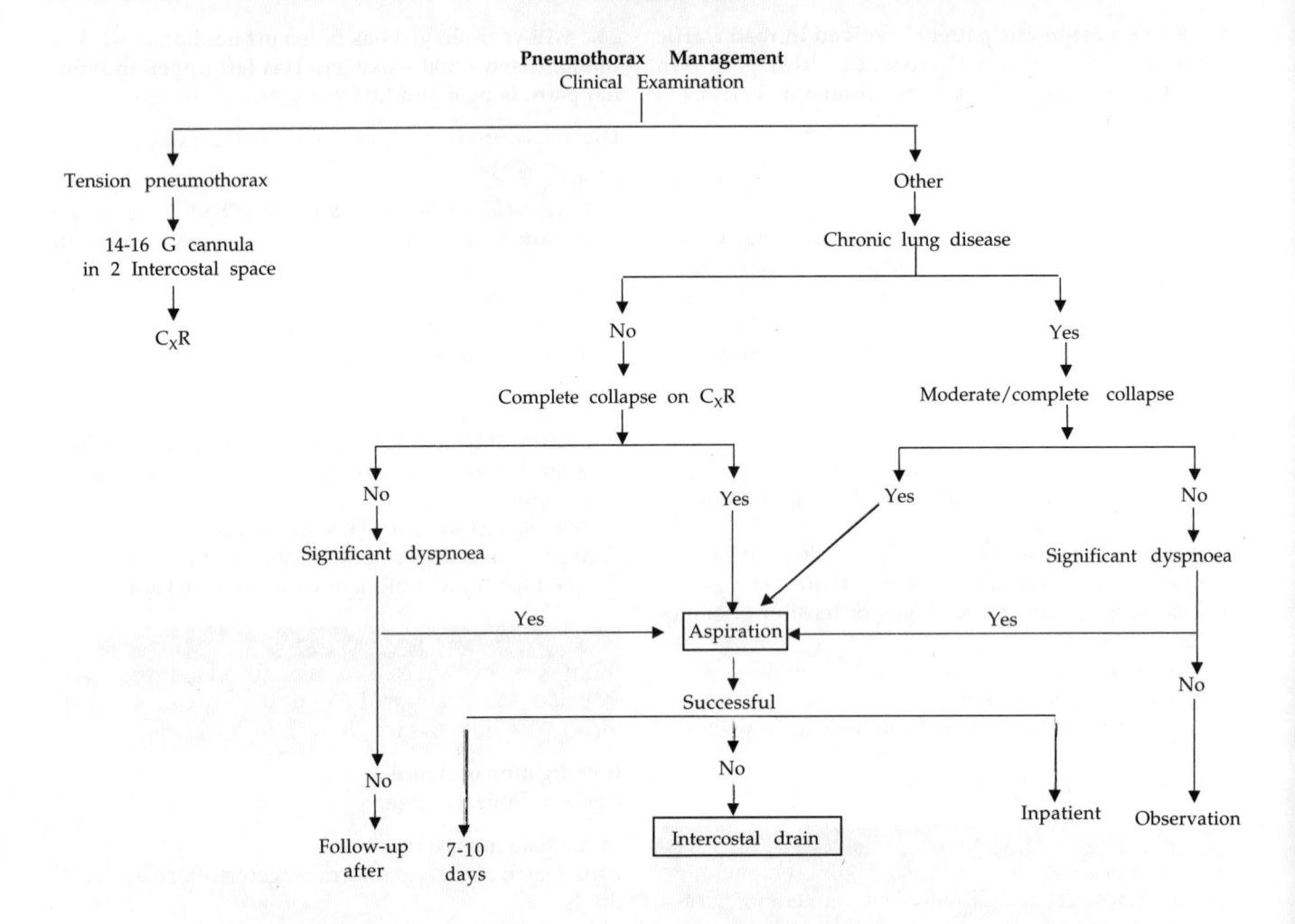

Pneumothorax Management
Clinical Examination

- Tension pneumothorax
  - 14-16 G cannula in 2 Intercostal space
  - C$_x$R

- Other
  - Chronic lung disease
    - No
      - Complete collapse on C$_x$R
        - No
          - Significant dyspnoea
            - Yes → Aspiration
            - No → Follow-up after 7-10 days
        - Yes → Aspiration
    - Yes
      - Moderate/complete collapse
        - Yes → Aspiration
        - No
          - Significant dyspnoea
            - Yes → Aspiration
            - No → Observation

Aspiration
- Successful
  - Yes → Inpatient
  - No → Intercostal drain

25. A 15-year-old girl has cut her wrist and bled profusely. She is pale, tachycardiac and does not want to live.

Diagnosis: Suicide attempt with hypovolemic shock.

Clinchers
- *Has cut her wrist:* Lacerations in this area frequently involve deep structures and accurate diagnosis is essential. History is usually unhelpful in suicide attempts.
- *Bled profusely:* This suggest a massive blood loss and so a search for features of hypotensive shock should be started.
- *Pale, tachycardiac:* This confirms the hypovolemic shock. Tachycardia is usually manifest after at least 15-30% loss of circulating blood.
- *Does not want to live:* She needs continuous monitoring and appropriate sedation as she may repeat the attempt to suicide.

CONFUSA
In wrist lacerations, a full assessment of the distal neurovascular function is essential. Test all tendons and nerves individually. Any positive finding of deep structure involvement must be discussed with a senior colleague at once. Further exploration must be carried out:
- In an operating theatre
- Under adequate anaesthesia (GA usually)
- With a bloodless field
- By an experienced surgeon

Note:
- A divided nerve may continue to conduct some sensation for several hours if the nerve ends are touching.
- Abductor pollices brevis is paralysed in T_1 root lesions but not in ulnar nerve lesions. To test this muscle the thumb is moved vertically upwards against resistance with the hand in supine position.

Investigation of choice
Urine output.

Immediate management
External compression to prevent further blood loss then start treating the shock

Treatment of choice
Microvascular surgery
+
Psychiatric referral later.

26. A 19-year-old female with complaint of a 1 year history of bloody diarrhoea and tenesmus. Has pale skin lesions. On examination-sigmoidoscopy shows inflammation and granulomata.

Diagnosis: Ulcerative colitis (UC).

Clinchers
- *19-year-old:* It is found in any age from infancy to elderly, but the maximum incidence is between the ages of 20 and 40 years.
- *Female:* Females are more often affected than males.
- *1 year history of bloody diarrhoea and tenesmus:* The most common presentation of ulcerative colitis is diarrhoea with blood and mucus. Oedema of rectal mucosa can lead to the symptom of tenesmus.
- *Pale skin lesions:* One of the several skin manifestation seen in UC.
- *Sigmoidoscopy shows inflammation and granulomata:* Sigmoidoscopy reveals oedema of the mucosa with contact bleeding in early mild cases, proceeding to granularity of the mucosa and ten frank ulceration with pus and blood in the bowel lumen. Biopsy will give confirming histological evidence of the diagnois.

CONFUSA
The changes in UC are confluent, with no unaffected "skip lesions" as found in Crohn's disease. Surprisingly, the inflamed colon does not become adherent to its neighbouring intra-abdominal viscera.

Investigation of choice
Sigmoidoscopy + biopsy.

Immediate management
Delineate family history.

Treatment of choice
Sulphasalazine.

Your Notes:

27. 65-year-old male with weight loss, right-sided pain, tenesmus. On examination-mass in the rectum

Diagnosis: Carcinoma rectum.

Clinchers
- *65-year-old male:* It occurs in any age group from the twenties onwards, but is particularly common in the age range 50-70 years. The sexes are equally affected.
- *Weight loss, right side pain and tenesmus:* Bowel disturbance (constipation and/or diarrhoea in 80%) and bleeding, which is almost 60% of patients. There may also be mucus discharge rectal pain and tenesemus.
- *Mass in rectum:* Rectal examination reveals the tumor in 90% of cases.

CONFUSA
Abdominal palpation is negative in early cases but careful attention must be paid to the detection of hepatomegaly, ascites or abdominal distension. Other general features that may be detected in lead cases are enlarged supraclavicular nodes, nodes in the groin or jaundice.

Investigation of choice
Sigmoidoscopy.

Immediate management
Rule out faecal impaction and plevic abscess.

Treatment of choice
Surgery
- Upper 1/3 tumors: Anterior resection
- Middle 1/3 tumors: Anterior resection if
  - female
  - satisfactory distal clearing
- Lower 1/3—Abdominal perineal resection.

Your Notes:

28. 18-year-old presents with frequent diarrhoea for about 3 weeks, relieved by defecation. Sigmoidoscopy is normal.

Diagnosis: IBS with diarrhoea (suspected).

Clinchers
- *18-year-old:* Patient is usually 20-40 years old and females are frequently affected than males.
- *Frequent diarrhoea:* Altered bowel habit i.e. constipation alternating with diarrhoea is a major feature and no cause can be found for it.
- *For 3 weeks:* Chronic symptoms, i.e. for more than 6 months are required for diagnosis of IBS (irritable bowel syndrome).
- *Relieved by defaecation:* There is central or lower abdominal pain in IBS which is characteristically relieved by defaecation.
- *Sigmoidoscopy is normal:* IBS is a diagnosis of exclusion, i.e. no pathology is found on examination and investigations.

CONFUSA
If diarrhoea is present send a stool culture and check the TSH. If the patient is young, with a classic history, check FBC, ESR, LFTs and urinalysis and perform a sigmoidoscopy and rectal biopsy.

Investigation of choice
Stool culture + TSH.

Immediate management
Reassruance and counselling.

Treatment of choice
Symptomatic (see page 237, OHCM, 5th edn).

Your Notes:

29. 80-year-old with complaint of diarrhoea and urinary retention.

Diagnosis: Faecal impaction.

Clinchers
- *80-year-old:* It occurs in the elderly with constipation.
- *Diarrhoea:* It may occur paradoxically wtih the overflow of liquid colonic contents around the impacted stool.
- *Urinary retention:* Chronic constipation or impaction of faeces can result in either urinary incontinence or retention is usually acute anal discomfort.

CONFUSA
Impaction of faeces give the classical characteristic sign of indentation on PR examination. The differential diagnosis is from a rectal tumor.

Investigation of choice
PR examination.

Immediate management
Find the cause of constipation.

Treatment of choice
Manual removal of impacted faeces.

Your Notes:

30. After an abdominal operation, a patient presents with subfebrile state and abdominal distention. There is associated abdominal tenderness, constipation. On auscultation no bowel sounds are heard.

Diagnosis: Paralytic ileus.

Clinchers
- *Abdominal operation:* Paralytic ileus is most commonly seen in the post-operative stage of peritonitis or of major abdominal surgery.
- *Subfebrile state:* It is quite common after major surgeries.
- *Abdominal distension, associated abdominal tenderness, constipation:* There is abdominal distension, absolute constipation and effortless vomiting. Pain is not present, apart from the discomfort of the laparotomy wound and the abdominal distension.

CONFUSA
The distension that occurs on the first and second post-operative day is probably produced by swallowed air. The air passes through the small intestine (where peristalsis usually returns quickly) to the colon, which is atonic and produces a functional hold up.

Investigation of choice
X-ray (usually not required).

Immediate management
Pethidine (as it has little effect on bowel motility).

Treatment of choice
Nasogastric suction (to remove swallowed air and prevent gaseous distension).

Your Notes:

First Aid for PLAB

31. A patient of multiple sclerosis has had urinary catheterisation for 4 years with intermittent obstruction.

Diagnosis: Multiple sclerosis (MS) with spinal cord lesions.

Clinchers
Sphincter disturbances such as urinary urgency or hesitancy which disappear after few days or weeks, to come again (relapsing/remitting disorder), weakness, numbness, tingling, or unsteadiness in a limb, unilateral optic neuritis are the symptoms of multiple sclerosis. First presentations are usually monosymptomatic MS consists of plaques of demyelination throughout the CNS.

> **CONFUSA**
> In MRI, initially individual plaques (e.g. in optic nerve, brainstem or cord) may cause diagnostic difficulty. They must be distinguished from compressive, inflammatory or vascular lesions.

Investigation of choice
In MS investigations only support and do not make the diagnosis. MRI is sensitive but not specific for plaque defection. It is the first line of investigation.

Treatment of choice
There is no curative treatment, but dietary polyunsaturated fats may help.

Your Notes:

---

32. 60-year-old with complaint of frequency, dysuria. PSA is 120 ng/ml, also has back pain.

Diagnosis: Carcinoma prostate.

Clinchers
- *60-year-old man:* Incidence of prostatic carcinoma increases with age. It is the most common malignant tumor in men over the age of 65 years. In England and Wales in 1998, 11000 men were registered and 8000 died from it.
- *Frequency, dysuria:* These are the symptoms of BOO, along with nocturia, hesitancy, poor stream and terminal dribbling. These symptoms can be seen in BPH, bladder neck stenosis, *prostate carcinoma*, urethral strictures, bladder neck hypertrophy and functional obstruction due to neuropathic conditions.
- *PSA is 120 ng/ml:* Prostate-specific antigen is good at following the course of advanced disease. Finding of a PSA > 10 ng/ml diagnostic of advanced prostate cancer.
  Decrease of PSA to the normal range following hormonal ablation is a good prognostic sign.
- *Back pain:* Bone pain, malaise, arthritis, anaemia are other clinical features of prostatic carcinoma. Weight loss and bone pain indicate metastatic disease, spread by the bloodstream.
- *Digital rectal examination:* May reveal hard, irregular prostate gland.

> **CONFUSA**
> These complaints may be present in BPH, but PSA value of 120 ng/ml is diagnostic of advanced carcinoma.

Investigation of choice
- Prostate-specific antigen (PSA)
- Transrectal ultrasound
- Bone X-ray/bone scan.

Treatment of choice
- *Local disease:* Nerve sparing radical prostatectomy (maintains erectile function) is widely used in USA, but there is a considerable defate over relative merits of prostatectomy, radiotherapy or watchful waiting with monitoring of PSA.
- *Metastatic disease:* Hormonal drugs (gonadotropin-releasing analogues) may give benefit for 1-2 years.

Your Notes:

33. Female patient with complaint of sever flank pain, is restless and the pain radiates to the groin.

Diagnosis: Ureteric colic.

Clinchers

- *Female:* Renal calculi is four times more common in males, than females (♀ : ♂ ≈ 4:1). And therefore female, cannot be excluded here. With peak age between 20-50 years.
- *Flank pain, restless, radiating to groin:* Stone in kidney cause loin pain. Stones in ureter cause ureteric colic. Here pain classically radiates from loin to the groin and is associated with nausea and vomiting.

Some important risk factors for renal calculi are: dehydration, UTI, hypercalcaemia, hypercalciuria, ↑ dietary oxalate.

CONFUSA
The diagnosis should be confirmed by abdominal KUB film and ultrasound. In KUB film 80% of stones are visible (97% on CT).

Investigation of choice
- Abdominal KUB film
- Ultrasound
- Blood: U and E, Ca^{2+}, PO_4^{3-}
- 24 h urine: creatinine, Ca^{2+}, oxalate, urate.

Immediate management
- IV fluids (if not accepting orally)
- Analgesia
- If evidence of obstruction, seek urological help urgently

Treatment of choice
Increase fluid intake. If no obstruction f/w attacks, manage conservatively.
- *Ureteric stones:* Usually pass spontaneously or remove endoscopically
- *Pelvicalyceal stones*
  - < 5 mm—no treatment, unless obstruction/infection
  - < 2 cm—lithotripsy
  - 2-4 cm—with normal collecting ducts—go for lithotripsy (take measure to prevent obstruction)
- *Renal colic:* IV fluids (oral if tolerating) + analgesia
- *Evidence of obstruction:* Seek urological help (retrograde stent insertion, nephrostomy and antegrade pyelography).

Your Notes:

34. 65-year-old man with history of frequency, urgency and decreased urinary flow.

Diagnosis: Benign prostatic hypertrophy (BPH).

Clinchers
- *65-year-old man:* BPH occurs in men over 50 years of age. By 60 years 50% of men home histological evidence of BPH.
- *Frequency, urgency, decreased urinary flow:* These are the symptoms of benign prostatic hypertrophy (BPH) due to bladder outflow obstruction (BOO).

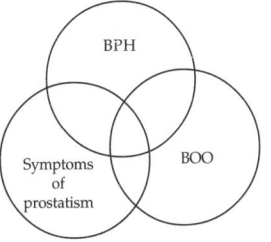

Relationships between BPH, BOO (urodynamically proven) and symptoms of prostatism
- *Rectal examination:* In benign enlargement, posterior surface of prostate is smooth, convex and elastic (sometimes firm because of fibrous element of prostate)
  - Rectal mucosa can be made to more over the prostate
  - Sometimes fluctuating swelling over the prostate (this is residual urine).

CONFUSA
All these symptoms of disturbed voiding in ageing men should not be always attributed to BPH causing BOO. These symptoms may owe to impairment of smooth muscles function and neurovesical coordination. Rule out prostatic carcinoma, refer to Q-32 (July 2001).

Investigation of choice
- PSA (rule out carcinoma)
- Flow rate measurement: Typical history and flow rate < 10 ml/second (for voided volume of > 200 ml) alarms treatment
- *Cystourethroscopy:* Before prostatectomy
- Serum creatinine/electrolytes

Treatment of choice
- Transurethral resection of the prostate (TURP)
- Transurethral incision of the prostate (TUIP)
- Retropubic prostatectomy
- Drugs (in mild cases
  - *α blockers (terazosin or indoramin):* Decrease smooth muscle tone (prostate and bladder)
  - *α reductase inhibitor (finasteride):* It ↓ conversion of testosterone to dihydrotestosterone.

35. A 39-year-old female presents with weakness of both legs, difficulty walking and urinary retention.

Diagnosis: Spinal cord lesion

Clinchers
- Bladder tone is lost immediately after spinal transection
- Distention leads to ureteric reflux and renal damage. Motor and sensory loss further support diagnosis of spinal cord lesion.

CONFUSA
Impairment of descending sympathetic pathways in the spinal cord leads to relative hypovolaemia and cardia. Any reduction of blood supply to the damaged cord will further impair its function. Bradycardia often responds to atropine.

Investigation of choice
MRI spine.

Immediate management
Intermittent catheterization may be the treatment of choice in the spinal unit but it is preferable to insert and retain a fairly thin catheter during the initial period of resuscitation and inter-hospital transfer. Catheterisation must be performed by an experienced member of staff using an aseptic technique.

Your Notes:

36. A young boy back from holiday in north Africa presents with night fever, weight loss. Began on antibiotics with minimal improvement. CSF shows: protein-960 mg/dL, glucose-2 mmol/L, cells-Lymphocytes.

Diagnosis: ZN staining

Clinchers
- *Young boy back from holiday in north Africa:* Africa especially the northern parts are endemic for tuberculosis infection.
- *Night fever and weight loss:* Tubercular meningitis commences with vague headache, low grade evening or night time pyrexia and weight loss due to loss of appetite (anorexia) and vomiting.
- *Began on antibiotics with minimal improvement:* Conventional or common antibiotics have insignificant effect on tubercle bacilli. A specific treatment (INH + Rmp) is required.
- *CSF shows protein—960 mg/dL; glucose—2 mmol/L; cells—lymphocytes:* Tuberculous meningitides have protein in CSF in range of 500-3000 mg/L; glucose < 1/3 blood glucose and 0-200/mm^3 polymorphs.

CONFUSA
Meningitic signs may take some weeks to develop in tubercular meningitis. Cryptococcal meningitis is the main differential diagnosis although syphilis, sarcoidosis and Behcet's syndrome can also cause chronic meningitis.

Investigation of choice
LP (Now: ZN staining).

Immediate management
CXR (to rule out pulmonary TB).

Treatment of choice
At least nine months treatment with anti TB drugs.

Your Notes:

37. An 8-year-old with acute leukemia is admitted in a comatose state. He is found to have lymphoblast depletion prevention of infectious diseases.

Diagnosis: Tumor lysis syndrome.

Clinchers
- *8-year-old:* leukemias are the most common type of childhood. Malignancies are over 95% of cases are of acute variety. In the acute series ALL accounts for 70-80% cases. The peak age of onset of ALL is 3-7 years.
- *Acute leukemia:* As his diagnosis is known he must be on some treatment. Usually chemotherapy is given for ALL.
- *Lymphoblast depletion:* Since lymphoblasts rapidly proliferate in ALL, their depletion should raise a suspicion of any treatment with chemotherapeutic drugs. Tumor lysis syndrome is due to rapid cell death on starting chemotherapy for rapidly proliferating tumors like ALL. It results in rise in serum urate, potassium and phosphate, precipitating renal failure, which can lead to comatose condition if not treated urgently.

CONFUSA
Coma can also occurs in ALL as leukaemic blast cells can infiltrate brain to produce leukaemic meningitis.

Investigation of choice
Serum urate level (increased).

Immediate management
Immediate hydration.

Treatment of choice
Haemodialysis.

Your Notes:

38. A 14-year-old boy presents with drowsiness and generalised headache. He is recovering from a bilateral parotitits. His CT scan is normal.

Diagnosis: Viral meningitis (aseptic meningitis)

Clinchers
- *14-year-old boy:* Mumps is generally a childhood disease caused by RNA paramyxovirus. Incidence of meningitis in males is three times more after mumps.
- *Drowsiness and generalised headache:* There are cardinal symptoms of increased ICP. Other symptoms can be:
  - Irritability
  - Vomiting
  - Fits
  - Bradycardia
  - BP increase
  - Impaired consciouness (confusion)
  - Coma
  - Irregular respiration
  - papilloedema (late sign)
- *Recovering from bilateral parotitis:* Meningitis secondary to mumps usually occur in convalescent phase. Mumps is characterised by painful swelling of the parotids, unilaterally at first, becoming bilateral in 70%.
- *CT scan is normal:* Rules out any space occupying lesion in the brain or ventricular dilatation, both of which are contraindication to lumbar puncture.

CONFUSA
In aseptic meningitis, CSF has cells but is Gram stain negative and no bacteria can be cultured on standard media. Mumps infection confers life-long immunity, so a documented history of previous infection excludes this diagnosis.

Investigation of choice
- *Screening:* Lumbar puncture, will show a picture of aseptic meningitis
- *Definitive:* Isolation of virus from CSF.

Immediate management
Symptomatic (hospital admission usually not required).

Treatment of choice
Bedrest in a quiet and dark room.

Your Notes:

39. An intravenous drug abuser presents with suspected meningitis. The organism is confirmed in the CSF by India ink preparation.

Diagnosis: Cryptococcal meningitis.

Clinchers
- *IV drug abuser:* He must be having an undiagnosed HIV infection resulting in immunodeficient state. Cryptococcal meningitis does not occur in immunocompetant people.
- *Suspected meningitis:* CNS infections in HIV positive people are usually by toxoplasmosis, CMV and *Cryptococcus*. Toxoplasmosis causes a SOL and CMV causes encephalitis. *Cryptococcus* is associated with meningitis usually.
- *Organism confirmed in CSF in India Ink preparation:* This is characteristic of *Cryptococcus neoformans* (a fungi) whose thick capsule resist staining and can only be demonstrated as translucencies against black background in India ink preparations.

CONFUSA
Cryptococcal meningitis have an insidious onset and is often without neck stiffness. The etiology of neck stiffness is inflammation and it is often absent in immunodeficients and neonates. Conditions (other than meningitis) which can produce neck stiffness are *Shigella* gastroenteritis and subarachnoid hemorrhage.

Investigation of choice
India ink staining of CSF.
or
Detection of cryptococcal antigen in blood/CSF.

Immediate management
Transfer to ITU.

Treatment of choice
Amphotericin/fluocytosine IV
Fluconazole can be given in milder cases (better tolerated).

Your Notes:

---

40. An anxious mother called you to say that her son's best friend in school has caught meningitis.

Diagnosis: Immediate 'contact' of meningitis.

Clinchers
Meningitis prophylaxis:
Talk to your consultant in community disease control. Offer prophylaxis is:
- Household/nurser contacts (i.e. within droplet range)
- Those who have kissed the patient's mouth.

CONFUSA
If the student suffering from meningitis is just a classmate and the best friend of her son, then there is no need of any chemoprophylaxis.

Investigation of choice
None required except screening the skin for any non-blanching petechiae.

Immediate management
Reassure mother

Treatment of choice
Rifampicin prophylaxis
- 600 mg/12 h PO for 2 days
- Children   > 1 yr 10 mg/kg/12 h
              < 1 yr 10 mg/kg/12 h

or
Ciprofloxacin
- 500 mg PO, 1 dose, adult only

Your Notes:

41. Patient stabbed in right chest. Ultrasound showed no free fluid perabdominally, patient is breathless, pale.

Diagnosis: Haemothorax.

Clinchers
- *Stabbed in right chest:* A stab wound may cause profound bleeding from the internal thoracic artery or other intrathoracic structures.
- *USG showed no free fluid per-abdominally:* This rules out intraperitoneal bleed after injury to any abdominal viscera.
- *Breathless:* Dyspnoea and reduced breath sounds are characteristic.
- *Pale:* It signifies blood loss and hence haemothorax.

CONFUSA
Haemothorax is usually a result of intercostal or internal thoracic vessel damage. The bleeding is often brisk and continuous from the high pressure of the intercostal arteries. In contrast, bleeding from the low-pressure pulmonary vessels usually stops with the collapse of the lung.

Investigation of choice
CXR (blunting of costophrenic angles).

Immediate management
High concentration oxygen by mask.

Treatment of choice
Chest drain (always required in a stab wound).

Your Notes:

42. Woman history of 8/52 amenorrhoea presents with abdominal pain rigidity and is pale. Pain radiating to tip of shoulder.

Diagnosis: Ruptured ectopic pregnancy

Clinchers
- *8 weeks amenorrhoea:* Ectopic pregnancy generally presents at around 8 weeks amenorrhoea, but it may present before a period is missed.
- *Abdominal pain, rigidity, pale:* Always think of ectopic in a sexually active women with abdominal pain and bleeding. Ectopic can rupture, and cause severe pain, may radiate to tip of shoulder (diaphragmatic irritation) abdominal rigidity (peritonitis) and shock, (excessive bleeding-hence pale).

Ectopic pregnancy is one outside the uterine cavity, the most common site being the fallopian tube.
The tubal pregnancy can terminate in following ways:
- *Absorption:* Embryo dies in the tube, with a small amount of bleeding and is partly absorbed.
- *Tubal abortion:* Part or all of the products of conception are expelled from the tube, into the peritoneal cavity.
- *Tubal rupture:* Most dramatic and best known termination of tubal pregnancy (there is acute intraperitoneal hemorrhage from erosion of an artery.
- *Secondary abdominal pregnancy:* Rare outcome. Here embryo gets attached in the peritoneal cavity. (In West Indies, many cases of children delivered from the peritoneal cavity by laparotomy has been reported).

CONFUSA
Other causes of abdominal pain to be kept in mind are: perforation of peptic ulcer, sigmoid diverticulum, or the appendix, acute pancreatitis, leaking aortic aneurysm; intra-abdominal sepsis with septic shock; acute salpingitis.

Investigation of choice
Ultrasonography

Immediate management
Patient must be taken immediately to the operation theatre. Do not waste time in attempting resuscitation which can prove useless and only increase bleeding step up IV drip and transfuse blood immediately and the affected tube should be removed.

Your Notes:

43. Patient with history of suggestive of atherosclerosis, now presenting with shock.

Diagnosis: Aortic aneurysm.

Clinchers
- *History suggestive of atherosclerosis:* Atheroma is the usual cause for arterial aneurysms. Other causes include:
  - Penetrating injuries
  - Infections
    - Endocarditis
    - Syphilis.
- *Shock:* Fifty percent of the patients of ruptured aortic aneurysm die from the initial rupture and never reach hospital. Those which do reach hospital are usually profoundly shocked (cold, clammy, tachycardia, hypotensive) with generalised abdominal tenderness.

CONFUSA
The ECG often shows ischemic changes as this group of patients has generalised atherosclerosis and coronary ischemia is worsened by hypotension. The main differential diagnosis is pancreatitis. If in doubt, assume a ruptured aneurysm. No investigation should delay the surgical referral.

Investigation of choice
USG.

Immediate management
Immediate surgical referral or take the patient to OT
+
Treat shock.

Treatment of choice
Surgery (aortic clamp + Dacron graft).

Your Notes:

44. Patient admitted with suspected tetanus and is given tetanus immunoglobulin and an antibiotic to which he is not allergic. 10 hours later the patient is breathless with tachycardia.

Diagnosis: Anaphylaxis.

Clinchers
- *Given tetanus Ig:* Tetanus Ig can produce anaphylaxis.
- *An antibiotic to which he is not allergic:* Anaphylaxis occurs via a different mechanism—it is due to induction of an IgE antibody response that causes a generalized release of mediators from mast cells.
- *Ten minutes later the patient is breathless:* Anaphylaxis is a life-threatening hypersensitivity reaction to contact with an allergen; it may appear within minutes to exposure to the offending substance. Manifestations include respiratory distress, pruritus, urticaria; mucous membrane swelling; GI disturbances including nausea, vomiting, pain and diarrhoea; and vascular collapse.
- *Tachycardia:* Its presence exclude a vasovagal syncope.

CONFUSA
Virtually any allergen may incite an anaphylactic reaction, but among the more common agents are proteins such as antisera, hormones, pollen extracts, hymenoptera venom, foods (peanuts), drugs (especially antibiotics), and diagnostic agents. Atopy does not seem to predispose to anaphylaxis from penicillin or venom exposures.

Investigation of choice
Purely clinical diagnosis.

Immediate management
Summon skilled anaesthetic help.

Treatment of choice
Parenteral adrenaline + IV hydrocortisone + IV chlorpheniramine.

Your Notes:

45. A known asthmatic on treatment with inhaled Beta-2-agonist and steroid. Now presents with hypotension, breathlessness and distended neck veins.

Diagnosis: Tension pneumothorax.

Clinchers
- *Asthmatic:* Asthma and other chronic lung diseases predispose to spontaneous pneumothorax. However, the most common disease implicated is COPD.
- *On treatment with inhaled beta-2 agonist and steroid:* This is the standard treatment to moderate to severe asthma. The presence of steroids in treatment regimen suggests a long-standing history and hence a comparatively higher risk of pneumothorax.
- *Hypotension, breathlessness and distended neck veins:* The six cardinal signs of a tension pneumothorax are:
  1. Air hunger + respiratory distress
  2. Pulse ↑ + BP ↓
  3. Tracheal deviation
  4. Breath sounds ↓ on one side
  5. Cyanosis
  6. Neck vein distension.

CONFUSA
Insertion of a needle does not always decompress a tension pneumothorax as the underlying pleura and lung are "sucked" into the needle and occlude it. If this happens, a second attempt should be made failure to achieve decompression at this point indicates the need to proceed immediately to rapid insertion of a chest drain.
Note: Never use nitrous oxide mixtures (e.g. Entonox) for pain relief in pneumothorax as it may result in expansion of a gas filled space.

Investigation of choice
CXR (after needle thoracocentesis).

Immediate management
Needle thoracocentesis (urgent).

Treatment of choice
Chest drain.

Your Notes:

46. A 60-year-old attends A and E and it is thought he may have aortic aneurysm.

Diagnosis: Unruptured aortic aneurysm (AA).

Clinchers
- *60-year-old:* Prevalence of AA is 3% of those above 50 years.
- *It is thought he may have aortic aneurysm:* The most common aortic aneurysms are abdominal between the renal and iliac arteries. They are usually due to atherosclerosis. The incidence increases with age, with men being affected four to five times more frequently. An ultrasound of the abdomen for evaluation of asymptomatic aneurysms will demonstrate the size of the aneurysm, the thickness of aortic wall and whether any leak has occurred.

CONFUSA
Angiography underestimates the size and extent of a true aneurysm, as it images the lumen, which is usually narrowed by thrombus. In addition, it may be dangerous, as the guide wire or cannual may perforate the aneurysm wall. It is useful in false aneurysm to identify the connection.

Investigation of choice
Abdominal ultrasound.

Immediate management
Evaluate for surgery.

Treatment of choice
Prophylactic surgery for aneurysm > 5.5-6 cm.

Your Notes:

47. A tall 34-year-old man develops severe central chest pain radiating to his back. He soon develops a dense hemiplegia.

Diagnosis: Dissecting aortic aneurysm (DAA)

Clinchers
- *Tall 34-year-old man:* Peak incidence of DAA occurs in sixth and seventh decade. Men are more commonly affected. DAA in young 34-year-old man (tall) may focus our attention towards Marfan's syndrome. Marfan's sydnrome is a dominent connective tissue disease with following criterias (diagnostic, e.g. > 2 criteria with positive family history)—lens dislocation, aortic dissection/dilatation, dural ectasia and skeletal features, e.g. arachnodactyly (long spidery fingers) armspan greater than height.
- *Severe central chest pain radiating to his back:* DAA presents with sudden onset, severe and tearing chest pain which may be localised to front or back. Other causes of chest pain are
  - *Cardiovascular:*
    - Angina
    - Myocardial infarction
    - Acute aortic dissection
    - Pericarditis.
  - *Gastrointestinal*
    - Oesophageal spasm
    - Reflux oesophagitis
    - Peptic ulcer disease
  - *Pulmonary*
    - Pneumonia
    - Pulmonary embolism
    - Pneumothroax
  - *Musculoskeletal*
    - Chest wall injuries
    - Costochondritis
    - Rib secondaries
    - Herpes zoster
  - *Emotional*
    - Depression
    - De Costa's syndrome
- *Develops dense hemiplegia:* Hemiplegia and hemianesthesia both are neurological findings in DAA due to carotid artery obstruction. It may also lead to spinal cord ischemia (paraplegia).

CONFUSA
Echocardiogram that shows no evidence of ischemia is helpful in distinguishing aortic dissection from myocardial infarction.

Investigation of choice
Chest X-ray/aortography or noninvasive techniques like two-dimentional echocardiography, CT scan or MRI (If haemodynamically compromised). MRI gives the best differentiation owing to high resolution.

Immediate management
Monitor hemodynamics and urine output. Unless hypotension is there, aim at reducing cardiac contractility and systemic arterial pressure.

Treatment of choice
For acute aortic dissection, beta-adrenergic blockers should be administered IV to achieve heart rate of about 60 beats/minute, followed by sodium nitroprusside infusion to lower systolic BP to 120 mmHg.

Long-term aim—control hypertension and reduce cardiac contractility.

Your Notes:

48. A patient is to have a repair of of his aortic aneurysm but also has severe myocardial ischemia.

Diagnosis: Risk of MI during surgery.

Clinchers
Coronary artery disease is common in the population who develop aortic aneurysms. It need to be ruled out before surgery as cross clamping the aorta during surgery dramatically increases the peripheral resistance against which the heart must work, and this extra stress, coupled with the metabolic stress that occurs when the legs are reperfused, may precipitate a myocardial infarct.

CONFUSA
Preoperative assessment includes evaluating the patient's operative risk by screening for coincident cardiac disease (by ECG, echocardiography or MUGA scan to assess the ventricular ejection fraction) and for carotid arterial disease.

Investigation of choice
Coronary angiography.

Immediate management
Refer surgery.

Treatment of choice
Symptomatic.

Your Notes:

49. Patient with aortic aneurysm has unstable angina.

Diagnosis: Dessecting aortic aneurysm (ascending aorta)

Clinchers
- *Aortic aneurysm:* The most common pathologic condition associated with aortic aneurysm is atherosclerosis. It is controversial whether atherosclerosis itself actually causes aortic aneurysm or develops as a secondary event in the dilated aorta. Causality is implied by studies that have shown that many patients with aortic aneurysms have coexisting risk factors and atherosclerosis in other blood vessels.
- *Unstable angina.* Unstable angina may be primary, i.e. occur in the absence of an extrathoracic condition that has intensified myocardial ischemia, or it may be precipitated by a condition extrinsic to the coronary vascular bed that has intensified myocardial ischemia, such as anaemia, fever, infection, tachyarrhythmias, emotional stress or hypoxaemia. Unstable angina may also develop shortly after MI.

CONFUSA
An ECG could be done urgently in this case as an ECG that shows no evidence of ischemia is helpful in distinjuishing aortic dissection from myocardial infarction. Rarely, the dissection involves the right or left coronary and causes acute myocardial infarction or unstable angina.

Investigation of choice
ECG + Aortography + concomitant coronary angiography.

Immediate management
Cross match > 6 units of blood + take to OT.

Treatment of choice
Surgery.

Your Notes:

50. Elderly patient suspected of having aortic dissection with complaint of abdominal pain yesterday, but is now hemodynamically stable.

Diagnosis: Aortic dissection (AD)—suspected.

Clinchers

> *Elderly:* The peak incidence of AD is in sixth and seventh decades. Men are more affected than women by a ratio of 2:1.
> *Suspected of having aortic dissection with complaint of abdominal pain:* Acute AD presents with a sudden onset of pain, which is often described as very severe and tearing and is associated with diaphoresis. The pain may be localized to the front or back of the chest, often the interscapular region, and typically migrates with preparation of dissection.
> *Now hemodynamically stable:* If hypotension is not present, therapy should be aimed at reducing cardiac contractility and systemic arterial pressure, and thereby shear stress.

CONFUSA
CT scan and MRI are each highly accurate in identifying the intimal flap and the extent of the dissection. They are useful in recognising intramural hemorrhage and penetrating ulcers. MRI also can detect blood flow which may be useful is characterizing antegrade versus retrograde dissection. These noninvasive tests are now becoming the diagnostic procedures of choice. Their relative utility depends on the availability and expertise in individual institutions as well as on the hemodynamic stability of the patient, with CT and MRI obviously less suitable for more unstable patients. Still trans-oesophageal echocardiography should be the first investigation.

Investigation of choice
Echocardiography (Trans-oesophageal).

Immediate management
Evaluation by a specialist.

Treatment of choice
As per the findings of echocardiography.

Your Notes:

51. A patient presents with intermittent abdominal Pain for about 30 minutes after meals. Also has history of abdominal pain radiating to the back. On examination-abdominal bruit. Also has intermittent claudication.

Diagnosis: Generalized atherosclerosis.

Clinchers

> *Intermittent abdominal pain for 30 minutes after meals:* Severe abdominal pain, often colicky, following meals, is seen in acute mesenteric ischemia. Other causes of acute abdomen are given in the confusa.
> *On examination abdominal bruit:* Abdominal bruits are often present in normal subjects. They should not necessarily be ascribed to an ischemic bowel, on this basis alone. It occurs due to partial obstruction to flow in the vessels.
> *Intermittent claudication:* It is a sign of chronic ischemia, almost always due to atherosclerosis.

CONFUSA
Differential diagnosis of acute abdomen—perforated viscus (especially peptic ulcer), acute cholecystitis, and biliary colic, acute intestinal obstruction, mesenteric vascular occlusion, Renal colic, myocardial infarction, dissecting aortic aneurysm.

Investigation of choice
If we go by the options in this question, mesenteric angiogram, should be the answer.

Immediate management
Go for tests to exclude diabetes mellitus, arteritis (ESR/CRP)
Do FBC (anemia, infection), lipids, ECG
Arteriography.

Treatment of choice
- Quit smoking
- ↓weight
- Exercise

If tests confirm any disease, treat it (e.g. treat DM, BP↑, hyperlipidaemia).

Your Notes:

52. Patient on antacids for extensive epigastric pain presents with acute abdominal pain, rigidity and is pale.

Diagnosis: Perforated peptic ulcer.

Clinchers

- *Patient on antacids for extensive epigastric pain:* Points forwards peptic ulcer disease. Epigastric pain is a characteristic feature of peptic ulcer disease. Both gastric and duodenal ulcers are helped by antacids.
- *Acute abdominal pain, rigidity, pale:* Since it is a case of peptic ulcer, these signs point towards perforation of peptic ulcer. Duodenal ulcer perforate more commonly than gastric ulcers, usually into the peritoneal cavity. Look for acute abdomenal conditions (e.g. cholecystitis, pancreatitis, etc).

CONFUSA
Check serum amylase to rule out pancreatitis. Avoid laparotomy if pancreatitis is diagnosed. Look for other acute gastrointestinal condition (e.g. cholecystitis). Non GI conditions (e.g. myocardial infarction).

Investigation of choice
- X-ray abdomen/USG
- Serum amylase
- ECG.

Immediate management
Investigage. If perofation diagnosed—laparotomy.

Treatment of choice
Immediate laparotomy.

Your Notes:

53. Female patient with 24 hours history of severe abdominal pain and vomiting. She is restless and afebrile. She has a history of chronic alcoholism.

Diagnosis: Acute pancreatitis.

Clinchers

- *Female:* Women are more affected than men. The patient is often obese and middle aged or elderly.
- *24 hours history of severe abdominal pain:* The pain is severe, constant usually epigastric and often radiates into the back.
- *Vomiting:* Vomiting is early, profuse and prominent sign. The patient often sits forward, and repeated setching is common.
- *Restless:* It is due to the severe pain which is relieved in certain positions, e.g. sitting forward.
- *Afebrile:* The temperature may either be subnormal or riased upto 39.5° C (103°F).
- *Chronic alcoholism:* The majority of non-gallstone pancreatitis is alcohol related. This is particularly common in France and North America. Alcohol is also the most common cause of recurrent pancreatitis. The mechanism is unlcear, and it may follow either chronic alcohol abuse or finge drinking.

CONFUSA

Causes of acute pancreatitis: mnemonic "GET SMASHED".
 G — Gallstones
 E — Ethanol
 T — Trauma
 S — Steroids
 M — Mumps
 A — Autoimmune (PAN)
 S — Scorpion venom
 H — Hyperlipidemia
       Hypercalcaemia
       Hypothermia
 E — ERCP
       Emboli
 D — Drugs = azathioprine
              = asparaginase
              = mercaptopurine
              = pentamidine
              = didanosine

Investigation of choice
Serum amylase > 1000 µ/mL.

Immediate management: Nil by mouth.

Treatment of choice: Symptomatic.

54. Patient with presenting complaint of severe flank pain. He is now restless. He says that the pain is radiating to the groin he is passing reddish urine.

Diagnosis: Ureteric colic

Clinchers
- *Severe flank pain:* Impaction of the stone at the pelvi-ureteric junction, or migration down the ureter itself, produces the deadful agony of ureteric colic.
- *Restless:* The pain is of great severity and is accompanied by typical restlessness of the patient, who is quite unable to lie still in bed.
- *Radiating to groin:* The pain typically radiates from groin to loin.
- *Reddish urine:* Haematuria, which may be microscopic or macroscopic, is frequently present so that detection of blood in the urine is an extremely helpful means of confirming the clinical diagnosis.

CONFUSA
Unlik the usual textbook description the pain is not usually intermittent, but is continuous, although quite often with sharp exacerbations on a background of continued pain. There is often accompanying vomiting and sweating. Pain is the presenting feature of the great majority of kidney stones, but if the calculus is embedded within the solid substance of the kidney it may be entirely symptom-free. Within the minor or major calyx system the stone produces a dull loin pain.

Investigation of choice
- *Screening:* Abdominal KUB film.
- *Definitive:* IVU.

Immediate management
See urgent urological help.
Analgesia: Diclofenac suppository 100 mg (single dose).

Treatment of choice
Lithotripsy or open surgery.

Your Notes:

55. A 50-year-old chronic alcoholic presents with a sudden onset difuse abdominal pain. It is radiating to the back. He has generalised abdominal tenderness with vomiting and rigidity.

Diagnosis: Acute pancreatitis.

Clinchers
Note: See Q 53 of this theme also
- *50-year-old:* The patient is often obese and middleaged or elderly.
- *Sudden onset:* The pain may be gradual or sudden onset but is severe and constant.
- *Diffuse abdominal pain:* The pain may be epigastric or central or diffuse.
- *Radiates to back:* It radiates to back characteristically.
- *Generalised abdominal tenderness with vomiting and rigidity:* On examination the abdomen reveals generalized tenderness and guarding.

CONFUSA
The symptoms of acute pancreatitis may be mild in severe disease. There may be periumbilical discoloration (Cullen's sign) or flank bruising (Grey turner's sign) later on. About 30% of cases have a tinge of jaundice due to oedema of the pancreatic head obstructing the common bile duct.

Investigation of choice
Serum amylase > 1000 μ/mL.

Immediate management
Nil by mouth.

Treatment of choice
Symptomatic.

Your Notes:

56. A 7-day-old baby cries whenever lifted. Labour was difficult.

Diagnosis: Fracture shaft femur.

Clinchers
- *7-day-old:* Since the baby is only of 7 days, he will not have any obvious features of fracture shaft femur (i.e. impaired mobility, etc.). It also suggest the fracture to be consequence of difficult labour.
- *Cries whenever lifted:* This may be the only feature of skeletal injuries in a newborn.
- *Labour was difficult:* Prolonged labour can produce fetal hypoxia and some powerful uterine contractions or bearing down efforts can cause fracture of clavicle or femur.

CONFUSA
Neonatal mortality rises with prolonged labour as does material mortality (especially with infection).

Investigation of choice
X-ray femur.

Immediate management
Splinting.

Your Notes:

57. Young girl tripped while holding mother's hand. Now cannot use arm at all.

Diagnosis: Pulled elbow.

Clinchers
- *Young girl:* This condition occurs in children between 1-4 years of age.
- *Tripped while holding mother's hand:* It occurs when pulled up by the arms, while being lifted in play. The head of the radius is pulled partly out of the annular ligament when a child is lifted by the wrist.
- *Now cannot use arm at all:* The child starts crying and is unable to move the affected limb. The forearm lies in an attitude of pronation. There may be mild swelling at the elbow.

CONFUSA
It is not possible to see the subluxated head on an X-ray because it is still cartilagineous. X-rays are taken only to rule out any other bony injury. Do not attempt to reduce a pulled elbow if there is any doubt about the diagnosis.

Investigation of choice
Entirely clinical diagnosis.

Immediate management
Refer to orthopaedics.

Treatment of choice
Elbow rotation (forced supination with a thumb over the radial head). A click will be heard on reduction. Final reassurance for the doctor, and doubling parents, is obtained by letting the child play and watching normal movements return. This may take sometime.

Your Notes:

58. Young boy fell off horse onto his hand. Now with complaint of mild tenderness over the clavicle but able to use forearm.

Diagnosis: Green stick injury.

Clinchers
- *Young boy:* Young soft bones may partially break after bending. This is called green stick fracture.
- *Fell off horse onto his hand:* Greenstick fractures of clavicle are common after childhood falls.
- *Mild tenderness over the clavicle but able to use forearm:* There may be minimal symptoms, i.e. little deformity and tenderness. There is also remarkably good movements of arm and shoulder girdle.

CONFUSA
In green stick fracture of clavicle, sometimes the child may refuse to use the whole arm on the affected side and thus mimic a pulled elbow.

Investigation of choice
Anteroposterior radiograph.

Immediate management
Appropriate analgesia.

Treatment of choice
Broad arm sling.

Your Notes:

59. Young child fell on outstretched hand and now has absent radial pulse.

Diagnosis: Supracondylar fracture.

Clinchers
- *Young child:* This injury occurs in older children (peak incidence at age 8 years). It is one of the most serious fractures in childhood as it is often associated with complications.
- *Fell on outstretched hand:* This is typical of supracondylar fracture. As the hand strikes the ground the elbow is forced into hyperextension resulting in fracture of the humerus above the condyles.
- *Absent radial pulse:* This implies vascular damage which is common in this injury. It suggests that the fracture is complicated with gross displacement (usually of the distal fragment posteriorly).

CONFUSA
Reduction under GA by the orthopaedic team and subsequent monitoring of distal neurovascular function is essential. Failure to do this may result in Volkmann's ischemic contracture of the forearm muscles with permanent disability in the hand. Some undisplaced fractures may be treated on an outpatient basis, but this decision should be left to the orthopaedic staff.

Investigation of choice
Radiography (AP + lateral view) with radiograph of opposite elbow for comparison.

Immediate management
Orthopaedics referral

Treatment of choice
Reduction under GA
Internal fixation if articular surface is implicated.

Your Notes:

60. A 12-year-old boy with left groin pain for 6 weeks is noticed to stand with the left leg externally rotated. Examination reveals negligible internal rotation of the hip.

Diagnosis: Slipped upper femoral epiphyses (SUFE).

Clinchers
- *12-year-old boy:* SUFE is found in older children. The child is frequently overweight and may have delayed sexual development
- *Boys > girls:* It is a bilateral in 24% of patients.
- *Left groin pain for 6 weeks:* Classically symptoms are insiduous in onset, as the displacement is gradual. It is often associated with a limp (like Perthes' disease).
- *Stand with the left leg externally rotated:* External rotation of the limb at rest is pathognomic. Also the limb may be slightly short.
- *Negligible internal rotation of the hip:* Passive internal rotation is characteristically diminished in SUFE.

CONFUSA
The condition may not be apparent in early stages on an AP X-ray, but is detectable on a lateral film. A line drawn through the centre of the femoral neck in any X-ray projection should pass through the centre of the head. If it does not then some displacement has occurred.

Investigation of choice
Special lateral X-ray view
(Findings: Posterior displacement of the upper femoral epiphysis)

Immediate management
Orthopaedics referral.

Treatment of choice
- *Acute symptoms*
  - Traction in internal rotation
  - Alternatively manipulation under GA
- *Chronic symptoms*
  - Pinning
  - If not possible—osteotomy.

Your Notes:

61. Known patient of multiple sclerosis now with complaint of urinary incontinence, weakness in all 4 limbs and difficulty walking.

Diagnosis (of anatomical site): Cervical spinal cord.

Clinchers
- *Known patient of multiple sclerosis:* Multiple sclerosis is characterised by chronic inflammation, and selective destruction of CNS myelin: sparing the peripheral nervous system. It presents a recurrent attacks of focal neurologic dysfunction.
- *Difficult walking:* The symptoms of multiple sclerosis often worsen with fatigue, stress, exercise or left.
- *Urinary incontinence:* Sensory system involves urinary urgency or frequency, visual difficulties, abnormalities of gate and coordination.
  Motor involvement presents as heavy, stiff, weak or clumsy limb.
- Difficulty in walking, Lhermitte's sign (paraesthesia in limbs on flexing legs) and urinary symptoms are common in spinal cord lesion.
- Paraparesis (weakness of both lower limbs) is characteristically diagnostic (not always) of spinal cord lesion.

CONFUSA
Initial individual plaques of MS (e.g. in optic nerve, brainstem or cord) must be distinguished from compressive, inflammatory, mass or vascular lesions. Other conditions that mimic the pattern of relapsing MS are CNS sarcoidosis, SLE and Behcet's syndrome.

Investigation of choice
MRI of the brain and spinal cord is the first line of investigation.

Immediate management
Refer to neurology.

Treatment of choice
When diagnosed, inform the patient of the diagnosis. There is no cure.
- *Polyunsaturated fats*—may help.
- *Methylprednisolone*—shortens relapses
- β-interferon 1b
  - ↓ relapse rate by 1/3
  - ↓ lesion accumulation on MRI
  - Slow accumulation of disability.

Your Notes:

62. Patient has nystagmus, diplopia, and positive past pointing.

Diagnosis (of anatomical site): Brainstem and its cerebellar connections

Clinchers
- *Nystagmus:* A rhythmic oscillation of the eye is a sign of disease of either the ocular or the vestibular system and its connection. In the lesions of brainstem and the cerebellum, long lasting horizontal or rotatory jerk and nystagmus are present.
- *Diplopia:* Diplopia in multiple sclerosis is the result of many different lesions—a sixth nerve lesion and the internuclear ophthalmoplegia (INO) are true examples.
- *Positive past pointing:* It is a sign of cerebellar lesion. Others include positive gait disturbances, nystagmus, dysarthria, etc.

CONFUSA
A typical picture of sole brainstem demyelination is sudden diplopia and vertigo with nystagmus, but without tinnitus or deafness.

Investigation of choice
MRI (magnetic resonance imaging).

Immediate management
Refer to neurology.

Treatment of choice
When diagnosed, inform the patient of the diagnosis. There is no cure.
- *Polyunsatured fats*—may help
- *Methylprednisolone*—shortens relapses
- β-interferon 1b
  - ↓ relapse rate by 1/3
  - ↓ lesion accumulation on MRI
  - Slow accumulation of disability.

Your Notes:

63. Patient has repeated attacks of multiple sclerosis, and now has pale temporal disc

Diagnosis (of anatomical site): Optic nerve

Clinchers
- *Pale temporal disc:* Disc pallor following an attack of multiple sclerosis is a sign of optic atrophy. It is first seen in temporal region.

The optic disc appearance depends upon the site of the plaque of multiple sclerosis, within the optic nerve. If the lesion is in the nerve head, there is disc swelling (optic neuritis). If the lesion is several millimeters behind the disc, there is generally no ophthalmoscopic feature. Here the doctor sees nothing and the patient sees nothing.

After the attack subsides, usually there is no residual symptom, but small scotoma or defects in colour vision can be demonstrated. Disc pallor is a late sequelae of multiple sclerosis and a sign of optic atrophy.

CONFUSA
Disc swelling from optic neuritis causes early and measurably visual acuity loss, thus distinguishing it from disc swelling from raised intracranial pressure.

Investigation of choice
MRI (magnetic resonance imaging)

Immediate management
Refer to neurology

Treatment of choice
When diagnosed, inform the patient of the diagnosis. There is no cure.
- *Polyunsatured fats*—may help.
- *Methylprednisolone*—shortens relapses
- β-interferon 1b
  - ↓ relapse rate by 1/3
  - ↓ lesion accumulation on MRI
  - Slow accumulation of disability.

Your Notes:

64. Patient with complaint of blurring of vision, papilledema and pain in eye.

Diagnosis (of anatomical site): Optic nerve

Clinchers
- *Blurring of vision:* Optic neuritis produces variable loss. It usually begins as blurring of the central visual field, which may remain mild or progress to severe visual loss, or rarely, to complete loss of light perception. In mild cases, the patient may complain only of a subjective loss of brightness in the affected eye. Symptoms are generally monocular, but attacks may be bilateral.
- *Papillodema:* This is due to optic neuritis fundoscopic examination in it may be normal or with swelling of optic disc.
- *Pain in eye:* Pain, localized to the orbit or supraorbital area is frequently present and may precede visual loss. The pain typically worsens with eye movement.

CONFUSA
Visual blurring in MS may result from optic neuritis or diplopia. They are distinguished by asking the patient to cover each eye sequentially and observing whether the visual difficulty clears. Diplopia in MS is often due to an internuclear ophthalmoplegia (INO) or to a sixth nerve palsy; ocular muscle palsies due to involvement of the third or fourth cranial nerve are rare.

Investigation of choice
MRI

Immediate management
Refer to neurology

Treatment of choice
When diagnosed, inform the patient of the diagnosis. There is no cure.
- *Polyunsatured fats*—may help
- *Methylprednisolone*—shortens relapses
- β-interferon 1b
  - ↓ relapse rate by 1/3
  - ↓ lesion accumulation on MRI
  - Slow accumulation of disability.

Your Notes:

65. A known patient of multiple sclerosis with unilateral facial paralysis with no loss of taste.

Diagnosis (of anatomical site): Facial nerve

Clinchers
- *Patient of multiple sclerosis with unilateral facial paralysis:* Facial paralysis, resembling idiopathic. Bell's palsy may be due to MS. It is a unilateral weakness of all the muscles of facial expression on the same site.
- *No loss of taste:* In MS, facial palsy is usually not associated with:
  - Ipsilateral loss of taste sensation
  - Retroaural pain at onset

Which are clinical characteristics of Bell's palsy.

CONFUSA
Chronic flickering contractions of the facial musculature, termed *facial myokymia*, is common in MS; it is thought to arise from involvement of corticobulbar tracts that deafferentation of the facial nucleus.

Investigation of choice
MRI

Immediate management
Refer to neurology

Treatment of choice
When diagnosed, inform the patient of the diagnosis. There is no cure.
- *Polyunsatured fats*—may help
- *Methylprednisolone*—shortens relapses
- β-interferon 1b
  - ↓ relapse rate by 1/3
  - ↓ lesion accumulation on MRI
  - Slow accumulation of disability

Your Notes:

66. Patient gets diplopia when he works very hard.

Diagnosis: Myasthenia gravis (MG)

Clinchers
- *Gets diplopia when he works very hard:* Fatiguability is the single most important feature of MG. Muscles are not commonly affected in the early stages:
  - Proximal limb muscles
  - Extraocular muscles
  - Muscles of mastication, speech and facial expression.

Complex extraocular palsies, ptosis and a typical fluctuating proximal weakness are found.

> **CONFUSA**
> The reflexes are initially preserved in MG but may be fatiguable. Muscle wasting is sometimes seen late in the disease. The clinical picture of fluctuating weakness may be diagnostic. Early symptoms of weakness and fatigue are frequently dismissed by attending doctors.

Investigation of choice
Tensilon test (only do if resuscitation facilities available)

Immediate management
Rule out
- Thymic tumor
- Hyperthyroidism
- Rheumatoid arthritis
- SLE

Treatment of choice
Pyridostigmine + prednisolone.

Your Notes:

67. Patient with attacks of numbness in left hand and right-sided headache.

Diagnosis: Space occupying lesion (SOL)

Clinchers
- *Attacks of numbness in left hand:* This suggests an evolving focal neurology. Usually focal neurology depends upon site of the tumor but the information provided in the question is insufficient to diagnose the site of SOL. Most probably it is a parietal lobe tumor (Hemisonsory loss, decreased two-point discrimination).
- *Right-sided headache:* It is a sign of increased ICP signs to space occupying property of the tumor. Other signs of ↑ ICP can be:
  - Vomiting
  - Papilloedema (only in 50% of tumors)
  - Altered consciousness.

> **CONFUSA**
> Evolving focal neurology must be differentiated from false localising signs which are produced by raised ICP. VI nerve palsy is the most common due to its long intracranial course.

Investigation of choice
CT (MRI is good for posterior fossa tumors).

Immediate management
Refer to neurology.

Treatment of choice
Complete removal if possible.

Your Notes:

68. This disease is characterised by neurofibrillary tangels and senil plaques.

Diagnosis: Alzheimer's dementia (AD)

Clinchers
- *Neurofibrillary tangles:* These are characteristic of AD and are composed of abnormally phosphorylated tan protein.
- *Senile plaques:* These are neuritic plaques composed of AB amyloid and other proteins.

CONFUSA
Risk factors for AD are old age, positive family history. The apolipoprotein E (apoE) gene (Chromosome 21) has a role in pathogenesis. Rare genetic causes of AD are:
- Down's syndrome (trisomy 21)
- Amyloid precursor protein (APP)
- Gene mutations (chromosome 21)
- ALL.

Investigation of choice
Neuroimaging (will help rule out frontal lobe dementia; Lewy body dementia and Picks's disease).

Immediate management
Counsel the relatives about taking care.

Treatment of choice
Donepezil.

Your Notes:

69. A 40-year-old female comes with complaints of headache, bitemporal hemianopia, increase in shoe size.

Diagnosis: Acromegaly

Clinchers
- *40-year-old female:* It typically presents between the ages of 30 and 50 years. It is equally prevalent in men and women.
- *Headache and bitemporal hemianopia:* Because of the pituitary tumor (responsible for growth hormone hypersecretion). Bitemporal hemianopia is characteristic of compression of optic chiasm (most common cause of it—pituitary tumor).
- *Increase in shoe size:* GH excess results in bony and soft tissue overgrowth. The features are insidious, chronic and debilitating, i.e.
  - Increased teeth spacing
  - Increased shoe size
  - Thick spade like hands
  - Large tongue
  - Prominent supraorbital ridge
  - Prognathism.

CONFUSA
Acromegalics are said to look more like each other than their family members. Presence of bitemporal hemianopia in it clinically corroborates the presence of a pituitary tumor and that acromegaly is not due to some ectopic secretion of growth hormone.

Ectopic (other than pituitary) tumors causing acromegaly
- GnRH secreting tumors
  - Bronchial carcinoids
  - Pancreatic islet cell tumors
  - Hypothalamic gangliocytomas
  - Harmatoma
  - Gliomas
- GH secreting tumors
  - Pancreatic islet cell tumor

Investigation of choice
MRI pituitary fossa.

Immediate management
Obtain old photographs for comparison.

Your Notes:

70.
A middle aged woman presents with recurrent nausea, weight loss and fever. She has pain, stiffness and weakness in her hips and shoulders. She does not have a rash, but the skin around the neck and shoulders appears thickened.

Diagnosis: Polymyositis

Clinchers
- *Middle-aged women:* Primary idiopathic polymyositis is twice as common in females as in males.
- *Recurrent nausea, weight loss and fever:* These are the systemic symptoms of polymyositis. These also include arthralgias and Raynaud's phenomenon.
- *Pain, stiffness and weakness in her hips and shoulders:* There is insidious, symmetrical, proximal muscle weakness which results from muscle inflammation. It is a presumed autoimmune disease in which skeletal muscle is damaged by an inflammatory process dominated by lymphocytic infiltration.
- *Skin around neck and shoulders appears thickened:* This can be scleroderma which is so frequently associated with this disease. Other associations usually are:
  - RA
  - SLE
  - MCTD
- *No rash:* This rules out dermatomyositis whose characteristics heliotrope rash usually precede muscle changes.

CONFUSA
Patients with dermatomyositis who have skin rash may not require muscle biopsy. In polymyositis, biopsy usually need to:
- Make a firm diagnosis
- Rule out other myopathies.

Investigation of choice
- Muscle enzyme (CK) levels (↓)
- EMG (fibrillation potentials)
- Muscle biopsy.

Immediate management
Refer to rheumatology.

Treatment of choice
High dose immune globulin + rest + prednisolone.

Your Notes:

71.
Patient after escaping from fire in a building has singed nostrils.

Diagnosis: Inhalation injury

Clinchers
- *After escaping from fire in a building:* Incapacity, which occurs quickly in domestic and industrial fires, is caused by a combination of
  - Hypoxia
  - Carbon monoxide poisoning (caused by incomplete combustion)
  - Hydrogen cyanide poisoning

  Soft furnishing are a particular hazard, producing many topic substances, including highly irritant and lethal hydrogen chloride.
- *Signed nostrils:* Burns around the lips, mouth, throat or nose, including singeing of nasal hairs invariably points towards associated inhalation injury.

CONFUSA
Beware of conventional blood gas analyser readings in patients who may have high carboxy or methemoglobin levels. The oxygen electrode measures oxygen dissolved in plasma only and oxygen saturation is then calculated assuming all hemoglobin to be normal. PaO_2 and oxygen saturation may thus appear to be satisfactory despite very low total blood oxygen content.

Investigation of choice
Carboxy hemoglobin (CoHb).

Immediate management
High concentration O_2 + early intubation.

Treatment of choice
Admit and observation for 24 hours (even if burns appear minimal).

Your Notes:

72. Patient has a large tense blister.

Diagnosis: Dermal burns

Clinchers
➤ *Large tense blister:* Small blisters can be left alone. Large ones can be slit open at the dependent edge to allow drainage. Alternatively they can be aspirated with a needle.

CONFUSA
Complete derooting of any blister is unnecessary and leaves a painful base. So avoid it. Blisters are absent in epidermal burns. Superficial dermal burns with blistering are usually dressed to absorb exudate, prevent desiccation, provide pain relief, encourage epithelialisation and prevent infection.

Investigation of choice
None required.

Immediate management
Drainage of blister/aspirate blister.

Treatment of choice
Regular dressing.

Your Notes:

73. An adult patient has partial thickness burns on the anterior chest and upper thighs.

Diagnosis: Significant burns requiring admission

Clinchers
➤ *Partial thickness burns:* They can be managed by clearning the wound and covering with a non adherent dressing such as paraffin gauze or with sliver sulfadiazine (flamazine cream)
➤ *On anterior chest and upper thighs:* According to Lund and Browder chart anterior chest is 7½ and upper thigh = $4\frac{3}{4}$. So the total area is 7½ + $4\frac{3}{4}$ + 4 = 17%. A burn of more than 15% in adults (>10% in children) require IV fluids and hence an admission to the hospital and treatment in a burns unit.

CONFUSA
Infection can easily convert a partial thickness burn to a full thickness burn, so ensure proper prevention from infection. For IV fluid resuscitation, the priming fluid can be isotolic saline. Thereafter a colloid is used. The choice of colloid includes synthetic sugars, gelatin and starch, albumin, plasma protein fraction and reconstitute plasma. Whole blood will be required if there is a significant element of full thickness skin loss.

Investigation of choice
Urine output.

Immediate management
Admit and refer to burns unit after starting IV fluids and maintaining airway.

Treatment of choice
- Regular dressing
- Grafting and contracture release after healing.

Your Notes:

74. An adult patient has full thickness circumferential burns (from the elbow to the fingers, covering them completely.

Diagnosis: Circumferential full thickness burns over limb.

Clinchers
- *Circumferential full thickness burns:* These can contract and impair blood flow to the hand and forearm. Such contractions must be excised acutely to save the limb (escharotomy).
- *From elbow to fingers:* Face, hands and the joint flexures and priority areas for immediate skin grafting as scanning or contractures at these sites will obviously produce considerable deformity and disability.

CONFUSA
Eschar is a completely burnt and coagulated skin. Apart from limbs they can cause mechanical obstruction is present around the chest (by restricting chest movements they impair respiration). Moreover, they become a culture medium for bacteria such as *Streptococcus pyogenes* and Pseudomonas aeruginosa.

Investigation of choice
Urine output.

Immediate management
Escharotomy

Treatment of choice
Immediate excision and split skin grafting.

Your Notes:

75. Man, slept while sunbathing comes with redness, and pain all over his body. Otherwise well.

Diagnosis: Sunburns.

Clinchers
- *Sunbathing:* It can cause sunburns if prolonged, but these are usually not serious.
- *Redness:* It is superficial erythema and is never taken into accounting when calculating the area of burn.
- *Pain:* Simple erythema is extremely painful. Even patients expected to go home after treatment may need parenteral analgesia.
- *Other wise well:* This rules out any other injury or fluid compromise. Since simple erythema do not require active treatment, he can be safely discharged home.

CONFUSA
Unprotected exposure to UV radiation can cause extremely painful, blistering, oedematous skin. In general the treatment is as for any other burn.

Investigation of choice
None required.

Immediate management
Oral analgesia if required.

Treatment of choice
Reassure and discharge
+
Regular application of hydrocortisone 1% cream

Your Notes:

76. Otosclerosis.

Diagnosis: Bilateral conductive deafness.

Clinchers
Otosclerosis is usually bilateral. Half of the patients have a family history. Symptoms usually occur in early adult life. In this disease, vascular spongy bone replaces normal bone around the oval window to which there is adherence of the stapes footplate. This produces conductive deafness.

CONFUSA
Sometimes tinnitus and vertigo are associated with conductive deafness. In conductive deafness hearing is better in background noise. Symptoms of otosclerosis are characteristically made worse by pregnancy.

Investigation of choice: Audiogram

Immediate management
Hearing aid

Treatment of choice
Replacement of stapes with an implant.

Your Notes:

77. Presbyacusis.

Diagnosis: Bilateral sensory neural deafness.

Clinchers
In presbyacusis there is loss of acuity for high frequency sounds. It starts before 30 years of age and the rate of loss of the higher frequencies is progressive thereafter. Deafness is due to loss of hair cells (sensory-neural). It is gradual in onset.

CONFUSA
Presbyacusis is senile deafness. In presbyacusis the hearing defect usually go unnoticed until hearing of speech is affected. This may occur with loss of high frequency sounds e.g. consonants at (~3-4 Hz are required for speech discrimination). Hearing is most affected in the present of background noise.

Investigation of choice Audiogram.

Immediate management Curtailment of smoking and stimulants like tea and coffee (to decrease associated tinnitus).

Treatment of choice
Hearing aids.

Your Notes:

78. Otitis media with effusion.

Diagnosis: Unilateral conductive deafness

Clinchers
- *Otitis media:* It can cause heaving loss by
  a. Conductive deafness: Due to fluid in middle ear
  b. Sensori-neural deafness: This is usually secondary to labyrinthitis due to ascending bacterial infection through niddle ear (tympanogenic) or through CSF (meningogenic)
- *Effusion:* This indicates the deafness is most probably conductive.

CONFUSA
Otitis media with effusion is commonly referred to as glue ear and is an insidious condition characterised by accumulation of non-purulent effusion in middle ear. Hearing loss is the presenting and sometimes the only symptoms. It is insiduous in onset and rarely exceds 40 dB. Deafness may pass unnoticed by the parents and may be accidentally discovered during audiometric screening tests.

Investigation of choice
Impedance audiometry.

Immediate management
Examine the other ear also.

Treatment of choice
Myringotomy and aspiration of fluid with grommet insertion.
Note: Uncomplicated or new cases can be managed by medical treatment also.

Your Notes:

79. Acoustic neuroma.

Diagnosis: Unilateral sensory deafness.

Clinchers
Acoustic neuroma is a slow growing neurofibroma. It often arises from the vestibular nerve and produces progressive ipsilateral tinnitus ± sensorineural deafness.

CONFUSA
Vertigo is rare with acoustic neuroma, giddiness is common. Big tumors may give ipsilateral above the tumor may give a facial numbness. Cranial nerves especially V, VI and VII may be affected.

Investigation of choice
MRI

Immediate management
Rule out ↑ ICP

Treatment of choice
Surgery (if possible).

Your Notes:

80. Noise-induced hearing loss (NIHL).

Diagnosis: Loss is not more than 60 dB.

Clinchers
- *Noise induced:* Hearing loss follows chronic exposure to less intense sounds for prolonged periods and is mainly a hazard of noisy occupations. It can cause:
  a. Temporary threshold shift: The hearing is impaired immediately after exposure to noise but recovers after an interval of a few minutes to a few hours.
  b. Permanent threshold shift: The hearing impairment is permanent and does not recover at all.
- Hearing loss: The damage caused by raise trauma depends on several factors (usually the hearing loss is not more than 60 dB):
  - Frequency: A frequency of 2000 to 3000 Hz causes more damage than lower or higher frequencies
  - Intensity and duration: As the intensity increases, permissible time for exposure is reduced
  - Continuous vs interrupted noise: Continuous noise is more harmful
  - Susceptibility of individual
  - Pre-existing ear disease.

CONFUSA
The single most successful way of reducing deafness is to limit damaging noise (<85 dB/8 h day) exposure at work and leisure—as indicated by finding talking difficult, ringing in the ears during exposure, or sounds appearing muffled after exposure.

Investigation of choice
Audiogram (shows a typical notch at 4 Hz, both for air and bone conduction).

Immediate management
Work to limit exposure.

Treatment of choice
Ear protectors should be used where noise levels exceed 85 dB. It hearing impairment has already occured work for rehabilitation and give hearing aids.

Your Notes:

81. The ability of a test to detect people who doe have the disease.

Answer: Sensitivity

Clinchers
Sensitivity is the percentage of the diseased people who are correctly detected or classified:

$$\text{Sensivity}: \frac{\text{number testing positive who have the disease}}{\text{total number tested who have the disease}} \times 100$$

So a test that is always positive for diseased individuals, identifying every diseased person, has a sensitivity of 100%. Therefore, a test that is insensitive leads to missed diagnosis (false negative results), whereas a sensitive test produces few false negative results.

CONFUSA
A sensitive test is obviously required in situations in which the consequence of a false negative result is serious, as in the case of a serious condition that is treatable or transmissible. High sensitivity is required of tests used to screen donated blood for HIV, or in the case of cytological screening tests for cervical cancer. Very sensitive tests are therefore used for screening or ruling out disease: if the result of a highly sensitive test is negative, it allows the disease to be ruled out with confidence.

Your Notes:

82. Measure of dispersion.

Answer: Standard deviation

Clinchers

Standard deviation is a measure of dispersion and is used most commonly in statistical analyses. It is computed by following six steps:
1. Calculate the mean.
2. Find the difference of each observation from the mean.
3. Square the differences of observation from the mean.
4. Add the squared values to get the sum of the squares.
5. Divide this sum by the number of observations minus one to get mean-squared deviation, called variance.
6. Find the square root of this varianace to get root-mean-squared deviation, called standard deviation.

CONFUSA

A large standard deviation shows that the measurement of the frequency distribution are widely spread out from the mean. Small standard deviation means the observations are closely spread in the neighbourhood of mean. Another measure of dispersion is mean-deviation.

Your Notes:

83. Relative risk can be obtained from these studies.

Answer: Cohort studies

Clinchers: The estimate of disease risk associated with exposure is obtained by an index known as "Relative Risk" (RR) or risk ratio, which is defined as the ratio between the incidence of disease among exposed persons and incidence among non-exposed. It is given by formula:

$$\text{Relative risk} = \frac{\text{incidence among exposed}}{\text{incidence among non-exposed}} \times 100$$

CONFUSA

A typical case control study does not provide incidence rates from which relative risk can be calculated directly, because there is no appropriate denominator or population at risk, to calculate there rates. In general, the relative risk can be exactly determined only form a cohort study. Because relative risk is a ratio of risks, it is sometimes called the risk ratio, or morbidity ratio. In the case of outcomes involving death, rather than just disease, it may also be called the mortality ratio.

Your Notes:

July—2001

84. The best indicator of central value when one or more of the lowest or the highest observations are wide apart or not so evenly distributed.

Answer: Median

Clinchers
When all the observations of a variable are arranged in either ascending or descending order, the middle observation is known as median. It implies the midvalue of series.

CONFUSA
Median is sometimes a better indicator than mean, e.g. in a study of duration of stay in a hospital in general or in a specific disease ward, or disease. In such cases it is better because the stay may be unduly long in some cases.

Your Notes:

85. The most frequently occurring observation in a series.

Answer: Mode

Clinchers
Mode is the most frequently occurring observation in a series, i.e. the most common or most fashionable, such as 8 mm in tuberculin test of 10 boys given below:
3,5,7,8,8,8,10,11,12

CONFUSA
Mode is rarely used in medical studies. Out of the three measures of central tendency, mean is better and utilized more often because it uses all the observations in the data and is further and in the tests of significance.

Your Notes:

86. The single largest cause of death in adults in the UK.

Diagnosis: Ischemic heart disease (IHD).

Clinchers
Coronary artery disease is the largest single cause of death in the UK. There are approximately 60 deaths per 100,000 (giving a standardized mortality rate of about 200 per 100,000).

> **CONFUSA**
> In UK, myocardial ischemia most commonly occurs as a result of obstructive coronary disease in the form of coronary atherosclerosis. In addition to this fixed obstruction, variations in the tone of smooth muscles in the wall of a coronary artery may add an important element of dynamic or variable obstruction.

Investigation of choice
Coronary angiography (definitive).

Immediate management
Cardiology referral.

Treatment of choice
As per the symptom profile.

Your Notes:

87. Warfarin decreases the incidence of stroke by about 30%.

Diagnosis: Atrial fibrillation

Clinchers
There is a direct relation between the duration of anticoagulation and the risk of recurrent thrombosis. Although recommendations vary somewhat, most patients with a single uncomplicated thromboembolic event have maximal benefit after 3 to 6 months of anticoagulation. About 10% of patients on an oral anticoagulant for 1 year have a serious complication requiring medical supervision, and 0.5 to 1% have a fatal hemorrhage event despite careful medical management.

> **CONFUSA**
> Patients with paroxysmal atrial fibrillation or a porcine bioprosthetic valve, who are taking a warfarin anticoagulant as a prophylactic measure, may be protected with an INR of 1.5 to 2. In contrast, patients with lupus like anticoagulants and thromboembolism or those patients with mechanical cardiac valves require more intense anticoagulation. Satisfactory control requires an INR of 3 to 4.

Investigation of choice
Echocardiography

Immediate management
Evaluation by an expert

Treatment of choice
For atrial fibrillation—anticoagulant therapy.

Your Notes:

88. Interfere with the function of vitamin K.

Diagnosis (Answer): Warfarin

Clinchers
The coumarin anticoagulants, which include warfarin and dicoumarol, present the reduction of vitamin K epoxides in liver microsomes and induce a state of analogous to vitamin K deficiency.

CONFUSA
Warfarin slows thrombin generation and clot formation by impairing the biologic activity of the prothrombin complex proteins and are used to prevent the recurrence of venous thrombosis and pulmonary embolism.

Investigation of choice
PT (prolonged)

Immediate management
Evaluate for any spontaneous bleed

Treatment of choice
Vitamin K supplements if toxicity is clinically confirmed.

Your Notes:

89. Probably most important public health problem in developed countries. Its ratio of frequency in women verses men increases from 0.6 to 0.7 at age 30 to 1.1 to 1.2 at age 65.

Diagnosis: Hypertension.

Clinchers
- Hypertension is the most important public health problem in the developed countries.
  It is common, asymptomatic, easily detectable, usually easily treatable, but may lead to lethal complications, if untreated.
- Increase in ratio of frequency in women with age
  In females the prevalence is closely related to age, with substantial increase occuring after age 50.
- The prevalance of hypertension depends upon the racial composition of the population studied, and criteria used to define the condition. In white-sufurban population like that in the Framingham study, nearly one fifth of individuals have BP>160/95, while almost one-half have pressures greater than 140/90. Even higher prevalence has been documented in non-white population.

Your Notes:

90. Its incidence in industrialized countries of the world has defined markedly. Peak age-relaged incidence is between 5 and 15 years.

Diagnosis: Rheumatic fever

Clinchers
- The incidence of rheumatic fever has declined remarkably in the industrialized countries of the world, where the disease has become rare. However, in many developing countries, which account for almost two-thirds of the world's population, strephococcal infection, rheumatic fever and rheumatic heart disease remain a very significant health problem today.

CONFUSA
Epidemiology fo rheumatic fever is similar to that of group-A streptococcal upper respiratory tract infection. Approximately 3 percent of individuals with untreated group A-streptococcal pharyngitis will develop rheumatic fever

Diagnosis of Rheumatic fever
- No specific laboratory tests available to establish the diagnosis of rheumatic fever. Thus diagnosis is essentially clinical, supported by clinical microbiology and clinical immunology laboratories. John's criteria's for rheumatic fever should be remembered here. There are five major and many minor criterias. Major criterias are Carditis, migratory polyarthritis, Sydenham's chorea, Subcutaneous nodules and erythema marginatum. Minor criterias include fever, arthralgia, elevated acute phose reactants, and prolonged PR interval.

Your Notes:

---

91. A patient who developed myocardial infarction one month ago is now breathless and has basal crackles.

Diagnosis: Pulmonary oedema (post MI).

Clinchers
- *Developed MI one month ago:* Left ventricular failure is an important complication of MI. For other complications of MI refer to page 108 (OHCM) 5th edn.
- *Breathlessness and basal crackles:* These are features of presenting with acute onset of dyspnoea (with history of recent MI), and on examination pulmonary rales, ronchi, fine lung crackles, is suggestive of pulmonary oedema.

CONFUSA
Look for cardiomegaly and signs of pulmonary edema on CXR [refer to figure in Q16 (July 2001)] and for signs of myocardial infarction on ECG to confirm the diagnosis.

Investigation of choice
- CXR and ECG
- ABG

Immediate management
- Sit patient upright and give oxygen.

Treatment of choice
Most appropriate management
- *Diuretics* (furosemide 40 mg LV) produce venodilation prior to diuresis.
- *Diamorphine* given 2.5-5 mg IV slowly increases venous capacitance and relieves anxiety.
- Sublingual or IV nitrates, phlebotomy and plasma pheresis are other methods of reducing left ventricular preload.

Your Notes:

92. Patient presents with one and a half hours of epigastric pain radiating to his arm. ECG shows acute inferior myocardial infarction. Oxygen + analgesia have already been given.

Diagnosis: Acute myocardial infarction.

Clinchers
- *Myocardial infarction:* Usually occurs from occlusion of coronary artery, resulting from rupture of the atheromatous plaque. It may occur due to coronary spasm, emboli or vasculitis.
- *Epigastric pain radiating to arm:* Acute prolonged (> 20 min) anterior chest discomfort, which may be associated with dysphonea, palpitations and nausea, are the symptoms of MI. Diagnosis confirmed by ECG, and raised cardiac enzyme levels (CK, AST, LDH). In 20% cases ECG may be normal initially.

CONFUSA
Differentiate if from angina, pericarditis, aortic dissection, myocarditis, pulmonary embolism and oesophageal reflux/spasm.

Investigation of choice
ECG and cardiac enzymes.

Immediate management
- High flow O_2 by mask (caution if COPD).
- Aspirin in 300 mg chewed.
- Analgesia (morphine 5-10 mg IV + antiemetic e.g. metoceopramide 10 mg IV.

Next step in management
Thyrombolysis is indicated after oxygen and analgesia in this patient, since his presentation is of only one and a half hour duration.

The British Heart Foundation advices that the time from the onset of pain to thrombolysis should be < 90 minutes (< 60 min if possible). Benefits of thrombolysis (reduces mortality) are seen if given upto more than 12 hours of onset of chest pain, but some benefit upto 24 hours.

Streptokinase (SK) is the usual thrombolytic agent. Do not repeat (SK) unless it is within 4 days of first administration. Use Alteplase if the patient has previously received SK.

Your Notes:

93. Patient recovering from myocardial infarction has a heart rate of 36/minute.

Diagnosis: Bradycardia/heart block.

Clinchers
- *Recovering from myocardial infarction:* Sinus bradycardia or heart block is complication of myocardial infarction. Other complications are:
  - Cardiac arrest/cardiogenic shock
  - Unstable angina
  - Tachyarrhythmias
  - Left ventricular failure
  - Right ventricular failure/infarction
  - Pericarditis, DVT, pulmonary embolism
  - Cardiac tamponade, mitral regurgitation
  - Ventricular septal defect
  - Left ventricular aneurysm
- *Heart rate of 36/minute:* May be due to sinus bradycardia of AV block. Sinus bradycardia is common in inferior infarction. First degree AV block does not require any treatment, but watch carefully as it progresses to higher degrees.

Mobitz type I form is often transient and requires treatment only if heart rate becomes slow enough to cause symptoms. Complete A-V block occurs in upto 5% of acute inferior infractions, usually preceded by second degree block. Treatment becomes necessary because of resulting hypotension and low cardiac output.

In anterior infarction, the site of block is distal below the AV node. Here urgent ventricular pacing is mandatory.

Investigation of choice
ECG

Immediate management
Atropine 0.6 to 1.2 mg IV or cardiac pacing as explained below.

Treatment of choice
In sinus bradycardia, observation or withdrawal of offending agent is usually sufficient. If associated with signs of low cardiac output, atropine 0.6-1.2 mg IV is usually effecting. Consider temporary *cardiac pacing* if not response.

Mobitz (type I) does not require pacing, unless poorly tolerated. Mobitz (type II), should be paced, as it carries risk of complete block.

Your Notes:

94. A 57-year-old man develops crushing pain in the chest associated with nausea and profuse sweating. The pain is still present when he arrives in hospital by an hour later.

Diagnosis: Myocardial infarction (MI)

Clinchers
- *Crushing pain in chest with nausea and sweating:* This is a typical presentation of myocardial infarction. The pain is acute in onset and lasts for more than 20 minutes.
  The diagnosis is supported by ECG changes and raised cardiac enzymes.
- *ECG changes in MI:* Hyper acute T wave, ST elevation or new LBBB occurs within hours of acute Q wave (transmural infarction). T wave inversion and development of Q waves follows over hour to days. In non Q wave (subendocardial) infarction, ECG findings are less specific, e.g. T wave inversion, ST depression.

Investigation of choice
ECG and cardiac enzymes.

Immediate management
High flow oxygen by mask and morphine (with metoclopromide).

Treatment of choice
Already discussed in Q 92 (July 2001).

Your Notes:

95. Not given in a chronic asthmatic after a myocardial infarction.

Diagnosis: β blockers

Clinchers
- *Chronic asthmatic:* β-blockers worsens chronic obstructive lung disease and can precipitate life threatening attack of bronchial asthma due to their bronchocontricting action. They are absolutely contraindicated in asthmatics.
- *Myocardial infarction:* They decreases heart rate, force of contraction (at relatively higher doses) and cardiac output. They prolong systole by retarding conduction so that synergy of contraction of ventricular fibres is disturbed. The effects on a normal resting subject are not appreciable, but becomes prominent under sympathetic overactivity e.g. exercise or emotion. Cardiac work and oxygen consumption are reduced as the product of heart rate and aortic pressure decreases. Total coronary blood flow is reduced because of blockade of dilator β-receptors, but this is largely restricted to the subepicardial region, while the subendocardial area (which is the site of ischaemia) is not affected. Overall effect in angina patients is improvement of O_2 supply) demand status and exercise tolerance is increased.

CONFUSA
The broncho-constriction effect is hardly discenible in normal individuals because sympathetic bronchodilator tone is minimal and β-blockers increase bronchial resistance by blocking $β_2$-receptors. In asthmatics, however, the condition is consistently worsened and a severe attact may be precipitated.

Your Notes:

96. Scabies.

Diagnosis (causation): Female mite

Clinchers

Scabies is a common disorder which particularly affects children and young adults. It tends to spread within families or those living in close contact. There are markedly itchy papula eruptions affecting:
- Finger webs (esp. first)
- Wrist flexures
- Axillae
- Abdomen (esp. around umbilicus) and waist band area)
- Buttocks
- Groins
- Palms and soles (in young infants)

Note: Itchy red penile or scrotal papules are virtually diagnostic.

> **CONFUSA**
> The eruption in scabies in a skin reaction to the saliva or faeces of the female mite. Scabies mites can sometimes be extracted from burrows and can be visualised microscopically. Similarly eggs can be visualised from skin scrapings. The rash and symptom of itch will take a few weeks to settle, occasionally longer.

Investigation of choice

The diagnosis is usually clinical. Demonstration of female mite is definitive.

Immediate management

Crotamin cream (relieves itching till anti-scaboidals have any effect)

Treatment of choice

Malathion/Permethrin

Note: Applied to all areas of skin, from neck down for 24 hours.

Your Notes:

97. Candidial nappy rash.

Diagnosis: (causation): Immunodeficiency

Clinchers
> *Nappy rash:* It is usually of 4 types:
>   1. Ammonia dermatitis
>   2. Candida dermatitis (thrush)
>   3. Seborrhoeic eczematous dermatitis
>   4. Isolated, psoriasis-like scaly plaques
> *Candidial:* It may be isolated from about half of all nappy rashes. Infections are red and often moist with satellite lesions.

> **CONFUSA**
> The hallmarks of candidal nappy rash are satellite spots beyond the main rash.

Investigation of choice

Microscopy (20% KOH skin scrapings).

Immediate management

Advise on clealiness to parents.

Treatment of choice

Nystatin or clotrimazole cream (± 1% hydrocortisone cream).

Your Notes:

98. Impetigo.

Diagnosis (causation)
Close community contact (that is why it is called Impetigo contagiosa)

Clinchers
Impetigo is a common superficial bacterial infection of skin caused by
- Group A beta-haemolytic streptococci
- Staphylococcus aureus

The primary lesion is a superficial pustule that ruptures and forms a characteristic yellow-brown "honey-coloured" crust. Lesions caused by staphylococci may be tense, clear bullae, and this less common form of the disease is called bullous impetigo. Lesions may occur on normal skin or in areas already affected by an other skin disease.

CONFUSA
Ecthyma is a variant of impetigo that generally occurs on lower extremities and causes punched out ulcerative lesions.

Investigation of choice:
Diagnosis is usually clinical but culture from wound swab may help in confirmation

Immediate management:
Gentle debridement of adherent crusts, which is facilitated by the use of soaks and topical antibiotics

Treatment of choice:
Oral antibiotics (flucloxacillin in case of staphylococci).

Your Notes:

99. Toxoplasmosis

Diagnosis (Causation): Animal to human

Clinchers
- The principle source of human toxoplasma infection remains uncertain. Transmission usually takes place by oral route and can be attributable to infestion of either sporulated oocysts from contaminated soil or bradyzoites from under cooked meat. During acute feline infection, a cat may excrete as many as 100 million parasites per day. These very stable sporozaite containing oocysts are highly infectious and may remain viable for many years in the soil. Human infected during a well-documented outbreak of oocyst-transmitted infection develop stage-specific antibodies to the oocyst/sporozoite.

CONFUSA
Though the actual transmission is through food or ingestion, amont the given list of options the choice "Animal to human" seem to be the most appropriate. Though "immunodeficiency" can also be a probable answer, the former choice is still a more valid answer.

Investigation of choice: Serology.

Immediate management: Rule out ocular toxoplasmosis by retinoscopy.

Treatment of choice:
Immunologically competent adults and older children who have only lymphadenopathy do not require specific therapy unless they have persistent and severe symptoms.

Your Notes:

July—2001

100. A first year university student develops headache, fever, photophobia, in the 1st week of term.

Diagnosis: Bacterial meningitis (probable)

Clinchers
- *A first year university student:* Overcrowded closed communities, schools, colleges, universities and day centres are risk factors for acquisition of infections meningitis.
- *Headache, photophobia:* These features along with stiff neck, Kernig's sign Brudzinskin's sign and ophisthotonus are constituents of "meningism".
- *Fever:* It signifies septicaemia and suggests bacterial infection. Other feature of septicaemia can be malaise, fever, arthritis, odd behaviour, rash, DIC, hypotension, tachycardia and tachypnoea.

CONFUSA
Any petechiae suggest meningococcus. If it is so, never delay treatment for any tests. This rash can be found in over 70% cases of meningococcal septicaemia if a careful examination is made. In early stages, the rash may be macular.

Investigation of choice
Lumbar puncture.

Immediate management
Give benzyl penicillin before anything (confirm if the GP has already given it).

Treatment of choice
Benzyl penicillin should be given by slow IV infusion immediately after the diagnosis of bacterial meningitis or suspected meningococcal septicaemia.

Causation: Close community contact.

Your Notes:

---

101. Male patient has nasal speech, snores at night. day time he is sleepy.

Diagnosis: Obstructive sleep apnoea

Clinchers
- *Male:* This condition occurs most often in over-weight middle-aged men and affects 1-2% of the population.
- *Nasal speech:* This signifies nasal obstruction i.e. nasal deformity, rhinitis, polyp or adenoid. It is a correctable factor and occurs in upto one-third of cases.
- *Snores at night:* Apnoeas occur when the airway at the back of the throat is sucked closed while breathing in during sleep. When awake this tendency is overcome by the action of opening muscles of upper airway which become hypotonic during sleep. Partial narrowing results in snoring, occlusion in apnoea and critical narrowing in hypoapnoeas.
- *Day time he is sleepy:* Patients are worked by the struggle to breathe against the blocked throat. The awakenings are so brief that the patient remains unaware of them but is woken thousands of times per night leading to day time sleepiness and impaired performance.

CONFUSA
It can occur in children also, particularly those with enlarged tonsils. In adults, apart from nasal obstruction, other associated correctable factors may be:
- Encroachment on pharynx—obesity, acromegaly, enlarged tonsils.
- Respiratory depressant drugs—alcohol, sedatives, strong analgesics.

Investigation of choice
- *Screening:* Noninvasive ear or finger oximetry (best performed at home).
- *Definitive:* Polysomnographic studies.

Immediate management
Nasal continuous positive airway pressure (CPAP) till definitive treatment is undertaken.

Treatment of choice
Correction of treatable factors (may be surgical).

Your Notes:

102. 2-year-old child has been keeping well, but now has decreased hearing. Motor function is normal.

Diagnosis: Hearing impairment.

Clinchers
- *2-year-old child   decreased hearing:* Hearing loss in a child may develop from causes
  - Prenatal
    - Genetic defects
    - Maternal infections
    - Drugs during pregnancy
    - Radiation to mother in first trimester
  - Perinatal
    - Prematurity
    - Birth injuries
    - Neonatal jaundice
    - Neonatal meningitis
    - Ototoxic drugs
  - Postnatal (most likely in this case)
    - Genetic
    - Nongenetic
- *Motor function is normal:* Rules out brain lesions as cause.

CONFUSA
Viral infections (measles, mumps, varicella, influenza) and meningitis and encephalitis are the most common causes of hearing loss postnatally. Genetic deafness may also present late as in familial progressive sensorineural deafness and in association with certain syndrome, e.g. Alport's, Klippel-fiel, Hurlers's, etc.

Investigation of choice
Hearing tests.

Immediate management
ENT referral.

Treatment of choice
As per the cause.

Your Notes:

103. An 18 months old patient is still says a few words, mother is worried.

Diagnosis: Speech delay (probable).

Clinchers
- *18-month-old:* The normal pattern of speech development is:
  - At 1 year—few meaningful words
  - At 18 months—2 word utterances
  - At 2 years—subject-verb-object sentences
  - At 3½ years—mastered thought, language, abstraction and elements of reason, with a 1000 word vocabulary.
- *Mother is worried:* If this is not her first child, she might be having knowledge of normal pattern of speech development as there will be a sound basis of her worries which require assessment.

CONFUSA
If a child reaches 3 years old with a vocabulary of less than 50 words one should suspect a pathology. In children presenting before that an assessment of developmental milestones is done. If that is satisfactory there is no need for detailed investigations usually.

Investigation of choice
Milestone assessment

Immediate management
Reassurance to mother

Treatment of choice
Usually none required except observation till 3 years of age.

Your Notes:

104. A 50-year-old male wakes up with a tingling and numbness in his right hand. This is accompanied by slurring of speech which recovers following about four hours.

Diagnosis: Transient ischemic attack (TIA) (left sided)

Clinchers
- *50-year-old:* Incidence of TIA increases with age as it is usually secondary to vascular diseases like atherosclerosis which are more prevalent in older age groups.
- *Wakes up with a tingling and numbness in his right hand:* Contralateral weakness and numbness is common carotid territory ischemia. It means that TIA has occurred in left side of cerebrum (hence carotid source is implicated)
- *Slurring of speech:* Dysphagia is typical of carotid territory ischemia. Dysarthria can occur in both carotid and vertebrobasilary territory ischemia.
- *Recovers in 4 hours:* By definition a TIA has no CNS signs after 24 hours.

CONFUSA
Presence of carotid bruits suggests a carotid source of emboli. Their absence does not rule it out. Tight stenosis often have no bruit.

Investigation of choice
Carotid Doppler

Immediate management
Aspirin (if not peptic ulcer)

Treatment of choice
Carotid endarterectomy (if carotid stenoses is present).

Your Notes:

105. A 3-year-old with a persistent and rough voice.

Diagnosis: Respiro-laryngeal dysfunction (RLD)

Clinchers
- *3 year old:* RLD affected child commonly present at this age as this disorder is noted after development of a good speech.
- *Loud and rough voice:* It is dysphonia from incorrect vocal fold vibration or air flow regulation.

CONFUSA
Other causes of speech disorder in a 3 years old child can be:
- Deafness
- Expressive dysphasia
- Speech dyspraxia
- Audio-premotor syndrome
- Congenital aphonia (rare)

Investigation of choice
Laryngeal airflow measurements

Immediate management
Exclude deafness (as child can be unduly loud in its presence) and refer to ENT.

Treatment of choice
- Voice training
- Surgical correction (rarely)

Your Notes:

106. Warts.

Diagnosis (transmission): Sexual contact (Most commonly).

Clinchers
Warts are caused by human papilloma virus (HPV) infection of keratinocytes. Warts can be clinically classified into four types:
1. Common warts
   - Most common in children and young adults
   - Often resolve spontaneously
   - Individual lesions can be stubbornly persistent
   - Treatment is destructive (i.e. keratolytics or cryotherapy)
2. Plantar warts
   - Large confluent lesions (mosaic warts)
   - Treatment curettage for large warts
   - Surgery contraindicated
3. Plane warts
   - Flat skin coloured or brownish lesions
   - Tend to keobnerise in scratch marks
   - Can be very resistant to treatment
4. Genital warts
   - Condylomata accuminata
   - Treatment with cryotherapy and/or podophyllin
   - Found in sexually active person

CONFUSA
Large number of warty lesions are often seen in the immunosuppressed, e.g. transplant patients.

Investigation of choice
Clinical diagnosis is usually sufficient.
Excision biopsy is definitive

Immediate management
Reassume and rule out immunosuppression

Treatment of choice
Depends upon type of wart (see clinchers)

Your Notes:

107. Typhoid fever.

Diagnosis (transmission): Faecal-oral

Clinchers
Typhoid is caused by *Salmonella typhi*. Its incubation period is 3-21 days. Patients usually present with malaise, headache, high fever with relative bradycardia, cough and constipation (or diarrhoea). Epistaxis, bruising, abdominal pain, and splenomegaly may occur. Complications can be osteomyelitis, DVT, GI bleed or perforation, cholecystitis, myocarditis, pyelonephritis, meningitis, abscess.

Note: Infection is said to have cleared when 6 consecutive cultures of urine and faeces are negative.

CONFUSA
CNS signs i.e. coma, delirium or meningism in typhoid fever are serious. Diarrhoea is more common after the first week. Rose spots occur on the trunk of 40% but may be very difficult to see. High fever with relative bradycardia is a very suggestive of typhoid fever.

Investigation of choice
- First 10 days—blood culture
- Later—urine/stool cultures.

Immediate management
Fluid replacement and good nutrition.

Treatment of choice
Chloramphenicol/ciprofloxacin
In encephalopathy ± shock, give dexamethasone 3 mg/kg IV stat, then 1 mg/kg/6 h for 48 h.

Your Notes:

108. Hepatitis C.

Diagnosis (transmission): Blood borne

Clinchers
It is caused by a RNA flavivirus. It spreads via:
- Blood products
- IVDU
- Sexual
- Unknown (40%).

Early infection is often mild and asymptomatic. About 85% develop chronic infection and 20-30% get cirrhosis within 20 years. It also increases the risk of hepatocellular carcinoma.

Investigation of choice
Anti HCV antibodies; RIBA; HCV-PCR
Liver biopsy if HCV-PCR +ve.

Treatment of choice
Interferon α + Ribavarin.

Your Notes:

109. HIV.

Diagnosis (Transmission): Sexual transmission or blood borne.

Clinchers
HIV infection is acquired by percutaneous exposure to bodily secretions, fluids and blood like semen, peritoneal fluid, pleural fluid or vaginal secretions.

CONFUSA
Tears and saliva have not been proved transmit HIV infection. Although HIV has been isolated from them but, is found in such minute quantities in them that it cannot effectuate a seroconversion reaction after exposure.

Investigation of choice
ELISA/PCR

Immediate management
Counselling

Treatment of choice
Prophylactic drug cocktail till AIDS develops.

Your Notes:

110. Lyme disease.

Diagnosis (Transmission): Tick borne.

Clinchers
Lyme disease is infection caused by Borrelia burgorferi. Although originally described in Lyme (connecticut) it is now widespread e.g. New forest in UK. It is transmitted by Ixoedes tick bite.

> **CONFUSA**
> Lyme disease is a frequently asked topic in PLAB exam, so read everything about it. Another GMC favourite about lyme disease is Erythema chronicum migrans, the cutaneous manifestation of lyme disease.

Investigation of choice
Clinical ± serology

Immediate management
Travel history

Treatment of choice
Doxycycline 100 mg/12 h PO (Amoxicillin or penicillin V if < 12 years)

Your Notes:

111. A schizophrenic who stabbed his mother's hand with a screw driver was recently admitted and treated with depot injection antipsychotic. He is now symptom-free and ready for discharge.

Diagnosis: Chronic schizophrenia

Clinchers
- *Schizophrenic:* It means that it is a previously diagnosed case.
- *Stabbed his mother's hand:* It must be an acute exacerbation of schizophrenic episode.
- *Recently admitted and treated with depot injection:* Patients who have had multiple episodes or persistent symptoms usually remain on medication for many years, though the need for it (and the effect of cautions reductions in dose) should remain under regular review. Medication is often given in depot form.

> **CONFUSA**
> The main specific psychological intervention is a form of family therapy. This arose from the finding that patients living with families who have high expressed emotion (EE) had a much higher chance of relapse than those exposed to low EE. EE is the intensity and amount of emotional involvement by the family with the patient. It was then found that high EE families could be taught to lower EE, and relapse rates fell.

Investigation of choice
None except observation.

Immediate management
Rule out tardive dyskinesia.

Treatment of choice
Family therapy.

Your Notes:

112. Patient (schizophrenia) has had about 8 admissions in the last 5 years. He is uncompliant with drugs.

Diagnosis: Chronic relapsing schizophrenia.

Clinchers
- *8 admissions in last 5 years:* Hospitalization in schizophrenia is indicated if there is:
  1. Neglect of food and water intake
  2. Danger to self or others
  3. Poor drug compliance
  4. Significant neglect of self care
  5. Lack of social support.
- *He is uncompliant with drugs:* To ensure drug compliance depot preparation with long duration of action can be used. Cognitive therapy is used to reduce symptoms and to increase treatment adherence (118, Lecture notes, psychiatry, 8th edn).

CONFUSA
Upto two-thirds will relapse if antipsychotic medication is discontinued within the first 5 years of treatment. So the best plan is to offer prophylaxis to everyone in the lowest effective dose and by depot infections if concordance/compliance is a problem.

Investigation of choice
None

Immediate management
Depot antipsychotic injections.

Treatment of choice
Cognitive therapy.

Your Notes:

113. Young patient now 25 years was diagnosed with schizophrenia at 15, but despite different medications has not recovered fully. The family is very supportive.

Diagnosis: Chronic schizophrenia

Clinchers
- *Young patient....diagnosed with schizophrenia at 15:* Onset of schizophrenia before 20 years of age is a poor prognostic factor.
- *Total duration: 10 years:* Course of disease more than 2 years is also a poor prognosis factor.
- *Not recovered fully:* In the presence of prognostic factors, the recovery is usually not fully possible.
- *Family is very supportive:* So this patient can be treated at home after educating the family regarding the nature of illness, its course and treatment.

CONFUSA
Apart from education, family is also given social skills training to enhance communication and decrease family tensions. Family is taught to decrease expectations and to give emotional over-involvement, critical comments and hostility.

Investigation of choice
None-required.

Immediate management
Rule out tardive dyskinesia (a side effect of antipsychotics).

Treatment of choice
Education of the patient and family.

Your Notes:

114. A 25-year-old patient is admitted. He is depressed and has not been eating/drinking for many days. Has lost weight.

Diagnosis: Severe depression (depressive stupor).

Clinchers
- *35-year-old:* In younger patient (<40 years old), psychomotor retardation is more common which is characterised by slowed thinking and activity, decreased energy and monotonous voice.
- *Has not been eating/drinking for many days:* Psychomotor retardation can increase to the point where the person sits motionless and mute—depressive stupor. The person does not eat or drink anything for many days and usually ends in death from dehydration. It calls for an emergency ECT.
- *Lost weight:* This corroborates the diagnosis.

CONFUSA
In older patients agitation is common with marked anxiety, restlessness (inability to sit still, hand-wriggling, picking at body parts or other objects) and subjective feeling of unease.

Investigation of choice
A routine screening for medical disorders before ECT.

Immediate management
Parenteral nutrition.

Treatment of choice
Emergency ECT.

115. 40-year-old patient with features of paranoid schizophrenia.

Diagnosis: Paranoid schizophrenia

Clinchers
- *40-year-old:* The onset of paranoid schizophrenia is usually insidious and occurs later in life (i.e. later 3rd and early 4th decade) as compared to other types of schizophrenia.
- *Paranoid schizophrenia:* The course is usually progressive and complete recovery usually does not occur. There may be frequent remissions and relapses. At times, the functional capability may be only slightly impaired.

CONFUSA
Differential diagnosis is from delusional (paranoid) disorders and paranoid personality disorders.

Investigation of choice
Purely clinical diagnosis however neuroimaging may be done especially in late onset of schizophrenia to rule out a brain lesion.

Immediate management
Admit (always in paranoid schizophrenia as the patient is a danger to self and others).

Treatment of choice
Antipsychotics
+
Benzodiazepine for paranoid episodes.

Your Notes:

Your Notes:

July—2001

116. Arachnophobia.

Diagnosis: Already stated as the question itself.

Clinchers
- Arachnophobia is irrational fear of spiders. Anticipatory anxiety leads to persistant avoidant behaviour, while confrontation with the avoided object or situation leads to panic attack. Gradually, the phobia may spread to other objects or situations. The disorder is diagnosed only if there is marked distress and/or disturbance in daily functioning in addition to fear and avoidance of the specified object or situation.

CONFUSA

Arachnophobia is a specific or simple phobia. Examples of simple a pbobia are:
- Acrophobia—fear of high places
- Zoophobia—fear of animals
- Xenophobia—fear of strangers
- Algopobia—fear of pain
- Claustrophobia—fear of closed placed.

In contrast to agoraphobia and social phobia where the stimuli are generalized, in specific phobia the stimulus is usually circumscribed.

These phobias are more common in women with an onset in late second decade or early third decade. Typically, the onset is sudden without any apparent cause. The cause is usually chronic with gradually increasing restriction of daily activities.

Investigation of choice
None

Immediate management
Rebreathing into paper bag if panic attack occurs.

Treatment of choice
Not well established; CBT or MAOI are used.

Your Notes:

117. Post-traumatic Stress Disorder (PTSD)

Diagnosis: Already stated as the question

Clinchers
PTSD is a delayed response to an exceptionally severe event (e.g. serious road accident, major disasters like earthquakes). The major symptoms are (according to components).
- Emotion—anxiety, irritability.
- Cognition—flashbacks, nightmares.
- Behaviour—avoidance (of situations associated with trauma).
- Bodily symptoms—exaggerated startle response.
- Associations—substance misuse, depression.

Onset of PTSD is usually after 6 months of the event.

CONFUSA

PTSD became topical in UK and USA because of its prevalence in Vietnam war veterans. It can be a legal basis for personal injury compensation claims. While diagnosing PTSD in PLAB EMQ never forget to ascertain whether the patient was personally involved in the event himself or not (If not, then it can never be PTSD).

Investigation of choice
A detailed psychiatric history

Immediate management
Exclude associated depression or substance misuse.

Treatment of choice
Cognitive behaviour therapy (CBT).

Your Notes:

118. Bereavement.

Diagnosis: Grief reaction

Clinchers
Bereavement induces a grief reaction as a normal response and a depressive illness as abnormal response. Three stages of grief have been described.
  I. Shock and disbelief
  II. Preoccupation and depression
  III. Acceptance and resolution.

Note: Recurrence of grief is common around anniversaries.

CONFUSA		
Before diagnosis grief reaction always exclude depression which may also follow bereavement.		

	Depression	*Grief*
Onset	Delayed	Immediate
Duration	Weeks to years	Weeks to months
Pattern	Denies loss	Gradually accepts loss
Adjustment	Absent	Ultimately ensues
Expression of grief	Difficult	Open
Guilt	Masked	Mild
Psychomotor retardation	+	Absent
Symptom course	Pervasive	Fluctuating
Suicidal thoughts	Common	Transient
Psychotic features	In severe cases	No

Investigation of choice
A detailed psychiatric history

Immediate management
Exclude associated depression and anorexia

Treatment of choice
No active intervention requires as it is a normal process, though counselling and support may be required. Antidepressants require only if there is associated depression.

Your Notes:

119. A female lawyer is becoming anxious when she has to speak in front of people. This is affecting her work as she needs to speak out in court.

Diagnosis: Anxiety.

Clinchers
➢ *Becoming anxious when she has to speak in front of people:* It is a type of performance anxiety and has a recognised anxiety provoking stimulus.
➢ *Affecting her work:* Anxiety is acceptable and require no treatment until and unless it becomes symptomatic, i.e.
  • Affect work/social life
  • Somatization symptoms

CONFUSA
If not treated, she may become less efficient because of her constant performance anxiety. This might lead to more interference with her work more and hence may be predisposed to develop anxiety neurosis.

Investigation of choice
A detailed psychiatric history.

Immediate management
Reassurance.

Treatment of choice
Desensitization, i.e. a graded exposure to the anxiety provoking stimulus (behaviour therapy). Anxiolytics may be needed to enable effective work to be done with the patient.

Your Notes:

120. This treatment is very effective in endogenous anxiety and phobias.

Diagnosis: Panick attacks associated with phobias.

Clinchers

The drug of choice of panic attacks associated with phobias is MAO inhibitor.

MAO inhibitors act on mono amine oxidase which is responsible for the degradation of catecholamines after reuptake. Their final effects is the same as tricyclic antidepressants, i.e. functional increase in the NE and/or 5HT levels at the receptor site. The increase in brain amine levels is probably responsible for their action.

CONFUSA

It takes 5-10 days before a MAO inhibitor has any evident action. Therefore it is useless to give it on a SOS basis. They must be administered regularly in sufficient doses to achieve desired effect.

Investigation of choice

A detailed psychiatric history.

Immediate management

Lorazepam if immediate agitation is present.

Treatment of choice

MAO inhibitors (phenelzine).

Your Notes:

121. Interferes with glutathione (reversible by methionine and acetyl cysteine).

Diagnosis: Paracetamol poisoning

Clinchers

- *Interferes with glutathione:* Paracetamol is partly converted into a toxic metabolite, N-acetyl-p-benzoquinonimine, which is normally inactivated with glutathione. After a large overdose, glutathione is depleted and the toxic metabolite binds covalently with sulphydryl groups on liver cell membranes, initiating a sequence of changes which leads to hepatocyte necrosis. Marked liver necrosis can occur with as little as 7.5 g (15 tablets), and death with 15 g.
- *Reversible by methionine and acetyl cysteine:* N-acetyl cysteine provides sulphydryl groups that increase the availability of hepatic glutathione. Oral methionine is an alternative and is significantly cheaper than N-acetyl cysteine but absorption and efficacy are unreliable if patient is vomiting (which is usual in such cases).

CONFUSA

Patients with lower reserve of glutathione are more susceptible to liver damage and should be treated in paracetamol poisoning if there plasma concentration is above the high risk treatment line. Such patients are:
- Malnourished people
- Have taken alcohol with overdose
- Alcohol dependent
- Taking enzyme-inducing drugs
- HIV positive or with AIDS.

Investigation of choice

Plasma paracetamol concentration.

Immediate management

Toxicology screen for associated poisons

Treatment of choice

N-acetylcysteine IV.

Your Notes:

122. Interferes with haemoglobin.

Diagnosis: Carbon monoxide poisoning

Clinchers

> *Interferes with hemoglobin:* Carbon monoxide (CO) combines readily with hemoglobin to form carboxy hemoglobin, thus preventing the formation of oxyhemoglobin. CO has a special affinity for fetal Hb and so babies and pregnant women present a special risk. This severity of poisoning is related to:
> - The concentration of CO inhaled
> - The length of exposure
> - The level of activity during the exposure.

CONFUSA

The classic pink colour of the skin due to carboxy-hemoglobin is rarely seen before death. (It is paradoxical to be pink despite hypoxemia). The symptoms of CO poisoning may persist or reoccur and are not well related to COHb level. This is probably because the intracellular half-life of CO is bound to the respiratory enzymes is upto 48 hours, as opposed to 280 minutes in the blood, as COHb. Patients with coexisting medical problems i.e.
- Heart disease
- Respiratory disease
- Anaemia.

and children are usually the worst affected. Usual treatment is with high concentration O_2 but hyperbaric O_2 should be given if:
- Symptoms of poisoning + COHb > 40%
- Last trimester of pregnancy + FCTG changes + COHb > 20%
- Loss of unconsciousness
- Severe cardiovascular complications
- Unresolved neurological signs after 2 hours of treatment with high-concentration O_2.

Investigation of choice

Early blood gas analysis (as levels may soon return to normal).

Immediate management

If the poisoning is severe, anticipate cerebral oedema and give mannitol IVI.

Treatment of choice

High concentration O_2 for 120 minutes given via endotracheal tube or tight-fitting mask.
 +
Consider hyperbrsic O_2 therapy (i.e. if COHb > 40%).

123. Anticholinergic effects, arrhythmias.

Diagnosis: Tricyclic antidepressant (TCA) poisoning

Clinchers

> *Anticholinergic effects:* The effects of TCA are largely related to their anticholinergic activity and so include:
> *Peripheral effects*
> - Blurred vision
> - Dry mouth
> - Dilated pupils
> - Urinary retention
> - Diverse GI symptoms
> - Tachycardia
> - Dysrhythmia
>
> *Central effects:*
> - Agitation
> - Anxiety
> - Hyperactivity
> - Disorientation
> - Confusion
> - Drowsiness
> - Lethargy
> - Hallucinations
> - Nystagmus
> - Dysarthria
> - Ataxia
> - Movement disorders
> - Hyper reflexia
> - Extensor plantar response
> - Hyperthermia
>
> *Arrhythmias:* Cardiac dysrhythmias are the most common cause of death. Tachycardia (rate > 120 bpm) is worrying, especially with ECG change. Prolongation of the QRS complex >100 ms suggests cardio-toxicity. A QRS duration of more than 160 ms is associated with a very high risk of life threatening dysrhythmia.

CONFUSA

Poisoning with TCAs is implicated in over one-fifth of all fatal ingestions. Dothiepin is the most common drug involved. Ingested amounts are usually significant as the patient who need TCAs will often have a mental state compatible with suicide. An ingestion of 35 mg/kg is the median lethal dose for an adult. TCAs are the most common cause of VF in children in UK. Anti-dysrhythmic drugs are best avoided in TCA poisoning as conduction deficits may make the ECG difficult to interpret. Moreover, some of these drugs will produce a synergistic cardiotoxicity. Mild hypotension usually responds to IV fluids; for more severe hypotension alkali therapy is required.

Investigation of choice
12 lead ECG

Immediate management
ICU admission
+
Gastric emptying (upto 8 hours)
+
Activated charcoal (may be repeated)
+
IV benzodiazepine (for agitation or convulsions)

Treatment of choice
IV sodium bicarbonate.

Your Notes:

124. Patient on treatment for atrial fibrillation, now has palpitations.

Diagnosis: Digoxin poisoning

Clinchers
- *On treatment for atrial fibrillation:* The patient is most probably on digoxin which is indicated in acute AF (i.e. ≤ 72 h) to control the ventricular rate.
- *Palpitations:* They represent to the patient the sensation of feeling his heart beat. Generally, they can be classified etiologically into four types (according to patient's description).
  - *Irregular fast palpitations:* due to:
    - paroxysmal AF (as in this case)
    - flutter with variable block.
  - *Dropped or missed beats*—related to rest, recumbency or eating, due to:
    - atrial/ventricular ectopics.
  - *Regular pounding:* due to anxiety
  - *Slow palpitations:* due to
    - drugs, i.e. β blockers
    - bigeminus

CONFUSA
The elderly and patients with hyperthyroidism are more prone to digoxin toxicity. But in patients with fluctuating renal function, digoxin, which is metabolized by the liver, may be preferable. The most common features of digoxin toxicity are:
- Anorexia, nausea, altered vision
- Arrhythmia (e.g. ventricular premature beats especially
  - bigeminy
  - VT
  - AV block)
- Digoxin levels >2.5 nmol/L

Investigation of choice
Serum digoxin level and potassium

Immediate management
Discontinue digoxin + management of arrhythmias

Treatment of choice
Digoxin antibodies (Fab fragments)
Dose: 60 × total digoxin load
[load (mg) = plasma digoxin concentration (ng/mL) × body weight (kg) × 0.0056].

Your Notes:

125. This interferes with metabolism at the mitochondrial level.

Diagnosis: Cyanide poisoning

Clinchers
Cyanide blocks electron transport, resulting in decreased oxidative metabolism and oxidative utilization, decreased ATP production and lactic acidosis.

Lethal dose
- Sodium cyanide 200-300 mg
- Hydrocyanic acid 500 mg

Early effects: Headache, vertigo, excitement, anxiety, burning of mouth and throat, dyspnoea, tachycardia, hypertension.

Later effects: Coma, seizures, opisthotonos, trismus, paralysis, respiratory, arrhythmia, hypotension and death.

Immediate management
100% O_2 and GI decontamination.

Treatment of choice
Amyl nitrite inhaled for 30 sec each min.
Sodium nitrite 3% solution IV, 2.5-50 ml/min then 50 ml of 25% sodium thiosulphate is given IV over 1-2 min, producing sodium thiocyanide, excreted in urine.

If symptom persist, repeat half the dose of sodium nitrite and sodium thiosulfate.

Your Notes:

126. Patient with atrophic gastritis has megaloblastic anemia.

Diagnosis: Pernicious anemia (PA)

Clinchers
- *Atrophic gastritis:* PA is a condition in which there is atrophy of gastric mucosa with consequent failure of intrinsic factor production and vitamin B_{12} malabsorption.
- *Megaloblastic anemia:* It is characterised by the presence in the bone marrow of erythroblasts with delayed nuclear maturation because of defective DNA synthesis (megaloblasts). Megaloblasts are large (>110 MCV) and have large immature nuclei. The nuclear chromatin is more finely dispensed than normal and has an open stippled appearance. It occurs in:
  - Vitamin B_{12} deficiency or abnormal B_{12} metabolism
  - Folic acid deficiency or abnormal metabolism
  - DNA synthesis defects, i.e.
    - Orotic aciduria
    - Drugs
      - hydroxyurea
      - azathioprine
      - AZT
  - Myelodysplasia due to dyserythropoiesis.

CONFUSA
Beware of diagnosing pernicious anemia in those under 40 years old: look for GI malabsorption with small bowel biopsy in them. Pernicious anemia must always be distinguished from other causes of vitamin B_{12} deficiency. Any disease involving the terminal ileum or bacter overgrowth in the small bowel can produce vitamin B_{12} deficiency. Gastrectomy can lead, in the long term, to vitamin B_{12} deficiency. A careful dietary history should be obtained.

Investigation of choice
Schilling test (expect it to show that < 7% of an oral administered dose of labelled B_{12} is excreted—unless concurrent intrinsic factor is given).

Immediate management
Rule out associated disease i.e.
- Thyroid disease
- Vitiligo
- Addison's disease
- Carcinoma stomach

Treatment of choice

Hydroxycobalamin (B_{12}) IM
- 1 mg alternate days
- For 2 weeks (or, if CNS signs, until improvement stops)
- Maintenance: 1 mg IM every 2 months for life.

Your Notes:

127. Patient who is a strict vegetarian has an MCV of 110.

Diagnosis: B_{12} deficiency anaemia

Clinchers
- *Strict vegetarian:* Vitamin B_{12} is synthesized by certain micro-organisms, and humans are ultimately dependent on animal sources. It is found in meat, fish, eggs and milk. No vegetable sources contain B_{12}. Strict vegetarians develop its deficiency if they do not even take milk or milk products.
- *MCV of 110:* This signifies a megaloblastic anemia (criteria: MCV $\geq$ 110). The peripheral blood film shows macrocytes with hypersegmented polymorphs with six or more lobes in the nucleus.

CONFUSA

Causes of vitamin B_{12} deficiency or abnormal metabolism:
I. Low dietary intake
   - Vegans (as is this case)
   - Alcoholics.
II. Impaired absorption
   A. Stomach
      - Pernicious anaemia
      - Gastrectomy
      - Congenital deficiency of IF.
   B. Small bowel
      - Ileal disease or resection
      - Bacterial overgrowth
      - Tropical sprue
      - Fish tapeworm (*Diphyllobrothrium latum*).
   C. Abnormal metabolism
      - Congenital transcobalamin II deficiency
      - Nitrous oxide (inactivates B_{12}).

Note:
- Malabsorption of B_{12} due to pancreatitis, coeliac disease or treatment with metformin is mild and does not usually result in significant vitamin B_{12} deficiency.
- Body stores of vitamin B_{12} are usually sufficient for 3 years.

Investigation of choice
- *Screening:* Deoxyuridine suppression test or Schilling's test.
- *Definitive:* Serum vitamin B_{12} (Normal: 160 ng/L).

Immediate management
Careful and detailed dietary history.

Treatment of choice
Replenish stores with hydroxyocobalamin (B_{12}) (Doses—see previous question).

128. Patient has both Iron and Folate deficiency Radiology sigmoidoscospy—normal, has pale stools which are difficult to flush away.

Diagnosis: Malabsorption (pancreatic insufficiency)

Clinchers
- *Both iron and folate deficiency* Malabsorption produces the signs of following deficiencies:
  - anemia (↓Fe, ↓B$_{12}$, ↓folate)
  - bleeding (↓vitamin K)
  - edema (↓protein).
- *Radiology and sigmoidoscopy normal:* This rules out other causes of malabsorption, e.g. Crohn's disease and coeliac disease.
- *Pale stools which are difficult to flush away:* This suggest pancreatic insufficiency to be the cause.

CONFUSA
Most common cause of malabsorption in UK are:
- Coeliac disease
- Crohn's disease
- Chronic pancreatitis (usually due to alcoholism).

Investigation of choice
USG (dilated biliary tree; stones)

Immediate management
Prescribe low fat diet + take alcohol history

Treatment of choice
As per the causation.

Your Notes:

---

129. Elderly patient with complaint of anemia and has bleeding gum.

Diagnosis: Scurvy

Clinchers
- *Elderly:* Vitamin C deficiency is seen mainly in infants fed with boiled milk and in the elderly and single people who cannot be bothered to eat vegetables. It can be seen in UK among Asian countries where people prefer to eat rice and chapatis and also in food faddists.
- *Anemia:* In scurvy the anemia is usually hypochronic but occasionally a normochromic or megaloblastic whether iron deficiency (owing to decreased absorption or loss due to hemorrhage) or folate deficiency (folate being largely found in green vegetables) is present.
- *Bleeding gums:* Swollen, spongy gums with bleeding and superadded infection and loosening of teeth are characteristic of scurvy.

CONFUSA
Humans, along with a few other animals (e.g. primates and the guinea pigs) are unusual in not being able to synthesize ascorbic acid from glucose. Vitamin C is present in all fresh fruits and vegetables. Unfortunately, ascorbic acid is easily leached out of vegetables when they are placed in water and it is also oxidised to dehydroascorbic acid during cooking, exposure to copper or alkalis. Potatoes is a good source and many people eat a lot of them, but vitamin C is lost during storage.

Investigation of choice
Plasma ascorbic acid level (Normal ≥ 11μmol/L)

Immediate management
Detailed dietary history

Treatment of choice
Ascorbic acid
- Initial: 250 mg daily
  - Maintenance: 40 mg daily

Your Notes:

130. Elderly patient in residential home a complaints of tiredness.

Diagnosis: Nutritional deficit (most probably)

Clinchers
- *Elderly:* Nutritional deficits in the elderly may be due to many factors such as:
  - Dental problems
  - Lack of cooking skills (particularly in widowers)
  - Depression
  - Lack of motivation
  - Disabilities.
- *Residential home stay:* This will result in vitamin D deficiency. In elderly patients who are confirmed to their houses, vitamin D supplements may be required because often these people do not go into sunlight.
- *Tiredness:* It is a common non-specific symptom of malnutrition.

CONFUSA
The daily energy requirement of elderly people (aged 60 and above, irrespective of age) has been set to approximately 1.5 × BMR. The BMR is reduced, owing to a fall in the fat-free mass, from an average of 60 kg to 50 kg in men and from 40 kg to 35 kg in women. The diet should contain the same proportions of nutrients, and essential nutrients are still required. Owing to the high prevalence of osteoporosis in elderly people, daily calcium intake should be 1-1.5 g.

Investigation of choice
Tests for various nutritional deficiencies

Immediate management
A detailed dietary history

Treatment of choice
Prescribe proper diet + treatment of any deficiency.

Your Notes:

131. 25-year-old patient now has to use inhaled β_2 agonists 2-3 times a day.

Best management: Inhaled steroids

Clinchers
For the management of chronic asthma, certain steps/guidelines have been formulated by the British Thoracic Society.

According to these guidelines, occasional short acting inhaled β_2 agonists is the first step for symptom relief. If used more than once daily, or night time symptoms present, add standard dose *inhaled steroids:* beclometasone or budesonide 100-400 μg/12h.

For British Thoracic Society Guidelines refer the high yield section of this book.

CONFUSA
Cromoglycate or nedocromil can also be tried after inhaled β_2 agonists, but they are no substitute to inhaled steroids, if symptoms are aggravate.

Investigation in chronic asthma
- PEFR monitoring
- CXR: hyperinflation
- Spirometry: obstructive defects ($\downarrow$ FEV_1/FVC, $\uparrow$ residual volume).

Investigations in acute asthma
PEFR, sputum culture, blood culture, FBC, U&E, CRP.

Your Notes:

132. 35-year-old uses β₂ agonist + low dose steroid but symptoms still uncontrolled.

Best management: Inhaled long acting β₂ agonist

Clinchers
According to British Thoracic Society Guidelines, if symptoms do not get relieved by inhaled short acting β₂ agonist + low dose steroids, then increase the dose of inhaled steroids. Alternatively we can try *long-acting β₂ agonist* (Salmeterol 50 mg/12h). For these guidelines refer page 172 (OHCM), 5th edn.

β₂ adrenoreceptor agonists relax bronchial smooth muscle, acting within minutes.

Salmeterol is a long-acting inhaled β₂ agonist, that can help nocturnal symptoms and reduce morning dips.

CONFUSA
If the symptoms still persist, give combination of drugs or add regular oral prednisolone (1 daily dose) and refer to asthma clinic.

Immediate management
Inhaled long-acting β₂ agonist.

Your Notes:

133. 37-year-old female presents with breathlessness, high RR.

Best management: Nebulized β₂ agonist

Clinchers
Features of acute attack of asthma are:
- *Breathlessness* (unable to complete sentences)
- *Respiratory rate* > 25/min
- Pulse rate > 110 beats/min
- Peak expiratory flow less than 50% of predicted or best.

Aerosolized (nabulized) β₂ agonists are the primary therapy of acute episodes of asthma. In emergency, give every 20 minute subsides for 3 doses, then every 2 hours until attack.

Nebulize with: Salbutamol 5 mg or terbutaline 10 mg made upto 5 ml with normal saline and nebulized in air.

Investigation of choice
PEFR, spirometry, CXR (rule out pneumothorax), sputum culture and full blood count.

Immediate management
- Sit patient up and give high dose O₂
- Nebulized β₂ agonist
- Hydrocortisone 200 mg IV or prednisolone 30 mg PO (both if very ill).

Your Notes:

134. A patient who was on 1000 microgram of beclomethasone has now developed oral thrush.

Best management: Reduce steroid

Clinchers
- *1000 mg of beclomethasone:* Standard dose of beclomethasone is 100-400 µg/12 hr. According to British Thoracic Society Guidelines, if the symptoms are not relieved by short-acting inhaled β_2 agonists and standard dose inhaled steroids, then high-dose inhaled steroids are given.
- *Developed oral thrush:* High-dose steroids can weaken host defence, hence susceptibility to infection increases. If high dose steroids create problems like in this question, reduce the dose of steroid and if symptoms persist, add either long-acting β_2 agonists or modified release oral theophylline.
Always rinse mouth after inhaled steroids to prevent oral candidiasis.

CONFUSA
Oral steroids are used acutely (high dose, short courses, e.g. prednisolone 30-40 mg/24 h PO for 7d) and longer term in lower doses (e.g. 5-10 mg/24 h), if control is not optimal on inhalers.

Immediate management
Reduce steroids

Your Notes:

135. An asthmatic patient of presents to A and E department with sudden onset, dyspnoea. On examination there is reduce, expansion, and diminished breathsounds on one side of chest. Trachea is deviated towards otherside.

Diagnosis: Tension pneumothorax

Clinchers
- *Asthmatic patient with sudden onset dyspnoea:* Patients with chronic lung disease are more prone to tension pneumothorax.
- *Reduce expansion, diminished breath sounds, and deviation of trachea* are all signs of tension pneumothorax. It is a medical emergency, and has to be dealt with immediately, else the patient may die.
CXR should not be performed if a tension pneumothorax is suspected, as it will delay immediate necessary treatment.

CONFUSA
Ensure that the suspected pneumothorax is not a large emphysematous bulla.

Investigation of choice
Arterial blood gas analysis

Immediate management
Aspiration of pneumothorax without waiting for CXR.

Treatment of choice
Surgical advice
- If bilateral pneumothoraces
- If lung fails to expose after intercoastal drain insertion
- If 2 or more previous pneumothoraces on the same side
- If history of pneumothorax on other side.

Your Notes:

136. A 70-year-old with complaint of malaise, weight loss, anorexia. Then develops sudden left-sided visual loss.

Diagnosis: Temporal arteritis (suspected)

Clinchers
- *70-year-old:* It occurs almost exclusively in individuals older than 55 years; however, well-documented cases have occured in patients 40 years old or younger.
- *Malaise, weightloss, anorexia:* The non-specific manifestations of temporal arteritis include malaise, fatigue, anorexia, weight loss, sweats and arthralgias.
- *Sudden left sided visual loss:* A well-recognised and dreaded complication of temporal arteritis, particularly in untreated patients, is ocular involvement due primarily to ischemic optic neuritis, which may lead to serious visual symptoms, even sudden blindness in some patients.

CONFUSA
Most patients have complaints relating to the head or eyes for months before objective eye involvement. Attention to such symptoms with institution of appropriate therapy will usually avoid this complication. In patients with involvement of the temporal artery, headache is the predominant symptom and may be associated with a tender, thickened or nodular artery, which may pulsate early in the disease but become occluded later. Scalp pain and claudication of the jaw and tongue may occur.

Investigation of choice
- *Screening:* ESR (elevated).
- *Definitive:* Temporal artery biopsy.

Immediate management
Steroid therapy

Treatment of choice
IV steroids immediately.

Your Notes:

137. 60-year-old develops tunnel vision. There is enlargement of the optic cup.

Diagnosis: Chronic simple glaucoma (CSG)

Clinchers
- *60-year-old:* The risk of CSG increases with increasing age.
- *Tunnel vision:* Isopter contraction is the earliest visual field defect occurring in glaucoma. It refers to mild generalized constriction of the central as well as peripheral field. However, it is of limited diagnostic value, as it may also occur in many other conditions.
- *Enlargement of optic cup:* Normal optic cups are similar (left and right) in shape and occupy less than 50% of the optic disc. In glaucoma these enlarge, especially along the vertical axis.

CONFUSA
Ocular hypertension is the term used when a patient has an IOT constantly more than 21 mm Hg but no optic disc or visual field changes. These patients should be carefully monitored by an ophthalmologist.

Investigation of choice
Visual field mapping

Immediate management
Refer to ophthalmologist

Treatment of choice
There is medical treatment to reduce IOT to less than 21 mmHg. Surgery is used if medical treatment fails.

Your Notes:

138. 50-year-old woman with history of symmetrical joint pains complains of eye symptoms and Schirmer's test is positive.

Diagnosis: Sjögren's syndrome

Clinchers

- *50-year-old woman:* The disease affects predominantly middle aged woman (female to male ratio 9:1), although it can be seen in all ages, including childhood.
- *History of symmetrical jiont pains:* Extraglandular (systemic) manifestations are seen in one-third of patients with Sjögren's syndrome, while they are very rare in patients with Sjögren's syndrome associated with rehumatoid arthritis. These patients complain more often to easy fatiguability, low grade fever, myalgias and arthralgias. Most patients with primary Sjögren's syndrome experience at least one episode of nonerosive arthritis during the course of their disease.
- *Eye symptoms:* Ocular involvement is a major manifestation of Sjögren's syndrome. Patient usually complains of dry eyes with a sandy or gritty feeling under the eyelids. Other symptoms include burning, accumulation of thick strands at the inter canthi, decreased tearing, redness, itching, eye fatigue and increased photosensitivity.
- *Schirmer's test is positive:* It is done by placing a strip of filter paper overlapping lower lid. Tears should soak more than 15 mm in 5 minutes normally (negative test). It is positive in dry eye syndromes (keratoconjunctivitis sicca) which includes Sjögren's syndrome/

CONFUSA
The differential diagnosis of Sjögren's syndrome includes other conditions that may cause dry mouth or eyes or parotid salivary gland enlargement. Human immunodeficiency virus (HIV) infection and sarcoidosis appear to produce a clinical picture indistinguishable from Sjögren's syndrome.

Investigation of choice
Schirmer's test (alread done in this case)

Immediate management
Ophthalmology referral

Treatment of choice
Artificial tears + other symptomatic treatment + steroids.

139. Woman, 30-year-old with complaint of blurred vision. CT is normal but she has bilateral papilledema.

Diagnosis: Pseudotumor cerebri (suspected)

Clinchers

- *Woman, 30-year-old:* Majority of its patients are young, obese, females.
- *Complaint of blurred vision:* Visual acuity is not affected by papilloedema, unless the papilloedema is severe, long-standing or accompanied by macular oedema or hemorrhage. So suspect there in this patient.
- *CT is normal:* Evaluation of papilloedema requires CT or MRI to exlcude a brain tumor. If none is found, MR angiography is appropriate in selected cases to investigate the possibility of a dural venous sinus occlusion or an arteriovenous shunt. If neuroradiologic studies are normal, the subarachnoid opening pressure should be measured by lumbar puncture to confirm that it is elevated. It if is elevated, without explanation, the diagnosis of pseudotumor cerebri is made by exclusion.
- *Bilateral papilloedema:* It connotes bilateral optic disc swelling from raised ICT.

CONFUSA
All forms of optic disc swelling, other than due to raised ICT is 'optic disc oedema'. This convention is arbitrary but serves to avoid confusion. Pseudotumor cerebri is also known as benign intracranial hypertension.

Investigation of choice
Lumbar puncture (opening pressure)

Immediate management
Ophthalmology referral

Treatment of choice
Acetazolamide

Your Notes:

140. A woman who is a Visual Display Operator develops headache when she works for several hours.

Diagnosis: Hypermetropia

Clinchers
- *Woman:* There is no as such sexual discrimination in the incidence.
- *Visual display unit operator develops headache when she works severel hours:* This is most probably an exacerbation of the asthenopic symptoms in a fully corrected hypermetropia due to sustained accomodative efforts. The vision is otherwise normal as the hypermetropia is fully corrected at all other times.

CONFUSA
Astheopic symptoms are
- Tiredness of eyes
- Frontal or fronto-temporal headache
- Watering
- Mild photophobia

These asthenopic symptoms are especially associated with near work and increase towards evening.

Investigation of choice
Test visual acuity

Immediate management
Refer to an opticians

Treatment of choice
Convex spectacle lenses.

Your Notes:

---

141. A 2-year-old boy ran and hit his forehead on the door. No history of loss of consciousness, and since then is playing well. No neurological signs.

Diagnosis: Head injury (minor)

Clinchers
- *2-year-old boy:* In young children minor head injuries are also important, even if they do not produce immediate major complications as repeated minor head trauma in children has been linked to lower IQ.
- *Hit his forehead on the door:* In the preschool are group the most common injuries are those which are sustained while playing or via household accidents. Nonaccidental injuries are also significant in this age group. In the school-going child the most common cause of death is a brain injury from a RTA.
- *No history of loss of consciousness:* Young children lose consciousness lesser readily than adults. Significant brain injury may thus occur without a history of unconsciousness.
- *Since then is playing well and no neurological signs:* These rule out any grave injury and the situation do not warrant a stay in hospital.

CONFUSA
Children are unique in invariably having a carer with them. This means that most can go home with their parents and a set of head injury instructions. They often sleep after trauma and should not be kept awake. Instead, they should be examined by their parents two or three times during the night. All that is required is for the parents to be confident that their child has a normal response to mild stimulation (verbal or tactile). Parents are much better judges of their children's night-time behaviour than hospital doctors or nurses.

Investigation of choice
Skull X-ray is unnecessary if all of the following apply:
- No LOC
- Occipital or frontal injury
- Low speed imapct or injuring agent flat and soft
- Normal neurological status at time of examination
- No scalp damage or laceration with no associated significant swelling.

So, No investigations are required in this case as it meet all of the above criterias.

Immediate management
Give a set of head injury instructions and explain (to parents)

Treatment of choice Discharge with advise.

142. An 8-year-old boy falls off a swing at his school. He is brought to Casualty by one of his teachers. He has a bruise over his right eye but the examination is otherwise normal. He is fully conscious with no history of blackouts since the accident. A skull X-ray is performed, which is normal.

Diagnosis: Insignificant head injury.

Clinchers

- *8-year-old boy:* Children are difficult to assess for head injury and their admission for monitoring is indicated.
- *Falls off a swing at his school:* A common mode of injury to a school going child. But the most common head injury is by RTA.
- *Brought to casualty by one of his teachers:* That means that no adult member of family is with him—a contraindication for discharge.
- *Bruise over his right eye:* Usually children do not suffer from fracture of skull bones as these are more pliable.
- *Examination is otherwise normal:* Rules out any cerebral injury GCS scoring should be done on adult scale and children. GCS if for < 5 years.
- *Fully conscious:* Also in favour of any cerebral injury but not that young children lose consciousness less readily that adults. Significant brain injury can occur without a history of loss of consciousness.
- *No history of blackouts since the accident:* Also a good prognostic sign.
- *Skull X-ray is normal:* Rules out any fracture which commands admission. But one should be aware of suture lines and normal anatomical variants while interpreting the X-rays.

CONFUSA
Assessment of consciousness in a child can be difficult. The best judge for minor alteration in consciousness in children are their parents.

Investigation of choice
Skull X-ray (already done in this case).

Immediate management
Antiseptic dressing of the bruise.

Treatment of choice
Admit and monitor.

Your notes:

143. A 19-year-old met with a road traffic accident (RTA). He is talking, responding and smells of alcohol.

Diagnosis: Suspected head injury.

Clinchers

- *19-year-old:* Head injury is a major cause of death in children and young adults.
- *Road traffic accident:* RTA is a leading cause of death through head injury and was responsible for 39% deaths from trauma in the UK in 1992.
- *He is talking, responding and smells of alcohol:* Although the patient might look normal at the time of assessment, he or she might have been unconscious or concurred at the time of injury. This is difficult to assess in an intoxicated person and require admission to hospital for proper assessment. A radiological investigation (at least a skull X-ray) is required in alcoholic cases for MLC purposes as such person might have been assaulted.

CONFUSA
Drunkenness increases the risk of sustaining a head injury and of that injury causing brain damage. Nevertheless, changes in conscious level must not be attributed to alcohol or other drugs except by exclusion and in retrospect. The plasma osmolality may be a useful investigation in this circumstance.

Investigation of choice
Skull X-ray

Immediate management
Admit to hospital

Treatment of choice
As per the X-ray findings.

Your notes:

144. A 74-year-old woman had a fall two weeks ago. She is brought into the A and E department with slowly increasing drowsiness. On examination you find mild hemiparesis and unequal pupils.

Diagnosis: Subdural hematoma.

Clinchers
- *74-year-old:* Bridging veins in the skull becomes more prone to rupture in old age. It is due to cortical atrophy producing gradual shrinkage of brain and thereby producing more traction on the veins.
- *Slowly increasing drowsiness:* It means that the hematoma which is now behaving like a SOL (space occupying lesion) is still expanding and there is danger if it is not evacuated urgently.
- *Two weeks ago:* Remember subdural hematomas are usually subdued in appearance i.e. they can occur weeks to months after the initial injury (as the bleeding is from very small veins).
- *Mild hemiparesis and unequal pupils:* Ipsilateral pupillary dilatation is a lagte sign. Focal neurological signs are an indication for urgent intervention.

CONFUSA
Do not rely on absence of ipsilateral pupillary dilatation as it is a late sign. Alteration in the conscious level is the cardinal feature; lateralising signs may be absent or minimal.

Investigation of choice
CT scan is diagnostic, showing a collection with an inner concave border (extradural—binconvex).

Immediate management
Urgent neurological opinion.

Treatment of choice
Surgical evacuation of the hematoma.

Your notes:

---

145. A 24-year-old patient presents with RTA. The pupil on the left side is dilated and the patient is obtunded. CT scan of the head reveals a binconvex hyperdense lesion on the temporal region.

Diagnosis: Extradural hemorrhage.

Clinchers
- *History of RTA:* Road traffic accidents produces maximum mortality due to head injuries.
- *Pupil on left side is dilated:* In cases of intracranial hematomas localising neurological symptoms (e.g. ipsilateral pupil dilatation, hemiparesis) occurs late (average 63 days in case of subdural hematoma). So the patient is in a critical stage warranting urgent surgical decompression).
- *Obtunded:* Deteriorating level of consciousness is caused by a rising ICP (due to the expanding hematoma).
- *Biconvex hyperdense lesion on the temporal region:* Fresh bleed on CT appears hyperdense. A binconvex hematoma is characterisitc of an extradural hematoma (lens-shaped). Its most common site is temporal region.

CONFUSA
In subdural hematoma, the CT appearance is usually concave on the inner side, most commonly in parietal region. Midline shift may be present.

Investigation of choice
CT scan (already done in this patient).

Immediate management
Urgent evacuation of the clot through multiple burr holes (as the patient is very critical and there is no spare time for transfer to a neurosurgical unit/centre).

Treatment of choice
Identification and ligation of the bleeding vessel (usually middle meningeal vessels).

Your notes:

146. A 40-year-old hypertensive male with complaint of left knee pain. Also history of similar attacks. Joint aspirate is cloudy.

Diagnosis: Gout

Clinchers

- *40-year-old-male:* Acute gout presents typically in a middle-aged made with sudden onset of agonizing pain in the joint.
- *Hypertensive:* Hypertension per se can impair uric acid excretion (Kumar and Clark, 483, 4th edn). This can lead to hyperuricemia and hence gout. Otherwise this person would've been on thiazide diuretics (a first line antihypertensive) which can precipitate gout in an already hyperuricemia state.
- *Left knee pain:* The most common joint to be involved is first MTP joint (podagra). In 25% of attacks, a joint other than the great toe is affected. Knee is frequently affected in these cases.
- *History of similar attacks:* Occasionally, individuals report a prodrome or previous episodes of milder pain lasting hours.
- *Aspirate is cloudy:* Urate crystals are precipitated in the synovial fluid only when it become supersaturated. Also neutrophils and other inflammatory residues are present in it. All this make the synovial fluid look cloudy when aspirated during an acute attack.

CONFUSA

After initial assessment and first parenteral dose of NSAIDs, the patient of acute gout should be referred back to the GP in order that he or she can:
- Assess progress
- Measure serum urate
- Exclude precipitating causes (FBC and EXR indicated)
- Consider Allopurinol therapy.

Note: Allopurinol is not given within 3 weeks of an acute attack.

Synovial fluid	Appearance	Colour	Viscosity
Normal	Clear	Colourless	High
Non-inflammatory	Clear	Straw	High
Hemorrhagic	Bloody	Xanthochromic	Variable
Acute inflammatory • Acute gout • Rheumatic fever • Rheumatoid arthritis	Turbid	Yellow	Decreased
Septic • TB • Gonorrhea • Septic (non-gonococcal)	Turbid	Yellow	Decreased

Investigation of choice
Synovial fluid microscopy.

Immediate management
A wool and crepe bandage required to protect the joint together with non-weight-bearing crutches. The inflamed area must be rested and elevated.

Treatment of choice
For an acute attack:
NSAID Ibuprofen/Naproxen)
- If NSAID contraindicated: Colchicine
- decreases if both NSAID and colchicine contraindicated (e.g. renal failure)

Steroids.

Your Notes:

147. A patient's ECG shows T wave inversion and ST depression.

Diagnosis: Ischaemic heart disease

Clinchers
- *T wave inversion:* It may signify previous MI. T wave inversions due to chronic ischaemia correlate with prolongation of repolarisation and are often associated with QT lengthening.
- *ST depression:* It is found in myocardial ischaemia, as a digoxin side effect or in the ventricular "strain pattern" which is found with right or left ventricular hypertrophy. The ST segments are also inverted in bundle branch blocks.

(*Note:* MI cannot be diagnosed from ECG in left bundle branch block).

CONFUSA
Negative T waves can be sign of a sub-endocardial myocardial infarction. They are found in the resolution phase of myocardial infarction and in ischaemic heart disease without evidence of myocardial death:
Note
- Horizontal depression of ST segment—ischaemia
- Downsloping depression of ST segment—digoxin

Investigation of choice
ECG

Immediate management
Specialist evaluation

Treatment of choice
As per the cause.

Your notes:

148. Three days of intravenous broad spectrum antibiotics beginning with induction of anaesthesia.

Diagnosis (Answer): Heart valve replacement

Clinchers
- The required prophylactic regimen is Amoxicillin 1g IV + Gentamicin 120 mg IV first dose is given at indcution of anaesthesia and is continued upto 3 days.

CONFUSA
Infection of valve post operating is a situation alcin to infective endocarditis of a native valve. For more detailed notes on chemoprophylaxis in various disease states refer to British national formularly or www.bnf.org.

Investigation of choice
As per the requirements of the operation.

Immediate management
Antimicrodial chemoprophylaxis

Treatment of choice
Stated as the question itself.

Your Notes:

149. A middle-aged woman with a history of rheumatoid arthritis develops sudden swelling in One of her knees. This knee is swollen and hot to touch.

Diagnosis: Pseudogout.

Clinchers

- *Middle-aged:* Though pseudogout occurs more commonly in old age, no age after thirties is exempt from it.
- *Woman:* There is a slight preponderance of female incidence.
- *Sudden swelling in one of her knees:* Knee is the main joint to get involved in it. A minority will have involvement of multiple joints.
- *This knee is swollen and hot to touch:* involved joint is erythematous, swollen, warm and painful.
- *History of rheumatoid arthritis:* Any existing arthritis is a risk factor for pseudogout. Other risk factors are old age, dehydration, intercurrent illness, hyperparathyroidism, myxoedema, diabetes mellitus, phosphate decrease, magnesium deficiency, hemochromatosis, acromegaly, gout, ochronosis, surgery.

CONFUSA

Acute pseudogout is less severe and longer lasting than gout and affects different joints. Pseudogout can even be secondary to gout. It cannot be septic arthritis also as there is no preceding history of joint trauma of presence of fever.

Investigation of choice

- *Screening:* Wrist X-ray (calcium deposition in triangular ligament or chondrocalcinosis)
- *Definitive:* Joint fluid aspiration and microscopy (positively birefringent calcium pyrophosphate crystals in plane polarised light).

Immediate management
Analgesia.

Treatment of choice
NSAIDs ± intra-articular injection of glucocorticoids ± colchicine.

Your Notes:

150. A 78-year-old woman complains of a stiff left hip joint after walking some distance. This is Most evident when she attempts to abduct the hip joint (limited abduction).

Diagnosis: Osteoarthritis (OA).

Clinchers

- *78-year-old woman:* The mean age of onset of OA is 5 years. OA is sympatomatic three times more in women.
- *Stiff hip joint after walking some distance:* Typically in OA, there is pain on movement. It is usually worse at end of day. There may be some background pain at rest.
- *Limited adduction of hip joint:* There can be stiffness of the joint which limits the movements (poor range of movements). There can be associated joint instability.

Joints affected in OA
  - Most commonly: DIP joints, first MCP joint, cervical and lumbar spine
  - Next most common: Hip joint
  - Other most common: Knee joint.

CONFUSA

Lets have a good look at the differentiating features of osteoarthritis and rheumatoid arthritis, the two most common arthritis of elderly females

	OA	RA
Joint stiffness	Late evening	Early evening
Palpable osteophytes	+	-
Skin redness	+/-	+
Swelling	+/-	+
Ligaments stretch	-	+
Age	Usually older	Usually adolescents
Arthrodesis use	Good	Poor
Fibrillation	+	-
Pannus	-	+
Bone around joint	Sclerotic	Osteoporotic
Joint deformity	Varus	Valgus

Investigation of choice
Joint X-ray (findings: Loss of joint space, Subchondral sclerosis, Subchondral cysts, Marginal osteophytes).

Immediate management: Paracetamol for pain.

Treatment of choice
Reduce weight + walking aid
  - Contralateral hand—for hip
  - Ipsilateral hand—for knee
- Joint replacement is done for end stage disease.
- If PCM does not bring relief from pain, then give
  - Day pain—NSAID
  - Night pain—TCA in low doses (tricyclic antidepressant)

151. A chronic alcoholic presents with increasing confusion and confabulation.

Diagnosis: Wernicke's-Korsakoff's syndrome (WKS)

Clinchers
- *Chronic alcoholic:* WKS can develop in heavy drinkers. The cause is severe, untreated, thiamine deficiency secondary to chronic alcohol use.
- *Increasing confusion:* The patient may be disoriented in WKS and is due to Wernicke's encephalopathy. Its patients are profoundly disoriented, indifferent, and inattentive, although rarely they have an agitated delirium related to ethanol withdrawal. If the disease is not treated stupor, coma and death may ensue.
- *Confabulation:* It is the component of Korsakoff's (or Korsakov's) psychosis in WKS. Severe loss of short term memory causes the patient to invent his or her immediate past and is called confabulation.

CONFUSA
The characteristic clinical trial of Wernicke's disease is that of ophthalmoplegia, ataxia and global confusion. However, only one third of patients with acute Wernicke's encephalopathy present with the classical clinical triad. As Korsakoff's psychosis often follows Wernicke's encephalopathy, these are together referred to as Wernicke's-Korsakoff's syndrome.

Investigation of choice
Red cell transketolase (↓)
Plasma pyruvate (↑)

Immediate management
Admit as it is a medical emergency

Treatment of choice
Urgent thiamine amine
- 200-300 mg/24 h PO

But this case is showing symptoms of Korsakoff's psychosis also, so give:
Pabrinex (High potency ampoules of thiamine)
- 2-3 pairs of ampoules/8 h IV over 10 minutes for ≤ 2 days, then daily for 5-7 days.

Your Notes:

152. An elderly patient presents with weight gain, hypothermia and confusion.

Diagnosis: Hypothyroidism (Myxoedema coma)

Clinchers
- *Elderly:* Incidence of myxoedema coma is maximum above 65 years of age.
- *Weight gain:* In the elderly the usual symptoms are fatigue, lethargy, constipation, cold intolerance, stiffness and cramping of muscles, carpal tunnel syndrome and menorrhagia. Intellectual and motor activity slows, appetite declines and weight increases.
- *Hypothermia:* If left untreated, the patient with long standing hypothyroidism may pass into a hypothermic, stuporous state (myxoedema coma) which may be fatal.
- *Confusion:* Although very rare, severe hypothyroidism, especially in the elderly, may present with confusion or even coma.

CONFUSA
In the elderly the symptoms of hypothyroidism may be erroneously attributed to ageing itself, Parkinson's disease, depression or Alzheimer's disease. In myxoedema coma the patient may have severe cardiac failure, hypoventilation, hypoglycemia and hyponatremia. Occasionally with severe hypothyroidism, the elderly patient may become frankly demented or psychotic, sometimes with striking delusions (Myxoedema madness). This may occur shortly after starting T_4 replacement.

Investigation of choice
Take
    venous blood for T_3, T_4, TSH, FBC, U&E, cultures
    arterial blood for PaO_2.

Immediate management
Admit in ICU
+
High flow O_2 if cyanosed

Treatment of choice
T_3 5-20 µg 12h/IV (slow).

Your Notes:

153. Elderly patient with complaint of fever and increasing confusion.

Diagnosis: Infection toxicity

Clinchers
- *Fever:* Infection, particularly of the central nervous system can cause an acute confusional state. Elderly patients with any infection (e.g. chest or urinary tract) can present in such a way that the underlying medical condition is completely masked.
- *Increasing confusion:* The diagnosis of sepsis is easily missed, particularly in the elderly when the classical signs may not be present. Mild confusion, tachycardia and tachypnoea may be the only clues, sometimes with unexplained hypotension, a reduction in urine output, a rising plasma creatinine and glucose intolerance.

CONFUSA
The clinical signs of sepsis are not always associated with bacteremia and can occur with noninfectious processes such as pancreatitis or severe trauma. In order to avoid confusion, the term systemic inflammatory response syndrome (SIRS) has been suggested to describe the disseminated inflammation that can complicate this diverse range of disorders.

Investigation of choice
Blood culture

Immediate management
Refer to ITU if possible for monitoring ± ionotropes

Treatment of choice
IV ceturoxine 1.5 g/8 h (after blood culture).

Your Notes:

154. A 57-year-old male comes to the A and E with his daughter, in a confused state. The daughter said that her father was started on some medication by his GP.

Diagnosis: Drug induced (Hypoglycemia-most probable)

Clinchers
- *57-year-old:* Mental disturbance caused by prescribed drugs is particularly common in elderly but may occur with central nervous system depressant drugs, beta blockers, digoxin and cimetidine at all ages.
- *Confused state:* Symptoms include fluctuating clouding of consciousness and restlessness with paranoid delusions and visual hallucinations in severe cases.
- *Started on some medication by his GP:* Although, drug induced psychiatric symptoms in elderly are usually a result of over dosage, there reactions may sometimes occur because of intolerance to the normal dose or after withdrawal of drug.

CONFUSA
It is often impossible to assess fully or manage a confused and distressed patient. Adequate sedation makes further therapy possible. IV diazepam or midazolam is effective and has a rapid onset of action but careful observation and monitoring are essential. Hypoglycemia is one of the few situations where rapid diagnosis and specific therapy obviate the need for sedation.

Investigation of choice
Blood glucose

Immediate management
If possible, contact GP

Treatment of choice
Symptomatic

Your Notes:

First Aid for PLAB

155. An elderly man found wandering aimlessly, brought to the A and E by neighbours, who inform that his GP had called on his yesterday.

Diagnosis: Acute psychiatric disturbances

Clinchers
- *Elderly man:* Episodes of acute psychiatric disturbance are much more common in the elderly patients who may have associated dementia or concurrent chronic medical problems or treatments which may precipitate it.
- *Wandering aimlessly:* This signifies disorientation and confusional state.
- *Brought to the A and E by neighbours:* This signifies lack of insight on the part o the patient and thus qualifies as a psychoses. Also it indicates lack of family support at home.
- *His GP had called on him yesterday:* This suggest that he is under some medical treatment. One should contact the GP immediately to enquire about it.

CONFUSA
Behaviour is influenced by the interplay between the environment and psyche and is modified by drugs. A disturbed patient may be suffering from a psychiatric condition, an organic brain lesion, a personality disorder or an emotional upset. The task of the emergency department is to:
- Identify those patients who need immediate therapy
- Support the coping strategies of the patient
- Liaise with the appropriate agency for further care

Investigation of choice
Blood glucose + EEG

Immediate management
Contact the GP

Treatment of choice
As per the diagnosis but mainly symptomatic

Your Notes:

---

156. Female on OCPs complains of postcoital bleeding.

Diagnosis: Cervical ectropion

Clinchers
- *OCP:* Ectocervix contain a transformation zone, where the stratified squamous epithelium of the vagina meets the columnar epithelium of the cervical canal. The anatomical site of this squamocolumnar junction fluctuates under hormonal influence, and the high turnover of this tissue is important in the pathogenesis of cervical carcinoma. The columnar epithelium is normally visible with the speculum during
  - Ovulatory phase of menstrual cycle
  - Pregnancy
  - OCP use
- *Postcoital bleeding:* It may give rise to postcoital bleeding, as fine blood vessels, within the columnar epithelium are easily traumatised.

CONFUSA
Cervical ectropion is sometimes termed as cervical erosion. Usually the main complaint of cervical ectropion is excessive nonpurulent discharge, as the surface area of the columnar epithelium containing mucus glands is increased. It may give rise to spotting during pregnancy in which case it is usually left untreated till after the pregnancy.

Investigation of choice
Per speculum exam (red ring around OS because the endocervical epithelium has extended its territory over the paler epithelium of the ectocervix).

Immediate management
Reassurance about cause and treatment.

Treatment of choice
Usually none required.
If symptoms are distressing
- Thermal cautery (sometimes confusingly called cold coagulation).

Your Notes:

157. A 55-year-old female develops a single episode of postmenopausal bleeding. She stopped menstruation 7 years ago. Ultrasound shows endometrial thickness.

Diagnosis: Endometrial carcinoma

Clinchers
- *55-year-old:* It usually presents after the menopause.
- *Single episode of postmenopausal bleeding:* Any post-menopausal vaginal bleeding must be investigated as the cause may be endometrial carcinomas.
- *Stopped menstruation 7 years ago:* Occasional bleeding is common upto 1 year after menopause but not upto 7 years.
- *USG shows endometrial thickness:* This clearly suggest endometrial growth and hence indicate a need to obtain the tissue diagnosis.

CONFUSA
Postmenopausal bleeding is an early sign and generally leads a woman to see her doctor, but examination is usually normal. Endometrial carcinoma is less common than carcinoma of cervix. Most endometrial tumors are adenocarcinomas and are related to excessive exposure to oestrogens unopposed by progesterone.

Investigation of choice
Uterine sampling or curettage

Immediate management
Take detailed history

Treatment of choice
- Stage I and II—total hysterectomy with bilateral salpingo-oophorectomy
- Inoperable cases—radiotherapy

Your Notes:

---

158. A 49-year-old woman with complaint of hot flushes, vaginal dryness and her menstruation become irregular 5 months ago.

Diagnosis: Menopause

Clinchers
- *49-year-old:* The menopause or cessation of periods, naturally occurs about the age of 45-55 years.
- *Hot flushes, vaginal dryness:* Features of oestrogen deficiency are hot flushes (which occur in most women and can be disabling), vaginal dryness and atrophy of the breasts. There may also be vague symptoms of loss of libido, loss of self-esteem, nonspecific, aches and pains, irritability, depression, loss of concentration and weight gain.
- *Menstruation become irregular 5 months ago:* Most women notice irregular scanty periods carrying on over a variable period, though in some sudden amenorrhoea or menorrhagia occur.

CONFUSA
Menopause may also occur surgically with radiotherapy to the ovaries and with ovarian disease (e.g. premature menopause).

Investigation of choice
Urinary FSH concentration (↑)—Just to reassure here that these are not symptoms of some pathology

Immediate management
Reassurance and counselling

Treatment of choice
Option of hormone replacement therapy

Your Notes:

159. A 14-year-old women with painless vaginal bleeding.

Diagnosis: Menarche

Clinchers
- *14-year-old:* Menarche usually occurs at age of 11-15 years.
- *Painless vaginal bleeding:* In this age group it most commonly represent menarche though any traumatic bleed must also be excluded.

CONFUSA
In girls events of puberty start age of 9-13 years with breast bud enlargement and continues to 12-18 years. Pubic hair commences at ages 9-14 years and is completed at 12-16 years. Menarche occurs relatively late (11-15 years) but peak height velocity is reached much earlier than in boys (10-13 years). Growth is completed earlier than in boys.

Investigation of choice
None required usually

Immediate management
Exclude traumatic bleed

Treatment of choice
None

Your Notes:

160. A 55-year-old lady with history of intermittent postmenopausal bleeding. Vaginal and speulum examinations are normal.

Diagnosis: Endometrial carcinoma

Clinchers
- *A 55-year-old:* Mean age of presentation is 56 years. It is rare under the age of 40.
- *Intermittent postmenopausal bleeding:* This symptom should always be assumed to be caused by carcinoma of endometrium until proven otherwise.
- *Vaginal and speculum examination are normal:* This has ruled out any local cause of bleeding (e.g. vaginal trauma) so this warrants examination of the endometrium now.

CONFUSA
Endometrial carcinoma is associated with hyperestrogenic states, i.e.
- Obesity
- Diabetes
- Late menopause
- Prolonged use of unopposed oestrogens
- Oestrogen secreting tumors

Investigation of choice
- *Screening:* Ultrasound (to assess dimensions of any tumor and to show endometrial thickness)
- *Definitive:* Uterine sampling or curettage

Immediate management
Perform staging to decide the line of treatment.

Treatment of choice
Usually surgical

Uterus	Tumor	Surgery
Small	Well differentiated	Total abdominal hysterectomy + bilateral salpingo-oophorectomy + internal iliac node frozen section biopsy
Enlarged	Confined to upper part of corpus	Extended hysterectomy + bilateral salpingo-oophorectomy + removal of a cuff of vagina + lymph node sampling
Cervix invaded		Wertheim's (Removal of upper lost half of the vagina and pelvic lymph node)

- *Radiotherapy*
  - If node is involved
  - If there is deep invasion of myometrium
- *Hormone therapy:* Progestogens inhibit the rate of growth and spread of endometrial carcinoma.

July—2001

161. A 39-year-old woman on thyroxine replacement comes for first check-up.

Diagnosis: Hypothyroidism (under treatment)

Clinchers

- *39-year-old:* Over replacement with thyroxine may increase the risk of atrial fibrillation in those over 60 years of age. Age of 39 years does not hold any unique significance.
- *Woman:* Overall females have a larger incidence of autoimmune diseases especially those of thyroid (most common: Hashimoto's)
- *Thyroxine replacement:* Replacement therapy with T_4 is given for life. The starting dose will depend upon the severity of the deficiency and on the age and fitness of the patient, especially cardiac performance. In the young and fit, 100 μg daily is suitable, while 50 μg daily is more appropriate for the small, old or frail. T_3 offers no significant advantage over T_4.
- *Comes for first check-up:* First review is suggested after 12 weeks of starting the treatment (6 weeks according to Kumar and Clark). It is done to assess the adequacy of replacement clinically. The aim is to restore TSH to well within the normal range. If serum TSH remain high, the dose of T_4 should be increased in 25-50 μg increments and the tests repeated six weeks later. This stepwise progression should be continued until TSH becomes normal.

CONFUSA
Thyroxine may precipitate angina especially in those with pre-existing heart disease. Osteoporosis is a theoretical risk of over replacement. The possibility of development of other autoimmune disease especially Addison's disease should be always considered in such patients. Clinical improvement on T_4 may not begin for two weeks or more, even though it is quicker on T_3, and full resolution of symptoms may take six months (although treatment is continued lifelong). During frequency about a 50 μg increase in T_4 dosage is required (due to ↑ TIBG levels).

Investigation of choice
TSH

Immediate management
A detailed clinical examination

Treatment of choice
T_4 dose adjustments according to TSH levels

---

162. 40-year-old woman, euthyroid (TSH normal) complains of palpitations, weight loss and diarrhoea.

Diagnosis: Pituitary TSH tumor

Clinchers

- *40-year-old women:* Pituitary adenomas are slightly more common in middle-aged women.
- *Euthyroid (TSH normal):* In such cases TSH may be normal or increased due to overproduction by the pituitary adenoma. Otherwise is all cases of hyperthyroidism TSH is invariably decreased. T_4 should be measured to reach an accurate diagnosis.
- *Palpitations, weight loss, diarrhoea:* These are the usual symptoms of a hyperthyroid state.

CONFUSA
In any case of suspected hyperthyroidism, ask for T_3, T_4 and TSH. A minority will have elevation of only one thyroid hormone, but all will have ↓ TSH—secretory pituitary adenoma. if TSH is normal and T_4 abnormal except for the rare phenomenon of a TSH, consider:
- hormone binding problems, e.g. pregnancy
- ↑ thyroid-binding globulin
- Amiodarone
- Pituitary TSH tumour

Investigation of choice
T_3 and T_4 assay, TIG assay

Immediate management
MRI skull

Treatment of choice
Surgery (if possible)

Your Notes:

163. 13-year-old woman, euthyroid has a soft diffuse swelling that moves with swallowing.

Diagnosis: Physiological goitre

Clinchers
- *13-year-old woman:* Incidence of thyroid disease is slightly more in females. The physiological goitre tends to occur at puberty (as in this case) and pregnancy.
- *Euthyroid:* Essentially the gland is euthyroid in this condition.
- *Soft diffuse swelling:* It is manifest as a smooth enlargement of the thyroid gland.
- *Moves with swallowing:* The characteristics of an enlarged thyroid are a mass in the neck on one or both sides of the trachea, which moves on swallowing, since it is attached to the larynx by the pre-tracheal fascia.

CONFUSA

This condition should be differentiated clinically from the common nodular goitre which also occurs with an euthyroid state. In it there is either a solitary nodule or multiple nodules.

Investigation of choice
TSH and T_4 (to rule out any derangement)

Immediate management
Rule out pregnancy

Treatment of choice
None required

Your Notes:

164. Elderly woman presents with a hard fixed lump ultrasound shows no cystic spaces.

Diagnosis: Anaplastic carcinoma thyroid

Clinchers
- *Elderly woman:* It occurs mainly in elderly women and is much less often diagnosed now than in the past when many thyroid lymphomas were mistakenly classified histologically as anaplastic carcinomas.
- *Hard fixed lump:* The tumor is histologically undifferentiated composed largely of spindle and giant cells (thus hard in consistency), fast growing and highly malignant, local infiltration (thus fixity) is an early feature of these tumors which spread by lymphatics and blood stream.
- *Ultrasound shows no cystic spaces:* This rules out any cyst which may produce this lump. Anaplastic carcinomas are invariably solid in consistency.

CONFUSA

Anaplastic thyroid carcinoma may be confused with lymphoma or sarcoma, and positive immunocytochemical stains for keratin or the cytoskeletal protein vimentin help to confirm the diagnosis. The lack of calcitonin immunoreactivity differentiates anaplastic carcinoma from undifferentiated medullary thyroid carcinoma.

Investigation of choice
Biopsy (Isthmusectomy)

Immediate management
Scan for metastases

Treatment of choice
If operable: radical thyroidectomy
If unoperable: palliative radiotherapy

Your Notes:

165. An elderly man presents with hoarse voice. On examination he have dilated chest vessels and engorged neck veins.

Diagnosis: Retrosternal goitre

Clinchers

- *Hoarse voice:* Recurrent nerve paralysis (producing hoarseness in this case), although rare in this condition, do exist especially if the goitre is malignant.
- *Dilated chest vessels and engorged neck veins:* This is "superior mediastinal syndrome." It is due to blockage of the venous return to the superior vena cava and consequential engorgement of the jugular veins and their tributaries and in oedema of the upper part of the body.

CONFUSA
A retrosternal goitre is often symptomless and is discovered on a routine chest radiograph. However there may be severe symptoms of dyspnoea, particularly at night, cough and stridor. Many of these patients may attend a chest clinic with a diagnosis of asthma before the true nature of the problem is discovered.

Investigation of choice
CXR

Immediate management
Rule out thyrotoxicosis (if present, antithyroid drugs are contraindicated).

Treatment of choice
Surgical resection

166. Patient with a pulsatile hard mass fixed under the upper 1/3 of the sternomastoid muscle.

Diagnosis: Chemodectoma

Clinchers

- *Hard mass:* Chemodectomas arise from carotid body and usually firm. Occasionally they are soft and pulsatile. It does not usually cause bruits.
- *Fixed:* These tumors more from side to side but not up and down. Most behave in a benign fashion, in a few patients the tumor becomes locally invasive and may metastasize.
- *Under the upper 1/3 of the sternomastoid muscle:* This tumor must be suspected in masses just anterior or under the upper third of sternomastoid.

CONFUSA
The tumor presents as a slowly growing enlarging mass in a patient over the age of 30 years. Occasionally, pressure on the carotid sinus from the tumor produces attacks of faintness. Extension of the tumor may lead to cranial nerve palsies (VII, IX, X, XI and XII), resulting in dysphagia and hoarseness.

Investigation of choice
Digital substraction angiography

Immediate management
Check the opposite side as the tumor is often bilateral.

Treatment of choice
Extirpation by vascular surgeon.

167. A 40-year-old male has a lump in the supero-posterior area of the anterior triangle.

Diagnosis: Parotid tumor.

Clinchers
- *40 years old:* Ninety percent parotid tumors present before the age of 50 although any age may be affected.
- *Male:* Sex distribution is equal.
- *Lump in superoposterior area of anterior triangle:* In a > 40 year old patient, a lump in this area is most likely to be a parotid tumor (498, OHCM, 5th edn). Although the swelling can be anywhere within the parotid gland, but usually in the lower pole and in the region of the angle of the jaw. The lump is well defined, usually firm or hard but sometimes cystic in consistency.

CONFUSA
The facial nerve is never involved in parotid tumors, except by frankly malignant tumors. Its integrity, however, should always be confirmed. Although slow growing, there tumors cannot be considered benign because of the lack of encapsulation, the occasional wide infiltration of the surrounding tissues and the tendency to recur.

Investigation of choice
Biopsy

Immediate management
Check the integrity of facial nerve

Treatment of choice
Superficial parotidectomy

Your Notes:

---

168. A 16-year-old female has a midline lump in the neck which moves on protrusion of the tongue and is below the hyoid bone.

Diagnosis: Thyroglossal cyst

Clinchers
- *16-year-old:* Thyroglossal cyst almost always presents before 20 years of age.
- *Female:* The sex ratio is nondiscriminatory.
- *Midline lump:* It is a fluctuant swelling in the midline of the neck.
- *Moves on protrusion of tongue:* It is diagnosed by its characteristic physical signs:
  - It moves upwards when the patient protrudes the tongue because of its attachment to the tract of the thyroid descent
  - It moves on swallowing because of its attachment to the larynx by the preitracheal fistula
- *Below the hyoid bone:* This is its most common location.

CONFUSA
Thyroglossal cyst may be present in any part of the thyroglossal tract. The common situations, in order of frequency are:
1. Beneath the hyoid
2. In the region of thyroid cartilage
3. Above the hyoid bone

Such a cyst occupies the midline, except in the region of the thyroid cartilage, where the thyroglossal tract is pushed to one side, usually to the left.

Investigation of choice
Entirely clinical diagnosis. USG may help.

Immediate management
Rule out an infected cyst which indicates a delay in surgery.

Treatment of choice
Excision (because infection is inevitable)

Your Notes:

169. **A 19-year-old male has a cystic mass under the anterior border of sternomastoid at the junction of upper 1/3 and middle 1/3 of the muscle. Aspiration revealed fluid containing cholesterol crystals.**

Diagnosis: Branchial cyst (BC).

Clinchers
- *19-year-old:* BC usually presents in early adult life.
- *Male:* The sex ratio is nondiscriminatary.
- *Cystic mass:* BC forms a soft swelling like a "half-filled hot water bottle."
- *Under the anterior border of sternomastoid at the junction of upper 1/3 and middle 1/3 of the muscle:* This is the typical location of the branchial cyst and it bulges forward from beneath the anterior border of sternomastoid.
- *Fluid containing cholesterol crystals:* This confirms the diagnosis of BC as it always contains pus like material, which is in fact cholesterol crystals. These are demonstrated under the microscope.

CONFUSA

BC often presents following an upper respiratory tract infection. Occasionally the cyst may be infected. It signifies the persistence of remnants of the second branchial arch. A rare first branchial arch cyst may present just below the external auditory meatus at the angle of the jaw, with extension closely related to VII nerve.

Investigation of choice
Aspiration and microscopy (already done in this case).

Immediate management
Rule out cyst infection but is an indication for delay in surgery.

Treatment of choice
Surgical excision.

Your Notes:

170. **An infant present with a transilluminant swelling in the lower third of neck.**

Diagnosis: Cystic hygroma (CH)

Clinchers
- *Infant:* CH usually manifests itself in the neonate or in early infancy and occasionally may be present at birth and be so large as to obstruct labour.
- *Transilluminant swelling:* The characteristic that distinguishes CH from all other neck swellings is that it is brilliantly transilluminant.
- *Lower third of neck:* Swelling in CH usually occurs in the lower third of the neck and as it enlarges it passes upwards towards the ear. Often the posterior triangle of the neck is mainly involved.

CONFUSA

As a result intercommunication of its many compartments, the swelling of CH is soft and partially compressible. It visibly increases in size when the child coughs or cries. The cheek, axilla, groin and mediastinum are other, although less frequent, sites for a cystic hygroma.

Investigation of choice
Transillumination test

Immediate management
Rule out infection of the cyst

Treatment of choice
Excision of all the cyst at an early stage.

Your Notes:

171. A 50-year-old woman underwent an anterior resection for carcinoma of the rectum one week ago. Has low grade fever and with complaint of pain in the calf + tenderness in the calf.

Diagnosis: Deep vein thrombosis

Clinchers
- *50-year-old:* Incidence of this complication is particularly more in:
  - Elderly
  - Obese
  - Those with malignant disease
  - Who have varicose veins
  - History of previous DVT
  - Those undergoing
    - Abdominal surgery
    - Pelvic surgery
    - Hip surgery (most common)
  - Women on
    - OCP
    - HRT
  - Presence of predisposing factors
    - Reduced levels of endogenous anticoagulants
      - protein C
      - protein S
      - antithrombin III
    - Possession of the Leiden mutation of coagulation factor V
- *Anterior resection for carcinoma of rectum:* Pelvic surgeries have the highest incidence of DVT post-operatively.
- *One week ago:* DVT typically occur in the second post operative week (see confusa also).
- *Low grade fever:* DVT is often associated with a mild pyrexia. The skin temperature of the affected calf is invariably raised (due to dilatation of the superficial veins of the leg and inflammatory reaction).
- *Complaint of pain in calf:* It is the major presenting feature and is usually associated with swelling and redness.
- *Tenderness in calf:* This confirm that pain is due to DVT only.

CONFUSA
DVT usually occurs during the second postoperative week. Earlier thrombosis particularly occurs when the patient has already been in hospital for sometime preoperatively. Radioiodine studies have confirmed that the thrombotic process usually commence at, or soon after, the operation. The classical Homan's sign (↑ resistance to forced foot dorsiflexion, which may be painful) is positive in less than 20% cases and cannot be relied upon. On the contrary, it may dislodge thrombus giving rise to thromboembolism.

Investigation of choice
Doppler USG/venogram

Immediate management
Enoxapain 1 mg/kg BD or 1.5 mg/kg OD

Treatment of choice
Heparin for 3 months

Your Notes:

172. A young woman underwent emergency appendicectomy 6 days ago for perforated appendix. She appeared to be making a good recovery but has developed intermittent pyrexia (up to 39°C). On examination—no obvious cause found, but she is tender anteriorly on rectal examination.

Diagnosis: Anterior pelvic abscess.

Clinchers
- *Appendicectomy:* A pelvic abscess may follow any general peritonitis, but it is particularly common after acute appendicitis (75%), or after gynaecological infections.
- *Perforated appendix:* This increases the chances of development of the abscess manifold as there is direct exposure of the septic load.
- *Good recovery:* Rules out any systemic involvement.
- *Intermittent pyrexia (upto 39°C):* This is the characteristic swinging pyrexia and points towards an abscess somewhere in body.
- *Tender anteriorly on rectal examination:* This suggests that the abscess in situated anteriorly between the uterus and posterior fornix of vagina.

CONFUSA
In the male the abscess lies between the bladder and the rectum, in the female between the uterus and posterior fornix of the vaginal anteriorly, and the rectum posteriorly (pouch of Douglas). An early pelvic cellulitis may respond rapidly to a short cause of chemotherapy, but there is the risk that the prolonged antibiotic treatment of an unresolved infection may produce a chronic inflammatory mass. It is safer therefore, where there is an established pelvic abscess, to withhold chemotherapy and await pointing into the vagina (as in this case) or rectum through which surgical drainage can be carried out.

Investigation of choice
USG/CT scan.

Immediate management
Chemotherapy (see confusa also).

Treatment of choice
Drainage of abscess.

Your Notes:

173. An elderly man underwent an emergency repair of an abdominal aortic aneurysm. Had been severely hypotensive before and during surgery. After surgery, his blood pressure was satisfactory, but urine output only 5 ml/hr in the first 2 hours.

Diagnosis: Acute tubular necrosis (Ischemic).

Clinchers
- *Emergency repair of an abdominal aortic aneurysm:* This means that the repair was undertaken after an aneurysmal rupture or acute aortic expansion. Either of these produce a severe hypotension. Moreover during the surgery the renal arterial ostia are often compressed when the aorta is clamped and are thus rendered ischemic for the duration of cross clamping. The left renal vein may be ligated and divided as part of the operative procedure. Hypotension pre-or post-operatively may exacerbate the renal injury.
- *Severely hypotensive before and during surgery:* Circulatory compromise produces renal hypoperfusion and thence ischemic necrosis of the tubules.
- *After surgery, his BP was satisfactory:* This rules out any continuing ischemia and a need for urgent intervention. Also it suggest a definitive injury to the kidney.
- *Urine output only 5 ml/hr in first 2 hours:* Urine output should be >30 mL/hr postoperatively. A value significantly lower than this suggest renal dysfunction (due to hypoperfusion or ATN).

CONFUSA
Low urine output (if there is no ATN) postoperatively is almost always due to inadequate infusion of fluid. One should check JVP, and review for sings of cardiac failure. Treat by increasing IVI rate unless patient is in heart or renal failure, or profusely bleeding (in that case, blood should be transfused). If in doubt a fluid challenge may be indicated: ½-1 L over 30-60 minutes, with monitoring of urine output. Then the IVI rate may be increased to 1 litre/h for 2-3 h. Only if output does not increase should a diuretic be considered; a CVP line may be needed if estimation of fluid balance is difficult. A normal value is 0-5 cm of water relative to the sternal angle.
Note: If not catheterised exclude retention.

Investigation of choice
Urinary sodium concentration (It differentiates whether the oliguria is prerenal and amenable to fluid therapy or a result of acute tubular necrosis—urinary Na >40 mmol/L.

Immediate management
Perform an aseptic catheterisation
 +
early specialist (nephrologist and internist) referral

Treatment of choice
Supportive until spontaneous recovery of renal function occurs.

Your Notes:

174. An elderly woman underwent emergency laparotomy for peritonitis. Fourth postoperative day she is noted to have serosanguinous discharge from the wound, but there is no erythema or tenderness around the wound.

Diagnosis: Impending burst abdomen.

Clinchers
- *Elderly women:* Incidence of wound dehiscence is more in elderly patients because of poor wound healing and weak abdominal muscles.
- *Peritonitis:* It implies a high septic load in the peritoneal cavity. It can have a significance in etiology of burst abdomen indirectly by inducing wound infection (not likely in this case).
- *Fourth postoperative day:* The abdomen usually dehiscence on about the 10th day. But the warning signs may be visible much before.
- *Serosanquinous discharge from the wound:* This is the blood tinged serous effusion (which is always present during the first week or two within the abdominal cavity after operation). It usually seeps through the breathing-down wound and serves as a warning of impending burst abdomen.
- *No erythema or tenderness around the wound:* this rules out wound infection and leaves us with only the above diagnosis.

CONFUSA
Sometimes, the deep layer of the abdominal incision gives way but the skin sutures hold; such cases result in a massive incisional hernia.

Investigation of choice
Clinical diagnosis, no investigation required.

Immediate management
Place a sterile dressing over the wound + call seniors.

Treatment of choice
Reassessment of wound in OT.

Your Notes:

175. A 60-year-old patient with features of septicaemia (warm peripheries, low BP, etc.) after an abdominal surgery.

Diagnosis: Postoperative septicaemia.

Clinchers
- *60-year-old:* Septicemia is a common postoperative complication among elderly and children because of incomplete immune system
- *Features of septicaemia after an abdominal surgery:* Gram negative septicaemia is particularly seen after colonic, biliary and urological surgery. The principal effect of endotoxins is to cause vasodilatation of the peripheral circulation together with increased capillary permeability. The effects are partly direct, and partly indirect due to activation of normal tissue inflammatory responses such as the complement system and mediators such as tumor necrosis factor.

CONFUSA
Septicemia is often overlooked as:
- The temperature may not be raised
- The WBC count may be normal or low
- Blood cultures may be negative.

The hallmark is impaired tissue perfusion.

Investigation of choice
Blood culture (take sample before starting antibiotics).

Immediate management
Colloid/crystalloid IVI + refer to ITU for monitoring ± ionotropes.

Treatment of choice
Cefuroxime 1.5 g/8h IV.
  +
Metronidazole 500 mg/6h IV.

Your Notes:

---

176. A 4-year-old boy gets hemarthrosis with trivial injury. He had similar episodes before maternal grandfather and uncle had a similar problem.

Diagnosis: Hemophilia (answer: X-linked recessive)

Clinchers
- *4-year old:* Severe deficiencies of factor VIII or IX are associated with frequent spontaneous bleeding from early life.
- *Boy:* Since it is a X-linked recessive disorder, it is manifest exclusively in males. Females who have this disorder are only carriers.
- *Hemarthrosis with trivial injury:* Bleeding into joints following insignificant injury is a usual mode of presentation. The episodes are recurrent. It is rare in von-Willebrand's disease.
- *Maternal grand father and uncle had a similar problem:* This pattern suggest an X-linked recessive trait and thus excludes von Willebrand's disease.

CONFUSA
In inherited coagulation disorders, deficiencies of all factors have been described. Those leading to abnormal bleeding are rare, apart from hemophilia A (factor VIII deficiency), hemophilia B (factor IX deficiency) and von Willebrand's disease. The prevalence of hemophilia A is about 1 in 5000 of male population and of hemophilia B is 1 in 30000. Both are inherited as X-linked recessive diseases.

Investigation of choice
Factor VIII and IX levels.

Immediate management
Seek expert advice
Avoid NSAIDs and IM injections.

Treatment of choice
Factor VIII/IX therapy.

Your Notes:

177. A young girl with complaint of prolonged bleeding following dental extraction. Father had a work-up for anemia and mother had multiple transfusions.

Diagnosis: von-Willebrand disease (answer: Autosomal dominant).

Clinchers
- *Young girl:* It usually presents at a young age. Females don't manifest hemophilia, so we are left with only von-Willebrand's disease (VWD).
- *Prolonged bleeding following dental extraction:* In VWD, bleeding follows minor trauma or surgery and epistaxis and menorrhagia often occur.
- *Father had a work-up for anemia and mother had multiple transfusions:* The condition has to be autosomally inherited as both parents are manifesting the symptoms (of blood loss and anemia). VWD is autosomal dominant (type 1 and 2) and autosomal recessive (type 3).

CONFUSA
Hemarthroses are rare in VWD. Type 3 VWD patients have more severe bleeding but rarely experience the joint and muscle bleeds seen in hemophilia A. The von-Willebrand's factor gene is located on chromosome 12 and numerous mutations of the gene has been identified. Consequently the disease has been classified into 3 types—VWD 1 to 3. The disease type in this question cannot be VWD type 3 as in it the parents are always phenotypically normally. Type 1 is the most common.

Investigation of choice
APTT (↑) ; VIII C (↓).

Immediate management
Liaise with a hematologist.

Treatment of choice
Factor VIII cryoprecipitate
 +
Vasopressin

Your Notes:

---

178. A 15-year-old girl with features of diabetes mellitus.

Diagnosis: IDDM (answer: Polygenic)

Clinchers
- *15-year old:* IDDM presents most commonly in childhood, with a peak at 10-13 years of age, but can present at any age.
- *Girl:* IDDM is slightly more common in girl as autoimmunity is implicated in its etiology (on the whole, any autoimmune disease is more prevalent in females).
- *Features of diabetes mellitus:* It has to be IDDM (type and diabetes) as NIDDM usually develops in older and obese persons. Both types of diabetes are polygenic in inheritance although in NIDDM environmental factors do play a role (i.e. obesity).

CONFUSA
IDDM is most common in populations of European extraction. The incidence rises as one moves north within Europe, with the highest rate in Finland and Scandinavian. The incidence of IDDM is rising in many parts of the world, and has doubled in Europe over the parts 20-30 years.

Investigation of choice
WHO criterias (Page 282, OHCM, 5th edn).

Immediate management
Delineate family history.
 +
Family counselling on genetics of IDDM

Treatment of choice
Insulin

Your Notes:

179. An 11-year-old boy presents with increasing difficulty walking, tremor and instability. Father died in his 40's with same disease.

Diagnosis: Huntington's disease (Answer: Autosomal dominant)

Clinchers
- *11-year-old boy:* Onset of Huntington's disease (HD) is usually in the fourth and fifth decade, but there is a wide range in age of onset, from childhood to greater than 70 years.
- *Increasing difficulty walking:* In HD, the gait is disjointed and poorly coordinated and has a so called dancing (choreic) quality. There is a steady progression, of both the dementia and chorea.
- *Tremor and instability:* There are frequent, irregular, sudden jerks and movement of any of the limbs or trunk. Early onset before the age of 20 (Juvenile HD) is associated with rigidity, ataxia, cognitive decline and more rapid progression, with a typical duration of about 8 years.
- *Father died in his 40's with the same disease:* Death usually occurs between 10 and 20 years after the onset (early in juvenile HD). Presence of disease in father of this boy also implies an autosomal disorder which infact is the case with HD.

CONFUSA
The prevalence of HD is about 5 in 100000. It occurs worldwide. Inheritance is as an autosomal dominant trait with full penetrance; the children of an affected parent have a 50% chance of inheriting the disease seizures are rare with adult onset HD but are more common with juvenile onset disease.

Investigation of choice
CT scan brain (atrophy of caudate nucleus).

Immediate management
Exclude other causes of chorea
+
Mutation analysis for presymptomatic testing of family members with genetic counselling.

Treatment of choice
No treatment arrests the disease
Phenothiazines (e.g. sulpiride) may reduce the chorea
Tetrabenazine helps control the movements.

180. An 18-year old female underwent caries tooth extraction and developed profuse bleeding. On taking history. She revealed menorrhagia. Her mother and her grand father had the same disease.

Diagnosis: Von Willebrand disease (type III) (Answer: Autosomal recessive)

Clinchers
- *Underwent caries torth extraction and developed profuse bleeding:* In mild cases, bleeding occurs only after surgery or trauma.
- *Menorrhagia:* More severely affected patients have spontaneous epistaxis or oral mucosal, gastro-intestinal, or genito-urinary bleeding.
- Mother and grand father had the same disease: Considering she is a female the inheritance is proven as autosomal. Since her grandfather had the same disease, but not the father, the disease is clearly recessive, as it needed another allede from mother to make herself homogenously inherited.

CONFUSA
This is an interesting question considering question 177 in this theme was also on this disease. The difference is that answer in that case was autosomal dominant. That was type I vWD. Type III vWD is very rare and is phenotypically recessive. Type III patients may inherit a different abnormality from each parent. In many cases the parents are very mildly affected or are a symptomatic (like the father in this case) but the patient have severe mucosal bleeding and no detectable vWF antigen or activity, and may have sufficiently low factor VIII that they have occasional haemorthroses like haemophiliacs.

Investigation of choice
APTT (↑) ; VIII C (↓).

Immediate management
Liaise with a hematologist.

Treatment of choice
Factor VIII cryoprecipitate
+
Vasopressin

Your Notes:

181. A 56-year-old woman who underwent mastectomy for a breast tumor four years ago, now complains of increasing breathlessness. On examination of her respiratory system, she is noted to have decreased movement of the left hemithorax which is dull to percussion and has absent breath sounds.

Diagnosis: Pleural effusion (left side).

Clinchers
- *56-year-old woman who underwent mastectomy for a breast tumor four years ago:* This implies a positive history of malignant breast disease and hence a high index of suspicion for recurrence or metastases should always be there for unexplained signs and symptoms later on.
- *Increasing breathlessness:* Pleural effusion can be asymptomatic or present with dyspnoea and pleuritic chest pains.
- *Decreased movement of the left hemithorax:* It is due to decreased expansion on the involved side.
- *Dull to percussion and absent breath sounds:* A stony dull percussion note and diminished breath sounds are hallmarks of pleural effusion.

CONFUSA
In pleural effusion tactile vocal tremitus and vocal resonance are decreased but they are inconstant and unreliable. Above the effusion, where lung is compressed, there may be bronchial breathing and aegophony. Breast carcinoma is often responsible for it so always look for mastectomy scars and radiation marks on chest in any suspected pleural effusion in an elderly female.

Investigation of choice
- *Screening:* CXR (blunting of costophrenic angles) or USG
- *Definitive:* Diagnostic aspiration or pleural biopsy.

Immediate management
Therapeutic aspiration.

Treatment of choice
Control of underlying malignancy.

Your Notes:

182. A 60-year-old woman is admitted to the accident and emergency department having fallen in the street. She is complaining of pain in the right hip and the right lower limb is lying in external rotation. She had breast conserving surgery, radiotherapy and chemotherapy eight years ago for breast cancer.

Diagnosis: Bony metastases.

Clinchers
- *60-year-old woman.... having fallen in street.... pain in right hip and right lower limb is lying in external rotation:* These all signify a fracture neck of the femur. It can be due to osteoporosis (since she is 60 years old) or bony metastasis (as in this case).
- *Breast conserving surgery, radiotherapy and chemotherapy eight years ago for breast cancer:* Since there is a positive history of breast cancer (which is known for osteolytic bony metastasis), the patient should be investigated for a recurrence and bony metastasis.

CONFUSA
Skeletal metastases in breast carcinoma occur via blood stream. In order of frequency they are found in:
1. Lumbar vertebrae
2. Femur (as in this case)
3. Thoracic vertebrae
4. Rib
5. Skull.

Investigation of choice
Bone scan (whole body).

Immediate management
Splinting.

Treatment of choice
- Open reduction and internal fixation
- Palliative treatment of breast carcinoma.

Your Notes:

183. A 43-year-old woman treated two years ago for a grade 3 axillary node positive breast cancer presents with increasing confusion, headache and vomiting. On examination, she is drowsy but has not focal neurological signs. She does have blurring of the optic disc margins.

Diagnosis: Cerebral metastases

Clinchers

- *43-year-old woman treated two years ago for a grade 3 axillary node positive breast cancer:* Presence of axillary lymph node metastasis in breast carcinoma is a poor prognostic factor. It signifies a high risk of recurrence of the carcinoma even if a block dissection of lymph nodes in axilla is done.
- *Increasing confusion, headache and vomiting:* These all are symptoms of increased ICT and suggest the presence of a space occupying lesion in brain.
- *Drowsy:* Due to ↑ ICT.
- *No focal neurological signs:* So any focal pathology of brain is excluded.
- *Blurring of optic disc margins:* it is due to papilloedema which suggests ↑ ICT.

CONFUSA
Although brain is a comparatively rare site of breast metastases, the presence of such symptoms with a positive history of breast carcinoma commands an intensive evaluation of the recurrence.

Investigation of choice
CT skull.

Immediate management
Mannitol IV.

Treatment of choice
Chemotherapy + Radiotherapy.

Your Notes:

184. A 35-year-old woman treated one year ago for a breast cancer with 12/20 nodes positive, presents with a two day history of increasing confusion. She is drowsy and disoriented. Her husband reports that she has been complaining of severe thirst for the past week.

Diagnosis: Hypercalcaemia.

Clinchers

- *35-year-old woman treated one year ago for a breast cancer with 12/20 nodes positive:* This status suggest a high risk of recurrence as nodal status is the best indicator of metastatic disease.
- *Two day history of increasing confusion...... severe thirst:* Signs and symptoms of hypercalcaemia of malignancy are:
  - Lethargy
  - Anorexia
  - Nausea
  - Polydipsia
  - Polyuria
  - Constipation
  - Dehydration
  - Confusion
  - Weakness.

CONFUSA
The signs and symptoms of hypercalcemia of malignancy are most obvious with serum calcium > 3 mmol/L. Diuretics should always be avoided in it. It is caused by:
- Lytic bone metastases
- Production of osteoclast activating factor by tumor
- PTH like hormones by tumor.

Investigation of choice
Serum calcium.

Immediate management
Bisphosphonate IV (if resistant: calcitonin).

Treatment of choice
Control of underlying malignancy.

Your Notes:

185. A 45-year-old woman treated three years ago for breast cancer is unable to walk. She complains of increasing weakness in her leg for the last seven days. She has been constipated and unable to pass urine for the last 24 hours.

Diagnosis: Spinal cord compression.

Clinchers
- *45-year-old woman treated three years ago for breast cancer:* Any positive history of breast cancer should raise suspicion of a recurrence or metastases if there are unexplained or new neurological symptoms.
- *Unable to walk:* It is due to weakness in both legs and sensory loss (a level may be present).
- *Constipated and unable to pass urine for last 24 hours:* Bowel and bladder dysfunction are pathognomonic of spinal cord compression if there is associated history of weakness in lower limbs.

CONFUSA
Causes of cord compression in a metastatic disease are usually:
- Extension of tumor from a vertebral body
- Direct extension of tumor
- Crush fracture (most likely in this case).

Investigation of choice
- *Screening:* X-ray spine
- *Definitive:* Myelogram.

Immediate management
Discuss with neurosurgeon and clinical oncologist immediately.

Treatment of choice
- Dexamethasone
  - 8-16 mg IV
  - then 4 mg/6 h PO
- Surgical decompression later on.

Your Notes:

186. A 65-year-old man presents with severe, retrosternal chest pain and sweating. An ECG shows an acute anterolateral myocardial infarction.

Diagnosis: Acute myocardial infarction (MI).

Clinchers
- *65-year-old man:* The incidence and severity of almost all the risk factors of MI increases with age, hence contributing to increase the risk for MI. Male sex is a definitive risk factor for MI.
- *Severe, retrosternal chest pain:* Pain is the most common presenting complaint. In some instances, the discomfort may be severe enough to be described as the worst pain the patient has even felt. The pain is deep and visceral; adjectives commonly used to describe it are heavy, squeezing and crushing, although occasionally it is described as stabbing or burning. It is similar in character to exertional angina, but usually is more severe and lasts longer (>20 minutes). Typically the pain involves the central portion of the chest and/or the epigastrium, and an occasion it radiates to arms (most commonly), abdomen, back, lower jaw and neck.
- *Severe retrosternal chest pain:* The pain of MI may radiate as high as the occipital area but not below the umbilicus. Painless infarcts also occur especially in:
  - Diabetes mellitus
  - Elderly (present as sudden onset breathlessness, which may progress to pulmonary oedema)
- *Vomiting and sweating:* Due to intense sympathetic stimulation.
- *Anterolateral MI:* If the infarction involves both the anterior and lateral surfaces of heart, a Q wave will be present in V_3 and V_4 and in the leads that look at the lateral surface—I, VL and V_{5-6}.

CONFUSA
Acute pancreatitis may present as a hypovalemic shock which may confuse a fresh SHO as there is no evident source of bleed or blood loss. Also the serum amylase levels should be more than 1000 IU/mL as many other disesae processes may produce mild rise in it.

Investigation of choice
12 lead ECG.

Immediate management
High flow O_2 by face mask (caution, if COPD).

Treatment of choice
IV opiate (5-10 mg), repeated every 5 min.

Your Notes:

187. A 70 year old man inoperable gastric cancer causing obstruction, and multiple liver metastases, is taking a large dose of oral analgesia. Despite this, his pain is currently unrelieved.

Diagnosis: Inoperable gastric carcinoma.

Clinchers
- *70-year-old man:* Gastric carcinoma can affect any age but particularly common in 50-70 year age groups (Incidence of most solid organ malignancies increases with age). In general men are more affected.
- *Inoperative gastric cancer:* Unequivocal evidence of incurability are
  - Hematogenous metastases
  - Involvement of distant peritoneum
  - N4 nodal disease
  - Disease beyond N4 nodes
  - Fixation to structures that cannot be removed (It is important to note that the involvement of another organ *per se* does not imply incurability provided it can be removed).
- *Causing obstruction:* The active medial management of malignant bowel obstruction includes:
  - The relief of intestinal colic using an antispasmodic such as hyoscine butylbromide 60-80 mg daily.
  - Treating continuous pain with adequate analgesia such as diamorphine.
  - Treating vomiting if nausea is a problem with a centrally acting antiemetic such as cyclizine 150 mg daily or haloperidol 5-10 mg daily.
- *Multiple liver metastases:* Liver metastases occur hematogenously and hematogenous spread implies inoperability.
- *Taking large dose of oral analgesia but ineffective pain relief:* It can be due to—non-absorption of oral dry due to obstruction

This necessiates the change of mode of administration. For cancer patients, who need long term analgesia, continuous subcutaneous infusion is the preferred route.

CONFUSA
Diamorphine is preferred for subcutaneous infusion because of its greater solubility. By subcutaneous or intramuscular injection, diamorphine is approximately twice as potent as morphine orally.

Investigation of choice
USG (for obstruction).

Immediate management
Subcutaneous opiate infusion (diamorphine).

Treatment of choice
In patients suffering from significant symptoms of either obstruction or bleeding, palliative resection is appropriate.

Your Notes:

188. A 25-year-old woman has just been diagnosed as having rheumatoid arthritis and her rheumatologist has begun giving her gold injections. She continues to complain of joint pain and stiffness, particularly for the first two hours of each day.

Diagnosis: Rheumatoid arthritis (RA).

Clinchers
- *25-year-old:* RA presents from early childhood (rare) to late old age. The most common age of onset is between 30 and 50 years.
- *Woman:* Women before menopause are affected three times more often than men. After the menopause the frequency of onset is similar between the sexes.
- *Gold injections:* gold is a disease modifying anti-rheumatic drug (DMARD). Usually DMARDs are used after symptomatic treatment, but in seropositive patients with a poor prognosis they should be used early, before the appearance of erosions on X-rays of hands and feet. DMARDs are only prescribed by a rheumatologist in UK. DMARDs exert minimal direct nonspecific anti-inflammatory or analgesic effects, and therefore NSAIDs must be continued during their administration (except in few cases when the true remissions are induced with them).
- *Continues to complain of joint pain and stiffness:* As already explained, DMARDs have very poor analgesic action and NSAIDs have to be given with them. Moreover NSAIDs produce symptomatic improvement in morning stiffness.
- *Particularly in the first two hours of each day:* This is an indirect way to describe the pathognomonic morning stiffness.

CONFUSA
The cheapest and most safe (in terms of propensity to cause GI bleed). NSAID is ibuprofen. Naproxen is an alternative and advantageous in having only twice daily dosage and being more anti-inflammatory. Diclofenac can also be given. NSAIDs should be combined with a gastroprotection agent (proton pump inhibitor or prostaglandin analogue misoprostol) if there is—
- History of
  - peptic ulcer disease
  - dyspepsia.
- Age > 70
- Taking
  - steroids
  - aspirin.

Note: Avoid NSAIDs if
- On harfarin
- Active peptic ulcer disease
- Asthma.

Investigation of choice
Rheumatoid factor (often negative initially, if positive at onset, the treatment plan differs—see above).

Immediate management
Physiotherapy referral for exercise programs.

Treatment of choice
Oral NSAIDs.

Your Notes:

189. A 50-year-old obese man with a known hiatus hernia, presents with recurrent, severe, burning retrosternal chest pain associated with acid regurgitation and increased oral flatulence.

Diagnosis: Gastro-oesophageal reflux disease (GORD)

Clinchers

- *50-year-old:* Hiatus hernia is most common in the elderly, but may occur in young fit people.
- *Obese:* Hiatus hernias probably represent a progressive weakening of the muscles of the hiatus. They occur in obese commonly.
- *Man:* Generally hiatus hernias are four times more common in females than males.
- *Known hiatus hernia:* Incompetence of cardiac sphincter is invariably present in the initial stages of hiatus hernia, but disappear as distortion of the cardia increases. This incompetence leads to GORD.
- *Recurrent, severe, burning retrosternal chest pain:* In GORD there is a burning, retrosternal discomfort that is related to:
  - Meals
  - Lying down
  - Stooping
  - Straining

It is typically relieved by antacids.

- *Acid regurgitation:* This is 'acid brash' and typical of GORD. It can also be due to bile regurgitation. Wather brash is also seen in GORD and is due to excessive salivation.
- *Increased oral flatulence:* This is due to unopposed release of intestinal gas through incomplete lower oesophageal sphincter.

CONFUSA

Gastro-oesophageal reflux occurs as a normal event, and the clinical features of GORD occurs only when the antireflux mechanisms fail sufficiently to allow gastric contents to make prolonged contact with the lower oesophageal mucosa. Hiatus hernia reduce acid clearance of oesophagus owing to trapping of acid within the hernial sac. Moreover a large hiatus hernia can impair the "pinchcork" mechanism of diaphragm. GORD can also occur with hiatus hernia.

Investigation of choice

- *Screening:* Endoscopy ± barium swallow (show hiatus hernia)
- *Definitive:* 24 hr oesophageal pH monitoring
  +
  Oesophageal manometry

Treatment of choice
Rule out gastric carcinoma (Common at this age).

Immediate management
Proton pump inhibitors,

Your Notes:

190. A 67-year-old woman reports severe paroxysms of knife-like or electric shock-like pain, lasting seconds in the lower part of the right side of her face.

Diagnosis: Trigeminal neuralgia (dic dcouloureux)

Clinchers
- *67 year old:* It is chiefly a condition of those over 50 years old.
- *Woman:* ♂/♀ > 1
- *Severe paroxysms of knife-like or electric shock like pain lasting seconds:* The patient suffers paroxysms of intense, stabbing pain, lasting only seconds in the trigeminal nerve distribution.
- *In the lower part of the right side of her face:* Pain is unilateral, affecting the mandibular and maxillary divisions most often, and the ophthalmic division only rarely. The face may screw up with pain (hence tic doloureux). Pain may recur many times in a day and can often by precipitated by.
  - touching the skin of affected area
  - washing
  - shaving
  - eating
  - talking
  - cold wind

CONFUSA
The pain characteristically do not occur at night (contraindication! OHCM, page 335, 5th edn, says it do occur at night; Kumar and Clark page 1021, 4th edn. on the contrary). Spontaneous remissions last for months or years before recurrence, which is almost inevitable)

Investigation of choice
Diagnosis is on clinical grounds alone.

Immediate management
Exclude structural causes, i.e.
- Multiple sclerosis (suspect when it present in young age)
- Vascular malformation
- Cerebello-pontine angle tumors.

Treatment of choice
- Drugs:
  - Carbamazepine
  - Alternatives: Phenytoin, clonazepam
- Surgical: Used when drug therapy fails
  - Radiofrequency ablation of ganglion
  - Neurovascular decompression
  - Sectioning of sensory root
  - Alcohol injection

191. A 20 year old married woman presents in the accident and emergency department with the onset of acute lower abdominal pain. Her past menstrual period was six weeks previously. She has pain radiating to the left shoulder.

Diagnosis: Ectopic pregnancy.

Clinchers
- *20-year-old married woman:* The diagnosis must be considered in any woman of child-bearing age with abdominal pain or unexplained collapse.
- *Acute lower abdominal pain:* Tenderness or pain in lower abdomen or iliac fossa is a frequent mode of presentation. Reason is tubal spasm.
- *Last menstrual period was six weeks previously:* A history of amenorrhoea in ectopic pregnancy can only be for a couple of weeks and not by any means essential for the diagnosis.
- *Pain radiating to left shoulder:* Pain may be referred to left shoulder via the phrenic nerve.

CONFUSA
The differential diagnosis is from any other abdominal catastrophe such as rupture of viscus or acute peritonitis. The clinical picture is so typical that in most cases diagnosis presents no difficulty. Other diagnosis which may confuse are:
- Incomplete miscarriage
- Bleeding with an ovarian cyst
- Pelvic appendicitis
- Acute salpingitis.

Investigation of choice
- *Screening:* USG
  (findings:
  - empty uterus with thickened decidua.
  - fluid (blood) in pouch of Douglas.
  - a multi-echo mass in the region of tube).
- *Definitive:* Laparoscopy.

Immediate management
IV infusion + cross match blood + refer the patient to a gynaecologist.

Treatment of choice
Urgent laparotomy
(sometimes laparoscopic surgery).

Your Notes:

192. A 15-year-old girl presents with a 24 hour history of central abdominal pain, followed by the right iliac fossa pain, worse on coughing. She has fever and rebound in the right iliac fossa.

Diagnosis: Appendicitis.

Clinchers

- *15-year-old girl:* It can occur at any age but is most common between the ages of 15 and 30 years and is uncommon under the age of 2 years.
- *Central abdominal pain:* Typically the pain commences as a central peri-umbilical colic, as it is referred to T_{10} dermatome.
- *Followed by right iliac fossa pain:* It shifts after approximately 6 hours to the RIF or more accurately to the site of the inflamed appendix as the adjacent peritoneum becomes inflamed.
- *Worse on coughing:* Typically, the pain is aggravated by movement of abdominal wall and the patient prefers to lie still with the hips and knees flexed. Coughing mimics the release test for rebound tenderness.
- *Fever:* During the first 6 hours there is rarely any alteration in temperature or pulse rate. After that time, slight pyrexia (37.2-37.3°C) with corresponding increase in the pulse rate to 80 to 90 is usual. However, in 20 percent of cases there is no pyrexia or tachycardia in early stages. In children a temperature greater than 38.5°C suggests other causes, for example mesenteric adenitis.
- *Rebound in RIF:* The abdomen shows localized tenderness in the region of the inflamed appendix. There is usually guarding of the abdominal muscles over this site with release tenderness.

CONFUSA

The classical visceral-somatic sequence of pain is present in only about half those patients. Subsequently proven to have acute appendicitis. Atypical presentations include pain which is predominantly somatic or visceral and poorly localised. Atypical pain is more common in the elderly in whom localisation to RIF is unusual. An inflamed appendix in the pelvis may never produce somatic pain involving the anterior abdominal wall, but may instead cause *suprapubic discomfort* and *tenesmus*. In this circumstance, tenderness may only be elicited on rectal examination and is the basis for the recommendation that a rectal examination should be performed on every case of lower abdominal pain.

Investigation of choice
None

Immediate management
Patient should be referred for admission. If the appendix is thought to be leaking, then IV metronidazole should be commenced.

Treatment of choice
Urgent appendicectomy
Except in
- Moribund patient
- Resolved attack (elective surgery done then)
- Appendix mass formed without evidence of general peritonitis
- Operation difficult/impossible.

Your Notes:

193. A 30-year-old woman has severe colic and upper abdominal pain radiating to her right scapula and is vomiting.

Diagnosis: Biliary colic.

Clinchers
- *30-year-old woman:* Always remember that incidence of gallbladder stones is more in fat, fertile, female in her fifties female sex as such is a risk factor for development of cholesterol stones in gallbladder.
- *Severe colic:* It is always sudden in onset and is due to impaction of stone in the gallbladder outlet (Hartmann's pouch) or cystic duct. Contraction of the smooth muscle in the wall of the gallbladder and the cystic duct for a short period, following which the calculus either falls back or is passed along the duct produce severe pain, usually rising to a plateau, which lasts for many hours.
- *Upper abdominal pain:* Pain is typically epigastric and right hypochrial (see above). It may also spread as a band across the upper abdomen.
- *Radiating to right scapula:* Pain from gallbladder may travel along the vagus, the sympathetic nerves, or along the phrenic nerves. It may be referred to different sites through these nerves as follows:
  i. Through the vagus to the stomach
  ii. Through the sympathetic nerves to the inferior angle of the right scapula
  iii. Through the phrenic nerve to the right shoulder.
- *Vomiting:* Any colicky pain is typically associated with vomiting and sweating due to intense activation of sympathetic system.

CONFUSA
Abdominal colic—causes
Biliary tract
- Stone in
  - Hartmann's pouch
  - Ampulla of vater
  - Cystic duct

Renal tract
- Ureteric colic, due to
  - Stone
  - Tumor
  - Blood clot

Intestinal tract
- Mechanical obstruction
- Appendicular colic

Uterus
- Parturition
- Ectopic pregnancy
- Menstruation

Investigation of choice
Early USG

Immediate management
Refer for admission

Treatment of choice
Morphine* 5-10 mg IM/4h + Prochlorperazine
Cholecystectomy later on or if pain unrelieved

* OHCM, Page 472, 5th edn

Your Notes:

194. A 12-year-old girl has central abdominal pain and is vomiting. On examination, her abdomen is found to be distended with no rebound and a tender lump in the right groin.

Diagnosis: Strangulated indirect inguinal hernia.

Clinchers

- *12-year-old girl:* Femoral hernia is rare before puberty. Also the external inguinal ring is common constricting agent for indirect inguinal hernia in children. Women practically never develop a direct inguinal hernia.
- *Central abdominal pain:* Sudden pain at first situated over the hernia is followed by generalised abdominal pain, colickly in character and often located mainly at umbilicus.
- *Vomiting:* Nausea and subsequently vomiting ensues in strangulated hernia cases.
- *Abdomen distended:* Due to paralytic ileus.
- *No rebound:* As there is no peritonitis before perforation (late complication)
- *Tender lump in right groin:* On examination, the hernia is tense, extremely tender and irreducible, and there is no expansible cough impulse.

CONFUSA

Although inguinal hernia may be 10 times more common than femoral hernia a femoral hernia is more likely to strangulated because of the narrowness of the neck and its rigid surrounds. In inguinal hernias, the indirect variety strangulates more commonly, the direct variety not so often owing to the wide neck of the sac.

Investigation of choice
Overtly clinical diagnosis.

Immediate management
Vigorous resuscitation with IV fluids + nasogastric aspiration + antibiotics + refer to surgery unit

Treatment of choice
Emergency operation.

Your Notes:

---

195. A 31-year-old woman has severe colic and upper abdominal pain. She is febrile and vomiting. Hematological investigations show a moderate leukocytosis.

Diagnosis: Acute cholecystitis

Clinchers

- *31-year-old woman:* Female sex, age and obesity are risk factors for formation of cholesterol stones. Risk factors for them is becoming symptomatic are smoking and parity.
- *Severe upper abdominal pain:* Acute cholecystitis follows stone impaction in the neck of the gall bladder, which may cause continuous epigastric or RUQ pain.
- *Febrile and vomiting:* Vomiting, fever, local peritonism or a GB mass usually accompany. The fever is in the range of 38-39° C with marked toxaemia.
- *Moderate leucocytosis:* The inflammatory component is pronounced in acute cholecystitis.

CONFUSA

The main confusion lies in differentiating a biliary colic and acute cholecystitis. The point to be noted here is that biliary colic is a preceding stage of acute cholecystitis.

Stone impaction in GB outlet
↓
Biliary colic
↓
Prolonged impaction
↓
Chemical cholecystitis
(due to irritation of GB wall by concentrated bile trapped within)
↓
Inflame GB
↓
Pus (sterile) in GB
↓
Pain persists and progressively intermites
↓
Fever + toxaemia + leukocytosis
↓
Acute cholecystitis

The main difference from biliary colic is the inflammatory component (local peritonism, fever, WCC ↑)

Other differential diagnosis is from:
- Acute appendicitis
- Perforated duodenal ulcer
- Acute pancreatitis
- Right sided basal pneumonia
- Coronary thrombosis

Investigation of choice
Early USG (thickened GBB wall, pericholecystic fluid, stones).

Immediate management
Nil by mouth + pain relief + admission.

Treatment of choice
Cefuroxime 1.5 g/8h IV.
In suitable candidates do cholecystectomy (laparoscopic surgery preferred if there is no question of GB perforation).

Your Notes:

196. You are the SHO on the psychiatry ward. Your consultant is having a sexual relationship with a widow he's been treated for depression. The lady is getting better and is awaiting discharge.

Diagnosis: Report him to trust managers.

Clinchers
> Any unprofessional conduct of practise by colleagues as serious shouldbe immediately reported to the hospital authorities N trust incharges who can then set an inquiry about the matter and have the power to take disciplinary action. she is received by low to report such occurrence if it is in his/her knowledge. Failure to report dispite knowledge may andity as abetment in the unprofessional conduct.

Your Notes:

197. A 34-year-old woman wants to have a sterilization. Her last born child has cerebral palsy and her partner strongly objects to the procedure. They are married.

Answer: Seek a judicial review

Clinchers
Legally only the consent of the partner to be sterilized is required but the agreement of both is desirable. But if the previous baby is not normal and health the case becomes complicated. One can apply for a judicial review to find a solution.

CONFUSA
Always confirm in case the woman that is she really wanting a hysterectomy or would she benefit from one. the sterilization most regretted and those carried out on the young and at times of stress, or immediately after pregnancy (termination or delivery). Reversal is only 50% successful in either sex and tubal surgery increases the risk of subsequent ectopics, so the couple should see sterilization on an irreversible step.

Your Notes:

198. A mother has siamese twins. One of the twins has no heart and liver and depends on the other for survival, and as such without an operation to save the one with major organs they will both perish. Since having the operation means certain death of one of the babies, the parents who are staunch christians oppose the operation. What should be done?

Answer: Seek a judicial review

Clinchers

Note: Catholic faith strictly prohibits contraception in any form. Patients have a right to decide whether or not to undergo any medical intervention even where a refusal may result in harm to themselves or in their own death. This right to decide applies equally to pregnany women as to other patients, and includes the right to refuse treatment where the treatment is intended to benefit the unborn child.

CONFUSA
Where a patient's capacity to consent is in doubt, or where difference of opinion about his or her best interest cannot be resolved satisfactorily, one should consult more experienced colleagues and where appropriate, seek legal advice on whether it is necessary to apply to the court for a ruling. One should seek the court's approval where a patient lacks capacity to consent to a medical intervention which is non-therapeutic or controversial, for example contraceptive sterilization or organ donation, withdrawal of life support from a patient in a persistent vegetative state. Where one decide to apply to a court one should, as soon as possible, inform the patient and his or her representative of the decision and of his or her right to be represented at the hearing.

Your Notes:

199. A 12-year-old girl wants oral contraceptive pills. She doesn't want her parents to know about this.

Answer: Give her the pills

Clinchers

Notes: A female of reproductive age group can have any form of contraception if she so opts for it. In this case one will have to disregard the parents completely but she should be told about all the risks and complications of the use of OCP.

CONFUSA
Problems may arise if you consider that the child is incapable of making decision because of immaturity, illness or mental incapacity. If such patients ask you not to disclose information to a third party, you should try to persuade them to allow an appropriate person to be involved in the consultation. If they refuse and you are convinced that it is essential, in their medical interests, you may disclose relevant information to an appropriate person or authority. In such cases you must tell the patient before disclosing any information.

Your Notes:

200. A 9-year-old girl wants to have a termination of pregnancy. She is 14 weeks pregnant. The procedure to terminate is not without complications. She doesn't want her mother informed about the termination.

Answer: Carry out the termination even without parental knowledge.

Clinchers

Note: You must assess a child's capacity to decide whether to consent to or refuse proposed investigation or treatment before you provide it. In general, a competent child will be able to understand the nature, purpose and possible consequences of the proposed investigation of treatment, as well as the consequences of non treatment. Your assessment must take account of the relevant laws or legal precedents in this area.

CONFUSA
• At the age of 16 a young person can be treated as an adult and can be presumed to have capacity to decide • Under age of 16 children may have capacity to decide, depending on their ability to understand what is involved231314

Your Notes:

Section 3
Data Base of High Yield Study Material

HIGH YIELD TOPIC ONE

CHILD IMMUNISATION CLINICS IN UK

AIMS
1. For all children aged 8 weeks to 4 years 3 months in the practice population to be fully immunised against:
   - Diphtheria
   - Tetanus
   - Whooping cough
   - HIB meningitis
   - Polio
   - Measles
   - Mumps
   - Rubella
2. For the provision of a smooth running, safe clinic, which is easily accessible to families, and in which waiting times are held to a standard. (Suggested standard: no longer than 20 minutes beyond appointment time).

TARGET GROUP
- All children aged between 8 weeks and 5 years.
- Those children over 5 years who for some reason have not been immunised yet.
- Parents of children in receipt of the polio vaccine who have not had a course of vaccine themselves at all.

In order to achieve this target, newly registered infants and children will have to have their immunisation status established at registration with practice.

IDENTIFICATION OF PATIENTS
Patients to be identified by:
1. Birth register held by health visitors and the clerical assistant
2. Practice computer search monthly.
3. Appointments will be made using an appointment book designed solely for use at the immunisation clinics
4. For new births, the appointment for first immunisation will be given to parents at the health visitor's primary visit or at the 6 week check.
5. Appointments for the second and third immunisations will be given following attendance at the clinic for the previous injection.
6. For the MMR, due at 13-15 months of age, the health visitor's clerical assistant will send patients an appointment by post, 7-14 days
7. For the pre-school booster dose of diphtheria, tetanus, polio and MMR, the health visitor's clerical assistant will send patients an appointment by post 7-14 days before hand.
8. Health visitors will give opportunistic advice about immunisation at antenatal visits and onwards. This advice is reinforced by good quality, easily understood information either in the book birth to five years or child health record.
9. Specific advice on the care of a child following immunisation will be given to parents, both verbally and in written form, following each immunisation.
10. Patients who fail to attend will be sent one further appointment by post by the clerical assistant. If this is not successful, the health visitor concerned will contact the family and negotiate a new appointment.

PROTOCOL

Consent
Consent must always be obtained before immunisation. It is the responsibility of the health visitor to ensure that this is informed consent and that all parents' questions have been answered and concerns about immunisation have been sensitively considered. Written consent provides a permanent record, but consent, either written or verbal is required at the time of each immunisation after the child's fitness and suitability have been established.

Consent before the occasion on which the child is brought for immunization is only an agreement for the child to be included in the programme.

Bringing a child for immunisation after an invitation to attend for this purpose will be viewed as acceptance that the child may be immunised. When a child is brought for this purpose, and fitness and suitability have been established, consent to immunisation will be implied in the absence of any expressed reservation to the immunisation proceeding at that stage.

Childhood Vaccinations
All Vaccinations
1. Child's name and date of birth.
2. Is the child well?-if you are uncertain or think the child is unfit for vaccination ask the doctor to see.
3. Have the child's notes available plus claim forms.
4. Check immunisation to be given
   - In notes. (Write in notes which batch no.)
   - In immunisation record
   - With parents

Before the administration of any injection, the contra indications and side effects must be discussed with the parents.

2nd & 3rd vaccinations and pre-school booster
1. Child's name and date of birth
2. Is child well? Any diarrhoes? (polio)
3. Was there any reaction to previous vaccination?
4. Has the child have been well since previous vaccination?
5. Any of polio vaccine contra-indications?

IMMUNISATION SCHEDULE IN UK

Primary Course	8 weeks 2 months	First Diphtheria Pertussis, Tetanus Polio, Hib and MenC	Hib, Diphtheria, Pertussis, Tetanus is given currently as a single injection, whilst Polio is given as drop of liquid on the tongue
	12 Weeks 3 months	Second Diphtheria, Pertussis, Tetanus, Polio, Hib and MenC	Triple
	16 Weeks 4 months	Third Diphtheria, Pertussis, Tetanus, Polio, Hib and MenC	
Measles, Mumps and Rubella (MMR)	13-15 months Not 9 months as in India	MMR vaccine	Given as a single injection
Pre School Booster	Age 4	Diphtheria, Tetanus, Polio and MMR + Acellular Pertussis Vaccine Since Oct 2001	Injections of Diphtheria Tetanus and MMR are given as two separate injections at the same clinic appointment. Polio is given as drops at liquid on the tongue. Children are sent appointments shortly after their fourth birthday.
	15-18 yrs	DT + Polio booster	
	>65 yrs	Flu vaccine (annually)	*Parents should get OPV at time of their children's vaccine

Polio
Contra-indications (Live)
1. Febrile illness.
2. Vomiting, and diarrhoea.
3. Suppression of immune system eg drugs, steroids, radiation, tumours, leukaemia, lymphoma and Hodgkin's disease.
4. Siblings of immuno-suppressed children, (but can have inactivated polio vaccine).
5. When live vaccine has been given if second live vaccine is needed, there must be an interval of 3 weeks.

Pertussis
Contraindications
1. Neonatal cerebral damage-evolving neurological problems until condition is stable.
2. Febrile illness.

Special Consideration-discuss with doctor
1. Severe local or general reaction to previous pertussis vaccination
2. Epilepsy in parents or siblings.
3. Personal or family history of febrile convulsion.

Measles, Mumps and Rubella
Contra-indications (Live)
1. Acute febrile illness

2. True egg allergy (anaphylaxis).
3. Immunosuppression-drugs, steroids, irradiation, malignancy.
4. Allergy to Neomycin or Kanamycin (would have had serious) had any illness to have these.
5. Within three weeks of previous live vaccination or 3 months of immunoglobulin.

Advice
"About 5-10 days after MMR vaccination some children are slightly unwell with fever and occasionally a rash. This is not serious. It is like a very mild form of measles and your child is not infections. It is important to give Paracetamol Paediatric suspension- one teaspoon four times a day to prevent a high temperature and keep your child cool".
NB You can give DPT and Polio or Polio or DT and Polio at the same time as MMR, i.e. if child comes late for 3rd DPT and Polio but is at least one year old. When recording- white batch no. of vaccine and injection site.

Convulsions
The parents of children with a tendency to have convulsions should be counselled on the management of any fever developing after immunisation. Febrile convulsions may occur 5-10 days after measles immunisation (or MMR) whereas

they may take place in the first 72 hours after pertussis immunisation. Suggestions may include paracetamol, sponge with repid water, give extra fluids, dress in thin clothing and place in a cool room. In high risk children, an antipyretic drug may be suggested routinely for the first 72 hours after immunisation. Where the tendency is severe, the parents may be instructed on rectal diazepam administration.

Therefore ask about:
1. Was the birth normal?
2. Did the baby need any special attention ?
3. Has the baby been well since birth?
4. Is there FH of epilepsy? In who?
5. Has the baby had any fits?

Discuss any queries with doctor or if parents are not happy about baby having pertussis vaccination, encourage parent to report any reaction to first vaccination and give Paracetamol Paediatric Suspension-leaflet and prescription.

Anaphylactic Shock
No Absolute contraindication to use adrenaline in life threatening conditions.

HIGH YIELD TOPIC TWO

WHAT IS NEW IN BNF NO. 43?

Note: BNF is *British National Formulary* and every PLAB giving student is required to keep himself aware of the latest developments and recent changes from here.

Vaccines

The Chief Medical Officer's letter (PL/CMO/2002/1 of 4 January 2002) gives details about extending meningococcal C vaccination to adults aged between 20 and 24 years because meningoccal infection occurs more frequently in these young adults than in order adults.

Pneumoccocal vaccinations is recommended for those at particular risk (because of immunodeficiency, diabetes, or heart, lung or liver disease). Unfortunately, the 2-3 valent pneumococcal vaccine is not suitable for children under 2 years. In order to protect younger children at particular risk, the CMO advises a 7-valent conjugated pneumococcal vaccine in those aged between 2 months and 2 years. Section 14.4 of the BNF reflects the CMO's advice.

BNF 43 also includes changes to the schedule for immunisation against pertussis (announced in CMO's letter PL/CMO/2001/5 of 15 October 2001). The new arrangement advises a booster dose of diphtheria, tetanus and acellular pertussis vaccine before starting school or nursery school. Using the acellular pertussis component (rather than the whole-cell pertussis components) as a booster minimises reactions)

Myasthenia gravis

Corticosteroids have an important role in the management of all the but milder forms of myasthenia gravis. Prednisolone is generally used but it should be introduced carefully to minimise the risk of an initial worsening of symptoms. Interestingly, summaries of product characteristics of some corticosteroids warm that they can reduce the effects of anticholinesterases in myasthenia gravis. Whereas this statement might be identified as an 'interaction' in some sources, the BNF, having taken expert advice, carefully omits it form High Yield Topic 1.

Notes on the use of drugs, including anticholinesterases, corticosteroids and immunosuppressants, have been revised in BNF 43 to better reflect their place in the management of myasthenia gravis (see section 10.2.1).

Aspirin and children

Healthcare professionals are aware of the association between Reye's syndrome and the use of aspirin in children. The incidence of this devastating condition –uncommon as it was- declined sharply when the use of aspirin in children under 12 years was restricted. The BNF has warned about the link between aspirin and Reye's syndrome since 1986.

Recent reports have linked Reye's syndrome with the use of aspirin in children older than 12 years (*BMJ* 2001; 322: 1591-2 and *N Engl J Med* 1999; 341: 845-7).In all, fewer than 20 cases have been reported in the UK in the last 15 years, but the reports suggest a tiny possibility of aspirin-associated Reys's syndrome in older children. BNF 43 (section 4.7.1) therefore advises that aspirin should preferably also be avoided in teenagers during a feverish illness.

Anthrax

The Public Health Laboratory Service has issued guidelines for action in case of deliberate release of the anthrax organism. Also, the marketing authorisation of ciprofloxacin now includes the treatment of inhalational anthrax in adults and children. BNF 43 contains advice on the management of anthrax as well as licensed and unlicensed doses of antibacterials used for the infection (see section 5.1.12).

Multiple sclerosis

BNF 43 summarises guidance from the National Institute for Clinical Excellence on interferon beta and glatiramer for multiple sclerosis. (Technology Appraisal Guidence No-32 issued in January 2002). NICE does not recommendal use of these drugs. In order to collect more data on the role of disease-modifying drugs for multiple sclerosis, the UK health departments have agreed to share the risk of research with manufacturers of interferon beta and glatiramer (Health Service Circular HSC 2002/004). More information is included in BNF 43 (section 8.2.4).www.bnf.org

HIGH YIELD TOPIC THREE

TUMOUR MARKERS (Reference 652-OHCM)

Marker	Generally Elevated in	May also cause elevation
α FP (AlphaFoeto Protein-adult)	Hepatoma, germ-cell tumour HCC, cirrhosis	Pregnancy, Neonates (call for data) Open neural tube defect
CA 125 (F)	Ca Ovary, Breast, Hepatoma, HCC	Pregnancy, Cirrhosis, Peritonitis
CA 15-3	Ca Breast	Benign Breast Disease
CA-19-9 (GIT)	Ca Pancreas, Colorectal Ca	Cholestasis
CEA (GIT)	Ca Colon & GI tract (Breast)	Cirrhosis, Pancreatitis, Smoking
hCG (urine)	Pregnancy, Germ-cell Tumour	
NSE (Neurone-Specific Enolase)	Small-Cell Ca Lung	
PLAP (Placental Alk. Phos'tase)	Seminoma, Ca ovary,	Smoking, Pregnancy
PSA (Prostate-Specific Antigen)	Ca Prostate	BPH, Digital Rectal Examination
SCC (Squamous Cell Ca)	Ca Cervix, Lung, Buccal Cavity	

HIGH YIELD TOPIC FOUR

EVIDENCE BASED CLINICAL PRACTICE IN PSYCHIATRY GUIDELINES (BRIEF VERSION)

PSYCHOLOGICAL THERAPIES AND COUNSELLING

Introduction
The recommendations in this guideline are relevant to the following presenting problems: depression, including suicidal behaviour, anxiety, panic disorder, social anxiety and phobias, post traumatic disorders, eating disorders, obsessive compulsive disorders, personality disorders, including repetitive self harm, and some somatic complaints (eg chronic pain, chronic fatgue).

The following condition for which psychological therapies may be helpful are excluded from this guideline: Disorders in childhood and adolescence, psychoses including schizophrenia, mania and bipolar disorder, alcohol and other drug addictions, sexual dysfunction and paraphilias, organic

Brain syndromes, and learning disabilities. The guideline does not consider pharmacological treatments, but in general, there is no reason

Why medication and psychotherapy should not be used together.

This document may be photocopied freely
The recommendations are weighted as follows:
A. Based on a consistent finding in a majority of studies in high quality systematic reviews or evidence from high quality studies.
B. Based on at least one high quality trial, a weak or inconsistent finding in high quality reviews or a consistent finding in reviews that do not meet all the criteria of "high quality".
C. Based on evidence from individual studies that do not meet all the criteria of 'high quality'.
D. Based on evdence from structured expert consensus.

General Principles
Effectiveness of all types of therapy depends on the patient and the therapist forming a good working relationship. (B) The patient's age, sex, social class or ethnic group should not determines access to therapy. (C)

In considering psychological therapies, more severe or complex mental health problems should receive secondary, specialist assessment. (D)

Therapies of fewer than eight sessions are unlikely to be optimally effective for most moderate to severe mental health problems. Often 16 sessions are required for symptomatic relief, and more for lasting change (C)

Counselling is not recommended as the main intervention for sever and complex mental health problems or personality disorders. (D) A co-existing personality disorder may take treatment of most disorders more difficult and possibly less effective; indications of personality disorder include forensic history, severe relationship difficulties, and recurrent complex problems. (D) Patient preference should inform treatment choice, particularly where the research evidence does not indicate a clear choice of therapy. (D) Interest in self-exploration and capacity to tolerate frustration in relationships may be particularly important for success in psychoanalytic and psychodynamic therapies.(C) The skill and experience of the therapist should also be taken into account. More complex problems, and those where patients are poorly motivated, require the more skilful therapist. (D) *Psychological Therapies and Counselling*

SESSIONAL REQUIRED
8 sessions   for any effect
16 sessions   for symptomatic relief
more   for lasting effect

PRINCIPAL RECOMMENDATIONS
Psychological therapy should be routinely considered as an option when assessing mental health problems. (B) Patients who are adjusting to life events, illness, disabilities or counselling losses may benefits from brief therapies such as counselling. (B) post traumatic stress symptoms may be helped by psychological therapy, with most evidence for cognitive behavioural methods. Routine debriefing following traumatic events is not recommended. (A) Depression may be treated effectively with cognitive therapy or interpersonal therapy. A number of other brief structured therapies for depression may be of benefit, such as psychodynamic therapy. (A) Anxiety disorders with marked symptomatic anxiety (panic disorder, agoraphobia, social phobia, obsessive compulsive disorders, generalised anxiety disorders) are likely to benefit from cognitive behavior therapy (A) Psychological intervention should be considered for somatic complaints with a psychological component with most evidence for CBT in the treatment of chronic pain and chronic fatigue. (C) Eating disorders can be treated with psychological therapy. Best evidence in bulimia nervosa is for CBT, IPT and family therapy for teenagers. Treatment usually includes psychoeducational methods. There is little strong evidence on the best therapy type for anorexia. (B) Structured psychological therapies delivered by skilled paractitioners can contribute to the longer-term treatment of personality disorders. (C)

- PTSD—Cognitive behavioral therapy (Psychological therapy)
- Depression-Cognitive therapy/Interpersonal/Psychodyn. therapy brief strd therapy)
- Anxiety disorders (Includes OCD) – Cognitive behaviour therapy.
- Somatic complaints – Psychological interven therapy with psychological components (max in –chronic pain)
- Chronic fatigue rating disorder-Psychological therapy

EVIDENCE

Psychological therapy shows benefits over no treatment for a wide range of mental health difficulties. There is evidence of counselling effectiveness is mixed anxiety/depression, most effective when used with specified client groups, e.g. postnatal mothers, bereaved groups. CBT has been found helpful. Some evidence of efficacy has been shown for other forms of psychological therapy. Single session debriefing appears to be unhelpful in preventing later disorders. CBT and IPT effectively reduce symptoms of depression. Benefits has also been found for other forms of psychological therapy, including focal psychodynamic therapy, Psychodynamic interpersonal therapy and counselling. CBT effectively reduces symptoms of panic and anxiety. Behaviour therapy and cognitive therapy both appear effective in treatment of obsessional problems. Psychological therapies have benefit in a range of somatic complaints including gastrointestinal and gynaecological problems. CBT has been found more effective than control in improving functioning in chronic fatigue and chronic pain. Etiology of CBT and IPT in bulimia has been established. Individual therapies have shown some benefit in anorexia, with little to distinguish treatment types. Early onset of anorexia may indicate family therapy, and later onset, broadly based individual therapy. A number of therapy approaches have shown some success with personality disorders, including dialectical behaviour therapy, psychoanalytic day hospital programme and therapeutic communities.

TYPES OF PSYCHOLOGICAL THERAPY

- **Cognitive behaviour therapy (CBT)** This refers to the pragmatic combination of concepts and techniques from cognitive and behaviour therapies, common in clinical practice. Cognitive techniques (such as challenging negative automatic thoughts) and behavioural techniques (such as graded exposure and activity scheduling) are used to relieve symptoms by changing maladaptive thoughts, beliefs and behaviour.
- **Psychoanalytic therapies** A number of different therapies draw on psychoanalytic theories. Focal psychodynamic therapy identifies a central conflict arising from early experience that is being re-enacted in adult life producing mental health problems. It aims to resolve this through the vehicle of the relationship with the therapist giving new opportunities for emotional assimilation and insight. Psychoanalytic psychotherapy is a longer-term process (usually a year or more) of allowing unconscious conflicts opportunity to be re-enacted and interpreted in the relationship with the therapist.
- **Systemic and family therapy** (whether treating individuals, couples or families) focuses on the relational context addresses patterns of interaction and meaning aims to facilitate personal and interpersonal resources within a system as a whole. Therapeutic work may include consultation to wider networks such as other professionals working with the individual or the family.
- **Other** This list is not comprehensive. Many others types of therapy are practised in the NHS including cognitive-analytic, existential, humanistic, feminist, personal construct, art therapy, drama therapy, Transactional analysis, group analysis and interpersonal therapy (IPT).
- **Counselling** A form of psychological therapy that gives individuals an opportunity to explore, discover, and clarify ways of living more resoucefully, with a greater sense of well being. Counsellors practise within the main therapeutic approaches listed above.

KEY IMPLEMENTATIONS POINTS

Recommendations are given to inform first treatment choice. Patients may choose not to accept this, and further treatment options may be considered if the first line treatment is unacceptable or inappropriate. Guidelines may be adapted to take account of the availability and organisation of local services, but not at the expense of changing the main recommendations. User involvement in local implementation and adult of the guideline is recommended.

Key Audit Criteria

Has access to the recommended range of psychological therapies been identified for the primary care group? Has psychological therapy been considered as one option for all patients with these presenting problems? Has patients preference and motivation been assessed? Do more severe and complex problems receive specialist assessment? Are adequate lengths of psychological therapies offered? Are patients' ethnic and cultural background considered? The full guideline is available at:

www.doh.gov.UK/mental health/treatment guideline

Psychological therapies are provided by mental health professionals from a range of disciplines, including clinical and counselling psychologists, psychiatrists, psychotherapists, art and drama therapists, and counsellors.

HIGH YIELD TOPIC FIVE

DETECTION OF DELIBERATE RELEASES- CARDINAL SIGNS FOR CASE DETECTION

Note: Although such questions have never been asked in PLAB exam, but with increasing threat of terrorism, these may be asked in future.

In a previously healthy person any of the following four clinical pictures requires urgent attention

1. **Inhalational (Pulmonary) Anthrax and Plague**
- Rapid onset severe sepsis with respiratory failure, not due to a predisposing illness
- Sudden, severe, unexplained febrile illness or febrile ddeath
Note: The cardinal sign for anthrax is mediastinal widening on Chest X Ray

2. **Cutaneous Anthrax**
- Commonly affects hands, forearms and head
- Cardinal feature is painless swelling of skin
- Originally a small bump which then ulcerates and becomes weepy
- Pronounced swelling (oedema of skin) frequently surrounds the lesion
- Ulcer develops a black centre in 2-6 days

For microbiologists the unexpected finding of non-motile positive bacilli in normally sterile or fluids or from wound sites require urgent consideration of the possibility of B. *anthracis*.

3. **Botulism**
- Acute onset of bilateral cranial nerve involvement
- Descending weakness or paralysis which may extend to complete flaccid paralysis, but the patient remains alert
- Fever is unusual, as is loss of sensation

4. **Smallpox**

In the events of a deliberate release in the UK population (mostly nonimmune), it is extremely unlikely that single, mild cases of feverish, pox-like illnesses will occur-it is much more likely that clusters of moderate to severe disease would be seen-ie. clusters of cases of:

- An abrupt onset moderate fever (up to 39C), with extreme prostration.
- A characteristic vesicular rash most dense on the extremities and face begins on the third to fourth day of illness. Skin lesions over one area of body are generally of the same stage of development. New and enlarging vesicles coalesce to form soft, flaccid bullae covered by skin, which easily rubs off.
- Less commonly, an erythematous or purpuric rash may appear earlier in the illness and is associated with a poorer prognosis.

If a patient is seen with any of these four pictures, expert clinical opinion should be sought urgently. In addition in England, Wales and Northern Ireland the local Consultant in Communicable Disease Control (or their counterpart in Scotland) and the CDSC Duty Doctor (020-8200-6868) should also be contracted urgently and given details.

HIGH YIELD TOPIC SIX
ASTHMA GUIDELINES—CHRONIC MANAGEMENT

- BTS Guidelines Thorax 1997;52 Suppl 11-21

Adults and School Children		Symptoms
Step 1 PEFR=100%	Occasional use of relief bronchodilators Inhaled short acting β agonists if > once daily—stage 2	Occasional symptoms less frequent than day
Step 2 (≤ 80%)	Regular inhaled anti-inflammatory agents Inhaled β agonist + Budesonide/beclomethasone 100-400 µg b.d. Or Cromoglycate, but start steroid if control not achieved	Daily symptoms
Step 3 (50-80%)	High dose inhaled steroids or low dose steroids + long acting β agonist e.g. Budesonide/beclomethasone 800-2000 µg daily Or Salmeterol 50*ug bd+ Budesonide/beclomethasone 100-400*ug	Severe symptoms
Step 4 (50-80%)	High dose inhaled steroids and regular bronchodilators Budesonide/beclomethasone 800-2000 µg daily plus • Inhaled long acting β agonist • SR theophylines • Inhaled ipratropium bromide • Long acting β agonist tablets • High dose inhaled bronchodilators • Cromoglycate	Severe symptoms uncontrolled with high dose inhaled corticosteroid
Step 5 (< 50%)	Addition of regular steroids tablets Education Inhaler technique Avoidance of provoking factors PEFR monitoring at home	Severe symptoms deteriorating
Step 6 (PEFR<30%)	Sever symptoms deteriorating inspite or oral Prednisolone	Hospital Admission

Children under 5 years old

Step 1	Occasional use of relief bronchodilators Short acting inhaled β-agonists prn Mild cases oral β-agonists prn	
Step	Regular inhaled preventer therapy Inhaled short acting β agonist+ Cromoglycate as powder via MDI Becotide/beclomethasone<400 µg FP<200 µg] Consider 5/7 oral prednisolone/high dose inhaled steroid to achieve control	

• Step 3	Increased dose inhaled steroids In haled β agonists + Becotide/beclomethasone < 800 mg [FP < 500 µg] Consider regular long acting β-agonists b.d.
• Step 4	High dose inhaled steroids and bronchodilators Inhaled steroids up to 200 µg Slow release xanthines or nebulised β-agonists

Leukotriene Antagonists
Oral treatment of atopic conditions

LT antagonists	montelukast and zafirlukast
5 lipoxygenase inhibitor	Zieluton

HIGH YIELD TOPIC SEVEN

FITNESS TO DRIVE

The patient must inform the DVLA, the doctor must advise the patient

- Vision
  - Acuity: 6/9 6/10 corrected 3/60 without correction
  - Monocular vision: No need to notify it field is full
  - Field defect: Banned if <120°
  - Diplopia: Banned unless mild
  - Night Blindness: Banned if fails to meet the field and acuity regulations at all times
  - Colour Blindness: No need to notify
- Neurology: All epileptics should inform the DVLA
  - Epilepsy
    - Single fit — Banned for 1 year
    - Awake — Fit-free for 2-years
    - Asleep — Fit-free for 3 years
    - HGV — 10 years fir-free, no treatment
  - LOC: Cease driving 1 year, restored until 70 years
  - CVA: Cease driving 3/12 if full clinical recovery
  - TIAs: Cease driving until 3/12 free from attacks
- Diabetes: All diabetics should inform the DVLA
  - IDDM/Type I: hypo awareness and visual acuity standards 1,2 or 3 year licence
  - NIDDM/Type II
    - Tablets — Limit by end-organ complications
    - Diet — No need to notify
  - Frequent Hypo's Cease driving
- Cadiology
  - Angina: If at the wheel cease driving
  - QMI: Cease driving for 4/52
  - Angioplasty: Cease driving for 4/52
  - PPM/Catheter: Cease driving for 4/52
  - CABG: Cease driving for 4/52
  - Transport: Cease driving for 8/52
  - Arrhythmias: Cease driving if ncapacitate restart 4/52 after control established
  - ICD: Cease driving
    - Re-issue if no discharge in 6/12
    - No incapacitating arrythmia in 5 years
- Drugs: Banned if any chemical, drug alcohol dependency

HIGH YIELD TOPIC EIGHT

DRUGS IN PREGNANCY

	I TM	II TM	III TM	Complications
ACE inhibitors	C/I	C/I	C/I	
Warfarin	C/I	safe	C/I	
Heparin	Safe	Safe	Safe	
Trimethoprim Sulfonamides			C/I	Kernictercus
Tetracycline	C/I	C/I/(safe?)	C/I	I-TM-bone & teeth III TM-Decompensation of liver
Gilibenclamide	Safe	Safe	C/I (late)	
Metformin	C/I	C/I	C/I	
Trimethoprim-sulflame thoxazole			C/I	
Chloramphemicol	C/I	C/I	C/I	Grey baby syndrome
Streptomycin	Restricted	restricted	restricted	To only complicated case of pregnancy
Erythromycin	Safe	Safe	Safe	
Penicillin	Safe	Safe	Safe	
Nitrofurantoin	Specific C/I	Specific C/I	Specific C/I	in G6PD defcy

* C/I = Contra Indication
  TM = Trimester

HIGH YIELD TOPIC NINE

BRITISH NOMENCLATURE FOR DRUGS

A number of drugs are known by different names in the UK to other countries, particularly the USA. Spellings often differ from accepted international spellings. Many of the British Approved Names are to be changed in line with the Recommended International Non-proprietary Names. There are a number of exceptions where the British name or spelling is so well established that either name may be used interchangeably. A few British names have been retained for drugs used in emergency settings, where confusion might be dangerous. In this book, I have mostly used the International name, except for emergency drugs. The lists below are not exhaustive but cover most drugs in common use. A full list may be found in the British National Formulary (BNF).

Drugs where the British Name has been retained

British approved name	Recommended International Non-proprietary name
adrenaline	epinephrine
bendrofluazide	bendroflumethiazide
chlorpheniramine	chlorphenamine
frusemide	furosemide
lignocaine	lidocaine
methylene blue	methylthioninium chloride
noradrenaline	norepinephrine

Drugs where the British spelling remains in common usage

British approved name	Recommended International Non-proprietary name
amoxycillin	amoxycillin
beclomethasone	beclometasone
cephalexin	cefalexin
chlormethiazole	chlomethiazole
cholecalciferol	colecalciferol
cholestyramine	colestyramine
corticotrophin	corticotropin
indomethacin	indometacin
phenobarbitone	phenobarbital
sodium cromoglycate	sodium cromoglicate
sulphasalazine	sulfasalazine

HIGH YIELD TOPIC TEN
GMC GUIDELINES ABOUT MEDICAL ETHICS

SERIOUS COMMUNICABLE DISEASES

Use of term 'serious communicable disease'
In this guidance the term serious communicable disease applies to any disease which may be transmitted from human to human and which may result in death or serious illness. It particularly concerns, but is not limited to, infections such as human immunodeficiency virus (HIV), tuberculosis and hepatitis B and C.

Providing a good standard of practice and care
1. All patients are entitled to good standards of practice and care from their doctors, regardless of the nature of their disease or condition.
2. You must not deny or delay investigation or treatment because you believe that the patient's actions or lifestyle may have contributed to their condition. Where patients pose a serious risk to your health or safety you may take reasonable, personal measures to protect yourself before investigating a patient's condition or providing treatment. In the context of serious communicable diseases these will usually be infection control measures. You must follow the guidance in paragraph 4 on consent to testing.
3. You must keep yourself informed about serious communicable diseases, and particularly their means of transmission and control. You should always take appropriate measures to protect yourself and others from infection. You must make sure that any staff for whom you are responsible are also appropriately informed and co-operate with measures designed to prevent transmission of infection to other patients.

Consent to testing for a serious communicable disease
4. You must obtain consent from patients before testing for a serious communicable disease, except in the rare circumstances described in paragraphs 6, 7, 9, 11 and 17 below. The information you provide when seeking consent should be appropriate to the circumstances and to the nature of the condition or conditions being tested for. Some conditions, such as HIV, have serious social and financial, as well as medical, implications. In such cases you must make sure that the patient is given appropriate information about the implications of the test, and appropriate time to consider and discuss them.

Children
5. When testing patients under 16 for a serious communicable disease, you must follow the guidance in paragraph 4 if you judge that they have sufficient maturity to understand the implications of testing.
6. Where a child cannot give or withhold consent, you should seek consent from a person with parental responsibility for the child. If you believe that that person's judgement is distorted, for example, because he or she may be the cause of the child's infection, you must decide whether the medical interests of the child override the wishes of those with parental responsibility. Whenever possible you should discuss the issues with an experienced colleague before making a decision. If you test a child without obtaining consent, you must be prepared to justify that decision.

Unconscious patients
7. You may test unconscious patients for serious communicable diseases, without their prior consent, where testing would be in their immediate clinical interests - for example, to help in making a diagnosis. You should not test unconscious patients for other purposes.

Injuries to health care workers
8. If you or another health care worker has suffered a needlestick injury or other occupational exposure to blood or body fluids and you consider it necessary to test the patient for a serious communicable disease, the patient's consent should be obtained before the test is undertaken. If the patient is unconscious when the injury occurs consent should be sought once the patient has regained full consciousness. If appropriate, the injured person can take prophylactic treatment until consent has been obtained and the test result is known.
9. If the patient refuses testing, is unable to give or withhold consent because of mental illness or disability, or does not regain full consciousness within 48 hours, you should reconsider the severity of risk to yourself, or another injured health care worker, or to others. You should not arrange testing against the patient's wishes or without consent other than in exceptional circumstances, for example where you have good reason to think that the patient may have a condition such as HIV for which prophylactic treatment is available. In such cases you may test an existing blood sample, taken for other purposes, but you should consult an experienced colleague first. It is possible that a decision to test an existing blood without consent could be challenged in the courts, or be the subject of a complaint to your employer or the GMC. You must therefore be prepared to justify your decision.
10. If you decide to test without consent, you must inform the patient of your decision at the earliest opportunity. In such cases confidentiality is paramount: only the patient and those who have been exposed to infection

may be told about the test and its result. In these exceptional circumstances neither the fact that test has been undertaken, nor its result, should be entered in the patient's personal medical record without the patient's consent.

11. If the patient dies you may test for a serious communicable disease if you have good reason to think that the patient may have been infected, and a health care worker has been exposed to the patient's blood or other body fluid. You should usually seek the agreement of a relative before testing. If the test shows the patient was a carrier of the virus, you should follow the guidance in paragraphs 21 - 23 of these guidelines on giving information to patients' close contacts.

Testing in laboratories

12. It is the responsibility of the doctor treating the patient to obtain consent to testing for diagnostic purposes. If you work in a laboratory you may test blood or other specimens for serious communicable diseases only for the purposes for which the samples have been obtained, or for closely related purposes which are in the direct interests of the patient. See paragraph 14 for guidance on testing undertaken for research purposes.

Unlinked anonymised screening

13. In unlinked anonymised surveillance programmes for serious communicable diseases, you should make sure that patients are provided with information which covers:
    - Their right to refuse inclusion of the sample in the programme.
    - The fact that their blood sample cannot be identified and there is no way of tracing it back to them.
    - The benefits of seeking a test if they think they have been exposed to infection.

Research

14. You may undertake research only where the protocol has been approved by the appropriate, properly constituted research ethics committee. It remains your responsibility to ensure that research does not infringe patients' rights.

Deceased patients

15. When a patient who is brain stem dead is being considered as an organ donor, you should explain to relatives that assessing the suitability of organs for transplantation will involve testing for certain infections, including HIV.

Post-mortem testing

16. Where a post-mortem has been authorised or ordered you may test the deceased patient for communicable diseases where relevant to the investigation into the causes of death.

17. You should not routinely test for serious communicable diseases before performing post-mortems; but you should take precautions to protect yourself and other health care workers. If you have reason to believe the deceased person had a serious communicable disease, you should assume the body to be infectious.

Confidentiality

Informing other health care professionals

18. If you diagnose a patient as having a serious communicable disease, you should explain to the patient:
    a. The nature of the disease and its medical, social and occupational implications, as appropriate.
    b. Ways of protecting others from infection.
    c. The importance to effective care of giving the professionals who will be providing care information which they need to know about the patient's disease or condition. In particular you must make sure that patient understands that general practitioners cannot provide adequate clinical management and care without knowledge of their patients' conditions.

19. If patients still refuse to allow other health care workers to be informed, you must respect the patients' wishes except where you judge that failure to disclose the information would put a health care worker or other patient at serious risk of death or serious harm. Such situations may arise, for example, when dealing with violent patients with severe mentally illness or disability. If you are in doubt about whether disclosure is appropriate, you should seek advice from an experienced colleague. You should inform patients before disclosing information. Such occasions are likely to arise rarely and you must be prepared to justify a decision to disclose information against a patient's wishes.

Disclosures to others

20. You must disclose information about serious communicable diseases in accordance with the law. For example, the appropriate authority must be informed where a notifiable disease is diagnosed. Where a communicable disease contributed to the cause of death, this must be recorded on the death certificate. You should also pass information about serious communicable diseases to the relevant authorities for the purpose of communicable disease control and surveillance.

21. As the GMC booklet Confidentiality makes clear, a patient's death does not of itself release a doctor from the obligation to maintain confidentiality. But in some circumstances disclosures can be justified because they protect other people from serious harm or because they are required by law.

Giving information to close contacts

22. You may disclose information about a patient, whether living or dead, in order to protect a person from risk of death or serious harm. For example, you may disclose

information to a known sexual contact of a patient with HIV where you have reason to think that the patient has not informed that person, and cannot be persuaded to do so. In such circumstances you should tell the patient before you make the disclosure, and you must be prepared to justify a decision to disclose information.

23. You must not disclose information to others, for example relatives, who have not been, and are not, at risk of infection.

Doctors' responsibilities to protect patients from infection

24. You must protect patients from unnecessary exposure to infection by following safe working practices and implementing appropriate infection control measures. This includes following the Control of Substances Hazardous to Health Regulations 1994 and other health and safety at work legislation. These regulations may require you to inform your employer, or the person responsible for health and safety in your organisation, if there are any deficiencies in protection measures in your work place. Failure to do so may amount to a criminal offence.

25. You must follow the UK Health Departments' advice on immunisation against hepatitis B. If you are in direct contact with patients you should protect yourself and your patients by being immunised against other common serious communicable diseases, where vaccines are available.

26. You must always take action to protect patients when you have good reason to suspect that your own health, or that of a colleague, is a risk to them.

27. You must consider how any infection you have may put patients at risk. You must take particular care if you work with patients for whom exposure to infection may be serious, for example pregnant women or immuno-suppressed patients.

28. You must comply promptly with appropriate requests to be tested for serious communicable diseases when there is an investigation into an outbreak of disease amongst patients.

Responsibilities of doctors who have been exposed to a serious communicable disease

29. If you have any reason to believe that you have been exposed to a serious communicable disease you must seek and follow professional advice without delay on whether you should undergo testing and, if so, which tests are appropriate. Further guidance on your responsibilities if your health may put patients at risk is included in our booklet Good Medical Practice.

30. If you acquire a serious communicable disease you must promptly seek and follow advice from a suitably qualified colleague - such as a consultant in occupational health, infectious diseases or public health on:
    - Whether, and in what ways, you should modify your professional practice.
    - Whether you should inform your current employer, your previous employers or any prospective employer, about your condition.

31. You must not rely on your own assessment of the risks you pose to patients.

32. If you have a serious communicable disease and continue in professional practice you must have appropriate medical supervision.

33. If you apply for a new post, you must complete health questionnaires honestly and fully.

Treating colleagues with serious communicable diseases

34. If you are treating a doctor or other health care worker with a serious communicable disease you must provide the confidentiality and support to which every patient is entitled.

35. If you know, or have good reason to believe, that a medical colleague or health care worker who has or may have a serious communicable disease, is practising, or has practised, in a way which places patients at risk, you must inform an appropriate person in the health care worker's employing authority, for example an occupational health physician, or where appropriate, the relevant regulatory body. Such cases are likely to arise very rarely. Wherever possible you should inform the health care worker concerned before passing information to an employer or regulatory body.

CONFIDENTIALITY: PROTECTING AND PROVIDING INFORMATION

The new guidance on confidentiality is the result of extensive discussion and debate with professional and patient groups. It places new responsibilities on doctors to keep patients informed about, and get agreement to, the disclosure of information. It sets out a framework for respecting patients' rights while ensuring that information needed to maintain and improve health care is passed to those who need it.

The additional duties to obtain consent and to anonymise data tie in with developments in the law, including the Data Protection Act 1998. The Data Protection Commissioner sees our guidance 'as a sound basis for establishing privacy-friendly relationships between patients and doctors assisting doctors in complying with their obligations under the Data Protection Act 1998'.

The guidance will have far-reaching effects on some areas of practice, for example, in research and public health and drug safety monitoring. The Medicines Control Agency's Yellow Card scheme, which has provided invaluable information on the safety of medicines in clinical use since 1964, asked doctors for identifiable data. The MCA said 'We recognise the need to adopt a privacy enhancing approach while maintaining the effectiveness of the scheme in the interests of public health. We are therefore introducing an updated Yellow Card which no longer requests patient personal identifiers, so that doctors can continue to report suspected adverse drug reactions with confidence'.

Dr Declan Mulkeen, of MRC, also welcomed the GMC's principles on disclosing information for medical research, as 'striking the right balance in a difficult area'. MRC will issue more detailed guidelines for research in the Autumn.

Frequently Asked Questions

Deciding whether to disclose information is often difficult. Our guidance sets out the principles which you should follow. The notes which follow explain how those principles apply in circumstances which doctors often meet, or find hard to deal with.

My health authority wants to conduct a post-payment verification (PPV) for claims I've made. Can I give them free access to the records?

Some disclosures, for example to the police or employers, may cause significant harm or distress to patients, but others, such as disclosures for audit or planning, are unlikely to affect patients. In these cases consent based on the patients' understanding and acceptance of the disclosure will be sufficient.

It is good practice to tell patients how their records might be used to help the running of the NHS or the development of medical care. You should make sure patients know they have a right to object to such disclosures and provide clear instructions about how they can do so. You can do this by providing leaflets for those attending the surgery, clinic or hospital; discussing the issues at a suitable consultation or at clinics or when new patients join a practice or attend a hospital for the first time; or by writing to your patients.

Where a health authority asks for access to your records for PPV you should:
- Review whether you have already given patients information about the use of records for audit and administration and about their right to object.
- Identify any patients who have expressed objections.
- If you are not satisfied that patients have had this information, ask your HA whether the patients whose records will be checked have been identified, and if so whether the HA has asked their permission to look at the records. If not, ask the HA to do so, or contact the patients yourself and ask whether they object to their records being examined.

When the PPV audit takes place:
- Make sure that you disclose only the minimum information necessary for the audit.
- Check with the health authority that staff have had training in confidentiality and have a contractual or professional duty to respect patients' privacy.

A patient of mine suffers from a serious mental illness. He is often erratic and unstable. I know that he drives, although I have warned him that it is often unsafe for him to do so. He insists that his illness does not affect his judgment as a driver. Should I tell the DVLA?

If you think the patient may be a danger to himself or others when driving and you cannot persuade him to stop driving or to inform the DVLA himself, then you should disclose the information to a Medical Adviser at DVLA. You should let him know of your decision.

I work with sex offenders who are transferred from prison to hospital during their custodial sentence. A patient has recently been discharged, but I know he does not intend to register his new address with the police, as he is required to do by law. Should I tell the police he has been discharged?

The Sex Offenders Act 1997 requires the offender to register his name and address with the police. However, disclosures without consent are justified when a failure to disclose information may put the patient, or someone else, at risk of death or serious harm. If you believe that the patient poses a risk to others, and you have good reason to believe that he does not intend to notify the police of his address, then disclosure of the patient's discharge would be justified.

Sometimes administrative staff in my practice need access to patients' records. At present they can call up the whole record on screen. Is that all right?

It is best practice to ensure that administrative staff have immediate access to information only on a need to know basis. When using computerised records, make sure that administrative data, such as names and addresses, can be accessed separately from clinical information, so that sensitive data is not automatically displayed. This will also help to reduce the risk of accidental breaches of confidentiality in reception areas or other areas to which patients have access. In addition, all staff who have access to clinical information must have a full understanding of their duty of confidentiality, and understand their responsibilities. Make sure new staff receive proper training.

A patient of mine is a doctor; I am concerned that he has a drinking problem which could affect his judgment. It has taken me a long time to get him to admit to any problems, and if I disclose the information to his employer or the GMC now he will probably deny everything and find another doctor. What should I do?

This patient has the same right to good care and to confidentiality as other patients. But, there are times when the safety of others must take precedence. If you are concerned that his problems mean that he is an immediate danger to his own patients, you must tell his employing authority or the GMC straight away. If you think the problem is currently under control, you must encourage him to seek help locally from counselling services set up for doctors or for the public generally. You must monitor his condition and ensure that if the position deteriorates you take immediate action to protect the patients in his care.

A child in my practice has recently been taken to hospital suffering serious injuries from abuse. His father is now being prosecuted. I've been asked to provide information about the child and her family for a Part 8 Review. I'm the GP to the child's father and he won't give consent to the release of information, what should I do?

Part 8 Reviews are intended to identify why a child has been seriously harmed, to learn lessons from mistakes and to improve systems and services for children and their families. The overall purpose can reasonably be regarded as serving to protect other children from a risk of serious harm. You should therefore co-operate with requests for information, even where the child's family does not consent, or if it is not practicable to ask for their consent. Exceptionally, you may see a good reason not to disclose information; in such cases you should be prepared to explain your decision to the GMC.

GMC Confidentiality: Key Principles
Confidentiality is central to trust between doctors and patients. Without assurances about confidentiality, patients may be reluctant to give doctors the information they need in order to provide good care. If you are asked to provide information about patients you should:
- Seek patients' consent to disclosure of information wherever possible, whether or not you judge that patients can be identified from the disclosure.
- Anonymise data where unidentifiable data will serve the purpose.
- Keep disclosures to the minimum necessary.

Are you complying with the Data Protection Act 1998?
The Act requires everyone who processes personal information about living individuals to notify the Commissioner. Gp practices, individual gps and other doctors who control records about patients or staff must notify the Commissioner and comply with the data protection principles.

To start the notification process telephone the Commissioner's notification department on 01625 545740 or visit http://www.dpr.gov.uk

Glossary: This defines the terms used within this document. These definitions have no wider or legal significance

Anonymised data: Data from which the patient cannot be identified by the recipient of the information. The name, address, and full post code must be removed together with any other information which, in conjunction with other data held by or disclosed to the recipient, could identify the patient. NHS numbers or other unique numbers may be included only if recipients of the data do not have access to the 'key' to trace the identity of the patient using this number.

Consent: Agreement to an action based on knowledge of what the action involves and its likely consequences.

Express consent: Consent which is expressed orally or in writing (except where patients cannot write or speak, when other forms of communication may be sufficient).

Health care team: The health care team comprises the people providing clinical services for each patient and the administrative staff who directly support those services.

Patients: Competent patients and parents of, or those with parental responsibility for, children who lack maturity to make decisions for themselves. (Adult patients who lack the capacity to consent have the right to have their confidentiality respected. Guidance on disclosure of information about such patients is included in paragraphs 38-39).

Personal information: Information about people which doctors learn in a professional capacity and from which individuals can be identified.

Public interest: The interests of the community as a whole, or a group within the community or individuals.

Section 1 - Patients' right to confidentiality
1. Patients have a right to expect that information about them will be held in confidence by their doctors. Confidentiality is central to trust between doctors and patients. Without assurances about confidentiality, patients may be reluctant to give doctors the information they need in order to provide good care. If you are asked to provide information about patients you should:
   a. Seek patients' consent to disclosure of information wherever possible, whether or not you judge that patients can be identified from the disclosure.
   b. Anonymise data where unidentifiable data will serve the purpose.
   c. Keep disclosures to the minimum necessary.
   You must always be prepared to justify your decisions in accordance with this guidance.

Protecting information
2. When you are responsible for personal information about patients you must make sure that it is effectively protected against improper disclosure at all times.
3. Many improper disclosures are unintentional. You should not discuss patients where you can be overheard or leave patients' records, either on paper or on screen, where they can be seen by other patients, unauthorised health care staff or the public. Whenever possible you should take steps to ensure that your consultations with patients are private.

Section 2 - Sharing information with patients
4. Patients have a right to information about the health care services available to them, presented in a way that is easy to follow and use.
5. Patients also have a right to information about any condition or disease from which they are suffering. This should be presented in a manner easy to follow and use, and include information about diagnosis, prognosis, treatment options, outcomes of treatment, common and/or serious side-effects of treatment, likely time-scale of treatments and costs where relevant. You should always give patients basic information about treatment

you propose to provide, but you should respect the wishes of any patient who asks you not to give them detailed information. This places a considerable onus upon health professionals. Yet, without such information, patients cannot make proper choices, as partners in the health care process.
6. It is good practice to give patients information about how anonymised information about them may be used to protect public health, to undertake research and audit, to teach or train medical staff and students and to plan and organise health care services.

Section 3 - Disclosure of information
Sharing information with others providing care
7. Where patients have consented to treatment, express consent is not usually needed before relevant personal information is shared to enable the treatment to be provided. For example, express consent would not be needed before general practitioners disclose relevant personal information so that a medical secretary can type a referral letter. Similarly, where a patient has agreed to be referred for an X-ray physicians may make relevant information available to radiologists when requesting an X-ray. Doctors cannot treat patients safely, nor provide the continuity of care, without having relevant information about the patient's condition and medical history.
8. You should make sure that patients are aware that personal information about them will be shared within the health care team, unless they object, and of the reasons for this. It is particularly important to check that patients understand what will be disclosed if it is necessary to share personal information with anyone employed by another organisation or agency providing health or social care. You must respect the wishes of any patient who objects to particular information being shared with others providing care, except where this would put others at risk of death or serious harm.
9. You must make sure that anyone to whom you disclose personal information understands that it is given to them in confidence, which they must respect. Anyone receiving personal information in order to provide care is bound by a legal duty of confidence, whether or not that they have contractual or professional obligations to protect confidentiality.
10. Circumstances may arise where a patient cannot be informed about the sharing of information, for example because of a medical emergency. In these cases you should pass relevant information promptly to those providing the patients' care.

Section 4 - Disclosure of information other than for treatment of the individual patient
Principles
11. Information about patients is requested for a wide variety of purposes including education, research, monitoring and epidemiology, public health surveillance, clinical audit, administration and planning. You have a duty to protect patients' privacy and respect their autonomy. When asked to provide information you should follow the guidance in paragraph 1, that is:
    a. Seek patients' consent to disclosure of any information wherever possible, whether or not you judge that patients can be identified from the disclosure.
    b. Anonymise data where unidentifiable data will serve the purpose.
    c. Keep disclosures to the minimum necessary.
12. The paragraphs which follow deal with obtaining consent, and what to do where consent is unobtainable, or it is impracticable to seek consent.

Obtaining consent
13. Seeking patients' consent to disclosure is part of good communication between doctors and patients, and is an essential part of respect for patients' autonomy and privacy.

Consent where disclosures will have personal consequences for patients
14. You must obtain express consent where patients may be personally affected by the disclosure, for example when disclosing personal information to a patient's employer. When seeking express consent you must make sure that patients are given enough information on which to base their decision, the reasons for the disclosure and the likely consequences of the disclosure. You should also explain how much information will be disclosed and to whom it will be given. If the patient withholds consent, or consent cannot be obtained, disclosures may be made only where they can be justified in the public interest, usually where disclosure is essential to protect the patient, or someone else, from risk of death or serious harm.

Consent where the disclosure is unlikely to have personal consequences for patients
15. Disclosure of information about patients for purposes such as epidemiology, public health safety, or the administration of health services, or for use in education or training, clinical or medical audit, or research is unlikely to have personal consequences for the patient. In these circumstances you should still obtain patients' express consent to the use of identifiable data or arrange for members of the health care team to anonymise records (see also paragraphs 16 and 18).
16. However, where information is needed for the purposes of the kind set out in paragraph 15, and you are satisfied that it is not practicable either to obtain express consent to disclosure, nor for a member of the health care team to anonymise records, data may be disclosed without express consent. Usually such disclosures will be made to allow a person outside the health care team to

anonymise the records. Only where it is essential for the purpose may identifiable records be disclosed. Such disclosures must be kept to the minimum necessary for the purpose. In all such cases you must be satisfied that patients have been told, or have had access to written material informing them:
   a. That their records may be disclosed to persons outside the team which provided their care.
   b. Of the purpose and extent of the disclosure, for example, to produce anonymised data for use in education, administration, research or audit.
   c. That the person given access to records will be subject to a duty of confidentiality.
   d. That they have a right to object to such a process, and that their objection will be respected, except where the disclosure is essential to protect the patient, or someone else, from risk of death or serious harm.
17. Where you have control of personal information about patients, you must not allow anyone access to them for the purposes of the kind set out in paragraph 15, unless the person has been properly trained and authorised by the health authority, NHS trust or comparable body and is subject to a duty of confidentiality in their employment or because of their registration with a statutory regulatory body.

Disclosures in the public interest
18. In cases where you have considered all the available means of obtaining consent, but you are satisfied that it is not practicable to do so, or that patients are not competent to give consent, or exceptionally, in cases where patients withhold consent, personal information may be disclosed in the public interest where the benefits to an individual or to society of the disclosure outweigh the public and the patient's interest in keeping the information confidential.
19. In all such cases you must weigh the possible harm (both to the patient, and the overall trust between doctors and patients) against the benefits which are likely to arise from the release of information.
20. Ultimately, the 'public interest' can be determined only by the courts; but the GMC may also require you to justify your actions if we receive a complaint about the disclosure of personal information without a patient's consent.

SECTION 5 - PUTTING THE PRINCIPLES INTO PRACTICE
21. The remainder of this booklet deals with circumstances in which doctors are most frequently asked to disclose information, and provides advice on how the principles in paragraphs 14 Ò 20 should be applied.

Disclosures which benefit patients indirectly
Monitoring public health and the safety of medicines and devices including disclosures to cancer and other registries
22. Professional organisations and government regulatory bodies which monitor the public health or the safety of medicines or devices, as well as cancer and other registries, rely on information from patients' records for their effectiveness in safeguarding the public health. For example, the effectiveness of the yellow card scheme run by the Committee on Safety of Medicines depends on information provided by clinicians. You must co-operate by providing relevant information wherever possible. The notification of some communicable diseases is required by law (see also paragraph 43), and in other cases you should provide information in anonymised form, wherever that would be sufficient.
23. Where personal information is needed, you should seek express consent before disclosing information, whenever that is practicable. For example, where patients are receiving treatment there will usually be an opportunity for a health care professional to discuss disclosure of information with them.
24. Personal information may sometimes be sought about patients with whom health care professionals are not in regular contact. Doctors should therefore make sure that patients are given information about the possible value of their data in protecting the public health in the longer-term, at the initial consultation or at another suitable occasion when they attend a surgery or clinic. Patients should be given the information set out in paragraph 16: it should be clear that they may object to disclosures at any point. You must record any objections so that patients' wishes can be respected. In such cases, you may pass on anonymised information if asked to do so.
25. Where patients have not expressed an objection, you should assess the likely benefit of the disclosure to the public and commitment to confidentiality of the organisation requesting the information. If there is little or no evident public benefit, you should not disclose information without the express consent of the patient.
26. Where it is not practicable to seek patients' consent for disclosure of personal information for these purposes, or where patients are not competent to give consent, you must consider whether disclosures would be justified in the public interest, by weighing the benefits to the public health of the disclosure against the possible detriment to the patient.
27. The automatic transfer of personal information to a registry, whether by electronic or other means, before informing the patient that information will be passed on, is unacceptable save in the most exceptional circumstances. These would be where a court has already decided that there is such an overwhelming public interest in the disclosure of information to a registry that patients' rights to confidentiality are overridden; or where you are willing and able to justify the disclosure, potentially before a court or to the GMC, on the same grounds.

Clinical audit and education

28. Anonymised data will usually be sufficient for clinical audit and for education. When anonymising records you should follow the guidance on obtaining consent in paragraphs 15-17 above. You should not disclose non-anonymised data for clinical audit or education without the patient's consent.

Administration and financial audit

29. You should record financial or other administrative data separately from clinical information, and provide it in anonymised form, wherever that is possible.
30. Decisions about the disclosure of clinical records for administrative or financial audit purposes, for example where health authority staff seek access to patients' records as part of the arrangements for verifying NHS payments, are unlikely to bring your registration into question, provided that, before allowing access to patients' records, you follow the guidance in paragraphs 15-17. Only the relevant part of the record should be made available for scrutiny.

Medical research

31. Where research projects depend on using identifiable information or samples, and it is not practicable to contact patients to seek their consent, this fact should be drawn to the attention of a research ethics committee so that it can consider whether the likely benefits of the research outweigh the loss of confidentiality. Disclosures may otherwise be improper, even if the recipients of the information are registered medical practitioners. The decision of a research ethics committee would be taken into account by a court if a claim for breach of confidentiality were made, but the court's judgement would be based on its own assessment of whether the public interest was served. More detailed guidance is issued by the medical royal colleges and other bodies.

Publication of case-histories and photographs

32. You must obtain express consent from patients before publishing personal information about them as individuals in media to which the public has access, for example in journals or text books, whether or not you believe the patient can be identified. Express consent must therefore be sought to the publication of, for example, case-histories about, or photographs of, patients. Where you wish to publish information about a patient who has died, you should take into account the guidance in paragraphs 40-41 before deciding whether or not to do so.

Disclosures where doctors have dual responsibilities

33. Situations arise where doctors have contractual obligations to third parties, such as companies or organisations, as well as obligations to patients. Such situations occur, for example, when doctors:
    a. Provide occupational health services or medical care for employees of a company or organisation.
    b. Are employed by an organisation such as an insurance company.
    c. Work for an agency assessing claims for benefits.
    d. Provide medical care for patients and are subsequently asked to provide medical reports or information for third parties about them.
    e. Work as police surgeons.
    f. Work in the armed forces.
    g. Work in the prison service.
34. If you are asked to write a report about and/or examine a patient, or to disclose information from existing records for a third party to whom you have contractual obligations, you must:
    a. Be satisfied that the patient has been told at the earliest opportunity about for the purpose of the examination and/or disclosure, the extent of the information to be disclosed and the fact that relevant information cannot be concealed or withheld. You might wish to show the form to the patient before you complete it to ensure the patient understands the scope of the information requested.
    b. Obtain, or have seen, written consent to the disclosure from the patient or a person properly authorised to act on the patient's behalf. You may, however, accept written assurances from an officer of a government department that the patient's written consent has been given.
    c. Disclose only information relevant to the request for disclosure: accordingly, you should not usually disclose the whole record. The full record may be relevant to some benefits paid by government departments.
    d. Include only factual information you can substantiate, presented in an unbiased manner.
    e. The Access to Medical Reports Act 1988 entitles patients to see reports written about them before they are disclosed, in some circumstances. In all circumstances you should check whether patients wish to see their report, unless patients have clearly and specifically stated that they do not wish to do so.
35. Disclosures without consent to employers, insurance companies, or any other third party, can be justified only in exceptional circumstances, for example, when they are necessary to protect others from risk of death or serious harm.

Disclosures to protect the patient or others

36. Disclosure of personal information without consent may be justified where failure to do so may expose the patient or others to risk or death or serious harm. Where third parties are exposed to a risk so serious that it outweighs the patient's privacy interest, you should seek consent to disclosure where practicable. If it is not practicable, you should disclose information promptly to an

appropriate person or authority. You should generally inform the patient before disclosing the information.

37. Such circumstances may arise, for example:
   a. Where a colleague, who is also a patient, is placing patients at risk as a result of illness or other medical condition. If you are in doubt about whether disclosure is justified you should consult an experienced colleague, or seek advice from a professional organisation. The safety of patients must come first at all times. (Our booklet Serious Communicable Diseases gives further guidance on this issue.)
   b. Where a patient continues to drive, against medical advice, when unfit to do so. In such circumstances you should disclose relevant information to the medical adviser of the Driver and Vehicle Licensing Agency without delay. Fuller guidance is given in High Yield Topic 2.
   c. Where a disclosure may assist in the prevention or detection of a serious crime. Serious crimes, in this context, will put someone at risk of death or serious harm, and will usually be crimes against the person, such as abuse of children.

Children and other patients who may lack competence to give consent

38. Problems may arise if you consider that a patient is incapable of giving consent to treatment or disclosure because of immaturity, illness or mental incapacity. If such patients ask you not to disclose information to a third party, you should try to persuade them to allow an appropriate person to be involved in the consultation. If they refuse and you are convinced that it is essential, in their medical interests, you may disclose relevant information to an appropriate person or authority. In such cases you must tell the patient before disclosing any information, and, where appropriate, seek and carefully consider the views of an advocate or carer. You should document in the patient's record the steps you have taken to obtain consent and the reasons for deciding to disclose information.

39. If you believe a patient to be a victim of neglect or physical, sexual or emotional abuse and that the patient cannot give or withhold consent to disclosure, you should give information promptly to an appropriate responsible person or statutory agency, where you believe that the disclosure is in the patient's best interests. You should usually inform the patient that you intend to disclose the information before doing so. Such circumstances may arise in relation to children, where concerns about possible abuse need to be shared with other agencies such as social services. Where appropriate you should inform those with parental responsibility about the disclosure. If, for any reason, you believe that disclosure of information is not in the best interests of an abused or neglected patient, you must still be prepared to justify your decision.

Disclosure after a patient's death

40. You still have an obligation to keep personal information confidential after a patient dies. The extent to which confidential information may be disclosed after a patient's death will depend on the circumstances. These include the nature of the information, whether that information is already public knowledge or can be anonymised, and the intended use to which the information will be put. You should also consider whether the disclosure of information may cause distress to, or be of benefit to, the patient's partner or family.

41. There are a number of circumstances in which you may be asked to disclose, or wish to use, information about patients who have died. For example:
   a. To assist a Coroner, Procurator Fiscal or other similar officer in connection with an inquest or fatal accident inquiry. In these circumstances you should provide relevant information (see also paragraph 19 of Good Medical Practice).
   b. As part of National Confidential Enquiries or other clinical audit or for education or research. The publication of properly anonymised case studies would be unlikely to be improper in these contexts.
   c. On death certificates. The law requires you to complete death certificates honestly and fully.
   d. To obtain information relating to public health surveillance. Anonymised information should be used unless identifiable data is essential to the study.

42. Particular difficulties may arise when there is a conflict of interest between parties affected by the patient's death. For example, if an insurance company seeks information in order to decide whether to make a payment under a life assurance policy, you should release information in accordance with the requirements of the Access to Health Records Act 1990 or with the authorisation of those lawfully entitled to deal with the person's estate who have been fully informed of the consequences of disclosure. It may also be appropriate to inform those close to the patient.

Section 6 - Disclosure in connection with judicial or other statutory proceedings

43. You must disclose information to satisfy a specific statutory requirement, such as notification of a known or suspected communicable disease.

44. You must also disclose information if ordered to do so by a judge or presiding officer of a court. You should object to the judge or the presiding officer if attempts are made to compel you to disclose what appear to you to be irrelevant matters, for example matters relating to relatives or partners of the patient, who are not parties to the proceedings.

45. You should not disclose personal information to a third party such as a solicitor, police officer or officer of a court without the patient's express consent, except in the circumstances described at paragraphs 36-37, 39 and 41.

46. You may disclose personal information in response to an official request from a statutory regulatory body for any of the health care professions, where that body determines that this is necessary in the interests of justice and for the safety of other patients. Wherever practicable you should discuss this with the patient. There may be exceptional cases where, even though the patient objects, disclosure is justified.

If you decide to disclose confidential information you must be prepared to explain and justify your decision.

SEEKING PATIENTS' CONSENT: THE ETHICAL CONSIDERATIONS

Introduction

1. Successful relationships between doctors and patients depend on trust. To establish that trust you must respect patients' autonomy - their right to decide whether or not to undergo any medical intervention even where a refusal may result in harm to themselves or in their own death1. Patients must be given sufficient information, in a way that they can understand, to enable them to exercise their right to make informed decisions about their care.

2. This right is protected in law, and you are expected to be aware of the legal principles set by relevant case law in this area2. Existing case law gives a guide to what can be considered minimum requirements of good practice in seeking informed consent from patients.

3. Effective communication is the key to enabling patients to make informed decisions. You must take appropriate steps to find out what patients want to know and ought to know about their condition and its treatment. Open, helpful dialogue of this kind with patients leads to clarity of objectives and understanding, and strengthens the quality of the doctor/patient relationship. It provides an agreed framework within which the doctor can respond effectively to the individual needs of the patient. Additionally, patients who have been able to make properly informed decisions are more likely to co-operate fully with the agreed management of their conditions.

Consent to investigation and treatment

Providing sufficient information

4. Patients have a right to information about their condition and the treatment options available to them. The amount of information you give each patient will vary, according to factors such as the nature of the condition, the complexity of the treatment, the risks associated with the treatment or procedure, and the patient's own wishes. For example, patients may need more information to make an informed decision about a procedure which carries a high risk of failure or adverse side effects; or about an investigation for a condition which, if present, could have serious implications for the patient's employment, social or personal life3.

5. The information which patients want or ought to know, before deciding whether to consent to treatment or an investigation, may include:
   - details of the diagnosis, and prognosis, and the likely prognosis if the condition is left untreated;
   - uncertainties about the diagnosis including options for further investigation prior to treatment;
   - options for treatment or management of the condition, including the option not to treat;
   - the purpose of a proposed investigation or treatment; details of the procedures or therapies involved, including subsidiary treatment such as methods of pain relief; how the patient should prepare for the procedure; and details of what the patient might experience during or after the procedure including common and serious side effects;
   - for each option, explanations of the likely benefits and the probabilities of success; and discussion of any serious or frequently occurring risks, and of any lifestyle changes which may be caused by, or necessitated by, the treatment;
   - advice about whether a proposed treatment is experimental;
   - how and when the patient's condition and any side effects will be monitored or re-assessed;
   - the name of the doctor who will have overall responsibility for the treatment and, where appropriate, names of the senior members of his or her team;
   - whether doctors in training will be involved, and the extent to which students may be involved in an investigation or treatment;
   - a reminder that patients can change their minds about a decision at any time;
   - a reminder that patients have a right to seek a second opinion;
   - where applicable, details of costs or charges which the patient may have to meet.

6. When providing information you must do your best to find out about patients' individual needs and priorities. For example, patients' beliefs, culture, occupation or other factors may have a bearing on the information they need in order to reach a decision. You should not make assumptions about patients' views, but discuss these matters with them, and ask them whether they have any concerns about the treatment or the risks it may involve. You should provide patients with appropriate information, which should include an explanation of any risks to which they may attach particular significance. Ask patients whether they have understood the information and whether they would like more before making a decision.

7. You must not exceed the scope of the authority given by a patient, except in an emergency4. Therefore, if you are the doctor providing treatment or undertaking an investigation, you must give the patient a clear explana-

tion of the scope of consent being sought. This will apply particularly where:
- treatment will be provided in stages with the possibility of later adjustments;
- different doctors (or other health care workers) provide particular elements of an investigation or treatment (for example anaesthesia in surgery);
- a number of different investigations or treatments are involved;
- uncertainty about the diagnosis, or about the appropriate range of options for treatment, may be resolved only in the light of findings once investigation or treatment is underway, and when the patient may be unable to participate in decision making.

In such cases, you should explain how decisions would be made about whether or when to move from one stage or one form of treatment to another. There should be a clear agreement about whether the patient consents to all or only parts of the proposed plan of investigation or treatment, and whether further consent will have to be sought at a later stage.

8. You should raise with patients the possibility of additional problems coming to light during a procedure when the patient is unconscious or otherwise unable to make a decision. You should seek consent to treat any problems which you think may arise and ascertain whether there are any procedures to which the patient would object, or prefer to give further thought to before you proceed. You must abide by patients' decisions on these issues. If in exceptional circumstances you decide, while the patient is unconscious, to treat a condition which falls outside the scope of the patient's consent, your decision may be challenged in the courts, or be the subject of a complaint to your employing authority or the GMC. You should therefore seek the views of an experienced colleague, wherever possible, before providing the treatment. And you must be prepared to explain and justify your decision. You must tell the patient what you have done and why, as soon as the patient is sufficiently recovered to understand.

Responding to questions
9. You must respond honestly to any questions the patient raises and, as far as possible, answer as fully as the patient wishes. In some cases, a patient may ask about other treatments that are unproven or ineffective. Some patients may want to know whether any of the risks or benefits of treatment are affected by the choice of institution or doctor providing the care. You must answer such questions as fully, accurately and objectively as possible.

Withholding information
10. You should not withhold information necessary for decision making unless you judge that disclosure of some relevant information would cause the patient serious harm. In this context serious harm does not mean the patient would become upset, or decide to refuse treatment.
11. No-one may make decisions on behalf of a competent adult. If patients ask you to withhold information and make decisions on their behalf, or nominate a relative or third party to make decisions for them, you should explain the importance of them knowing the options open to them, and what the treatment they may receive will involve. If they insist they do not want to know in detail about their condition and its treatment, you should still provide basic information about the treatment. If a relative asks you to withhold information, you must seek the views of the patient. Again, you should not withhold relevant information unless you judge that this would cause the patient serious harm.
12. In any case where you withhold relevant information from the patient you must record this, and the reason for doing so, in the patient's medical records and you must be prepared to explain and justify your decision.

Presenting information to patients
13. Obtaining informed consent cannot be an isolated event. It involves a continuing dialogue between you and your patients which keeps them abreast of changes in their condition and the treatment or investigation you propose. Whenever possible, you should discuss treatment options at a time when the patient is best able to understand and retain the information. To be sure that your patient understands, you should give clear explanations and give the patient time to ask questions. In particular, you should:
- use up-to-date written material, visual and other aids to explain complex aspects of the investigation, diagnosis or treatment where appropriate and/or practicable;
- make arrangements, wherever possible, to meet particular language and communication needs, for example through translations, independent interpreters, signers, or the patient's representative;
- where appropriate, discuss with patients the possibility of bringing a relative or friend, or making a tape recording of the consultation;
- explain the probabilities of success, or the risk of failure of, or harm associated with options for treatment, using accurate data;
- ensure that information which patients may find distressing is given to them in a considerate way. Provide patients with information about counselling services and patient support groups, where appropriate;
- allow patients sufficient time to reflect, before and after making a decision, especially where the information is complex or the severity of the risks is great. Where patients have difficulty understanding information, or there is a lot of information to absorb, it may be appropriate to provide it in manageable amounts, with

appropriate written or other back-up material, over a period of time, or to repeat it;
- involve nursing or other members of the health care team in discussions with the patient, where appropriate. They may have valuable knowledge of the patient's background or particular concerns, for example in identifying what risks the patient should be told about;
- ensure that, where treatment is not to start until some time after consent has been obtained, the patient is given a clear route for reviewing their decision with the person providing the treatment.

Who obtains consent

14. If you are the doctor providing treatment or undertaking an investigation, it is your responsibility to discuss it with the patient and obtain consent, as you will have a comprehensive understanding of the procedure or treatment, how it is carried out, and the risks attached to it. Where this is not practicable, you may delegate these tasks provided you ensure that the person to whom you delegate:
    - is suitably trained and qualified;
    - has sufficient knowledge of the proposed investigation or treatment, and understands the risks involved;
    - acts in accordance with the guidance in this booklet.
    You will remain responsible for ensuring that, before you start any treatment, the patient has been given sufficient time and information to make an informed decision, and has given consent to the procedure or investigation.

Ensuring voluntary decision making

15. It is for the patient, not the doctor, to determine what is in the patient's own best interests. Nonetheless, you may wish to recommend a treatment or a course of action to patients, but you must not put pressure on patients to accept your advice. In discussions with patients, you should:
    - give a balanced view of the options;
    - explain the need for informed consent.
    You must declare any potential conflicts of interest, for example where you or your organisation benefit financially from use of a particular drug or treatment, or treatment at a particular institution.
16. Pressure may be put on patients by employers, insurance companies or others to undergo particular tests or accept treatment. You should do your best to ensure that patients have considered the options and reached their own decision. You should take appropriate action if you believe patients are being offered inappropriate or unlawful financial or other rewards.
17. Patients who are detained by the police or immigration services, or are in prison, and those detained under the provisions of any mental health legislation may be particularly vulnerable. Where such patients have a right to decline treatment you should do your best to ensure that they know this, and are able to exercise this right.

Emergencies

18. In an emergency, where consent cannot be obtained, you may provide medical treatment to anyone who needs it, provided the treatment is limited to what is immediately necessary to save life or avoid significant deterioration in the patient's health. However, you must still respect the terms of any valid advance refusal which you know about, or is drawn to your attention. You should tell the patient what has been done, and why, as soon as the patient is sufficiently recovered to understand.

Establishing capacity to make decisions

19. You must work on the presumption that every adult has the capacity to decide whether to consent to, or refuse, proposed medical intervention, unless it is shown that they cannot understand information presented in a clear way5. If a patient's choice appears irrational, or does not accord with your view of what is in the patient's best interests, that is not evidence in itself that the patient lacks competence. In such circumstances it may be appropriate to review with the patient whether all reasonable steps have been taken to identify and meet their information needs (see paragraphs 5-17). Where you need to assess a patient's capacity to make a decision, you should consult the guidance issued by professional bodies6.

Fluctuating capacity

20. Where patients have difficulty retaining information, or are only intermittently competent to make a decision, you should provide any assistance they might need to reach an informed decision. You should record any decision made while the patients were competent, including the key elements of the consultation. You should review any decision made whilst they were competent, at appropriate intervals before treatment starts, to establish that their views are consistently held and can be relied on.

Mentally incapacitated patients

21. No-one can give or withhold consent to treatment on behalf of a mentally incapacitated patient7. You must first assess the patient's capacity to make an informed decision about the treatment. If patients lack capacity to decide, provided they comply, you may carry out an investigation or treatment, which may include treatment for any mental disorder8, that you judge to be in their best interests. However, if they do not comply, you may compulsorily treat them for any mental disorder only within the safeguards laid down by the Mental Health Act 19839, and any physical disorder arising from that mental disorder, in line with the guidance in the Code of Practice of the Mental Health Commission10. You should seek the courts' approval for any non-therapeutic or controversial treatments which are not directed at their mental disorder.

Advance statements

22. If you are treating a patient who has lost capacity to consent to or refuse treatment, for example through onset or progress of a mental disorder or other disability, you should try to find out whether the patient has previously indicated preferences in an advance statement ('advance directives' or 'living wills'). You must respect any refusal of treatment given when the patient was competent, provided the decision in the advance statement is clearly applicable to the present circumstances, and there is no reason to believe that the patient has changed his/her mind. Where an advance statement of this kind is not available, the patient's known wishes should be taken into account - see paragraph 25 on the 'best interests' principle.

Children

23. You must assess a child's capacity to decide whether to consent to or refuse proposed investigation or treatment before you provide it. In general, a competent child will be able to understand the nature, purpose and possible consequences of the proposed investigation or treatment, as well as the consequences of non-treatment. Your assessment must take account of the relevant laws or legal precedents in this area11. You should bear in mind that:
    - at age 16 a young person can be treated as an adult and can be presumed to have capacity to decide;
    - under age 16 children may have capacity to decide, depending on their ability to understand what is involved12;
    - where a competent child refuses treatment, a person with parental responsibility or the court may authorise investigation or treatment which is in the child's best interests. The position is different in Scotland, where those with parental responsibility cannot authorise procedures a competent child has refused. Legal advice may be helpful on how to deal with such cases.

24. Where a child under 16 years old is not competent to give or withhold their informed consent, a person with parental responsibility may authorise investigations or treatment which are in the child's best interests13. This person may also refuse any intervention, where they consider that refusal to be in the child's best interests, but you are not bound by such a refusal and may seek a ruling from the court. In an emergency where you consider that it is in the child's best interests to proceed, you may treat the child, provided it is limited to that treatment which is reasonably required in that emergency.

'Best interests' principle

25. In deciding what options may be reasonably considered as being in the best interests of a patient who lacks capacity to decide, you should take into account:
    - options for treatment or investigation which are clinically indicated;
    - any evidence of the patient's previously expressed preferences, including an advance statement;
    - your own and the health care team's knowledge of the patient's background, such as cultural, religious, or employment considerations;
    - views about the patient's preferences given by a third party who may have other knowledge of the patient, for example the patient's partner, family, carer, tutor-dative (Scotland), or a person with parental responsibility;
    - which option least restricts the patient's future choices, where more than one option (including non-treatment) seems reasonable in the patient's best interest.

Applying to the court

26. Where a patient's capacity to consent is in doubt, or where differences of opinion about his or her best interests cannot be resolved satisfactorily, you should consult more experienced colleagues and, where appropriate, seek legal advice on whether it is necessary to apply to the court for a ruling. You should seek the court's approval where a patient lacks capacity to consent to a medical intervention which is non-therapeutic or controversial, for example contraceptive sterilisation, organ donation, withdrawal of life support from a patient in a persistent vegetative state. Where you decide to apply to a court you should, as soon as possible, inform the patient and his or her representative of your decision and of his or her right to be represented at the hearing.

Forms of consent

27. To determine whether patients have given informed consent to any proposed investigation or treatment, you must consider how well they have understood the details and implications of what is proposed, and not simply the form in which their consent has been expressed or recorded.

Express consent

28. Patients can indicate their informed consent either orally or in writing. In some cases, the nature of the risks to which the patient might be exposed make it important that a written record is available of the patient's consent and other wishes in relation to the proposed investigation and treatment. This helps to ensure later understanding between you, the patient, and anyone else involved in carrying out the procedure or providing care. Except in an emergency, where the patient has capacity to give consent you should obtain written consent in cases where:
    - the treatment or procedure is complex, or involves significant risks and/or side effects;
    - providing clinical care is not the primary purpose of the investigation or examination;
    - there may be significant consequences for the patient's employment, social or personal life;
    - the treatment is part of a research programme.

29. You must use the patient's case notes and/or a consent form to detail the key elements of the discussion with the patient, including the nature of information provided,

specific requests by the patient, details of the scope of the consent given.

Statutory requirements

30. Some statutes require written consent to be obtained for particular treatments (for example some fertility treatments). You must follow the law in these areas.

Implied consent

31. You should be careful about relying on a patient's apparent compliance with a procedure as a form of consent. For example, the fact that a patient lies down on an examination couch does not in itself indicate that the patient has understood what you propose to do and why.

Reviewing consent

32. A signed consent form is not sufficient evidence that a patient has given, or still gives, informed consent to the proposed treatment in all its aspects. You, or a member of the team, must review the patient's decision close to the time of treatment, and especially where:
    - significant time has elapsed between obtaining consent and the start of treatment;
    - there have been material changes in the patient's condition, or in any aspects of the proposed treatment plan, which might invalidate the patient's existing consent;
    - new, potentially relevant information has become available, for example about the risks of the treatment, or about other treatment options.

Consent to screening

33. Screening (which may involve testing) healthy or asymptomatic people to detect genetic predispositions or early signs of debilitating or life threatening conditions can be an important tool in providing effective care. But the uncertainties involved in screening may be great, for example the risk of false positive or false negative results. Some findings may potentially have serious medical, social or financial consequences not only for the individuals, but for their relatives. In some cases the fact of having been screened may itself have serious implications.

34. You must ensure that anyone considering whether to consent to screening can make a properly informed decision. As far as possible, you should ensure that screening would not be contrary to the individual's interest. You must pay particular attention to ensuring that the information the person wants or ought to have is identified and provided. You should be careful to explain clearly:
    - the purpose of the screening;
    - the likelihood of positive/negative findings and possibility of false positive/negative results;
    - the uncertainties and risks attached to the screening process;
    - any significant medical, social or financial implications of screening for the particular condition or predisposition;
    - follow up plans, including availability of counselling and support services.

If you are considering the possibility of screening children, or adults who are not able to decide for themselves, you should refer to the guidance at paragraphs 19-25. In appropriate cases, you should take account of the guidance issued by bodies such as the Advisory Committee on Genetic Testing 14.

Consent to research

35. Research involving clinical trials of drugs or treatments, and research into the causes of, or possible treatment for, a particular condition, is important in increasing doctors' ability to provide effective care for present and future patients. The benefits of the research may, however, be uncertain and may not be experienced by the person participating in the research. In addition, the risk involved for research participants may be difficult to identify or to assess in advance. If you carry out or participate in research involving patients or volunteers, it is particularly important that you ensure:
    - as far as you are able, that the research is not contrary to the individual's interests;
    - that participants understand that it is research and that the results are not predictable.

36. You must take particular care to be sure that anyone you ask to consider taking part in research is given the fullest possible information, presented in terms and a form that they can understand. This must include any information about possible benefits and risks; evidence that a research ethics committee has given approval; and advice that they can withdraw at any time. You should ensure that participants have the opportunity to read and consider the research information leaflet. You must allow them sufficient time to reflect on the implications of participating in the study. You must not put pressure on anyone to take part in research. You must obtain the person's consent in writing. Before starting any research you must always obtain approval from a properly constituted research ethics committee.

37. You should seek further advice where your research will involve adults who are not able to make decisions for themselves, or children. You should be aware that in these cases the legal position is complex or unclear, and there is currently no general consensus on how to balance the possible risks and benefits to such vulnerable individuals against the public interest in conducting research. (A number of public consultation exercises are under way.) You should consult the guidance issued by bodies such as the Medical Research Council and the medical royal colleges16 to keep up to date. You should also seek advice from the relevant research ethics committee where appropriate.

HIGH YIELD TOPIC ELEVEN

6DEVELOPMENT (DENVER SCREENING) AND MOTOR MILE STONES

Mean age	Eye/hand coordination	Locomotor skills	Speech/communication skills	Social/personal skills
6 weeks	Follow a moving face with eyes	Holds head but some head lag	Cooing noise begins	Smiles when spoken to
3 months	Hand regard brings hand to midline Follows horizontally and vertically	Minimal or no head-lag Lift head upon prone	Stills to mother's voice. Coos reciprocally with mother	Friendly response to attention Initiates smile
6 months	Transfers cube from one hand to others Reaches nut and grasps a rattle or toy	Up on extended forearms in prone. Sits without lateral support	Squeals and starts to bubble (blow bubbles)	Discriminates family from stangers. Laughs out loud
9 months	Picks up cube with fine pincer grasp Looks for a fallen body	Stands holding on to furniture. Pulls self to stand	Babbles Ma-Ma/Da-Da/Ba-Ba. understands 'No' and shakes head for 'No'	Waves good-bye. Finger feeds self
1 years	Bangs bricks together when shown. Picks up pellet with pincer grasp	Cross round the furniture. Pulls self to stand	Mama, Dada and Baba with meaning 2-3 other words reported	Finds toy under cup. Claps hands. Begins to point
15 months	Holds two 1" cubes in one hand Stop casting toys	Walks with one hand held. Walk unsupported	3-4 clear words heard Beginning to point to what he wants	Manages cup or transfer cup Helps with dressing
1½ years	Scribbles freely on paper. Builds 3 × 1" cube tower when shown	Climbs up stairs, (hand held). Kneels with support	Points to three parts of the body. Single word vocabulary 6-20 words	Spoon feeds self Manages cup on own. Know parts of body like eye and nose
2 years	Vertical line/circular scrible Builds 6 7 × 1"cube tower	Up and down stairs, hand held, two feet per step. Runs and kick a ball	Simple 3-4 word combinations. Names 6-8 familiar pictures/toys	Aware when wet/dirty May use potty Worries if mother leave room
3 years	Builds a brige of 3 cubes Copies line	Walk on tip toes. Walks up stairs, one foot per step	Talks in 6-syllable sentences. Able to give name, age and sex	Washes hands/undresses self imagenative play/ cooperates with friends
4 years	Draws a recognisable man. Copies a square	Hops on one foot. Walks down stairs, one foot per step.	Clear, grammatical conversation. Knows primary colours and big/small	Dresses self (not laces/ fastenings) Play with friends separate from parents
	WARNING SIGNS: 1. Presistent fisting of hands. 2. Handedness before 15 months 3. Casting all toys after 18 months	*WARNING SIGNS:* 1. Scissoring at any age 2. Mark hypotonia 3. Persistent moro reflex reflex after 4 months 4. Unexpected limp	*WARNING SIGNS:* 1. No babble at 8 months 2. Persistent drooling after 18 months 3. No comprehension of situation of single command by 18 months 4. No words by 18 months 5. Marked echolalia after 2½ years 6. Speech unintelligible by 3 years	*WARNING SIGNS:* 1. Persistent high pitched screaming 2. Marked eye contact avoidance 3. Persistent hand regard 5 months 4. Repetitive movement (stereotypes) 5. Persistent mouthing after 18 months 6. Persistent tantrums after 3 years

NOTE: Not all children develop at same rate.

Index

A

ABCM regimen 391
Abdominal bruits 650
Abdominal distension 385, 639
Abdominal mass 181
Abdominal pain 160, 169, 246, 322, 384, 385, 391, 396, 398, 630, 635, 645, 650-652, 678, 724-727
Abdominal striae 106, 162
Abdominoperineal resection 384, 638
Abruption 183
ABVD regimen 392
Acamprosate 136
Accidental injury 89, 421, 539
Acetazolamide 371, 388, 440, 626, 695
Achalasia 507
Aciclovir 170, 179, 225, 401
Acid brash 723
Acidosis 371, 438
Acoustic neuroma 224, 553, 664
Acral lentiginous melanoma 132
Acrodermatitis enteropathica 397
Acrolein 157
Acromegaly 106, 143, 162, 285, 659, 675
Acrophobia 683
Actinic keratosis 133, 134
Actinomyces israelii 363
Activated charcoal 687
Acute adrenal insufficiency 438, 521
Acute appendicitis 161
Acute atrial fibrillation (AF) 282, 583
Acute bronchitis 137
Acute cholecystitis 161, 178, 424, 510, 650, 727
Acute gastroenteritis (GE) 291
Acute intermittent prophyria 159
Acute lymphoblastic leukaemia (ALL) 154, 390, 425, 563, 659
Acute mucopurulent conjunctivitis 492
Acute myocardial infarction (AMI) 534, 570
Acute on chronic PID 101
Acute pancreatitis 93, 178, 318, 651, 652
Acute pericarditis 283, 584
Acute phase reactants 670
Acute renal failure 369, 624
Acute severe asthma 231
Acute suppurative otitis media (ASOM) 130

Acute tubular necrosis 103, 381, 713
Adair-Dighton syndrome 87, 419
Addison's disease 119, 320, 688, 707
Addisonian crisis 438
Adenocarcinoma of the ethmoids 227
Adrenal hyperplasia 106
Adrenal insufficiency 438
Adrenaline 121
AFB microscopy 456
Africa 141
Agnosia 251, 367
Agoraphobia 167
Agranulocytosis 111, 255
AIDS 368, 685
AIDS-dementia complex 368
Air hunger 647
Akathisia 253
Alanine aminotransferase (ALT) 438
Alcohol abuse 136
Alcohol addiction 315
Alcohol dependence 136
Alcohol intoxication 256, 633
Alcoholic liver disease 275
Alcoholics anonymous 136
Alcoholism 161, 173, 410, 651, 690, 702
Algopobia 683
Alkalosis 233, 238, 417
Allergic bronchopulmonary Aspergillosis 152
Allogenic transplantation 391
Alloimmunization 390
Allopurinol 97, 144
Alopecia 370, 624
Alport's 676
Alteplase 671
Altered bowel habit 180, 385, 638
Alzheimer's dementia (AD) 87, 251, 256, 367, 420, 453, 659
Amaurosis fugax 89
Amenorrhoea 151, 162, 441
Amiloride 164
Aminoglycoside antibiotics 371
Aminophylline 232
Amiodarone 321, 707
Amitriptiline 179, 401
AML 98
Ammonia dermatitis 673
Amnesia 122, 251
Amoebiasis 141, 631
Amoebic dysentery 141

Amoxicillin 158, 229, 364, 428, 458, 700
Amphetamines 393
Amphotericin 155, 426, 439, 644
Ampicillin 137, 428
Ampula of Vater 159
Amputation 172
Amyl nitrate 240
Amyl nitrite 395, 688
Amylase 161, 423, 651, 652
Amyloid angiopathy 251
Amyloidosis 110, 118
Anaemia 143, 384, 391, 451, 452, 558, 689, 690
Analeptics 229
Anankastic personality disorder 357
Anaphylactic shock 121
Anaphylactoid reactions 121
Anaphylaxis 244, 376, 592, 646
Anaplastic carcinoma thyroid 320, 516, 708
Androgen deficiency 451
Angina 179, 422, 672, 707
Angioedema 121
Angiography 105, 647
Angle closure glaucoma (ACG) 388
Ankle branchial pressure index (ABPI) 172
Ankylosing spondylitis 187
Anorexia 96, 136, 392, 418, 434, 456, 642, 694
Anorexia nervosa 296, 434
Antenatal care 433
Antepartum hemorrhage 150
Anterior ischaemic optic neuropathy (AION) 364
Anterior resection 384, 638
Anterograde amnesia 122
Anticholinergic activity 686
Anticoagulant overdose 226
Anticoagulant therapy 159, 668
Anticoagulants 366
Anticoagulation 148, 159, 394, 414, 668
Antihypertensive 430
Antinuclear antibodies 90
Antiphospholipid syndrome 148, 150
Antiplatelet drug 95
Antithrombin III 379
Antitubercular therapy (ATT) 456
Anxiety 165, 166, 632, 684

Anxiety neurosis 116
Anxiolytics 165, 166, 684
Aortic aneurysm (AA) 646, 647
Aortic dissection (AD) 455, 533, 650
Aortic insufficiency 414
Aortography 104, 649
Aortoiliac bypass grafts 172
Aphasia 127, 251
Aplasia 451
Apolipoprotein E 659
Appendicectomy 162, 248, 380, 460, 590, 713
Appendicitis 161, 725
Appendicular colic 159
Appendicular mass 143
Appendix 713
Apple core' appearance 141
Apple jelly nodules 119
Apraxia 251, 367
Arabs 322
Arachis oil enema 157
Arachnodactyly 146, 648
Arachnophobia 683
ARDS 631
Argon laser trabeculoplasty 90
Arrhythmia 370, 686, 687
Arterial ulcers 312
Arteriography 171, 172, 650
Arteriosclerosis 388
Arthralgia 106, 445, 447, 660, 694
Arthritis 97, 396, 443, 640
Asbestosis 527
Ascorbic acid 690
Aseptic meningitis 155, 425, 643
Asia 141
Asparaginase 651
Aspartate transaminase 438
Aspergillosis 362
Aspergillus 363
Aspiration pneumonia 531, 633
Assertiveness training 359
Asthma 151-153, 230-232, 374-376, 529, 632, 647, 672
Ataxia 96, 136, 235, 702, 717
Alpha-thalassemia 452
Atherosclerosis 105, 127, 172, 646, 647, 649, 650, 677
Atopic infantile eczema 271
Atopy 646
Atrial fibrillation 171, 448, 668, 687
Atrophic gastritis 688
Atrophic vaginitis 309, 574
Atropine poisoning 395
Atropine 228, 366, 671
Audiogram 663, 665
Audio-premotor syndrome 677
Augmentin 428
Autonomic neuropathy 360, 515

Autosomal dominant 717
AVPU scoring 102
Avulsion of renal pedicle 259
Axial compression injury 174
Azathioprine 651, 688

B
Beta blockers 672
B_{12} 367
B_{12} deficiency anaemia 558, 689
Beta2 adrenoreceptor agonists 230
Bacillary angiomatosis 133
Bacillary dysentery 141
Backache 187, 390, 391
Baclofen 403
Bacterial meningitis 675
Bacterial vaginosis 101, 168
Bacteroides 94
Balloon dilatation 104
Barbiturates 114
Barium enema 143, 384, 396, 434
Barium swallow 148, 723
Barium 398
Barret's oesophagus 318
Bartonella 133
Basal body temperature 176
Bat wing appearance 631
Battered baby syndrome 87, 88, 419, 421, 538,
Battle's sign 237
Bazin's disease 119
Becker muscular dystrophy 109
Beclomethasone 691, 693
Bedwetting 421
Bee sting 121
Beet root 159
Behaviour therapy 116, 165, 167, 357, 359, 684
Behcet's syndrome 444, 642, 655
Belching 455
Bell's palsy 657
Bence-Jones proteins 441
Bendrofluazide 164
Benign prostatic hypertrophy (BPH) 159, 641
Benzodiazepine addiction 135
Benzodiazepine withdrawal 135
Benzodiazepines 114, 682, 687
Benzyl penicillin 111
Bereavement 684
Beta thalassemia 452
Beta-lactum antibiotics 229
Bigeminus 687
Bilateral adrenalectomy 162
Bilateral basal consolidation 140
Bilateral cavitating bronchopneumonia 140
Bilateral crepitation 139

Bilateral interstitial infiltrates 139
Biliary calculi 178
Biliary colic 650, 726, 727
Biliary peritonitis 377
Bilirubinuria 313
Binconvex hematoma 124
Beta-interferon 1b 96, 390, 655-657
Bioprosthetic valve 668
Biphasic P-wave 415
Bipolar affective disorder 115
Birth marks 88, 421
Bisphosphonate 96, 324
Blackouts 697
Bladder neck hypertrophy 640
Bladder neck stenosis 640
Bladder outflow obstruction (BOO) 288, 569, 627, 641
Bladder training 404
Bleeding gums 690
Bleeding per rectum 141
Bleeding per vaginum 420
Blindness 364, 694
Blister 661
Bloating 423
Blood borne 679
Blood culture 169, 181, 191, 387, 715
Blood glucose 235, 447
Blood loss 173, 587
Blood slime 384
Blood transfusions 437
Bloody diarrhoea 142, 384
Bloody stools 396
Blue extremities 172
Blue sclerae 87, 419
Blurring of vision 254, 390, 657, 695
Boerhaave's syndrome 180, 454
Bone marrow biopsy 390
Bone marrow transplantation 452
Bone pain 390, 391, 451, 640
Bone scan 718
Bony metastases 718
Borrelia burgdorferi infection 447
Borrelia burgdorferi sensu lato 447
Bounding pulse 411
Box splint 145
Bradycardia 155, 321, 425, 643, 671, 678
Brain biopsy 154, 424
Brainstem ischaemia 402
Branchial arch 711
Branchial cyst (BC) 541, 711
Break through bleeding 182, 521
Breast cancer 96
Breast carcinoma 323-325, 406, 718
Breast mass 406, 408
Breathlessness 166, 234, 454, 633, 718, 670, 692
Breavment 136
Breech 399

Index

Bridging veins 173
British Heart Foundation 671
British National Formulary 243
British Thoracic Society guidelines 231, 232, 376, 691-693
Brittle bone syndrome 87, 419
Broad arm sling 654
Bronchial asthma 635
Bronchial carcinoids 118, 458
Bronchial carcinoma 117, 281, 456, 529, 107
Bronchial obstruction 458
Bronchial rattles 303
Bronchiectasis 107, 457
Bronchiolitis 118
Bronchoalveolar lavage 363
Bronchoconstriction 153, 458
Bronchodilators 457
Bronchopneumonia 362
Bronchopulmonary fistula 635
Bronchoscopy 107, 240, 456
Brucellosis 412
Bruch's membrane 91
Brudzinskin's sign 675
Bruising 678
β-thalassemia major 452
Budesonide 691
Buerger's disease 171
Buffalow hump 162
Bulimia nervosa 116
Bullous impetigo 674
Burns 241, 242, 542, 661
Burr holes 123, 236, 239, 372, 698
Burst abdomen 382, 714
Buserelin 181
Busulfan 97, 442

C

C peptide assay 411
C difficile 142
Cadavaric renal transplantation 438
Caecal carcinoma 143
Caesarean section 121, 436
Calcitonin 96
Campylobacter 631
Campylobacter enteritis 443
Cancer cervix, 450
Candida 97, 148, 363
Candida albicans 168, 169
Candida dermatitis 673
Candidiasis 107, 133, 168, 182, 506
Capillary refill time 634
Captopril 369, 624
Carbamazepine 111, 401, 403, 724
Carbamizole 448
Carbimazole 322
Carbon monoxide poisoning 240, 394, 686, 499

Carboxyhemoglobin (COHb) 394, 660, 686
Carcinoid syndrome 105, 118, 458
Carcinoma larynx 108
Carcinoma oesophagus 507
Carcinoma of colon 141, 143, 434, 504
Carcinoma of maxillary antrum 227, 561
Carcinoma of rectum 638, 712
Carcinoma of tail of pancreas 446
Carcinoma pancreas 446
Carcinoma prostate 442, 640
Cardiac enzymes 672
Cardiac pacing 671
Cardiac syndrome X 422
Cardiac tamponade 259, 671
Cardiogenic shock 121, 671
Cardiomegaly 379, 670
Cardiotocogram 185
Carditis 187, 670
Carotid artery stenosis 284
Carotid bruits 188, 677
Carotid Doppler 95, 125, 677, 188
Carotid endarterectomy 95, 677
Carotid territory ischaemia 95, 127
Carpal tunnel syndrome (CTS) 106, 301, 702
Cataract 90, 579
Catheterisation 360
Catholic 729
Caudate nucleus 717
CBD obstruction 509
CBT 683
CDH 109
Cefixime 428
Cefotaxime 111
Cefuroxime 137, 178, 383, 424, 428, 633, 703, 715, 728
Central abdominal pain 161
Central chest pain 146, 648
Central cyanosis 117, 457
Central retinal artery occlusion (CRAO) 366, 495
Central serous retinopathy 365
Cephalexin 317
Cerebellar syndrome 117
Cerebello-pontine angle tumors 401, 724
Cerebral edema 123, 185, 325, 433
Cerebral haemorrhage 365, 494
Cerebral metastases 325, 719
Cerebral oedema 394
Cerebral toxoplasmosis 154, 424
Cervical biopsy 450
Cervical carcinoma 449
Cervical cytological screening 449
Cervical ectropion 169, 296, 297, 575
Cervical erosion 169

Cervical OS 149
Cervical spine injury 174
Chaga's disease 416
Champagne bottle leg 311
Charcot-Bouchard aneurysms 98
Charcot-Layden crystals 152
Chemodectoma 539, 709
Chemoprophylaxis 459, 644
Chest drain 373, 645, 647
Chest pain 146-148, 246, 414, 416, 445, 454, 456, 633, 635, 720, 723, 781
Chest trauma 373
Chickenpox 93, 401
Chlamydia 101, 137, 169, 181
Chlamydial UTI 308
Chlamydia-trachomatis 177
Chloasma 249
Chlorambucil 370, 624
Chloramphenicol 111, 678
Chlordiazepoxide 135
Chlorpheniramine 646
Chlorpromazine 115, 253
Cholchicine 144
Cholecystectomy 160, 178, 379, 728
Cholecystitis 160, 178, 314, 377, 378, 423, 424, 651
Choledocholithiasis 378
Cholelithiasis 92, 160, 313
Cholesterol crystals 711
Cholesterol stones 424
CHOP regimen 393
Chorea 368, 717
Chorioretinitis 424
Choroidal haemorrhage 389
Choroiditis 389
Chrome salts 226
Chronic bronchitis 404
Chronic intestinal ischaemia 307
Chronic myeloid leukaemia (CML) 98, 305, 391, 564
Chronic non-specific diarrhoea 397
Chronic pancreatitis 93, 423
Chronic renal failure 233
Chronic simple glaucoma (CSG) 90, 578, 694
Chronic suppurative otitis media 131
Cimetidine 156, 703
CIN 448, 449
Ciprofloxacin 142, 156, 426, 427, 644, 678
Circumcorneal congestion 186, 366, 389
Cirrhosis 128, 679
Clarithromycin 319
Claudication distance 171, 361
Claustrophobia 683
Clavicle 654
Clear plan kit 176
Clindamycin 168, 458

Clomipramine 357
Clonazepam 724
Clostridium difficile 142
Clotrimazole 168, 673
Clozapine side effects 502
Clozapine 255
Clubbing 448
Clue cells 168
CML *see* Chronic myeloid leukaemia
CMV 148, 155, 426, 438, 644
Coagulation factor V 712
Co-amoxiclav 428
Coarctation of aorta (CoA) 104, 278
Coarse hair 321
Coarse tremor 136
Cobblestone pattern 142
Cocaine abuse 240
Cocaine 137, 226, 393, 414
Coccidioidomycosis 362
Codiene 157
Coeliac disease 100, 272, 299, 396, 446, 690
Cognitive behaviour therapy (CBT) 683
Cognitive therapy 116, 681
COHb *see* Carboxy-haemoglobin
Cohort studies 666
Colchicine 143, 444
Cold intolerance 434
Cold sores 170
Colic 159
Coloboma of the choroid 389
Colon carcinoma 141, 143, 292, 383, 434, 504
Colonic hypotonia 157
Colonoscopy 142, 384, 398
Colorectal surgery 459
Colour Doppler ultrasound 158
Coloured haloes 186
Colposcopy 150, 450
Coma 113, 154, 155, 393, 395, 425, 633, 643, 678
Common bile duct obstruction 313
Common bile duct 160
Compartment syndrome 170
Complete abortion 150
Compression stockings 310
Condoms 437, 443
Conductive deafness 663, 664
Condylomata accuminata 678
Confabulation 136, 702
Confusion 136, 154, 155, 239, 254, 324, 325, 361, 643, 702, 703, 719
Congenital aphonia 677
Congenital dysplasia 109
Congenital heart disease 458
Congenital naevus 88, 421

Congenital transcobalamin II deficiency 689
Conjunctival cytology 389
Conjunctivitis 158, 366, 389, 444
Conn's syndrome 277
Consent 729
Consolidation 362-364
Constipation 96, 141, 157, 160, 180, 254, 324, 383, 384, 390, 398, 433-435, 639, 678
Constitutional delay 110
Continuous positive airway pressure (CPAP) 675
Contraception 730
Contraceptive pill 125, 168, 169, 182
Convulsions 154, 245
COPD 228, 635, 647
Cord compression 174
Corneal anaesthesia 224
Corneal edema 366, 388
Coronary angiography 649, 668
Coronary artery aneurysm 179
Coronary artery disease 668
Cortical blindness 402
Cortical dysfunction 367
Corticosteroid induced cataract 90
Costochondritis 648
Co-trimoxazole 139, 363, 437
Cotton wool spots 364
Cough 108, 362, 363, 369, 374, 404, 709
Crackles 670
Cramp 385
Cranial arteritis 89, 188
Cranial nerve palsies 390, 709
Cranial nerve 224
Creatine kinase 147
Creatine phosphokinase (CK) 109
Creatinine 369, 438
Crohn's disease (CD) 142, 384, 396, 505, 574, 690
Crohn's involvement of the colon 141, 142
Cromoglycate 232, 374, 691
Cromolyn 376
Crotamin 673
CRP 190
Crushing pain 455, 672
Crusted scabies 412
Cryotherapy 133, 187, 678
Cryptococcal meningitis 154, 155, 424, 426, 642, 644
Cryptococcosis 133, 362
Cryptococcus neoformans 155, 644
Cryptococcus 363, 426
Cryptosporidium 631
CT scan 446
CTG 183, 185, 430

Cullen's sign 652
Curschmann's spirals 152
Cushing's disease 162
Cushing's syndrome 106
CVP 234
Cyanide poisoning 395, 688
Cyanosis 247
Cyanotic heart disease 117, 457
Cyclopentolate 390
Cyclophosphamide 157, 370, 624
Cyclosporin 99
Cyclothymia 115
Cyproheptadine 118, 458
Cystectomy 157
Cystic duct 159
Cystic fibrosis 118, 140, 362, 423, 457
Cystic hygroma (CH) 541, 711
Cystitis 159, 404, 405, 624
Cystoscopy 370, 624
Cystourethroscopy 641
Cytomegalovirus (CMV) disease 438, 522

D

Dacron graft 646
Dalteparin 117
Danazol 181
Day 21 progesterone 176
De Costa's syndrome 146, 648
Deaddiction 114, 135, 137
Deafness 224, 663, 664, 677
Debulking 458
Decreased urinary flow 641
Deep dyspareuria 169
Deep transverse 399
Deep vein thrombosis 158, 379, 712
Defence mechanisms 358
Dehydration 113, 141, 238, 410, 441, 586, 587, 629, 641
Delirium tremens (DT) 256
Delirium 252, 257, 395, 702
Delusion 136, 702
Dementia 252, 367-369, 717
Demyelination 390, 640, 656
Deoxyuridine suppression test 689
Dependent personality disorder 359
Depovera 250
Depression 114-116, 136, 251, 258, 682
Depressive stupor 682
Dermatitis 673
Dermatomyositis 444, 660
Desensitization 165, 166, 684
Desmopressin 421
Dessecting aortic aneurysm 649
Detrusor instability 404
Diabetes mellitus 162, 164, 165, 187, 403, 433, 447, 716

Index

Diabetic dermopathy 447
Diabetic ketoacidosis (DKA) 112, 161, 411, 586, 113, 410
Diagnostic laparoscopy 161
Diamorphine 157, 670, 721
Diaphoresis 650
Diaphragm 250
Diarrhoea 141-143, 160, 180, 234, 248, 322, 383, 384, 396, 434, 446, 458, 638, 678, 707
Diazepam 135, 149, 395
Diclofenac 652
Dicoumarol 669
Didanosine 651
Diffuse oesophageal spasm 508
Digoxin poisoning 687
Dilated CBD 378
Dilated pupils 393
Diloxanide furoate 141
Dilutional hyponatraemia 439
Dilutional hyponatremia with nephrotic syndrome 523
Diphtheric myocarditis 416
Diphyllobrothrium latum 689
Diplopia 96, 656, 657, 658
Dipstick test 403
Disinhibition 252
Dispersion 666
Dissecting aortic aneurysm (DAA) 146, 648
Dissociation 358
Disulfiram 136
Diuretics 144
Diurnal steroid 162
Diverticulitis 160
Diverticulosis of colon 434
Dizziness 166
DLE 99
DMSA scintigraphy 92
Donepezil 251, 659
Doppler flow studies 150
Doppler of umbilical circulation 185
Doppler ultrasound 158
Doppler USG 361, 712, 380
Dorzolamide 90
Double vision 185
Down's syndrome 453, 659
Doxapram 229
Doxycycline 412
DPT 243
Dramatization 358
Drowsiness 361, 698
Drug abuser 114, 127, 413, 426, 435
Drug addict 137, 409
Drug addiction 393
Drug dependency teams 137
Drug induced thyrotoxicosis 321, 517

Drug reactions 133
Drusen 91
Dry cough 137, 139, 140, 363, 364
Dry mouth 166
Duchenne muscular dystrophy (DMD) 109
Dumping 419
Duodenal ulcers 651
Duplex USG 361
Dural vein tears 124
DVT 117, 150, 158, 394
Dye reduction tests 418
Dysarthria 95, 127, 435, 656, 677, 686
Dysentery 396, 443
Dysmenorrhoea 250
Dysmotility 630
Dyspareunia 309
Dyspepsia 455
Dysphagia 180, 320, 444, 677, 709
Dysphasia 95, 127
Dysplasia 448
Dyspnoea 117, 140, 147, 166, 178, 179, 246, 247, 373, 395, 414, 416, 445, 456, 688, 693, 709, 718
Dysuria 309, 317, 413, 418, 627, 630, 640

E

E. coli 94, 413, 427, 627, 631
Ear protectors 665
Ear toilet 131, 428
Ear wax 552
Earache 130, 131
Eastern European descent 171
Eatan-Lambert syndrome 117
Echovist 177
Eclampsia 184, 430
ECT 682
Ecthyma 674
Ectopic pregnancy 100, 645, 724
Eczema 271, 272, 311, 408
Edema in pregnancy 431
Egg allergy 244
Elderly abuse 87, 420, 537
Electric burns 241
Electric shock like pain 401, 403
Electroconvulsive therapy (ECT) 114
Elephantiasis 317
ELISA 135, 401
Embolectomy 171
Embolisation 458
Emphysema 454
Emphysematous cholecystitis 359
Emphysematous pyelonephritis 359
Encephalitis 155, 426, 644, 676
Encephalopathy 678
End diastolic 185

Endobronchial tumor 456
Endocarditis 458, 646
Endocervical swabs 101
Endocrine abnormalities 438
Endometrial cancer 450
Endometrial carcinoma 295, 576, 577, 705, 706
Endometriosis 169, 181, 519
Endometritis 101
Endomysial antibodies (IgA) 446
Eneuresis 421
Enoxapain 380, 712
Enterobius vermicularis 397
Enterococcus faecalis 413
Entonox 103, 647
Enucleation 389
Eosinophilia 152
Eosinophilic folliculitis 133
Epicanthic folds 453
Epidermidis 413
Epididymo-orchitis 315, 316, 511
Epidural anaesthesia 398, 399, 400
Epigastric pain 313, 361, 422, 423, 430, 651, 671
Epigastric 319
Epilepsy 95
Epileptic seizure 294
Episodic diarrhoea 384, 398
Epistaxis 226, 227, 560, 678, 716
Ergometrine 149, 172
Erythema ab ignes 319, 423
Erythema chronicum migrans (Lyme disease) 273, 445, 447
Erythema marginatum 670
Erythema multiforme 158, 364
Erythema nodosum 396, 445
Erythematous annular rash 445
Erythematous lesion 447
Erythematous rash 179, 444
Erythroderma 93
Erythromycin 140, 364, 428, 429
Eschar 662
Escharotomy 241, 662
Escherichia coli 413
ESR 188, 190, 364, 387, 650, 694
Essential hypertension (EH) 183, 429
Estradiol 156
European 716
Evisceration 389
Excision biopsy 134
Excretion urography 159
Exercise ECG 422
Exercise induced asthma 232, 374
Exertional angina 720
Exertional dyspnoea 139, 363
Exophthalmos 321, 322
Explorative laparotomy 173

Expressive dysphasia 677
Extradural hematoma 236
Extradural hemorrhage (EDH) 124, 372, 498, 698
Extraocular palsies 658
Extrapyramidal symptoms 255
Exudative retinopathy of Coat's 389

F

Facial hirsutism 106
Facial nerve palsy 262
Facial nerve 710
Facial pain 401, 402
Facial palsy 657
Factor IX deficiency 715
Factor VIII deficiency 715
Faecal impaction 638, 639
Faeco-oral transmission 631
Failed induction 183
Failure to thrive 266
Faints 253
False localising signs 111
False neurological signs 112, 411
Familial hypercholesterolemia 414
Familial occurrence 111
Family counselling 716
Fasciotomy 170
Fasting glucose 162, 164, 433
Fat necrosis 408
Fatiguability 658
Fatigue 370, 390-392, 416
Fatty meals 160
Fava beans 418
Febrile convulsions 243, 245, 292, 293, 591, 592
Fecal impaction 289
Fecal incontinence 420
Felty's syndrome 145
Femoral artery emboli 171
Femoral bruits 105
Femoral hernia 727
Femoral shaft fracture 102, 103
Fetal alcohol syndrome 110
Fetal death 150
FEV_1 151, 153
Fiberoptic bronchoscopy 117, 456
Fibrillation potentials 660
Fibrocystic breast disease (FCBD) 409
Fibromuscular dysplasia 105
Filtration surgery 388
Finasteride 627, 641
Finger oedema 186
Finland 716
Fish tapeworm 689
Fishy smelling discharge 168
Flamazine 661
Flank bruising 652

Flank pain 418, 641, 652
Flap valve trabeculectomy 90
Flashing lights 185
Flat femoral head 189
Flattened T waves 415
Flatulence 723
Flatus 180, 398
Flavivirus 679
Fleeting paresis 367
Flexor plantar 367
Flucloxacillin 93, 101, 139, 140, 191, 362, 387, 674
Fluconazole 155, 426, 644
Fluid loss 585
Fluid overload 234, 526
Flumazenile 114
Fluocytosine IV 426, 644
Fluorescein angiography 91
Fluorescent antibody to membrane antigen (FAMA) 401
Fluoroscent antibody tests 225
Fluoxetine 116
Fluticasone 428
FNAC 408
Fogarty catheter 171
Folate deficiency 690
Foley's catheter 104
Food allergy 273
Food fear 384
Foot ulcers 361
Forceps delivery 399
Foreign body in ear 131
Forgetfulness 369
Formalin 157
Fortification specta 125
Foul smelling vaginal discharge 169
Fractional curettage 450
Fracture femur 372
Fracture neck of femur 145, 386, 582
Fracture rib 178
Fracture scaphoid 263, 265
Fracture shaft femur 634, 653
Fragilitas ossium 87, 419
Fragmented epiphyses 189
Frail 434
France 651
Frequency 162, 166, 317, 360, 404, 418, 630, 640, 641
Frontal dementia 252
Frontal lobe dementia (FLD) 256, 257, 659
Fructosamine 164
Frusemide 164, 235, 370, 439, 526, 625
Full thickness burn 661, 662
Fulminant hepatitis 413
Fulminating PIH 183, 430
Fundoscopy 373

Fungal pneumonia 363, 437, 439
Fungating breast carcinoma 304

G

G6PD deficiency 418
Galactorrhoea 151
Gallbladder perforation 119
Gallstones 93, 161, 178, 411, 651
Gamete intrafallopian transfer (GIFT) 177
Gamma GT 136
Ganciclovir IV 438
Gangliolysis 403
Gangrene 172
Gas gangrene 93
Gastrectomy 689
Gastric carcinoma 570, 721
Gastric emptying 687
Gastric lavage 238
Gastric reflux 629
Gastric ulcer 148
Gastroenteritis 631
Gastrograffin swallow 180
Gastrojejunostomy 419
Gastro-oesophageal reflux disease (GORD) 630, 723
GB perforation 424
General anaesthesia 400
General peritonitis 377
Generalised tonic clonic seizure (GTCS) 270
Genital prolapse 307
Genital warts 678
Gentamicin 223, 371, 625, 700
Genuine stress incontinence (GSI) 404
Gestational diabetes mellitus 431
Gestational diabetes 165
Gestational ring 149
Gestrinone 181
Giant cell arteritis (GCA) 89, 285, 578
Giardia lamblia 396
Giardiasis 631
Glasgow Coma Scale 102, 103, 123, 124, 237
Glaucoma 186, 366, 388, 694
Global confusion 702
Glomerular function 441
Glomerulonephritis 278, 370
Glucagon 411
Glue ear 130, 664
Gluen free diet 396
Glutathione 685
Gluten sensitive enteropathy 272
Gluten 396
Glycosuria 165, 403-405
Glycosylated hemoglobin (HbA1c), 164

Index

Goitre 106, 708
Gonioscopy 388
Gonococcus 169, 177
GORD 572
Goserelin 181
Gout 143, 144, 301, 581, 699
Gram negative septicaemia 383
Graves' disease 322, 448, 518
Green stick injury 654
Greenstick fractures 654
Grey Turner's sign 652
Grief reaction 684
Grommet 664
Group psychotherapy 136, 358, 359
Guarding 160, 161, 424, 652
Guillain-Barré syndrome 364
Gum hypertrophy 99
Gynaecomastia 156, 451

H

H mole 185
H influenzae 111, 130, 243, 402, 428, 460
Haematocrit 442
Haematopoiesis 452
Haematuria 317, 370, 413, 418
Haemetemesis 454
Haemochromatosis 315, 413, 423
Haemodialysis 154, 425, 643
Haemodilution 441
Haemoglobin 452
Haemoglobin A1c 164
Haemoglobinuria 159
Haemolysis 418, 451
Haemophilia 159, 436, 715
Haemopneumothorax 102
Haemoptysis 107, 108, 117, 118, 137, 362, 456,
Haemorrhage 390
Haemorrhagic cystitis 157, 370
Haemorthroses 715-717
Haemosiderosis 452
Haemothorax 173, 178, 645
Haemotympanum 237
Hairy mole 134
Haloperidol 721
Halothane 400
Haorseness 109
Hartmann's pouch 159
Hashimoto's thyroiditis 321, 517
Hb electrophoresis 451
Head injury 103, 113, 122, 123, 239, 267, 410, 696, 697
Headache 125, 136, 154, 185, 188, 236, 249, 325, 364, 391, 395, 399, 402, 412, 424, 642, 643, 658, 675, 696, 719
Hearing aids 663, 665

Hearing impairment 132, 676
Hearing loss 664, 665
Heart block 281, 416, 583, 671
Heart valve replacement 459
Heel prick test 110
Helicobacter pylori 319
Heliotrope rash 660
Hemianopia 365
Hemiarthroplasty 145, 386
Hemiparesis 95, 96, 127, 698
Hemiplegia 126, 146, 648
Hemisonsory loss 658
Hemolysin 627
Hemolysis 451
Hemoptysis 633
Hemorrhagic cystitis 624
Henoch-Schölein purpura 88, 420
Heparin 150, 380, 454, 457, 633
Hepatic encephalopathy 299
Hepatitis A 129, 413, 549
Hepatitis B 127-129, 313, 435, 436, 509
Hepatitis C 679
Hepatocellular carcinoma 128, 679
Hepatomegaly 391, 392
Hereditary haemochromatosis (HHC) 143, 315, 423, 511
Heroin addiction 135, 137
Herpes labialis 309, 575
Herpes simplex 158, 170
Herpes type II 170
Herpes zoster 132, 179, 225, 401, 554
Hesitancy 166, 640
Hiatus hernia 148, 160, 723
Hib vaccine 244
Hiccups 233
High contrast ultrasonography (HyCoSy) 177
High vaginal swab 101, 182
Hip girdle weakness 125, 444
Hip pain 145, 189, 386, 387
Hippocratic facies 377
Hirsutism 152, 162
Histoplasmosis 362
Histrionic personality disorder 358
HIV transmission 437
HIV 129, 133, 139, 154, 155, 179, 243, 368, 424, 426, 435, 436, 437, 644, 679, 685
HLA-B5 171
HMMA 105
Hoarseness 108, 709
Hodgkin's disease (HD) 392
Holter monitoring 95
Homan's sign 379, 712
Homonymous hemianopia 127, 188, 365
Homosexual 141, 413

Horizontal nystagmus 136
Hormone replcement therapy 182
Hot flushes 705
HSV 133
Human bite 274
Human papilloma virus (HPV) 449, 678
Huntington's chorea (HC) 251, 368, 717
Hurlers's 676
Hutchinson's sign 132, 225
Hydralazine 183, 433
Hydrocortisone sodium 438
Hydrocyanic acid 395
Hydrogen cyanide poisoning 240, 660
Hydrosalpinx 169
Hydroxycobalamin (B12) 320, 689
Hydroxyurea 97, 98, 391, 688
Hymenoptera venom 121, 646
Hyper reflexia 686
Hyperacute T wave 147, 379, 672
Hyperaldostereonism 417
Hypercalcaemia 96, 164, 287, 302, 370, 433, 535, 568, 641, 651, 719
Hypercalcemia of malignancy 324
Hypercalciuria 641
Hyperchloremia 439
Hypercoagulability 148, 441
Hyperglycaemia 162, 360, 403, 447, 514
Hyperkalemia 624
Hyperkeratotic 443
Hyperlipidemia 147, 651
Hypermetropia 696
Hyperparathyroidism 423, 434
Hyperreflexia 185, 432
Hypersexuality 252
Hypertension 227, 253, 441, 562, 669, 699
Hyperthermia 255, 686
Hyperthyroidism 448, 658, 707
Hypertriglyceridaemia 361
Hypertrophic pulmonary osteoarthritis 117
Hyperventilation syndromes 116, 166, 417
Hyperviscosity 391
Hypoalbuminaemia 384, 417
Hypocalcaemia 417
Hypogammaglobulinaemia 118, 157
Hypoglycaemia 112, 164, 165, 235, 359, 410, 411, 438, 633
Hypokalaemia 233-235, 370, 371, 439, 440, 525, 526, 625
Hyponatraemia 414, 438-440
Hypopyon 444
Hypotension 174, 381, 395, 646, 647, 713
Hypotensive shock 93, 260, 635, 637

Hypothermia 415, 651, 702
Hypothyroidism 110, 254, 321, 702, 707
Hypovolemic shock 121, 173, 178, 637
Hypoxaemia 139, 649
Hysterectomy 148, 234, 400, 705
Hysterosalpingogram 177

I

IBS with diarrhoea 638
Ibuprofen 145
IDDM 360, 716
Idiopathic haemorrhagic sarcoma 133
Ifosphamide 157
Iliotibial bands 109
Imidazole pessary 168
Imipramine 115
Immunocompromised 363
Immunosuppressed 139
Impedance audiometry 664
Impending burst abdomen 382
Impetigo contagiosa 674
Impotence 156, 162, 253
Incisional hernia 383
Incomplete abortion 99, 150
Incontinence 390, 655
Increased intracranial tension 111
India Ink preparation 644
India ink staining 155, 426
India 141
Indigestion 455
Individual psychotherapy 358, 359
Indoramin 641
Inevitable abortion 99, 149
Infection toxicity 703
Infertility 175, 177, 370
Inflammatory bowel disease (IBD) 291, 396
Influenza 140, 676
Inhalation injury 240, 542, 660
Inhaled bronchodilators 375
Inhaled foreign body 279
Inherited clotting abnormality 443
INR 226
Insignificant head injury 497
Insulin assay 411
Insulin deficiency 447
Insulin sliding scale 410
Insulin 112, 360
Interferon alpha 413
Intermenstrual spotting 182
Intermittent catheterization 642
Intermittent claudication 361, 515, 650
International normalized ratio 394
Internuclear ophthalmoplegia (INO) 656, 657
Interstitial nephritis 370, 625
Intestinal adhesions 384
Intestinal colic 384
Intestinal hurry 419
Intestinal obstruction 161, 650
Intracerebral haemorrhage 98, 563
Intractable dysphagia 297
Intractable hiccups 302
Intradermal melanoma 134
Intraocular foreign bodies (IOFB) 491
Intrauterine device 181
Intrauterine growth retardation 150
Intrauterine infections 110
Intravenous drug users 140, 155, 644
Intussusception 629
Invasive carcinoma 450
In-vitro fertilization (IVF) 177
Involucrum 191, 387
Ipratropium bromide 228
Iridocyclitis 186, 366, 388, 389
Irritability 322
Irritable bowel syndrome (IBS) 100, 180, 290, 385, 398, 506, 519
Irritable hip syndrome (transient synovitis) 190, 191, 556
Ischaemic heart disease (IHD) 416, 668, 700
Isoniazid 119
Isopter contraction 694
Isotope cystography 626
Ispaghula husk 157
Isthmusectomy 708
Itch 446
Itchy blisters 446
IUCD 249
IVU 92, 627, 652
Ixodes dammini 447
Ixodid ticks 447
Ixoedes 680

J

J waves 415
Jaundice 160, 314, 424, 451, 652
Jaw claudication 188
Jejunal biopsy 396
Jews 322
John's criteria 670
Joint aspiration 190, 386
Joint stiffness 701
Judicial review 729
Junctional naevi 134
Juvenile HD 717
JVP 234

K

Kaposi's sarcoma 133, 456
Kartageneger's syndrome 118, 457
Karyotyping 451, 453
Keratic precipitates (KP) 366
Keratoconjunctivitis sicca 314, 695
Kernig's sign 126, 675
Ketanserin 118, 458
Ketoacidosis 361
Ketotic breath 113, 410
Klebsiella aerogenes 413
Klinefelter's syndrome 451
Klippel-fiel 676
Koch-Weeks bacillus 389
KOH examination 408
Korsakoff's psychosis 136, 702
Kulchitsky cell 118
Kveim test 445
Kyphosis 106

L

Labetalol 183, 186, 433
Labyrinthitis 664
Lactic acidosis 361, 516
Lamivudine 436
Lansoprazole 148
Laparoscopy 100, 101, 177, 181
Laparotomy 93, 377, 635, 651
Large tongue 106, 110
Laryngeal airflow measurements 677
Laryngeal edema 121
Laryngoscopy 108, 109
Laxatives 141, 157, 160, 383, 384
LBBB 379
Left atrial hypertrophy (LAH) 415
Left ventricular aneurysm 671
Left ventricular dilatation 379
Left ventricular failure 671
Left ventricular hypertrophy 416
Left-sided appendicitis 160
Legg-Calve-Perthes disease 189, 385
Legionella pneumophila 140
Legionella serology 140
Leiden mutation 379, 712
Leptospirosis 129
Lethargy 440
Leucocoria 389
Leucocytosis 424
Leucoerythroblastic anemia 97
Leukaemia 97, 140, 439
Leukaemic meningitis 154, 643
Leukopenia 438
Levodopa 369
Lewy body dementia 256, 659
Lexipafant 93
LFTs 136
Lhermitte's sign 655
Libyan 389
Lichen planus 133
Lidocaine 395
Lidocaine gel 170
Lipodermatosclerosis 311, 312

Index

Lithium side effects 503
Lithium 115, 254
Lithotripsy 424, 652
Liver function tests 112
Lobar consolidation 137
Loin pain 413
Long saphenous vein 446
Loperamide 118, 458
Lorazepam 167, 685
Lordosis 109
Loss of appetite 418
Loss of consciousness 94, 696
Loss of libido 156
Loss of vision 125, 186, 187, 365, 366
Low fertility 175
Low urine output 713
Lucid interval 236
Lumbar fracture 175
Lumbar puncture 111, 155, 239, 643, 675, 695
Lund and Browder chart 661
Lung fibrosis 187
Lung function tests 108
Lupus plasma marker 150
Lupus vulgaris 119
Luque operation 110
Luteal rise 176
Lyme disease 445, 447, 680
Lymphadenopathy 97, 99, 117, 390, 393, 445, 447
Lymphangiography 323
Lymphoblast depletion 154, 425, 643
Lymphocytic infiltration 444
Lymphoedema 323
Lymphoma 97, 140, 319, 393
Lytic metastases 96

M

Macrocytes 689
Magnesium sulfate 186, 433
Malabsorption 396, 419, 423, 558, 690
Malabsorption syndrome 322
Malaena 383
Malaise 441
Malaria 159, 305
Malathion 673
Malaysia 140
Male prostitute 179
Malignancy 442
Malignant external otitis 359
Malignant hypertension 364
Malignant melanoma (MM) 132, 389
Mallory-Weiss syndrome (MWS) 454
Malnutrition 691
MALT lymphoma 319
Mammography 406
Manic depressive illness (MDI) 115

Manning criteria 385
Mannitol 123, 239, 366, 394, 719
Mantoux test 119
MAO inhibitors 116, 167, 683, 685
Marfan's sydnrome 146, 648, 455
Marginal osteophytes 144, 701
Mask like face 369
Mastalgia 249
Maxillary carcinoma 227
Mean 666
Measles 676
Mebendazole 397
Median 667
Mediastinal adenopathy 393
Mediastinal gas 180
Mediastinal shift 246
Megacolon 157
Megakaryocytes 97
Megaloblastic anemia 306, 320, 688
Megaloblasts 688
Melanoma 134
Melphalan 391
Menarche 577, 706
Meningeal artery rupture 124
Meningism 239, 675
Meningitis 97, 111, 119, 155, 274, 425, 426, 642-644, 675, 676
Meningitis photophobia 239
Meningitis prophylaxis 156, 426, 644
Meningococcal meningitis 111, 239
Meningococcus 675
Meningoencephalitis 364, 444
Menopause 576, 705
Menorrhagia 702, 705, 716, 717
Menstrual irregularities 162
Menstruation 182, 705
Mental retardation 453
Mercaptopurine 651
Mesalazine 384
Mesenteric angiogram 650
Metabolic acidosis 233, 439
Metabolic alkalosis 233, 234, 524
Metastases to liver 442
Metastatic disease 287
Metastatic prostate carcinoma 569
Metformin 361
Methergin 99
Methionine 685
Methyl alcohol amblyopia 365
Methyldopa 186, 433
Methylprednisolone 657
Meticulous bowel preparation 459
Metoclopramide 148, 671, 672
Metronidazole 141, 142, 168, 383, 427, 633, 715, 725
Mexico 141
MIBG scan 105

Microangiopathy 187
Microcephaly 110
Micturating cystourethrogram 626
Micturition cystouretherography 405
Mid systolic click 166
Midcycle mucus test 176
Migraine 95, 125, 172, 248, 565
Migratory polyarthritis 670
Migratory superficial vein thrombophlebitis 171
Milpar 160
Mini labour 99
Minimal change disease 370
Mirena coil 250
Mite 412, 673
Mitral regurgitation 671
Mitral valve prolapse syndrome 166
Mixed incontinence 404
MMR 243, 244
Mobitz type I 671
Mode 667
Molluscum contagiosum 133
Monoarthritis 144, 190
Monoilial vaginitis 101, 182
Morning stiffness 187
Morphine 157, 161
Mortality ratio 666
Mosaic warts 678
MRC menu 367
Mucocutaneous lesions 443
Mucopurulent conjunctivitis 389
Multiinfarct dementia (MID) 251, 253, 367
Multiparous 430, 431
Multiple myeloma (MM) 95, 306, 391, 433, 439, 441
Multiple pregnancy 185

Multiple sclerosis (MS) 96, 390, 493, 640, 655, 656, 724
Mumps 155, 425, 651, 676
Murphy's sign 424
Muscle cramps 370
Mutation analysis, 368
Myalgia 140, 412
Myasthenia gravis (MG) 286, 658
Mycoplasma pneumoniae 137, 364
Mydriasis 166
Myelodysplasia 157, 688
Myelofibrosis 97, 562
Myelogram 720
Myeloid leukemia 144
Myobacterium tuberclosis 456
Myocardial infarction (MI) 147, 179, 227, 231, 247, 379, 414, 455, 651, 671, 672, 720
Myocarditis 416

Myoglobinuria 159
Myopathy 125
Myringotomy 664
Myxoedema 143, 448, 701
Myxoedema coma 702

N
N-acetyl cysteine 121, 685
Naevi 134
Naloxone 114, 393, 400, 409, 411
Naltrexone 136
Nappy rash 673
Naproxen 145, 699, 722
Narcotic drug abuse 137
Narcotic overdose 114
Narcotic withdrawal 135
Nasal decongestants 402
Nasal perforation 226
Nasal speech 675
Nasogastric suction 639
Nasopharyngeal bleeding 237
Nausea 660, 672
Nebulisation 374
Nebulised beta2 agonist 231
Neck pain 374
Neck stiffness 97, 155, 426
Neck vein distension 647
Necrobiosis lipoidica (NL) 447
Nedocromil 376, 691
Needle exchange programme 114, 135
Needle thoracocentesis 373, 635, 647
Neisseria 101
Neopterin 368
Nephrotic syndrome (NS) 370, 439, 417, 624
Nephrotoxic drugs 235
Nephrotoxicity 371, 625
Neurofibrillary tangles 251, 659
Neurofibroma 664
Neurogenic bladder 404
Neurogenic shock 174
Neuroleptic malignant syndrome (NMS) 255, 501
Neutropaenia 99, 390
NIDDM 403, 447, 716
Nigerian 183
Night fever 642
Night pain 144, 701
Night sweats 392, 393, 412, 418
Nitrous oxide 102, 398
Nocardia asteroides 363
Nocturia 640
Noise-induced hearing loss (NIHL) 665
Non-accidental injury (NAI) 238, 266, 268, 419
Non-Hodgkin's lymphoma (NHL) 322, 392, 393

Nonketotic (HONK) coma 112, 411
Non-Q wave MI 414
Non-small cell tumors 107, 456
Norfloxacin 427
Normochromic macrocytic anemia 321
Normocytic anaemia 418
Normocytic normochromic anaemia 391
North Africa 642
North America 651
Norwegian scabies 412
Nutritional deficit 559, 691
Nystagmus 136, 656, 686
Nystatin 673

O
Obesity 447
Obsessive compulsive personality disorder (OCD) 357
Obstructive jaundice 178
Occipital lobe infarct 188
Occipitoanterior 399
Occipitoposterior 399
Occult blood test 143
Ochronosis 143, 701
OCP 117, 248, 454
Octreotide 118, 458
Oculomotor 261
Oesophageal carcinoma 508
Oesophageal manometry 723
Oesophageal rupture 454
Oesophageal spasm 146, 648
Oesophagitis 148
Offal 144
Offensive discharge 168
Offensive vaginal discharge 182
Ofloxacin 427
Olfactory 261
Oliguria 103, 233
Oncogenesis 157
Ophthalmoplegia 136, 322, 702
Ophthalmoscopy 365, 389
Opiate overdosage 269, 409, 411
Opioid 241
Opioid poisoning 393, 502
Opioid withdrawal 269
Opisthotonus 395
Optic atrophy 656
Optic nerve 656
Optic neuritis 96, 365, 390, 640, 656, 657, 694
Ora serrata 318
Oral cholecystography (OCG) 424
Oral contraceptive pill 101, 158, 443
Oral glucose tolerance test (OGTT) 106, 162, 164

Oral hairy leukoplakia 133
Oral thrush 693
Orchitis 424
Orf 225
Organophosphates 393
Orotic aciduria 688
Osteoarthritis (OA) 144, 189, 581, 701
Osteogenesis imperfecta 87, 537, 419
Osteomyelitis 191, 387, 452, 557, 678
Osteonecrosis 189
Osteophytes 701
Osteoporosis 150, 162, 386, 718
Osteoporotic fracture 175
Osteotomy 190
Otitis externa 131
Otitis media 664, 428
Otosclerosis 663
Otoscopy 130, 131
Ototoxic drugs 223
Ototoxicity 223, 371, 552, 625
Outpatient withdrawal programmes 137
Ovarian cyst 100
Overcrowding 413
Overflow diarrhoea 289
Ovulation 176
Ovulatory mucus 176
Oxytocin 99

P
P antigen 627
Pabrinex 136, 702
Pacemaker 95
Paget's disease 408
Palliative surgery 408
Palpitation 147, 166, 254, 416, 448, 632, 687, 707
Pancreatectomy 161
Pancreatic duct obstruction 423
Pancreatic insufficiency 423, 690
Pancreaticojejunostomy 161, 423
Pancreatin 423
Pancreatitis 94, 160, 161, 319, 423, 424, 646, 651, 652
Panhypopituitarism 151
Panic attacks 116, 166, 167, 270, 530, 632, 683, 685, 701
Panophthalmitis 389
Pap smear 448, 449
Papanicolaou test (Pap smear) 450
Papillary muscle rupture 283
Papilledema 123, 154, 155, 325, 373, 424, 425, 643, 657, 658, 695
Paracetamol poisoning 238, 500, 685
Paraesthesiae 166, 170, 632, 655
Paraffin gauze 661
Parainfluenza virus 376

Index

Paralytic ileus 298, 377, 639, 727
Paramyoxovirus 155, 425, 643
Paraneoplastic syndromes 118, 458
Paranoia 136
Paranoid personality disorder 357, 682
Paranoid schizophrenia 357, 682
Paraparesis 655
Paraplegia 146, 175, 648
Parkinsonism (Shy-Drager syndrome) 251, 253, 369, 435
Parotid tumor 540, 710
Parotidectomy 710
Parotitis 161, 425, 643
Paroxysmal 687
Paroxysmal atrial fibrillation 668
Partial thickness burns 661
Past pointing 656
Pasteurization 412
Pathological fracture 325
PCR antigen 135
Peanuts 646
PEFR 151, 153, 232, 375
Peg view 174
Pelvic abscess 248, 380, 713
Pelvic floor exercises 404
Pelvic fracture 103, 104
Pelvic inflammatory disease (PID) 101, 169, 181, 520
Pelvic pain 169
Pelvicalyceal stones 641
Pentamidine 139, 651
Peptic ulcer (PU) 422
Percutaneous drainage 377
Percutaneous nephrostomy 92
Perforated appendix 380
Perforated gallbladder 92
Perforated peptic ulcer 161, 651
Performance anxiety 165, 684
Perianal rash 397
Pericardial effusion 147
Pericardial rub 147
Pericardiocentesis 147
Pericarditis 147, 648
Perihilar infiltration 139
Peri-lunate dislocation 264
Periorbital puffing 448
Peripheral iridectomy 186, 388
Peripheral polyneuropathy 360
Peripheral vascular disease (PVD) 172
Peritoneal lavage 173
Peritonitis 94, 162, 380, 382, 645, 714
Periumbilical discoloration 652
Permethrin 412, 673
Pernicious anaemia (PA) 320, 448, 557, 688, 689
Perthes disease 189, 190, 385, 554, 655

Pertussis 457
Pertussis immunization 245
Pethidine 93, 161, 400, 639
Petit mal epilepsy (absence seizures) 294
Petrous temporal bone fracture 224, 553
Phaeochromocytoma 105, 183, 276, 429
Phenelzine 167, 685
Phenobarbitone 149, 159
Phenothaizines 157, 368, 717
Phenoxymethyl penicillin 460
Phenytoin 99, 403, 564
Pheochromocytoma 162
Philadelphia chromosome 97, 391
Phobia 167, 683, 685
Photocoagulation 91
Photophobia 675, 696
Physiotherapist 441
Physostigmine 395
Pick's disease 256, 257, 659
Picolax 141
PID 177, 182-184
PIH 183, 430
Pill rolling movement 369
Pilocarpine 388
Pinchcork" mechanism 723
Pinning 387
Pinpoint pupil 114, 393, 411
Pituitary adenoma 162, 707
Pizotifen 125
Placenta accreta 400
Placental hydrops 185
Placental insufficiency 150
Placental thrombosis 150
Plane warts 678
Plantar fascitis 187
Plantar warts 678
Plasma osmolality 410
Platelet transfusions 390
Plethoric appearance 442
Pleural biopsy 718
Pleural effusion 377, 718
Pleural rub 117
Pleuritic chest pain 117, 148, 442, 457
Pleuritic pain 453
Plevic abscess 638
Pneumococcal 111
Pneumococcus 389, 460
Pneumocystis 97
Pneumocystis carinii pneumonia (PCP) 139, 363, 437
Pneumocystis carinii 137, 363
Pneumomediastinum 454
Pneumonia 107, 137, 363, 391
Pneumothoraces 453
Pneumothorax 102, 146, 151, 180, 230, 373, 453, 398, 453, 635, 647, 692, 693

Podagra 699
Poikilocytes 97
Polycystic kidney disease (PKD) 277
Polycystic ovary syndrome (PCOS) 295
Polycythaemia vera 442
Polycythaemia 95, 144
Polycythemia rubra vera (PCRV) 442
Polydipsia 96, 162, 433
Polymyalgia rheumatica (PMR) 125, 565
Polymyositis 117, 125, 444, 660
Polysomnographic studies 675
Polytrauma 170
Polyuria 162, 164, 324, 360, 433
Poor stream 640
Popliteal pulse 172
Post herpetic neuralgia prophylaxis 179
Postcoital test 176
Postgastrectomy 419
Postictal confusion 94
Postmenopausal bleeding 705
Postpartum haemorrhage 400
Post-traumatic amnesia 122
Post-traumatic Stress Disorder (PTSD) 683
Postural hypotension 399, 417
Postvagotomy 419
Pouch of Douglas 248, 380, 713
Pox viruses 225
PR interval 670
Prazosin 627
Pre-eclampsia 183-185, 399, 432, 429, 430, 431, 432
Pre-eclamptic toxaemia 186
Pregnancy induced hypertension (PIH) 184, 431
Pregnancy 441
Premenstrual migraine 125
Pre-menstrual syndrome (PMS) 409
Presbyacusis 663
Pretibial myxedema 322
Priapsim 391
Primary biliary cirrhosis (PBC) 314, 510
Primary survey 102, 103, 372, 374, 634
Primigravida 431
Probable Crohn's disease (CD) 308
Probable osteoarthritis (OA) 300
Prochlorperazine 93
Proctosigmoidoscopy 384, 396
Productive cough 414
Prognathism 106
Progressive relaxation training 166
Projectile vomiting 629
Prolapse 573
Proliferative glomerulonephritis 417

Prolonged labour 653
Prostate carcinoma 288, 289, 568
Prostatectomy 627
Prostate-specific antigen 640
Prostatism 641
Prosthetic heart valve 226
Protein C 379
Protein S 379
Proteinuria 184, 185, 417, 430, 431, 441
Proteus mirabilis 413
Prothrombin time 394
Proton-pump inhibitor 422
Proximal myopathy 117
Proximal RTA 371, 626
Pruritus 314, 392
Pseudodementia 252
Pseudogout 143, 580, 701
Pseudomembrane 142
Pseudomembranous colitis 142, 427
Pseudomonas aeruginosa 662
Pseudomonas 245
Pseudopolyps 384
Pseudotumor cerebri 695
Psoriasis 133
Psychoanalysis 115, 358
Psychoanalytic psychotherapy 358
Psychometric testing 367
Psychomotor retardation 682
Ptosis 136, 658
Pudendal block 399
Pudendal nerve block 399
Pulled elbow 653, 654
Pulmonary angiogram 117, 457
Pulmonary angiography 148, 633
Pulmonary collapse 246, 247
Pulmonary embolism (PE) 117, 146, 148, 247, 280, 282, 312, 454, 457, 528, 531, 584, 633
Pulmonary fibrosis 157
Pulmonary oedema 117, 369, 457, 624, 670, 631
Pulmonary tuberculosis (PTB) 280, 297, 527, 528
Pulmonary venous thromboembolism (PE) 454
Pulse oximetry 247
Puncture marks 393, 409
Pupil dilatation 698
Pupillary dilatation 126, 372
Purine rich foods 144
Purpura 111
Purulent cough 137, 139, 140
Purulent sputum 414
Purulent vaginal discharge 182
Pyelitis 413
Pyelonephritis 370, 413, 625, 626
Pyloric stenosis 233, 629

Pyonephrosis 92
Pyosalpinx 169
Pyramidal lesion 367
Pyrazinamide 119
Pyridostigmine 658
Pyrimethamine 154, 424

Q
Q wave 147, 379, 414
QT lengthening 416
Queer 358
Quinine overdose 500
Quinine 393

R
Racoon or panda eyes 237
Radiation proctitis 303
Radical prostatectomy 640
Radioisotope bone scanning 391
Radiotherapy 450
Raised intracranial pressure (ICP) 325, 536, 656
Ramstedt's pyloromyotomy 629
Random blood glucose 162
Ranitidine 148
Rattles 634
Raynaud's disease 172
Raynaud's phenomenon 171, 660
Reactive arthritis 191
Rebound tenderness 161, 424, 725
Rebreathing 166, 167, 417
Rectal bleeding 160
Rectal carcinoma 384, 504
Rectal tumor 639
Recurrent acute otitis media 131
Recurrent nerve paralysis 709
Red cell transketolase 136
Red-currant jam 629
Reflux oesophagitis 146, 148, 648
Reiter's syndrome 443
Relative risk (RR) 666
Release test 725
Renal artery stenosis 105
Renal calculi 92
Renal colic 159, 641
Renal failure 233, 525, 625
Renal scars 626
Renal stones 144, 154
Renal tubular acidosis 371, 439, 440, 626
Renal vein thrombosis 159
Respiratory depression 371, 400
Respiratory syncytial virus 376
Respiro-laryngeal dysfunction (RLD) 677
Restless 651, 652
Retained placenta 400

Retinal detachment (RD) 187, 365, 366, 494
Retinitis 444
Retinoblastoma 389, 492
Retinopathy 391
Retinoscopy 438
Retrograde amnesia 122
Retrolental fibroplasia 389
Retropubic prostatectomy 641
Retrosternal goitre 709
Retrosternal pain 455
Rh disease 185
Rhabdomyolysis 103
Rheumatic fever 190, 414, 670
Rheumatoid arthritis (RA) 143, 145, 300, 571, 582, 658, 701, 722
Rheumatoid factor 145, 722
Rheumatoid 658
Rhinocerebral mucormycosis 359
Rhinorrhoea 130
Rib notching 104
Rifampicin prophylaxis 156, 249, 426, 644
Rifampicin 119, 159
Right bundle branch block 117
Right ventricular failure 671
Rigors 248
Rigors 424
Ring enhancing lesions 154, 424
Rinne test 223
Risk ratio 666
Rose spots 678
Rotavirus 631
Rough voice 677
Rouleaux formation 391
Ruptured aneurysm 646
Ruptured ectopic pregnancy 645
Ruptured oesophagus 180

S
S hematobium 550
Sabouraud's medium 168
Sacroiliac pain 187
SAH 98
Salbutamol 151, 153, 228, 692
Salicylate poisoning 238
Salmeterol 232
Salmonella typhi 678
Salmonella 631
Salt baths 170
Sarcoidosis 445, 530, 642, 655
Scabies 133, 412, 673
Scalp tenderness 188
Scandinavian 716
Schilling test 688
Schirmer's test 695
Schistosomiasis 159

Index

Schizoid personality disorder 358
Schizophrenia 251, 253, 255, 268, 369, 680-682
Schizotypal personality disorders 358
Scleral silicone implants 187
Scleroderma 660
Sclerotherapy 311
Scotomata 90
Scurvy 559, 690
Sebaceous cyst 317, 513
Seborrheic dermatitis 133
Secondary dysmenorrhoea 169
Secondary survey 102, 372, 374
Semen analysis 176
Senile deafness 663
Senile keratosis 133
Senile macular degeneration (SMD) 580, 91
Senile plaques 251, 659
Senna 159
Sense of incomplete defecation 384
Sensitivity 665
Sensorineural deafness 664
Sensory deafness 664
Sensory neural deafness 663
Septal perforation 226
Septic abortion 182
Septic abortion 520
Septic arthritis 190, 191, 386, 387, 555
Septic shock 119, 120
Septicaemia 298, 383, 675, 715
Sequesterum 191, 387
Serosanquinous discharge 382
Serotonin 152
Serous otitis media 130
Serum amylase 93
Serum calcium 433, 434
Serum urate 154
Severe asthma 375
Severe blood loss 634
Severe earache 428
Severe ulcerative colitis (UC) 505
Sewage workers 129
Sexual abuse 267, 420, 538, 88
Sheehan's syndrome 151
Sheep farmer 412
Shellfish 413
Shigella 631
Shingles 179
Shock 438, 646
Shoulder girdle weakness 125
Shy-Drager syndrome 435
SIADH 414
Sickle cell disease (SCD) 159, 451, 452
Sickle cell 95
Sigmoid carcinoma 141
Sigmoid colectomy 459

Sigmoidoscopy 100, 141, 142, 160, 180, 385, 398, 434, 638, 690
Signed nostrils 660
Silver sulphadiazine 241
Simmonds disease 151
Singeing 242
Sinunasal cancer 227
Sinus bradycardia 415, 671
Sinus tachcycardia 117, 632
Sinusitis 130, 402
Sixth nerve palsy 657
Sjögren's syndrome 439
Sjögren's syndrome 695
Skin dimpling 408
Skin nodules 393
Skip lesions 637
Skull fractures 124
Skull traction 174
SLE 90, 655, 658, 660
Sleep apnoea 106, 675
Slipped femoral epiphyses 387
Slipped upper femoral epiphyses (SUFE) 190, 655
Sliver sulfadiazine 661
Slurring 677
Small bowel enema 384
Small bowel lymphoma (probable) 322
Small bowel lymphoma 518
Small cell carcinoma 118
Small cell lung cancer 439
Small cell tumor 456
Smith's arthritis 190
Smoking 249
Social phobia 683
Sodium bicarbonate 687
Sodium cromoglycate 232, 374-376
Sodium nitrite 395, 688
Sodium nitroprusside 146
Sodium thiosulfate 395, 688
Solar keratoses 133
Somatization symptoms 684
Somatization 165
South America 141
Space occupying lesion (SOL) 126, 286, 658
Specific phobia 683
Speech delay 676
Speech discrimination 663
Speech dyspraxia 677
Sperm count 156
Sphincter disturbances 640
Sphincter of Oddi spasm 161
Sphincterectomy 378
Spidery fingers 146
Spiking fever 248
Spinal accessory 262

Spinal cord compression 324, 720
Spinal osteotomy 187
Spinal shock 174
Spiral CT 117, 148
Spirometry 118, 151, 457, 691, 692
Splenectomy 460, 589
Splenic infarction 452
Splenic rupture 120, 258, 260, 635
Splenomegaly 98, 145, 390, 391, 392, 442, 678
Spontaneous pneumothorax 647
Spotting 182
Spurious diarrhoea 384
Sputum culture 362, 456
Sputum microscopy 414, 423
Sputum 362
Squamous cell carcinoma (SCC) 134
ST depression 415, 700
ST elevation 147, 379, 645, 672
Stabbing pain 403
Stable angina 422
Standard deviation 666
Staphylococcal pneumonia 139, 140
Staphylococcal scalded skin syndrome 93
Staphylococcal toxic shock syndrome (TSS) 101
Staphylococcus aureus 93, 245, 362, 389, 674
Staphylococcus saprophyticus 413
Staphylococcus 631
Staphyloma 389
STDs 248
Steam inhalation 402
Steatorrhoea 423
Sterile pyuria 418
Sterilization 249
Steroid 230
Steven-Johnson syndrome 158, 364
Stiff neck 126
Still's disease 190
Stokes-Adams attacks 95
Stone impaction 178
Stone in common bile duct 378
Stone 159
Stony dull percussion note 718
Stool microscopy 141
Strangulated indirect inguinal hernia 727
Strangulation 388
Strangury 159, 317
Strawberry angioma 88, 421
Streptococcal pharyngitis 429
Streptococci 674
Streptococcus faecalis 245
Streptococcus pneumoniae 137, 402, 633

Streptococcus pyogenes 93, 662
Streptococcus 169, 389
Streptokinase (SK) 671
Streptomycin 412
Stridor 634, 709
ST-segment elevation, 414
Subacute hypothermia 415
Subarachnoid haemorrhage (SAH) 126, 566
Subchondral cysts 144, 701
Subchondral sclerosis 144, 701
Subconjunctival haemorrhage 237, 388, 491
Subcutaneous emphysema 180
Subdural hematoma 102, 113, 122, 124, 126, 173, 235, 239, 251, 372, 410, 498, 566, 633, 698
Subendocardial infarction 672
Subepidermal eruption 446
Suboccipital craniectomy 403
Subperiosteal reaction 191, 387
Subphrenic abscess 92, 377
Sudden blindness 188
Suicide 637
Sulfadiazine 154, 424
Sulfasalazine 384, 396
Sulfonamides 158
Sulfonylurea 112
Sulphasalazine 637
Sulpiride 368
Sunbathing 242
Sunburns 242, 544, 662
Superficial head injury 496
Superior mediastinal syndrome 709
Superior vena cava (SVC) obstruction 304
Supportive counselling 136
Supportive psychotherapy 357
Supracondylar fracture 654
Suspected testicular tumor 512
S-wave 415
Swinging fever 362
Swinging pyrexia 713
Swinging 413
Sydenham's chorea 670
Sympathetic stimulation 166
Syncope 94, 148
Synovial fluid microscopy 144
Syphilis 642, 646
Syringing 223
Systemic inflammatory response syndrome (SIRS) 703
Systolic murmur 166

T
T wave inversion 379
T wave 379
T gondii 154, 424
Tachyarrhythmias 649, 671
Tachycardia 173, 395, 454, 457
Tachycardia 637, 646, 703
Tachypnoea 117, 166, 454, 457, 675, 703
Tamponade 147
Tardive dyskinesia 681
TB 137, 159, 368
Tear-drop forms 97
Technetium labelled leucocyte scan 384
Temporal arteritis (TA) 125, 402
Temporal arteritis 364, 493, 694
Temporary threshold shift 665
Tenesmus 141, 248, 398, 637, 638, 725
Tensilon test 658
Tension pneumothorax 102, 260, 373, 635, 693, 647
Terazosin 641
Terbutaline 692
Terminal dribbling 640
Testicular tumor 316
Testosterone 438
Tetanus Ig 646
Tetrabenazine 368, 717
Tetracycline 364
Thalassemia 451
Theophylline 633
Thiamine 136, 702
Thiazides 370
Third space sequestration 178
Thoractomy 180
Threatened abortion 149, 150
Thromblysis 379
Thromboangiitis obliterans 171
Thrombocytopenia 159
Thromboembolism 249, 380, 394, 442, 633, 712
Thrombolysis 147, 455
Thrombophlebitis migrans 446
Thrombophlebitis 446
Thrush 168, 169
Thyroglossal cyst 540, 710
Thyroglossal tract 710
Thyroid acropachy 322
Thyroid bruit 322
Thyroidectomy 708
Thyrombolysis 671
Thyrotoxicosis 162, 709
Thyroxine 707
TIA 127, 567
Tic douloureux 401, 724
Tick borne 680
Timed vital capacity 151
Timolol 90
Tinnitus 663, 664
Torsion of testis 316, 512
Torted ovarian cyst 100
Total pancreatectomy 423
Toxic epidermal necrolysis (TEN) 93
Toxocara endophthalmitis 389
Toxoplasmosis 154, 155, 424, 426, 644, 674
Tracheal deviation 647
Transbronchial biopsy 445
Transient ischaemic attack (TIA) 95, 677
Transient synovitis 191
Transillumination test 711
Transmural infarct 414
Transmural infarction 672
Trans-oesophageal echocardiography 650
Transrectal ultrasound 640
Transurethral incision of the prostate (TUIP) 641
Traumatic pneumothorax 373
Travel history 412
Tremor 322
Trendelenburg's sign 387
Trichomonas vaginalis 168
Trichomonas 101
Tricyclic antidepressant (TCA) poisoning 686
Tricyclic antidepressant 144
Tricyclic antidepressants overdose 395, 501, 503
Trigeminal neuralgia (TN) 401, 403, 572, 724
Trigger zone 403
Trimethoprim 230, 405, 413, 427, 626, 627, 628, 630
Triple assessment 409
Triple therapy 422
Trisomy 21 (Down's syndrome) 453
Trophozoites 141
Tropical sprue 689
True incontinence 405
Trycyclic antidepressants 115
TSH 707
Tubal dysfunction 177
Tubal infertility 101
Tubal patency test 177
Tubal pregnancy 645
Tubercular meningitis 642
Tuberculosis (TB) 119, 139, 177, 414, 418, 423, 456
Tumor lysis syndrome 154, 425, 643
Tunnel vision 694
Turner's syndrome 104
TURP 627
T-wave inversion 416
Two-point discrimination 658

Index

Tympanic membrane 131
Tympanometry 130
Type I renal tubular acidosis (Distal RTA) 522
Type II renal tubular acidosis (Proximal RTA) 524
Typhoid 678
Tzanck preparation 401
Tzank smears 132, 225

U
Ulcerative colitis (UC) 142, 384, 396, 398, 637
Ulcerative pancolitis 142
Ultrasonography 645
Unconscious 236, 238, 409, 415
Undulating fever 412
Unstable angina 649, 671
Ureteric colic 641, 652
Ureteric reflux 642
Ureteric stones 641
Urethral strictures 640
Urethral swabs 169, 181
Urethral syndrome (US) 405
Urethritis 159
Urethrogram 104
Urge incontinence (UI) 404
Urgency 360, 640, 641
Urinary incontinence 639
Urinary retention 254, 324, 399
Urinary tract infection (UTI) 276, 317, 413, 427, 513, 630
Urodynamic studies 404
Uterine atonia 121
UTI 573, 626, 628
UV radiation 242
Uveitis 187, 366, 495

V
V/Q scan 148, 454, 457, 633
Vaccination 460, 591
Vaginal bleeding 99, 150, 706
Vaginal discharge 101, 168-170
Vaginal dryness 705
Valproate 293
Vancomycin resistant enterococcus (VRE) 245
Vancomycin 142, 427
Varicella zoster 133
Varicella 676
Varicose veins 310-311
Vascular dementia 367
Vasogenic cerebral edema 497
Vasopressin 716
Vasovagal syncope 94, 646
Venogram 712, 380
Venography 158, 312
Venous thromboembolism 158
Venous ulcer 312
Ventricular "strain pattern" 416, 700
Ventricular arrhythmia 395
Ventricular septal defect 671
Ventricular tachyarrhythmias 416
Vertebral compression fracture 324, 535
Vertebrobasilar territory ischaemia 95
Vertigo 395, 656, 663, 664, 688
Vibrio cholerae 631
Villous adenoma 234
Villous atrophy 396
Vimentin 708
Viral meningitis 155, 425, 643
Visual field charting 365
Visual field mapping 364, 694
Visual loss 91, 127, 188, 364, 366, 367, 694
Vital capacity 151
Vitamin B12 689
Vitamin C deficiency 690
Vitamin K deficiency 378, 394, 669
Vitiligo 688
Vitrectomy 91
Vitreous haemorrhage 91, 365, 366, 579
VMA 105
Vocal cord trauma 108, 109
Vocal nodules 108
Voice training 677
Vomiting 233, 651
Von Willebrand disease 715-717

W
Waldeyer's 392
Warfarin 117, 150, 394, 457, 499, 633, 668, 669
Warts 678
Wasting 396, 658
Water's view 402
Watery brown vaginal discharge 181
Watery diarrhoea 142
Wax impaction 223
Wechsler scale 367
Wedge-shaped opacities 633
Weight gain 162, 254, 702
Weight loss 143, 322, 384, 393, 418, 456, 638, 642, 660, 694, 707
Welsh farmer 447
Wernicke's encephalopathy 136, 702
Wernicke's-Korsakoff's syndrome (WKS) 702
Wet microscopy 168
Wheeze 232
Wheeze 374, 375
Whiplash injuries 374
White curds 168
Whooping cough 388
Wickham's striaes 133
Wound dehiscence 373, 382
Wound infection 245
Writhing movements 368

X
Xenophobia 683
Xylometazoline 428

Y
Young's syndrome 118

Z
Zidovudine 368, 436
Zinc deficiency, 397
ZN staining 642
Zoophobia 683

READER SUGGESTIONS SHEET

Please help us to improve the quality of our publications by completing and returning this sheet to us.

Title/Author: **First Aid for the PLAB by Himanshu Tyagi and Ankush Vidyarthi**

Your name and address:

E-mail address,
Phone and Fax:

How did you hear about this book? [please tick appropriate box (es)]

- ☐ Direct mail from publisher   ☐ Conference   ☐ Bookshop
- ☐ Book review   ☐ Lecturer recommendation   ☐ Friends
- ☐ Other (please specify)   ☐ Website

Type of purchase: ☐ Direct purchase   ☐ Bookshop   ☐ Friends

Do you have any brief comments on the book?

Please return this sheet to the name and address given below.

JAYPEE BROTHERS
MEDICAL PUBLISHERS (P) LTD
EMCA House, 23/23B Ansari Road, Daryaganj
New Delhi 110 002, India